Basics of Anesthesia

Second Edition

Basics of Anesthesia

Second Edition

Robert K. Stoelting, M.D.

Professor and Chairman
Department of Anesthesia
Indiana University School of Medicine
Indianapolis, Indiana

Ronald D. Miller, M.D.

Professor and Chairman
Department of Anesthesia
Professor
Department of Pharmacology
University of California, San Francisco
School of Medicine
San Francisco, California

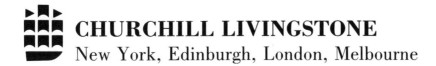

CHURCHILL LIVINGSTONE
New York, Edinburgh, London, Melbourne

Library of Congress Cataloging-in-Publication Data

Stoelting, Robert K.
    Basics of anesthesia / Robert K. Stoelting, Ronald D. Miller. —
2nd ed.
    p.   cm.
    Includes bibliographies and index.
    ISBN 0-443-08571-4
    1. Anesthesia.   I. Miller, Ronald D., date. II. Title.
    [DNLM: 1. Anesthesia.   WO 200 S872b]
RD81.S86   1989
617′.96—dc19
DNLM/DLC
for Library of Congress   89-921
                                                       CIP

Second Edition © Churchill Livingstone Inc.   1989
First Edition © Churchill Livingstone Inc. 1984

Distributed in the United Kingdom by Churchill Livingstone, Robert
Stevenson House, 1–3 Baxter's Place, Leith Walk, Edinburgh EH1
3AF, and by associated companies, branches, and representatives
throughout the world.

Accurate indications, adverse reactions, and dosage schedules for
drugs are provided in this book, but it is possible that they may
change. The reader is urged to review the package information data
of the manufacturers of the medications mentioned.

The Publishers have made every effort to trace the copyright holders
for borrowed material. If they have inadvertently overlooked any,
they will be pleased to make the necessary arrangements at the first
opportunity.

Acquisitions Editor: *Toni M. Tracy*
Copy Editor: *Marian Ryan*
Production Designer: *Marci Jordan*
Production Supervisor: *Sharon Tuder*

Printed in the United States of America

First published in 1989

Second printing in 1989

Third printing in 1989

Preface to the Second Edition

Since publication of the first edition of *Basics of Anesthesia* in 1984, new drugs, techniques, and concepts have found a place in our specialty that require even an introductory textbook to undergo revision. For example, organ transplantation and pain management receive increased attention in the second edition. In addition, many new figures and tables are included, which are intended to graphically emphasize important concepts. As a result, the size of the second edition is larger than that of the first, but the book still remains, in our opinion, the most concise presentation of essential information for the practice of anesthesiology available to the trainee and practitioner.

We wish to acknowledge the excellent secretarial support provided by Deanna Walker of Indiana University and Barbara Turner of the University of California, San Francisco. The staff of Churchill Livingstone provided the ingredients necessary for timely publication. In particular, we thank Toni Tracy, President of Churchill Livingstone, for her continued support of and contributions to this textbook.

Robert K. Stoelting, M.D.
Ronald D. Miller, M.D.
1989

Preface to the First Edition

Basics of Anesthesia is intended to provide the student and beginning trainee with introductory information pertinent to the wide spectrum (operating room, intensive care, pain management, cardiopulmonary resuscitation) of the practice of anesthesiology. Likewise, the advanced trainee and practitioner should find the concise but thorough description of anesthetic practice a useful review as well as a reference source for fundamental questions.

An in-depth and highly referenced presentation is not the goal of *Basics of Anesthesia*. Nevertheless, we believe it is possible, in a concise manner, to achieve an accurate and pertinent presentation of essential information for the practice of anesthesiology. References are limited in number but should direct the reader to classic articles or more detailed discussions of the specific topic.

The editors wish to acknowledge the superb editorial and technical assistance of Deanna Walker of Indiana University and Susan M. S. Ishida of the University of California, San Francisco. The staff of Churchill Livingstone provided the necessary encouragement and flexibility to ensure timely progression of the textbook to its final form. In particular, Donna Balopole guided this project through the important publication steps.

Robert K. Stoelting, M.D.
Ronald D. Miller, M.D.
1984

Contents

SECTION IV Special Anesthetic Considerations

SECTION V Recovery Period

SECTION VI Consultant Anesthetic Practice

Section

I

Introduction

Chapter 1

History and Scope of Anesthesia

Since its beginning in 1842, anesthesiology has evolved into a recognized medical specialty providing continuing improvement in patient care based on the introductions of new drugs and techniques made possible in large part by research in the basic and clinical sciences (Table 1-1). The scope of anesthesiology extends beyond the operating room to include respiratory therapy, treatment of acute postoperative pain, management of chronic pain problems, and the care of acutely ill patients in intensive care units. As for other medical specialties, anesthesiology is represented by professional societies, scientific journals, a Residency Review Committee that establishes compliance of anesthesia residency programs with published standards, and a board that establishes criteria for becoming a certified specialist in anesthesiology (Table 1-1).

DISCOVERY OF ANESTHESIA

Discovery of anesthesia represents a totally American contribution to medicine.[1] Dr. Crawford W. Long, a medical practitioner in rural Georgia, was the first physician known to administer the vapor of ether by inhalation to produce surgical anesthesia, in 1842. This finding was not publicized. Thus 4 years later a dentist, Dr. William T. Morton, from Hartford, Connecticut, administered the vapor of ether to Mr. Gilbert Abbott for the removal of a tumor from below the mandible by the well-known surgeon Dr. John C. Warren. The successful anesthesia took place at Massachusetts General Hospital on Friday, October 16, 1846 in front of an audience that included surgeons, medical students, and a newspaper reporter. Indeed, an account of the "ether demonstration" appeared the next day in the *Boston Daily Journal*. Within a few weeks, the entire civilized world knew the discovery of surgical anesthesia.

In England, Dr. James Y. Simpson, a highly respected obstetrician, administered ether to a parturient in 1847 to relieve the pain of labor. The use of chloroform in England for obstetrical analgesia gained public acceptance when another English physician, Dr. John Snow administered this drug to Queen Victoria during the birth of Prince Leopold in 1853. Dr. Snow qualifies as the first anesthesiologist because he was the first to devote his medical practice to the administration of anesthetics.

Another American dentist, Dr. Horace Wells, was the first to recognize the potential of nitrous oxide as an anesthetic. Although nitrous oxide was isolated in 1772 and its anesthetic properties described in 1799, it was not until 1844—when Dr. Wells allowed nitrous oxide to be administered to him by Gardner C. Colton (an itinerant showman) while a fellow dentist painlessly extracted one of Dr. Well's teeth—that the anesthetic potential of

1

Table 1-1. History of Anesthesia

1842	Diethyl ether used by Long to produce surgical anesthesia
1844	Nitrous oxide used by Wells to produce dental analgesia
1846	Diethyl ether used publicly by Morton to produce surgical anesthesia
1847	Chloroform popularized for surgical anesthesia in England
1853	Chloroform administered by Snow to Queen Victoria for the birth of Prince Leopold; this removed the stigma attached to pain relief for child birth
1854	Hollow metallic needle invented by Wood
1868	Administration of nitrous oxide with oxygen introduced by Andrews
1871	Cylinders of compressed nitrous oxide introduced by Brothers
1884	Cocaine used by Koller to produce topical anesthesia
1885	Nerve block and infiltration anesthesia by injection of cocaine introduced by Halsted Epidural block anesthesia introduced by Corning
1893	London Society of Anaesthetists founded
1898	Spinal block anesthesia introduced by Bier
1904	Buchanan appointed first professor of anesthesia in the United States at the New York Medical College
1905	Procaine synthesized by Einhorn Long Island Society of Anesthetists founded by Erdmann
1911	Long Island Society of Anesthetists becomes the New York Society of Anesthetists
1914	*American Journal of Anesthesia and Analgesia* first published as a quarterly supplement to the *American Journal of Surgery*
1917	Oxygen mask developed by Poulton
1919	National Anesthesia Research Society founded by McMechan
1920	Gudel published data on signs of anesthesia Tracheal tubes for delivery of inhaled anesthetics introduced by Magill
1922	The journal *Current Researches in Anesthesia and Analgesia* first published
1923	Mary A. Ross, M.D. becomes the first postgraduate trainee (Iowa) in anesthesiology in the United States *British Journal of Anaesthesia* first published
1924	Lundy organized a Department of Anesthesia at the Mayo Clinic
1925	National Anesthesia Research Society becomes the International Anesthesia Research Society
1926	*American Journal of Anesthesia and Analgesia* ceases publication
1927	Waters appointed as the first university professor of anesthesia in the United States at the University of Wisconsin Anesthetists' Travel Club founded
1930	Circle anesthetic breathing and carbon dioxide absorption system described by Sword

(continued)

this gas was realized. Unfortunately, the use of nitrous oxide for medical purposes temporarily fell into disrepute when Dr. Wells, who did not appreciate the lack of potency of nitrous oxide, failed in an attempt to produce anesthesia for surgery during a demonstration before a group of his colleagues at the Massachusetts General Hospital. It was not until 1868 when a Chicago surgeon, Dr. Edmond W. Andrews, popularized the use of nitrous oxide with oxygen that the full value of this gas as an anesthetic began to be appreciated. Between 1844 and 1868, nitrous oxide continued to be used by itinerant showmen who staged public displays of the exhilarating effects of this gas on the sensorium. Likewise, ether was often used for nonmedical purposes described as "ether frolics."

Indeed, it is likely that Dr. Long saw ether used in this way during his medical student days in Philadelphia before 1842.

ANESTHESIA AFTER ETHER

The discovery of the anesthetic properties of ether, chloroform, and nitrous oxide satisfied the immediate needs to provide analgesia during surgery. Indeed, no significant new inhaled anesthetics were introduced during the next 80 years (Fig. 1-1).[2] The search for new inhaled anesthetics began in the 1920s when the expanding scientific basis of anesthesia and surgery demanded drugs with greater flexibility and fewer side effects than currently provided by ether and chloroform. As such,

Table 1-1. (*continued*)

1932	Association of Anaesthetists of Great Britain and Ireland founded
1933	Cyclopropane used by Waters to produce surgical anesthesia
1934	Thiopental used by Lundy for induction of anesthesia
1935	Rovenstine organized a Department of Anesthesia at Bellevue Hospital in New York
	New York Society of Anesthetists becomes the American Society of Anesthetists
1938	American Board of Anesthesiology founded
1940	The journal *Anesthesiology* first published
1942	d-Tubocurarine used by Griffith and Johnson to produce skeletal muscle relaxation during general anesthesia
1943	Lidocaine synthesized by Lofgren
1945	American Society of Anesthetists becomes the American Society of Anesthesiologists
1946	The journal *Anaesthesia* first published
1949	Succinylcholine used clinically by Phillips and Fusco
1952	The journal *Der Anaesthetist* first published
1953	Association of University Anesthetists founded
	Residency Review Committee in Anesthesiology established
1954	*Canadian Anaesthetists' Society Journal* first published
	Anesthetists' Travel Club becomes the Academy of Anesthesiology
1956	Halothane used clinically by Johnson
1957	The journal *Survey of Anesthesiology* first published
	The journal *Acta Anesthesiologica Scandinavica* first published
	Current Researches in Anesthesia and Analgesia becomes *Anesthesia and Analgesia, Current Researches*
1958	"Audio Digest Anesthesiology" first recorded
1959	Methoxyflurane used clinically by Artusio and Van Poznak
1968	Society of Academic Anesthesia Chairman founded
1972	Enflurane used clinically
1973	The journal *Critical Care Medicine* first published
1975	In-training examination in anesthesiology initiated
	American Society of Regional Anesthesia refounded
1976	The journal *Regional Anesthesia* first published
1979	*Anesthesia and Analgesia, Current Researches* becomes *Anesthesia and Analgesia*
1981	Isoflurane used clinically
1985	Anesthesia Patient Safety Foundation established
1986	Foundation for Anesthesia Education and Research established

(Information in part derived from a chart prepared by William H. G. Dornette, M.D., for the Ohio Chemical and Surgical Equipment Company, Madison, WI, 1962.)

cyclopropane, because of its low blood solubility and support of the circulation, became the most important new inhaled anesthetic in the 1930s.

Until the 1950s, all the available inhaled anesthetics possessed at least one of two defects: being explosive in oxygen (ether, ethylene, vinethene, cyclopropane) or being toxic (chloroform, vinethene, trichloroethylene). The evolution of fluorine technology, stimulated originally by the need to separate uranium isotopes for the development of the atomic bomb, led to a new generation of fluorinated inhaled anesthetics in the 1950s. For example, combining fluorine with carbon decreased flammability while the stability of this bond tended to reduce metabolism and thus organ toxicity. The first of the new fluorinated inhaled anesthetics introduced in 1954 was fluroxene. Fluroxene had several desirable characteristics, including low blood solubility and a minimal tendency to depress cardiovascular function or sensitize the heart to exogenous epinephrine. Fluroxene, however, frequently caused nausea and vomiting and at higher anesthetic concentrations was flammable. Later work also suggested this inhaled anesthetic could on rare occasions be hepatotoxic and might also be carcinogenic.[3] Fluroxene was voluntarily withdrawn from the market in 1975, mainly because of its flammability.

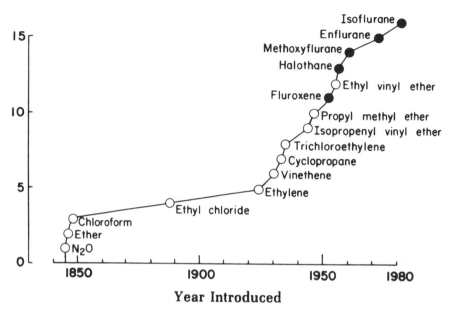

Fig. 1-1. Anesthetics used in clinical practice. The history of anesthesia began with the introduction of nitrous oxide, ether, and chloroform. After 1950, all introduced drugs, with the exception of ethyl vinyl ether, have contained fluorine (closed circles). (From Eger,[2] with permission.)

Modern Inhaled Anesthetics

Presently, one gas (nitrous oxide) and the vapors of three volatile liquids (halothane, enflurane, isoflurane) represent the commonly used inhaled anesthetics. These drugs differ in their physical and chemical characteristics (see Chapter 2) and their pharmacology (see Chapters 4 and 5).

Halothane

Halothane was introduced in 1956 after pharmacologists had predicted that its halogenated chemical structure would provide nonflammability, low blood solubility, molecular stability (trifluorocarbon molecule), and anesthetic potency (chlorine and bromine) (Fig. 1-2).[4] This drug was found to produce a rapid and pleasant induction of anesthesia, bronchodilation, skeletal muscle relaxation, a prompt return to consciousness, and minimal postoperative nausea and vomiting. These attributes and the subsequent clinical popularity of halothane temporarily halted the search for new

inhaled anesthetics. With continued use of halothane, however, its limitations (depression of ventilation and circulation, enhanced dysrhythmogenic effects of epinephrine, rare potential to produce hepatotoxicity) led to renewed interest in the search for other inhaled anesthetics.[5]

Methoxyflurane

The search for new inhaled anesthetics focused on methyl ethyl ethers, since ether derivatives do not increase the incidence of cardiac dysrhythmias. Methoxyflurane, introduced in 1959, was the first of the methyl ethyl ethers to be used clinically (Fig. 1-2).[6] This drug did not increase myocardial irritability and seemed to be less depressant to the circulation than halothane. Methoxyflurane, however, was extensively metabolized particularly to fluoride, introducing the potential for fluoride nephrotoxicity (see Chapter 5). In addition, its high blood and tissue solubility resulted in slow induction of anesthesia and in the potential for delayed awakening, especially after prolonged ad-

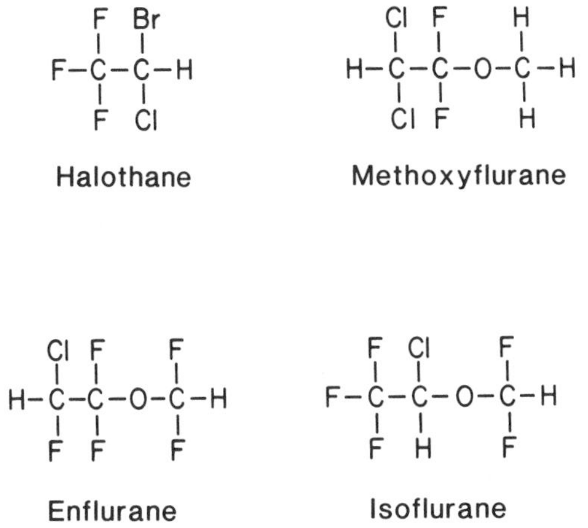

Fig. 1-2. Chemical structure of volatile anesthetics. Halothane is an alkane derivative while the other volatile anesthetics are derivatives of methyl ethyl ether. Isoflurane is the chemical isomer of enflurane.

Characteristics of an Ideal Inhaled Anesthetic

Absence of flammability

Easily vaporized at ambient temperature

Potent

Low blood solubility to assure rapid induction and recovery from anesthesia

Minimal metabolism

Compatible with epinephrine

Skeletal muscle relaxation

Suppresses excessive sympathetic nervous system activity

Not irritating to airways

Bronchodilation

Absence of excessive myocardial depression

Absence of cerebral vasodilation

Absence of hepatic and renal toxicity

ministration. These undesirable characteristics have led to the infrequent use of methoxyflurane despite its continued clinical availability.

Enflurane

Enflurane, introduced in 1972, was the next methyl ethyl ether derivative to become available for use as an inhaled anesthetic (Fig. 1-2).[7] This drug provided stable cardiac rhythm, produced excellent skeletal muscle relaxation, and underwent minimal metabolism, which made organ toxicity unlikely. Rapid induction and recovery from anesthesia was predictable because of the low blood solubility of enflurane. As a result of these desirable characteristics, enflurane has become a popular and frequently administered anesthetic.

Isoflurane

Isoflurane was introduced for patient use in 1981 (Fig. 1-2).[8] This inhaled anesthetic is the chemical isomer of enflurane but, in contrast to enflurane, undergoes less metabolism, does not stimulate the central nervous system, and is less soluble in blood. In many respects, isoflurane possesses the characteristics considered important for the ideal inhaled anesthetic.

Regional Anesthesia

The introduction of regional anesthesia awaited the development of a hollow metal needle in 1854 and the discovery of local anesthetics. Dr. Carl Koller in 1884 discovered the local anesthetic effects of cocaine when applied topically to the eye. In 1885, Dr. William S. Halsted, a surgeon, introduced the concept of nerve block and infiltration anesthesia by the injection of cocaine. Also, in 1885, Dr. Leonard Corning, a neurologist, was the first to produce lumbar epidural block by the injection of cocaine. Dr. August Bier in 1898 demonstrated the feasibility of spinal block by the injection of cocaine into the subarachnoid space of a patient undergoing a foot amputation. Procaine, synthesized in 1905 by Einhorn, replaced cocaine for producing regional anesthesia. Today the most frequently used local anesthetics are tetracaine (topical anesthesia, spinal block), lidocaine (topical anesthesia, infiltration anesthesia, peripheral nerve block, epidural block, spinal block), and bupivacaine (peripheral nerve block, epidural block, spinal block) (see Chapter 7).

Injected Drugs

Induction of anesthesia with the intravenous injection of thiopental was introduced by Dr. John S. Lundy in 1934. Subsequently, the introduction of d-tubocurarine into clinical anesthesia in 1942 revolutionized the methods by which skeletal muscle relaxation during surgery was produced.[9] Finally, opioids, used for many years in combination with nitrous oxide to produce general anesthesia, can also be used as the sole anesthetic (high-dose fentanyl) for critically ill patients who cannot tolerate even minimal cardiac depression produced by inhaled drugs.[10]

ANESTHESIA AS A MEDICAL SPECIALTY

Anesthesia as a medical specialty evolved differently in England and the United States. Chloroform, the standard anesthetic in England, was a potent ventilatory and cardiac depressant requiring great skills in its administration. As a result, only physicians were considered competent to administer chloroform. In contrast, ether remained the dominant anesthetic in the United States. Unlike chloroform, ether stimulated ventilation and maintained the circulation. For these reasons, ether was thought to have a built-in protection for the patient, and its administration was often relegated to an inexperienced physician or nurse. Indeed, it was more than 60 years after the demonstration of ether anesthesia by Dr. Morton before American physicians began to devote full-time medical practice to the administration of anesthetics. For example, the first department of anesthesia was created in 1904 at the New York Medical College, with Dr. Thomas D. Buchanan as professor and chairman. Dr. Arthur E. Gudel, a 1908 graduate of Indiana University School of Medicine, described the stages and planes of anesthesia in a monograph published in 1920. In 1923, Dr. Mary A. Ross became the first formal postgraduate trainee in anesthesiology in the United States, receiving a certificate from the University

of Iowa for her year of training after graduation from medical school. Dr. John S. Lundy organized a department of anesthesia at the Mayo Clinic in 1924, and Dr. Ralph M. Waters arrived at the University of Wisconsin for the same purpose in 1927. Graduates of the training programs directed by Drs. Lundy and Waters continued to expand the scope of anesthesiology. Among those graduates was Dr. Emory A. Rovenstine who in 1935 left Wisconsin to develop a department of anesthesia at Bellevue, the teaching hospital of New York University. During the next 25 years, over 30 graduates of Dr. Rovenstine's program became chairmans of departments of anesthesia.

American Society of Anesthesiologists (ASA)

The first anesthesia organization in the United States was the Long Island Society of Anesthetists started in 1905 by Dr. A. Frederick Erdmann and eight physician colleagues from the New York City area. The stated goal of this society was to "promote the art and science of anesthesia," and annual dues were $1.00. Only the London Society of Anaesthetists, founded in 1893, preceded this first society in the United States. The Long Island Society of Anesthetists grew in membership, becoming the New York Society of Anesthetists in 1911. This society became the American Society of Anesthetists in 1935, with 487 members and annual dues of $5.00. In 1945, the name was changed to the American Society of Anesthesiologists. This name change was intended to reflect more accurately the membership of the society, which consists of physicians with postgraduate training in anesthesia, (anesthesiologists) in contrast to nonphysicians (anesthetists) who also administer anesthesia (see the section *Certified Registered Nurse Anesthetist*). This semantic distinction is observed most consistently in the United States, whereas in other areas of the world the terms tend to be used interchangeably. Today, the American Society of Anesthesiologists has over 26,000 members, making anesthesia the sixth largest among the American medical specialties.

Anesthesiology, the official journal of the American Society of Anesthesiologists, was first published in July 1940, with Dr. Henry S. Ruth as the editor. This initial issue was sent to 568 members of the society and 300 additional nonmember subscribers. Today this highly respected journal has a monthly worldwide circulation that exceeds 35,000.

International Anesthesia Research Society (IARS)

At the same time that the New York Society of Anesthetists was evolving into the American Society of Anesthesiologists, another important organization was developing under the direction of Dr. Francis H. McMechan, a physician practicing in Cincinnati, Ohio. In 1919, Dr. McMechan established the National Anesthesia Research Society. This society held annual meetings, and in August 1922 the first medical journal devoted entirely to the specialty of anesthesiology, *Current Researches in Anesthesia and Analgesia*, appeared with Dr. McMechan as editor. Previously, the only other source of scientific information for anesthesiology was the *American Journal of Anesthesia and Analgesia*, published since 1914 as a quarterly supplement to the *American Journal of Surgery*. In 1925, the National Anesthesia Research Society was renamed the International Anesthesia Research Society, which today continues to sponsor an annual scientific meeting and publish the journal *Anesthesia and Analgesia*.

American Society of Regional Anesthesia (ASRA)

The American Society of Regional Anesthesia was founded in 1923 to provide a forum for those physicians interested in regional anesthesia. This society was absorbed into the American Society of Anesthetists in 1941 only to again become an independent organization in 1975. The official journal of this society, *Regional Anesthesia*, was first published in October 1976.

American Board of Anesthesiology (ABA)

The American Board of Anesthesiology was incorporated as an affiliate of the American Board of Surgery in 1938. After the first voluntary examinations, 87 physicians were certified as Diplomates of the American Board of Anesthesiology. The American Board of Anesthesiology was recognized as an independent board by the American Board of Medical Specialties in 1941. To date, over 17,000 anesthesiologists have been certified

as Diplomates of the American Board of Anesthesiology.

Certified Registered Nurse Anesthetist

In the past, nearly 50 percent of the anesthetics given in the United States each year were administered by certified registered nurse anesthetists (CRNA). To become a CRNA, the candidate must earn a Registered Nurse degree, followed by 2 years of anesthesia training in an approved nurse anesthesia training program. At present, the American Association of Nurse Anesthetists (AANA) remains responsible for the curriculum of the majority of nurse anesthesia training programs, as well as establishment of criteria for certification as a nurse anesthetist. The activities of nurse anesthetists are usually confined to the operating room, where they often work under the supervision of an anesthesiologist. This supervised team approach is consistent with the concept that the administration of anesthesia is the practice of medicine.

Postgraduate (Residency) Training in Anesthesiology

Postgraduate training in anesthesiology consists of 4 years of supervised experience in an approved program after the degree of Doctor of Medicine or Osteopathy has been obtained. The first year of postgraduate training in anesthesiology consists of nonanesthesia experience (Clinical Base Year) in patient-care related specialties, such as internal medicine, surgery, or pediatrics. The second, third, and fourth postgraduate years (Clinical Anesthesia Years 1–3) are spent in learning all aspects of clinical anesthesia, including subspecialty experiences in obstetrical anesthesia, pediatric anesthesia, cardiac anesthesia, neuroanesthesia, pain management, and critical care medicine. A maximum of 6 months during the Clinical Anesthesia Years may be elected by the resident for pursuit of research interests.

The content of the educational experience during the clinical anesthesia years reflects the wide-ranging scope of anesthesiology as a medical specialty. At present, anesthesiology is defined in the booklet of information of the American Board of Anesthesiology as a practice of medicine dealing with but not limited to

1. The assessment of, consultation for, and preparation of patients for anesthesia.
2. The provision of insensibility to pain during surgical, obstetrical, therapeutic and diagnostic procedures, and the management of patients so affected.
3. The monitoring and restoration of homeostasis during the perioperative period, as well as homeostasis in the critically ill, injured, or otherwise seriously ill patient.
4. The diagnosis and treatment of painful syndromes.
5. The clinical management and teaching of cardiac and pulmonary resuscitation.
6. The evaluation of respiratory function and application of respiratory therapy in all its forms.
7. The supervision, teaching, and evaluation of performance of both medical and paramedical personnel involved in anesthesia, respiratory, and critical care.
8. The conduct of research at the clinical and basic science levels to explain and improve the care of patients insofar as physiologic function and the response to drugs are concerned.
9. The administrative involvement in hospitals, medical schools, and outpatient facilities necessary to implement these responsibilities.

This definition emphasizes the continued major role of the anesthesiologist in the operating room. Indeed, the anesthesiologist should function as the clinical pharmacologist and internist or pediatrician in the operating room. Furthermore, this definition emphasizes that the scope of anesthesiology extends beyond the operating room to include pain management (see Chapter 33), cardiopulmonary resuscitation (see Chapter 34), respiratory therapy (see Chapter 31), critical care medicine (see Chapter 32), and research. Indeed, much remains to be learned, and even the mechanism of general anesthesia remains unknown.

Approximately 160 postgraduate training programs in anesthesiology are approved by the Accreditation Council for Graduate Medical Education of the American Medical Association. These training programs offer more than 4200 postgraduate positions in anesthesiology. Approved post-graduate training programs are visited periodically by a representative of the Residency Review Committee to assure continued compliance with the published standards of quality medical education. The Residency Review Committee consists of members appointed by the American Medical Association, American Society of Anesthesiologists, and American Board of Anesthesiology.

After completion of the required postgraduate training in anesthesiology, the physician can voluntarily enter the examination system of the American Board of Anesthesiology. Successful completion of a written and then an oral examination results in the issuance of a certificate confirming that the physician is a Diplomate ("Board certified") of the American Board of Anesthesiology. A certificate of special qualifications in Anesthesiology Critical Care Medicine is available to Diplomates of the American Board of Anesthesiology who meet additional training and written examination requirements (see Chapter 32).

REFERENCES

1. Greene NM. Anesthesia and the development of surgery (1846–1896). Anesth Analg 1979;58:5–12.
2. Eger EI II. Isoflurane (Forane). A compendium and reference. Madison WI, Anaquest, a division of BOC, Inc. 1985:1–4.
3. Baden JM, Kelley M, Wharton RS, Hitt BA, Simmon VF, Mazze RI. Mutagenicity of halogenated ether anesthetics. Anesthesiology 1977;46:346–50.
4. Raventos J. Action of Fluothane—New volatile anesthetic. Br J Pharmacol 1956;11:394–410.
5. Summary of the national halothane study. JAMA 1966;197:775–88.
6. Artusio JF, Van Poznak A, Hunt RE, Tiers FM, Alexander M. A clinical evaluation of methoxyflurane in man. Anesthesiology 1960;21:512–7.
7. Dobkin AB, Heinrich RG, Israel JS, Levy AA, Neville JF, Ounkasem K. Clinical and laboratory evaluation of a new inhalation agent. Compound 347 (CHF_2OCF_2CHFCl). Anesthesiology 1968;29:275–87.
8. Vitcha JF. A history of Forane. Anesthesiology 1971;35:4–7.
9. Griffith HR, Johnson GG. Use of curare in general anesthesia. Anesthesiology 1942;3:418–20.
10. Stanley TH, Webster LR. Anesthesia requirements and cardiovascular effects of fentnayl-oxygen and fentanyl-diazepam-oxygen anesthesia in man. Anesth Analg 1975;57:411–6.

Section II

Pharmacology

Basic Principles

Basic principles of pharmacology are derived from an understanding of pharmacokinetics and pharmacodynamics.[1] Pharmacokinetics describe the absorption, distribution, metabolism, and excretion of inhaled or injected drugs. Pharmacodynamics describes the responsiveness of receptors to drugs and the mechanism by which these effects occur (i.e., potency of a drug). Receptors are the component of the cell that interacts with drugs to initiate a chain of events leading to pharmacologic effects. Selectivity of drug action is also determined by receptors that recognize specific drugs. Termination of a drug's effect is by metabolism, excretion, and/or its redistribution to inactive tissue sites.

TERMINOLOGY AND DEFINITIONS

Drugs that activate receptors are called agonists (e.g., isoproterenol). Antagonists are drugs that bind to receptors without activating the receptors while at the same time preventing agonists from stimulating these same receptors (e.g., propranolol). Competitive antagonism is present when increasing concentrations of an antagonist (e.g., nondepolarizing muscle relaxants) progressively inhibit responses to unchanging concentrations of agonist (e.g., acetylcholine). High concentrations of agonist, however, can overcome competitive antagonism. Noncompetitive antagonism is present when even high concentrations of agonist cannot completely overcome antagonism.

An additive effect means that a second drug acting with the first drug will produce an effect equal to algebraic summation. For example, the anesthetic effects of two inhaled anesthetics are additive as reflected by minimum alveolar concentration (MAC) equivalents[2] (see the section *Minimum Alveolar Concentration*). Synergistic means that two drugs interact to produce an effect greater than algebraic summation. For example, aminoglycoside antibiotics do not produce clinically significant neuromuscular blockade by themselves but greatly enhance that produced by nondepolarizing muscle relaxants.

Hyperactive and hyporeactive describe individuals in whom the usual dose of drug produces exaggerated or reduced effects, respectively. Hyporeactivity acquired from chronic exposure to a drug is often termed tolerance. Cross-tolerance commonly develops between drugs of different classes that produce similar pharmacologic effects (e.g., inhaled anesthetics and chronic alcohol ingestion). Tolerance that develops acutely with only a few doses of a drug such as ephedrine is termed tachyphylaxis. Idiosyncrasy is present when an unusual effect of a drug occurs in uniquely susceptible and often small groups of patients regardless of the dose. More correctly, idiosyncrasy should be attributed to likely or documented mech-

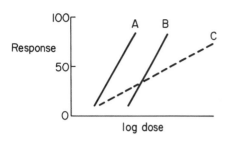

Fig. 2-1. Schematic dose-response curves that illustrate parallelism (curves A and B) and deviation from parallelism (curve C compared with A or B). A potency ratio can be derived only when the dose-response curves for two drugs are parallel. Conversely, when the curves deviate from parallelism, a potency ratio cannot be derived. For example, at 20 percent response, the drug represented by curve C is more potent than the drug represented by curve B. At 90 percent response, however, the potency of these two drugs is reversed.

$$P_A \leftrightharpoons P_a \leftrightharpoons P_{br}$$

Fig. 2-2. The alveolar partial pressure (PA) of an inhaled anesthetic is in equilibrium with partial pressure of the arterial blood (Pa) and brain (Pbr). Therefore, the PA is an indirect measure of the anesthetic partial pressure at the site of action, the brain.

anisms such as hypersensitivity (i.e., allergy) or genetic differences.

Dose-response curves plot the dose of drug administered (or the resulting plasma concentration) against the pharmacologic response evoked by that dose. A potency ratio can be derived when dose response curves are parallel (Fig. 2-1). For example, the relationship is similar between the dose that produces a 90 percent response (effective dose 90 or ED_{90}) and the dose that produces a 20 percent response (ED_{20}). Drugs that produce parallel dose-response curves are generally thought to have identical, or at least similar, mechanisms of action. When dose response curves deviate from parallelism, the potency must be described individually at each level of response. Drugs that produce dose-response curves that deviate from parallelism generally have different mechanisms of action.

PHARMACOKINETICS OF INHALED ANESTHETICS

Pharmacokinetics of inhaled anesthetics describes their uptake (absorption) from alveoli into the systemic circulation, distribution in the body, and eventual elimination via the lungs or metabolism in the liver.[3] By controlling the inspired partial pressure (PI) (same as concentration when refer-

ring to the gas phase) of an inhaled anesthetic, a gradient is created such that the anesthetic is delivered from the anesthetic machine to its site of action, the brain. The primary objective of inhalation anesthesia is to achieve a constant and optimal partial pressure of the anesthetic in the brain (Pbr).

The brain and all other tissues equilibrate with the partial pressure of the inhaled anesthetic delivered to them by the arterial blood (Pa) (Fig. 2-2). Likewise, the blood equilibrates with the alveolar partial pressure (PA) of the anesthetic (Fig. 2-2). Therefore, maintaining a constant and optimal PA becomes an indirect but reliable method for controlling the Pbr. The fact that the PA of an inhaled anesthetic mirrors its Pbr is the reason the PA is used as an index of anesthetic depth, reflection of the rate of induction and recovery from anesthesia, and measure of equal potency (see the section *Minimum Alveolar Concentration*).

Understanding those factors that determine the PA and thus the Pbr allows the anesthesiologist to skillfully control the dose of inhaled anesthetic delivered to the brain.

Factors that Determine the Alveolar Partial Pressure

The PA and ultimately Pbr of an inhaled anesthetic is determined by input (delivery) into the alveoli minus uptake (loss) of the drug from the alveoli into the arterial blood. Input of the inhaled anesthetic is dependent on three factors: PI, alveolar ventilation (VA), and characteristics of the anesthetic breathing system. Likewise, uptake of the inhaled anesthetic is dependent on three factors: solubility, cardiac ouput (CO), and the alveolar to venous partial pressure difference (A−vD). These six factors act simultaneously to determine the PA. Metabolism and percutaneous loss of inhaled anesthetics do not significantly influence

---

Summary of Factors Determining Partial Pressure Gradients Necessary for Establishment of Anesthesia

Transfer of inhaled anesthetic from anesthetic machine to alveoli
    Inspired partial pressure
    Alveolar ventilation
    Characteristics of anesthetic breathing system

Transfer of inhaled anesthetic from alveoli to arterial blood
    Blood:gas partition coefficient
    Cardiac output
    Alveolar to venous partial pressure difference

Transfer of inhaled anesthetic from arterial blood to brain
    Brain:blood partition coefficient
    Cerebral blood flow
    Arterial to venous partial pressure difference

PA during induction and maintenance of anesthesia.

Inspired Anesthetic Partial Pressure

A high PI is necessary during initial administration of an inhaled anesthetic. This initial high PI (input) offsets the impact of uptake and thus accelerates induction of anesthesia as reflected by the rate of rise in the PA. This effect of the PI is known as the concentration effect.

With time, as uptake into the blood decreases, the PI should be decreased to match the reduced anesthetic uptake. Indeed, decreasing the PI to match decreasing uptake with time is crucial if one is to achieve the goal of maintaining a constant and optimal Pbr. For example, if the PI were maintained constant with time (input constant), the PA (and Pbr) would progressively increase as uptake diminished.

Second Gas Effect. The second gas effect is a distinct phenomenon that occurs independently of the concentration effect.[4] The ability of the large volume uptake of one gas (first gas) to accelerate the rate of rise of the PA of a concurrently administered companion gas (second gas) is known as the second gas effect. For example, the initial large volume uptake of nitrous oxide accelerates the uptake of companion gases such as volatile anesthetics and oxygen. Indeed, the transient increase (about 10 percent) in PaO_2 that accompanies the early phases of nitrous oxide administration reflects the second gas effect. This increase in PaO_2 has been designated as alveolar hyperoxygenation. Increased tracheal inflow of all inhaled gases (i.e., first and second gases) and concentration of the second gases in a smaller lung volume (concentrating effect) due to the high volume uptake of the first gas are the explanations for the second gas effect.[5] Although the second gas effect may produce detectable alterations in the PA, it probably should not be considered clinically significant.

Alveolar Ventilation

Increased VA, like PI, promotes input of inhaled anesthetics to offset uptake. The net effect is a more rapid rate of rise in the PA and induction of anesthesia. Predictably, hypoventilation has the opposite effect, acting to slow the induction of anesthesia.

Controlled ventilation of the lungs that results in hyperventilation and decreased venous return accelerates the rate of rise of the PA by virtue of increased input (increased VA) and decreased uptake (decreased CO) (see the section *Cardiac Output*). As a result, the risk of anesthetic overdose may be increased during controlled ventilation of the lungs. For this reason, it may be appropriate to reduce the PI of volatile anesthetics when ventilation of the lungs is changed from spontaneous to controlled so as to maintain the PA similar to that present during spontaneous ventilation.

Another effect of hyperventilation is decreased cerebral blood flow due to reductions in the $PaCO_2$. Conceivably, the impact of increased input on the rate of rise of the PA would be offset by decreased delivery of anesthetic to the brain. Furthermore, coronary blood flow may remain unchanged, such that increased input produces myocardial depression, and decreased cerebral blood flow prevents a concomitant onset of anesthesia.

Anesthetic Breathing System

Characteristics of the anesthetic breathing system that influence the rate of rise of the PA include the (1) volume of the system, (2) solubility of inhaled anesthetics in the rubber or plastic components of the system, and (3) gas inflow from the anesthetic machine. The volume of the anesthetic breathing system acts as a buffer to slow achievement of the PA. High gas inflow from the anesthetic machine negates this buffer effect. Solubility of inhaled anesthetics in the components of the anesthetic breathing system initially slows the rate at which the PA rises. At the conclusion of an anesthetic, reversal of the partial pressure gradient in the anesthetic breathing system results in elution of the anesthetics that slows the rate at which the PA decreases. Furthermore, re-use of the same anesthetic breathing system results in exposure of the patient to that anesthetic, even if another drug or technique has been selected.

Solubility

Solubility of inhaled anesthetics in blood and tissues is denoted by partition coefficients (Table 2-1). A partition coefficient is a distribution ratio describing how the inhaled anesthetic distributes itself between two phases at equilibrium (i.e., when the partial pressures are identical). For example, a blood:gas partition coefficient of 10 means that the concentration of the inhaled anesthetic is 10 in the blood and 1 in the alveolar gas when the partial pressures of that anesthetic in these two phases are identical. It is important to recognize that partition coefficients are temperature-dependent. For example, solubility of a gas in a liquid is increased when the temperature of the liquid decreases. Unless otherwise stated, partition coefficients are for 37° Celsius.

Blood:Gas Partition Coefficients. Based on their blood:gas partition coefficients (i.e., solubilities) inhaled anesthetics are traditionally considered as soluble (methoxyflurane), of intermediate solubility (halothane, enflurane, isoflurane), and poorly soluble (nitrous oxide) (Table 2-1). High blood solubility means that a large amount of inhaled anesthetic must be dissolved in the blood before equilibrium is reached with the gas phase. For example, the high solubility of methoxyflurane slows the rate at which the PA and Pa rise such that the induction of anesthesia is slow (Fig. 2-3). The blood can be considered a pharmacologically inactive reservoir, the size of which is determined by the solubility of the anesthetic in the blood. When the blood:gas partition coefficient is high,

Table 2-1. Comparative Characteristics of Inhaled Anesthetics

	Methoxyflurane	Halothane	Enflurane	Isoflurane	Nitrous Oxide
Blood:gas partition coefficient[a]	12	2.4	1.9	1.4	0.47
Brain:blood partition coefficient[a]	2	2.6	2.6	3.7	1.1
Oil:gas partition coefficient[a]	970	224	98	98	1.4
MAC (volumes percent, 30–55 years old)	0.16	0.75	1.68	1.15	105–110
Vapor pressure (mmHg)					
18° Celsius	20	224	156	219	
20° Celsius	23	244	172	240	
22° Celsius	26	267	189	262	
Molecular weight	165	197.4	184.5	184.5	
Commercial preparation contains preservative	Yes	Yes	No	No	
Stable in soda lime	No	No	Yes	Yes	
Reacts with metal	Yes	Yes	No	No	

[a] 37° Celsius.

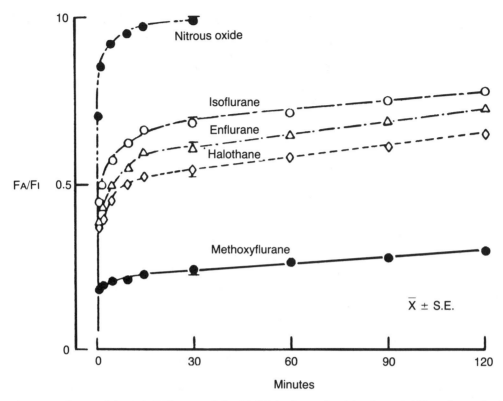

Fig. 2-3. The rate of rise of the PA (FA) toward the PI (FI) is determined by the solubility of anesthetics in the blood. (From Carpenter et al.,[7] with permission.)

a large amount of anesthetic must be dissolved in the blood before the Pa equilibrates with the PA. Clinically, the impact of high blood solubility on the rate of rise of the PA can be offset to some extent by increasing the PI. When blood solubility is poor, as with nitrous oxide, minimal amounts of the anesthetic have to be dissolved in the blood before equilibrium is reached such that the rate of rise of the PA and thus that of the Pa and Pbr are rapid (Fig. 2-3).

Tissue:Blood Partition Coefficients. Tissue:blood partition coefficients determine the time necessary for equilibration of the tissue with the Pa. This time can be predicted by calculating a time constant (amount of inhaled anesthetic that can be dissolved in the tissue divided by tissue blood flow) for each tissue. Brain:blood partition coefficients for volatile anesthetics are approximately 2.5, resulting in

a time constant equal to roughly 5 minutes (Table 2-1). Complete equilibration of any tissue, including the brain, with the Pa requires at least three time constants. This is the rationale for maintaining the PA of volatile anesthetics constant for about 15 minutes before assuming that the Pbr is similar. Three time constants for nitrous oxide amount to about 6 minutes, reflecting its low brain solubility (Table 2-1).

Nitrous Oxide Transfer to Closed Gas Spaces. The blood:gas partition coefficient of nitrous oxide (0.47) is 34 times greater than nitrogen (0.014). This differential solubility means that nitrous oxide can leave the blood to enter an air-filled cavity 34 times more rapidly than nitrogen can leave the cavity to enter the blood.[6] As a result of this preferential transfer of nitrous oxide, the volume or pressure of the air-filled cavity in-

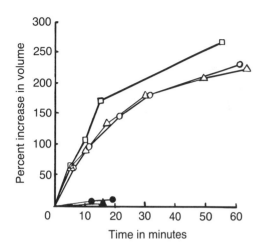

Fig. 2-4. Inhalation of 75 percent nitrous oxide in oxygen (open symbols) but not oxygen alone (solid symbols) rapidly increases the volume of a pneumothorax. (From Eger and Saidman,[6] with permission.)

creases. The entrance of nitrous oxide into an air-filled cavity surrounded by a compliant wall (intestinal gas, pneumothorax, pulmonary blebs, air embolism) causes the gas space to expand. Conversely, entrance of nitrous oxide into an air-filled cavity surrounded by a noncompliant wall (middle ear, cerebral ventricles, supratentorial subdural space) causes an increase in pressure.

The magnitude of volume or pressure increase is influenced by the PA of nitrous oxide, blood flow to the air-filled cavity, and duration of nitrous oxide administration. In an animal model, the inhalation of 75 percent nitrous oxide doubles the volume of a pneumothorax in 10 minutes (Fig. 2-4).[6] Therefore, the presence of a closed pneumothorax is a contraindication to the administration of nitrous oxide. Indeed, decreasing pulmonary compliance during administration of nitrous oxide to patients with histories of chest trauma may reflect nitrous-oxide-induced expansion of a previously unrecognized pneumothorax.

In contrast to the rapid expansion of a pneumothorax, the increase in bowel gas volume produced by nitrous oxide is slow. The question of whether to administer nitrous oxide to patients with a bowel obstruction is of little importance if the operation is short. Limiting the inhaled con-

centration of nitrous oxide to 50 percent, however, may be a prudent recommendation when bowel gas volume is increased preoperatively. Following this guideline, bowel gas volume, at most, would double even with prolonged operations.[6]

Postoperative manifestations of nitrous oxide passage into the middle ear include altered hearing acuity, serous otitis, tympanic membrane rupture, and disruption of prior ossicle reconstructive surgery (see Chapter 25).

Cardiac Output

The CO influences uptake and therefore, PA, by carrying away more or less anesthetic from the alveoli. A high CO (fear) results in more rapid uptake such that the rate of rise in the PA, and thus the induction of anesthesia, is slowed. A low CO (shock) speeds the rate of rise of the PA since there is less uptake to oppose input. Indeed, a common clinical impression is that induction of anesthesia in patients in shock is rapid.

Right-to-Left Shunt. A right-to-left intracardiac or intrapulmonary shunt slows the rate of induction of anesthesia. This slowing reflects the dilutional effect of shunted blood containing no anesthetic on the partial pressure of anesthetic in blood coming from ventilated alveoli. Although shunt will slow the induction of anesthesia, the magnitude of this change is small and probably would not be apparent clinically.

Alveolar to Venous Partial Pressure Difference

The $A-vD$ reflects tissue uptake of inhaled anesthetics. Highly perfused tissues (brain, heart, kidneys, liver) account for less than 10 percent of body mass but receive about 75 percent of the CO (Table 2-2). As a result, these tissues equilibrate rapidly with the Pa. Indeed, after three time constants (about 15 minutes for volatile anesthetics) about 75 percent of the returning venous blood is at the same partial pressure as the PA. For this reason, uptake of volatile anesthetics from the alveoli is greatly decreased after 15 minutes, as reflected by a narrowing of the PI to PA difference. After this time, the inhaled concentrations of volatile anesthetic should be reduced so as to maintain a constant PA in the presence of decreased uptake.

Table 2-2. Body Tissue Compartments

	Body Mass (Percent of 70-kg Adult)	Blood Flow (Percent of Cardiac Output)
Vessel-rich group	10	75
Muscle group	50	19
Fat group	20	5
Vessel-poor group	20	1

Skeletal muscle and fat represent about 70 percent of the body mass but receive less than 25 percent of the CO (Table 2-2). Therefore, these tissues continue to act as inactive reservoirs for anesthetic uptake for several hours. Indeed, equilibration of fat with inhaled anesthetics in the arterial blood probably never occurs.

Recovery from Anesthesia

Recovery from anesthesia can be defined as the rate at which the PA decreases with time (Fig. 2-5).[7] In many respects, recovery is the inverse of induction of anesthesia. For example, VA, solubility, and CO determine the rate at which the PA decreases. Conversely, recovery from anesthesia is also influenced by factors unique to this phase of the anesthetic.

Differences from Induction

Recovery from anesthesia differs from induction of anesthesia with respect to (1) the absence of a concentration effect on recovery (the PI cannot be less than zero), (2) variable tissue concentrations of anesthetics at the start of recovery, and (3) the potential importance of metabolism on the rate of decline in the PA.

Tissue Concentrations. Tissue concentrations of inhaled anesthetics serve as a reservoir to maintain the PA when the partial pressure gradient is reversed by reducing the PI to near zero at the conclusion of anesthesia. The impact of tissue storage will depend on the duration of anesthesia and solubility of the anesthetics in various tissue components. The variable concentrations of anesthetics in different tissues at the conclusion of anesthesia contrasts with induction of anesthesia when all tissues are at the same zero concentration.

Metabolism. An important difference between induction of anesthesia and recovery from anesthesia is the potential impact of metabolism on the rate of decline in the PA at the conclusion of anesthesia (Fig. 2-5).[7] In this regard, metabolism is a principal determinant of the rate of decline in the PA of highly lipid soluble methoxyflurane. Metabolism and VA are equally important in the rate of decline in the PA of halothane, whereas the rate of decrease in the PA of less lipid soluble enflurane and isoflurane is principally due to VA.[8]

Diffusion Hypoxia. Diffusion hypoxia may occur at the conclusion of nitrous oxide administration if patients are allowed to inhale room air. The initial high volume outpouring of nitrous oxide from the blood into the alveoli when inhalation of this gas is discontinued can so dilute the PAO_2 that the PaO_2 decreases.[3] The occurrence of diffusion hypoxia is prevented by filling the patient's lungs with oxygen at the conclusion of nitrous oxide administration.

PHARMACODYNAMICS OF INHALED ANESTHETICS

Minimum Alveolar Concentration

MAC is the minimum alveolar concentration (partial pressure) of an inhaled anesthetic at 1 atmosphere that prevents skeletal muscle movement in response to a noxious stimulus (surgical skin incision) in 50 percent of patients.[9] As such, MAC represents one point on the dose-response curve of effects produced by inhaled anesthetics. The fact that MAC reflects the partial pressure at the anesthetic site of action (Pbr) has made MAC the most important index of anesthetic equal potency.

Use of equally potent doses (i.e., comparable MAC concentrations) of inhaled anesthetics is mandatory for comparing effects of these drugs on vital organ function. For example, 1 MAC enflurane (1.68 percent) depresses cardiac output more than an equally potent concentration of isoflurane (1.15 percent) (see Chapter 4). The fact that the dose-response curves for different inhaled anesthetics are not parallel with respect to vital organ depression is an important observation. Specifically, a therapeutic index may be characterized for the inhaled anesthetics with respect to any

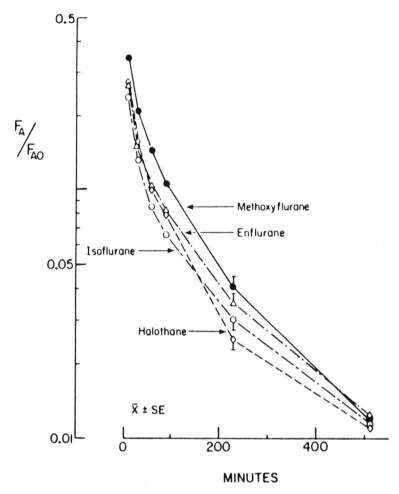

Fig. 2-5. Recovery from anesthesia is reflected by a decline in the PA (FA) expressed as a ratio (FA/FAo) of the PA at any given time to the PA at the conclusion of anesthesia (FAo). (From Carpenter et al.,[7] with permission.)

untoward or undesired side effects (e.g., respiratory or cardiac depression; neuromuscular blockade; cerebral, renal, hepatic, or coronary blood flow). The denominator in this ratio is MAC. Each anesthetic possesses unique qualities with respect to these anesthetic side effects, yet similar MAC concentrations all produce equivalent depression of the central nervous system. Such information is vital for the safe and rational selection of specific inhaled anesthetics for individual patients, as well as the dose of drug that is administered.

MAC values for combinations of inhaled anesthetics are additive. For example, 0.5 MAC nitrous oxide plus 0.5 MAC isoflurane has the same effect at the brain as either drug alone at a 1 MAC concentration. The fact that nitrous oxide MAC is above 100 percent, however, means that this anesthetic cannot be used alone at 1 atmosphere and still provide a minimum of 21 percent oxygen. Therefore, 50 percent to 75 percent inhaled nitrous oxide is commonly administered with the remaining anesthetic requirement being provided by volatile anesthetics and/or opioids. A guideline is that MAC for volatile anesthetics is reduced about 1 percent for every 1 percent alveolar nitrous oxide concentration. An important reason for administering nitrous oxide with volatile anesthetics is the observation that depression of ventilation and circulation is less when nitrous oxide is substituted for an equivalent MAC dose of the volatile drug (see Chapter 4).

Clinically, a MAC concentration of inhaled anesthetic greater than 1 is necessary, because, as noted earlier, 50 percent of patients would move with surgical stimulation at a 1 MAC concentration. Administration of approximately 1.3 MAC prevents movement in nearly all patients during surgery.

In addition to its value as an index of equal potency, the MAC concept also allows a quantitative analysis of the impact of various pharmacologic and physiologic factors on anesthetic requirements.[2] Likewise, factors that do not influence MAC can be determined.[2] Finally, MAC is useful as a tool to understand better the mechanism by which anesthetics produce anesthesia.

Theories of Anesthesia

Inhaled anesthetics produce reversible inhibition of synaptic transmission in several areas of the central nervous system. A decrease in dorsal horn activity produced by low partial pressures of inhaled anesthetics interferes with synaptic transmission in the spinothalamic tract and presumably produces some degree of analgesia (Stage 1). At a higher Pbr, blockade of inhibitory neurons plus facilitation of excitatory transmission accounts for the disinhibitory effects of inhaled anesthetics, manifesting as patient excitement before the onset of unconsciousness (Stage 2). The ascending pathways in the reticular activating system are progressively depressed with a further increase in the Pbr of the inhaled drugs, leading to unconsciousness (Stage 3). Occurring at the same time as unconsciousness, suppression of spinal reflex activity produces skeletal muscle relaxation. At an even higher Pbr (i.e., overdose), there is depression of vital medullary centers, manifesting as profound cardiorespiratory depression (Stage 4).

Impact of Physiologic and Pharmacologic Factors on Minimum Alveolar Concentration

No change in MAC
  Duration of anesthesia
  Hyperkalemia or hypokalemia
  Magnitude of anesthetic metabolism
  Thyroid gland dysfunction
  Male or female
  $PaCO_2$ 15 mmHg to 95 mmHg
  PaO_2 above 38 mmHg
  Blood pressure above 40 mmHg

Increase MAC
  Hyperthermia
  Hypernatremia
  Drugs that increase CNS catecholamine levels (monoamine oxidase inhibitors, tricyclic antidepressants, acute cocaine ingestion, acute amphetamine ingestion)
  Chronic ethanol abuse

Decrease MAC
  Hypothermia
  Hyponatremia
  Pregnancy
  Lithium
  Pancuronium (?)
  Lidocaine
  Alpha-2 agonists
  PaO_2 below 38 mmHg
  Blood pressure below 40 mmHg
  Increasing age
  Preoperative medication
  Drugs that decrease CNS catecholamine levels (alpha-methyldopa, clonidine, chronic amphetamine ingestion)
  Acute ethanol ingestion

Proposed Theories of Anesthesia

The mechanism by which inhaled anesthetics produce progressive and sometimes selective depression of the central nervous system (anesthesia) is not known. Inhaled anesthetics have multiple effects including alterations in membrane properties, neurotransmitter activity, receptor responsiveness, and chemical- and voltage-gated ion channels and enzymes.[10,11] With all these possible effects, it is difficult to define precisely the mechanisms of general anesthesia. Although a single theory to explain the mechanism of anesthesia seems unlikely, several unitary theories have been proposed to explain the production of anesthesia by inhaled drugs.

Meyer-Overton Theory (Critical-Volume Hypothesis). This theory recognizes the close correlation between the lipid solubility of inhaled anesthetics (oil:gas partition coefficient) and their potencies (MAC) (Table 2-1). Such a correlation suggests that anesthesia occurs when a sufficient number of anesthetic molecules dissolve (critical volume) in crucial hydrophobic sites, such as lipid cell membranes. Conceptually, expansion of hydrophobic membranes by dissolved anesthetic molecules could exert pressure on ionic channels necessary for sodium flux and the subsequent development of action potentials necessary for synaptic transmission. Indeed, membrane expansion by a critical volume of 0.4 percent results in anesthesia. Furthermore, high pressures (40 atmospheres to 100 atmospheres) partially antagonize the action of inhaled anesthetics (pressure reversal), presumably by returning (compressing) lipid membranes to their "awake" contour.[12] Universal acceptance of this theory, however, is prevented by the observation that some lipid soluble compounds are not anesthetics and, in fact, may be convulsants.

Protein (Receptor) Hypothesis. This theory proposes hydrophobic regions of specific proteins (receptors) in the central nervous system as the site of action of inhaled anesthetics. Evidence to support this theory includes the steep nature of anesthetic dose-response curves (i.e., 1 MAC prevents movement in 50 percent of subjects, whereas 1.3 MAC is effective in about 95 percent), suggesting a crucial receptor occupancy. Receptor specificity is also suggested by conversion of an anesthetic to a nonanesthetic by increasing the molecular weight despite corresponding increases in lipid solubility.

In animals, the dextro isomer of medetomidine,

an alpha-2 agonist, produces dose-dependent and stereospecific reductions in halothane MAC.[13] The stereospecificity of this MAC-reducing property suggests an effect on a homogenous receptor population such as alpha-2 receptors in the central nervous system. It is possible that alpha-2 stimulation supplements the anesthetized state by producing an increase in potassium conductance (hyperpolarizes) with subsequent depresssion of neuronal excitability.

Alteration in Neurotransmitter Availability. Inhaled anesthetics may interfere with the metabolic breakdown of the inhibitory neurotransmitter, gamma-aminobutyric acid (GABA). This inhibition leads to increased brain concentrations of GABA and the speculation that anesthesia may reflect enhanced synaptic inhibition by GABA.

PHARMACOKINETICS OF INTRAVENOUS DRUGS

Pharmacokinetics of intravenous drugs are influenced by the volume of distribution for that drug (Vd) and the clearance (CL) of that drug from the body. The rate at which the plasma concentration of a drug declines with time (i.e., elimination half-time) is directly related to the Vd and inversely related to CL. It must be recognized that pharmacokinetic characteristics of drugs measured in healthy and ambulatory adults may be different in patients with chronic diseases (especially renal and/or hepatic dysfunction) and in various extremes of age, hydration, nutrition, and skeletal muscle mass.

Knowledge of the pharmacokinetics and pharmacodynamics of intravenous drugs clearly defines the drug-response relationships of a drug and its comparisons to other drugs.[14] Furthermore, the influence of altered physiologic states (e.g., aging) on drug effect can be determined. Finally, new approaches to drug administration (e.g., computer-driven infusion pumps, patient controlled analgesia) can be established.

Volume of Distribution

Vd is a calculated number (dose of drug administered intravenously divided by the plasma concentration) that reflects the apparent volumes of

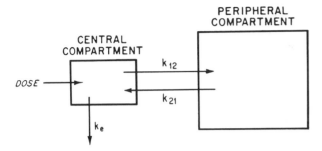

Fig. 2-6. A two compartment pharmacokinetic model. K12 and K21 are rate constants for transfer of drugs between compartments and Ke is the rate constant for clearance of drug from the body. (From Stanski and Watkins,[1] with permission.)

the compartments that constitute the compartmental model for that drug (Fig. 2-6).[1] Binding to plasma proteins, a high degree of ionization, and poor lipid solubility limit passage of drugs to tissues (peripheral compartments), thus maintaining high plasma concentrations (i.e., central compartment) and a small calculated Vd. Examples of drugs with a small Vd similar to extracellular fluid are muscle relaxants. Nonionized lipid soluble drugs readily pass into tissues (peripheral compartments) from the circulation (central compartment) such that plasma concentrations are low and the calculated Vd is large. Examples of such drugs are thiopental and diazepam. It is important to recognize that Vd does not refer to absolute anatomic volumes.

Clearance (CL)

CL is the volume of plasma (central compartment) cleared of drug (ml·min^{-1}) by renal excretion and/ or metabolism in the liver or other organs. CL is one of the most important pharmacokinetic variables to be considered when defining a constant rate of intravenous drug infusion. When the rate of drug infusion exceeds CL, the plasma concentration rises progressively and cumulative drug effects occur.

Renal Elimination

The kidneys are the most important organs for CL of unchanged drugs or their metabolites. Water soluble compounds that are not bound to proteins are excreted more efficiently than protein-bound, lipid soluble drugs. This emphasizes the important role of metabolism in converting lipid soluble drugs to water soluble metabolites. Creatinine clearance or serum creatinine concentrations are useful clinical indicators of the ability of the kidneys to eliminate drugs. The magnitude of elevation of these indices provides an estimate of the downward adjustment in drug dosage required to prevent accumulation of drug in the plasma.

Metabolism

Metabolism (principally in the liver but to some extent also in the kidneys, lungs, and gastrointestinal tract) converts pharmacologically active lipid soluble drugs to water soluble and often inactive metabolites. Increased water solubility reduces the Vd of a drug and enhances its renal excretion. A lipid soluble drug is poorly excreted because of the ease of reabsorption from the lumens of renal tubules into pericapillary fluid.

Microsomal enzymes that participate in the metabolism of many drugs are located principally in hepatic smooth endoplasmic reticulum. The term microsomal enzymes is derived from the fact that centrifugation of homogenized hepatocytes concentrates fragments of the disrupted smooth endoplasmic reticulum in what is designated as the microsomal fraction. The microsomal fraction contains the cytochrome P-450 system, which is likely to be a large number of protein enzymes responsible for metabolism of many foreign compounds. Enzyme induction is stimulation of microsomal enzyme activity by drugs (classically phenobarbital) leading to accelerated metabolism of other drugs. The principal determinant of microsomal enzyme activity, however, is likely to be genetic, emphasizing the predictable large individual variation in rate of metabolism of drugs among patients.

Plasma Concentration Curves

A graphic plot of the logarithm of the plasma concentration of drug versus time following rapid intravenous (bolus) injection characterizes the distribution half-time and elimination half-time of that drug (Fig. 2-7).[1] Two distinct phases are present on this graphic plot. The first phase is designated the distribution (alpha) phase corre-

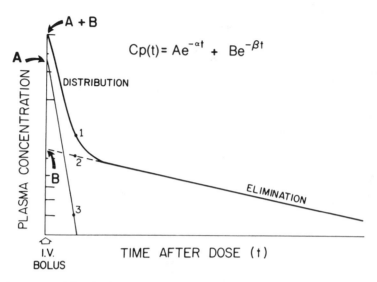

Fig. 2-7. Schematic depiction of the decline in the plasma concentration of drug with time following rapid intravenous injection into the central compartment (see Fig. 2-6). The initial rapid decrease in plasma concentration reflects distribution to tissues, whereas the subsequent slow decline in plasma concentration reflects drug elimination by the liver and kidneys. The time necessary for the plasma concentration to decline 50 percent during the distribution or elimination phase is the corresponding distribution or elimination half-time for that drug. (From Stanski and Watkins,[1] with permission.)

sponding to the initial distribution of drug from the circulation to tissues (peripheral compartments). The second phase is designated the elimination (beta) phase. This phase is characterized by a gradual decline in the plasma concentration of drug and reflects its elimination from the central vascular compartment by renal and hepatic mechanisms.

Elimination Half-Time

Elimination half-time is the time necessary for the plasma concentration of drug to decline 50 percent during the elimination phase (Fig. 2-7).[1] Five elimination half-times are required for almost complete elimination of a drug. Repeated doses of drug equivalent to the initial dose at intervals more frequent than five elimination half-times will result in cumulative drug effects. Drug accumulation continues until the rate of drug elimination equals the rate of drug administration. As with drug elimination, the time necessary for a drug to achieve a steady state plasma concentration (Cpss)

with intermittent doses is about five elimination half-times. A common practice is to administer a large initial dose (loading dose) of drug to rapidly achieve a therapeutic concentration followed by continuous or intermittent injections of reduced doses of drug to match the rate of elimination and thus maintain an optimal and unchanging plasma concentration. In most circumstances, this is most reliably achieved by continuous intravenous infusion techniques. The maintenance dose must be adjusted downward in the presence of renal or hepatic dysfunction so as to prevent drug accumulation due to a prolonged elimination half-time.

Ionization

The pharmacokinetics of drugs is highly dependent on the characteristics of the nonionized and ionized fraction of that drug (Table 2-3). The nonionized drug fraction tends to be pharmacologically active and lipid soluble, whereas the ionized fraction is inactive and water soluble. Lipid

Table 2-3. Characteristics of Nonionized and Ionized Drug Molecules

	Nonionized	Ionized
Pharmacologic effect	Active	Inactive
Solubility	Lipids	Water
Cross lipid barriers (renal tubules, gastrointestinal tract, placenta, blood-brain barrier)	Yes	No
Renal excretion	No	Yes
Hepatic metabolism	Yes	No

or water solubility also determines absorption and elimination characteristics of drugs.

The degree of ionization of a drug is a function of its pK and the pH of the surrounding fluid. When pK and pH are identical, 50 percent of the drug exists in the ionized form. Small changes in pH can result in large changes in the degree of ionization, especially if the pH and pK values are similar. Acidic drugs, such as barbiturates, tend to be highly ionized at an alkaline pH, whereas basic drugs, such as opioids and local anesthetics, are highly ionized at an acid pH.

Route of Administration

Intravenous administration of drugs ensures achievement of predictable plasma concentrations. Absorption of drugs after oral or intramuscular injection is often unpredictable and dependent on local blood flow. Drugs absorbed from the gastrointestinal tract (principally the small intestine) enter the portal venous blood and thus pass through the liver before entering the systemic circulation for delivery to tissue receptors (Fig. 2-8). This is known as the first-pass hepatic effect, and, for drugs that undergo extensive hepatic metabolism (e.g., propranolol, lidocaine), this is the reason for large differences between effective oral and intravenous (drug delivered to receptors before passing through the liver) doses.

Redistribution

Following systemic absorption of drugs, the highly perfused tissues (brain, heart, kidneys, liver) receive a proportionally large amount of the total dose (Table 2-2). For example, approximately 75 percent of the cardiac output is delivered to about 10 percent of the total body mass. This is consistent with the rapid onset of central nervous system effects of lipid soluble drugs (barbiturates, opioids) after their intravenous administration. As the plasma concentrations of drugs decline below that in highly perfused tissues, drugs leave these tissues to be delivered to less well perfused sites, such as skeletal muscles and fat. This transfer of drug to inactive tissue sites, such as skeletal muscles, is known as redistribution. Redistribution of thiopental from the brain to inactive tissue sites is principally responsible for awakening after a single dose of this drug. Repeated doses of thiopental can saturate inactive tissue sites leading to delayed awakening until metabolism can reduce plasma concentrations. Similarly, the normal short duration of action of fentanyl that is due to redistribution becomes a prolonged effect when repeated

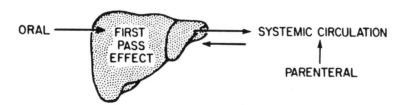

Fig. 2-8. Drugs administered orally are absorbed from the gastrointestinal tract into the portal venous blood and pass through the liver (first-pass hepatic effect) before entering the systemic circulation for distribution to receptors. Conversely, intravenously administered drugs gain rapid access to the systemic circulation for delivery to receptors without an initial impact of metabolism in the liver.

doses or continuous infusions saturate inactive tissue sites.

PHARMACODYNAMICS OF INTRAVENOUS DRUGS

The pharmacologic effects evoked by intravenous drugs reflects their interaction with specific protein macromolecules in cell membranes known as receptors (see Chapter 3).

Receptors

The drug–receptor interaction alters the function or conformation of a specific cellular component that initiates or prevents a series of changes characteristic of the pharmacologic effects of the drug. Regulation of intracellular concentrations of cyclic adenosine monophosphate (cAMP) is a common function of receptors (see Fig. 3-3). Other receptors may act by opening or closing channels, thus altering ion movements and electrical gradients across cell membranes. For example, acetylcholine attaches to nicotinic receptors at the neuromuscular junction causing transmembrane channels to open and leading to a flux of potassium and sodium and generation of an action potential. Nondepolarizing muscle relaxants attach to these receptors and prevent changes in the transmembrane channel so that ion flux and an action potential cannot occur (i.e., skeletal muscle paralysis is present).

Receptors are identified and subsequently classified (e.g., alpha, beta, histamine, mu) primarily on the basis of effects of specific antagonists and agonists. Such a classification serves to summarize the pharmacologic effects of agonist drugs and the likely effects of antagonist drugs (see Chapter 3). Multiple subtypes of receptors (alpha-1, alpha-2, beta-1, beta-2, histamine-1, histamine-2, mu-1, mu-2) may exist.

Number of Receptors

The number of receptors in lipid cell membranes is dynamic, either increasing (up-regulation) or decreasing (down-regulation) in response to specific stimuli. For example, prolonged administration of beta agonists, as in the treatment of asthma, is associated with tachyphylaxis and a concomitant decrease in the number of beta receptors. Con-

versely, chronic interference with activity of receptors as produced by beta antagonists may result in increased numbers of beta receptors such that an exaggerated response occurs if the blockade is abruptly reversed by discontinuation of drug therapy as might occur in the preoperative period. Changes in responsiveness of receptors in the absence of an increase or decrease in the number of receptors may occur with aging. Indeed, more isoproterenol is necessary to increase heart rate in the elderly compared with younger patients despite an unchanged number of receptors with aging (see Chapter 28). Variable pharmacologic responses evoked by drugs in individual patients become more predictable when dynamic changes in concentrations of receptors or alterations in responsiveness of receptors are considered.

Relationship Between Receptor Concentration and Drug Effect

During steady state conditions, plasma concentrations of drugs are probably proportional, if not equal, to receptor concentrations of drugs. Certainly, pharmacokinetic factors that influence plasma concentrations of drugs (tissue uptake, renal excretion, hepatic metabolism) will also influence the concentration of drugs at receptors. Pharmacodynamics are usually expressed by relating the plasma concentration of a drug to the pharmacologic response elicited. For example, demonstration that the Cpss of a nondepolarizing muscle relaxant that produces 50 percent depression of twitch response (ED_{50}) is similar in young adults and elderly patients suggests that pharmacodynamics of the neuromuscular junction do not change with aging (see Chapter 8).

REFERENCES

1. Stanski DR, Watkins WD. Drug Disposition in Anesthesia. Orlando, FL, Grune & Stratton, 1982.
2. Quasha AL, Eger EI II, Tinker JH. Determination and application of MAC. Anesthesiology 1980;53: 315–34.
3. Eger EI II. Uptake of inhaled anesthetics: The alveolar to inspired anesthetic difference. In: Eger EI II, ed. Anesthetic Uptake and Action. Baltimore, Williams & Wilkins, 1974:77–96.
4. Epstein RM, Rackow H, Salanitre E, Wolfe GL.

Influence of the concentration effect on the uptake of anesthetic mixtures: the second gas effect. Anesthesiology 1964;25:364–71.

5. Stoelting RK, Eger EI II. An additional explanation for the second gas effect. Anesthesiology 1969;30:273–7.

6. Eger EI II, Saidman LJ. Hazards of nitrous oxide anesthesia in bowel obstruction and pneumothorax. Anesthesiology 1965;26:61–6.

7. Carpenter RL, Eger EI II, Johnson BH, Unadkat JD, Sheiner LB. Pharmacokinetics of inhaled anesthetics in humans: Measurements during and after simultaneous administration of enflurane, halothane, isoflurane, methoxyflurane, and nitrous oxide. Anesth Analg 1986;65:575–82.

8. Carpenter RL, Eger EI II, Johnson BH, Unadkat JD, Sheiner LB. The extent of metabolism of inhaled anesthetics in humans. Anesthesiology 1986;65:201–5.

9. Merkel G, Eger EI II. A comparative study of halo-thane and halopropane anesthesia. Including method for determining equipotency. Anesthesiology 1963;24:346–57.

10. Harris RA, Groh GI. Membrane disordering effects of anesthetics are enhanced by gangliosides. Anesthesiology 1985;62:115–9.

11. Elliott JR, Haydon RA. Mapping of general anesthetic target sites. Nature 1986;319:77–8.

12. Halsey MJ, Smith B. Pressure reversal of narcosis produced by anesthetics, narcotics and tranquilizers. Nature 1975;257:811–3.

13. Segal IS, Vickery RG, Walton JK, Doze VA, Maze M. Dexmedetomidine diminishes halothane anesthetic requirements in rats through a postsynaptic alpha-2 adrenergic receptor. Anesthesiology 1988;69:818–23.

14. Stanski DR. The contribution of pharmacokinetics and pharmacodynamics to clinical anaesthesia care. Can J Anaesth 1988;35:542–5.

Chapter 3

Autonomic Nervous System

The pharmacologic effects of catecholamines, sympathomimetics, antihypertensives, beta-adrenergic agonists, beta-adrenergic antagonists, anticholinergics, and anticholinesterases involve the actions of these drugs on the central and peripheral autonomic nervous system. An appreciation of the anatomy and physiology of the peripheral autonomic nervous system is important for understanding the effects of these drugs and predicting potential adverse drug interactions in the perioperative period.

ANATOMY AND PHYSIOLOGY OF THE PERIPHERAL AUTONOMIC NERVOUS SYSTEM

The peripheral autonomic nervous system is divided into the sympathetic and parasympathetic nervous systems (Fig. 3-1).[1] Preganglionic fibers of the sympathetic nervous system arise from cells in the thoracolumbar portions of the spinal cord, whereas craniosacral cells are the origin of preganglionic fibers of the parasympathetic nervous system. A number of cell bodies form the autonomic ganglion, which acts as the site of synapse between preganglionic and postganglionic fibers. The preganglionic fibers are myelinated. The postganglionic fibers of the sympathetic nervous system are distributed throughout the body, whereas distribution of parasympathetic nervous system postganglionic fibers is more limited. The para-

sympathetic nervous system has its terminal ganglia near the organs innervated and thus is more discrete in its discharge of impulses than is the sympathetic nervous system (Fig. 3-1).[1]

Sympathetic Nervous System

Postganglionic fibers of the sympathetic nervous system that release norepinephrine as the neurotransmitter are adrenergic, and receptors that respond to norepinephrine are adrenoceptive (Table 3-1). Postsynaptic adrenoceptive receptors are classified as beta-1, beta-2, and alpha-1 (Fig. 3-2).[2] Alpha-2 receptors are usually presynaptic and function in a negative freeback loop such that their activation inhibits subsequent release of neurotransmitter (Fig. 3-2). Stimulation of alpha- and beta-adrenergic receptors by endogenous catecholamines or synthetic adrenergic agonists produces predictable pharmacologic responses (Table 3-1). An important factor in the pharmacologic responses elicited by drugs that act on these receptors is the density and sensitivity of alpha and beta receptors to neurotransmitters. Furthermore, there is an inverse relationship between circulating concentrations of neurotransmitters and the number of receptors. For example, increased plasma concentrations of norepinephrine result in decreases in the density or sensitivity (down-regulation) of beta receptors in cell membranes. The effects of alpha- and beta-adrenergic antagonists

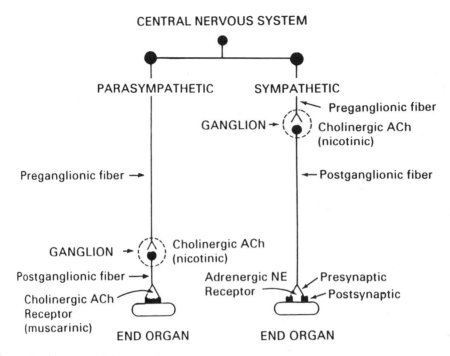

Fig. 3-1. Schematic diagram of the peripheral autonomic nervous system. Preganglionic fibers and postganglionic fibers of the parasympathetic nervous system and preganglionic fibers of the sympathetic nervous system release acetylcholine (ACh) as the neurotransmitter. Postganglionic fibers of the sympathetic nervous system (exceptions are fibers to sweat glands, which release ACh) release norepinephrine (NE) as the neurotransmitter. (From Lawson and Wallfisch,[1] with permission.)

are predictable based on a knowledge of responses evoked by stimulation of affected receptors.

Termination of action of norepinephrine on adrenoceptive receptors is principally by uptake (re-uptake) of this neurotransmitter from the receptors back into the postganglionic nerve ending. Following uptake, a small amount of norepinephrine is deaminated in the cytoplasm by the enzyme monoamine oxidase. Most of the norepinephrine, however, escapes breakdown and can be stored for subsequent release.

Parasympathetic Nervous System

Postganglionic fibers of the parasympathetic nervous system that release acetylcholine as the neurotransmitter are cholinergic and receptors that respond to acetylcholine are cholinoceptive (Table 3-1). These postsynaptic receptors are classified as nicotinic and muscarinic. Stimulation of nicotinic

or muscarinic receptors by acetylcholine or synthetic cholinergic agonists produces predictable pharmacologic responses (Table 3-1). The effects of cholinergic antagonists are predictable based on a knowledge of responses evoked by stimulation of cholinoceptive receptors. The action of acetylcholine at cholinoceptive receptors is terminated by hydrolysis of this neurotransmitter by the enzyme acetylcholinesterase.

Transmembrane Signaling Systems

The traditional concept of receptors as the mechanism for converting external stimuli to intracellular signals is overly simplistic. In fact, it is likely that transmembrane signaling systems involve three components—receptors, effectors and coupling proteins (Fig. 3-3).[3] The receptor is a specific molecule that faces the external surface of cell membranes and acts as a recognition site for

Table 3-1. Characteristics of the Autonomic Nervous System

Receptors	Effector Organ	Response to Stimulation	Synthetic Drugs	
			Agonist	Antagonist
Beta-1	Heart	Increased heart rate Increased contractility Increased automaticity Increased conduction velocity	Dobutamine Dopamine Isoproterenol[a]	Metropolol Atenolol Esmolol Propranolol[a] Timolol[a]
	Fat cells	Lipolysis		

Beta-2	Blood vessels (especially
	  skeletal and coronary
	  arteries)
		Dilation	Terbutaline
			Ritodrine
			Albuterol
			Metaproterenol
			Isoetharine
			Isoproterenol[a]
				Propranolol[a]
				Timolol[a]

	Bronchioles	Dilation		
	Uterus	Relaxation		
	Kidney	Renin secretion		
	Liver	Glycogenolysis Gluconeogenesis		
	Pancreas	Insulin secretion		
Alpha-1	Blood vessels	Constriction	Phenylephrine Methoxamine	Prazosin Phentolamine[b]
	Pancreas	Inhibit insulin secretion		
	Intestine and bladder	Relaxation Constriction of sphincters		

Alpha-2	Postganglionic
	  sympathetic nerve
	  ending
		Inhibit norepinephrine
		  release
			Clonidine	Yohimbine
				Phentolamine[b]

	Platelets	Aggregation		
Dopamine-1	Blood vessels	Dilation	Dopamine	Droperidol

Dopamine-2	Postganglionic
	  sympathetic nerve
	  ending
		Inhibit norepinephrine
		  release
			Dopamine	

Muscarinic	Heart	Decreased heart rate Decreased contractility Decreased conduction velocity	Methacholine Carbachol	Atropine Scopolamine Glycopyrrolate
	Bronchioles	Constriction		
	Salivary glands	Stimulate secretions		
	Intestine	Contraction Relaxation of sphincters Stimulate secretions		
	Bladder	Contraction Relaxation of sphincter		

(*continued*)

Table 3-1. (*continued*)

Receptors	Effector Organ	Response to Stimulation	Synthetic Drugs	
			Agonist	Antagonist
Nicotinic	Autonomic ganglia	Sympathetic nervous system stimulation		Hexamethonium
	Neuromuscular junction	Skeletal muscle contraction	Succinylcholine	d-Tubocurarine Metocurine Gallamine Pancuronium Atracurium Vecuronium

[a] Produces mixed beta-1 and beta-2 effects.
[b] Produces mixed alpha-1 and alpha-2 effects.

interaction with ligands such as neurotransmitters, hormones, or drugs. Effectors are enzymes, such as adenylate cyclase and phospholipase C, that face the cytoplasmic (interior) surface of the cell. Effectors may also be ion channels. Interposed between receptors and effectors are coupling proteins known as guanine nucleotide regulatory proteins or G proteins. G proteins are necessary for receptor mediated activation or inhibition of effectors. cAMP acts as the second messenger to stimulate events characterized as beta-adrenergic stimulation (Table 3-1).

CATECHOLAMINES

Catecholamines are compounds with hydroxyl groups on the 3 and 4 positions of the benzene ring of phenylethylamine (Fig. 3-4). Endogenous catecholamines are dopamine, norepinephrine, and epinephrine. Catecholamines that do not occur endogenously are isoproterenol and dobutamine.

Pharmacologic effects produced by catecholamines reflect the ability of these substances to stimulate adrenoceptive receptors. Clinically, cate-

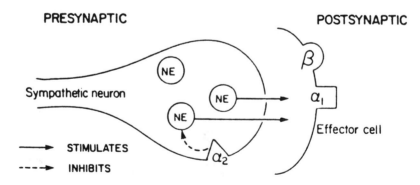

Fig. 3-2. Schematic depiction of the postganglionic sympathetic nerve ending. Release of the neurotransmitter, norepinephrine (NE), from the nerve ending results in stimulation of postsynaptic receptors that are classified as alpha-1, beta-1, and beta-2. Stimulation of presynaptic alpha-2 receptors results in inhibition of NE release from the nerve ending. (Modified from Ram and Kaplan,[2] with permission.)

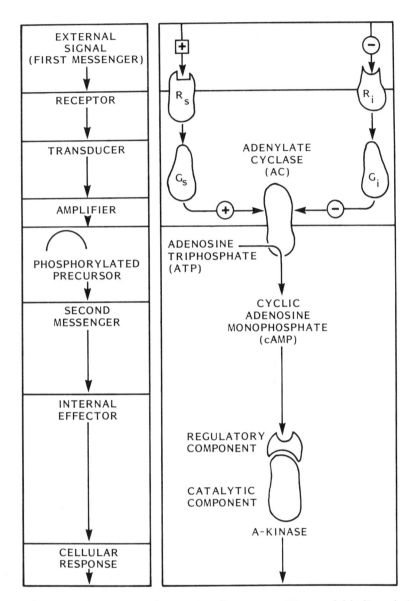

Fig. 3-3. Schematic diagram of a transmembrane signaling system. Water-soluble ligands (neurotransmitters) attach to stimulating (Rs) or inhibitory (Ri) receptors in the membranes of cells. Signals from these receptors converge on the amplifier enzyme, adenylate cyclase (AC), which converts adenosine triphosphate (ATP) to cyclic adenosine monophosphate (cAMP). Convergence of signals from receptors to AC is modulated by guanine (G) proteins. cAMP binds to the regulatory components of protein kinase, liberating the catalytic component, which is then free to phosphorylate specific proteins that regulate a cellular response. (From Berridge,[3] with permission.)

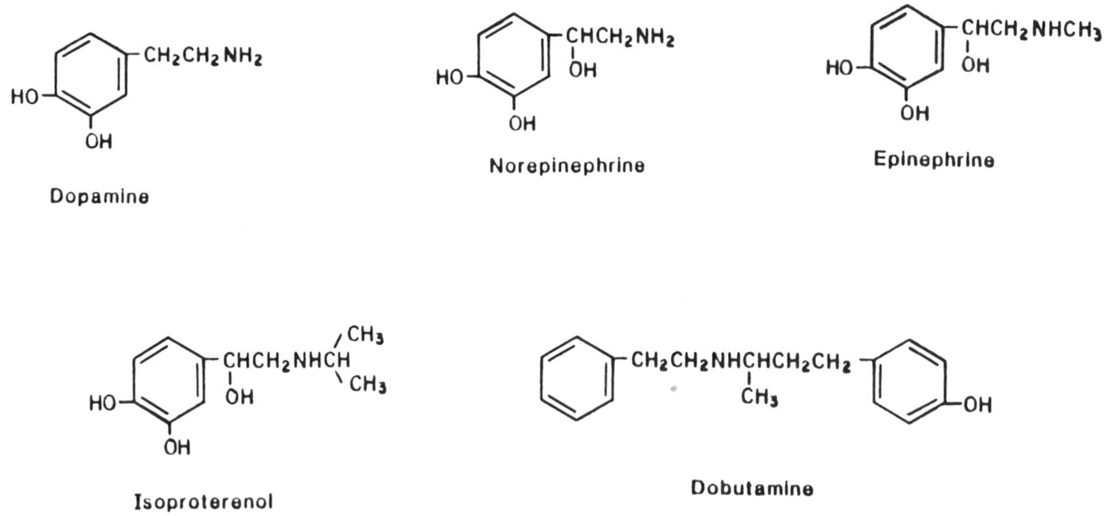

Fig. 3-4. Chemical structure of endogenous (dopamine, norepinephrine, epinephrine) and exogenous (isoproterenol, dobutamine) catecholamines.

cholamines are administered as continuous intravenous infusions to produce desirable pharmacologic effects manifesting predominantly on the cardiovascular system (Table 3-2).

Dopamine

Dopamine, depending on the dose, directly stimulates dopaminergic, beta- and alpha-adrenergic receptors. This catecholamine is unique among this class of drugs in its ability to stimulate dopaminergic receptors and redistribute blood flow to the kidneys. These renal effects predominate when the rate of continuous intravenous infusion of dopamine is less than $3 \mu g \cdot kg^{-1} \cdot min^{-1}$. This dose can also inhibit secretion of aldosterone, which, along with dopaminergic stimulation, results in increased urine output. Beta-adrenergic stimulation characterized by increased myocardial contractility without marked changes in heart rate and blood pressure occurs when the rate of dopamine infusion is $3 \mu g \cdot kg^{-1} \cdot min^{-1}$ to $10 \mu g \cdot kg^{-1} \cdot min^{-1}$. Some residual dopaminergic stimulation persists up to doses of $5 \mu g \cdot kg^{-1} \cdot min^{-1}$. Dopamine also exerts part of its inotropic effect by releasing endogenous stores of norepinephrine, which predisposes to cardiac dysrhythmias. Furthermore, this indirect stimulation may be an unreliable mechanism when cardiac catecholamine stores are depleted as with chronic congestive heart failure. Beta- and alpha-adrenergic agonist effects occur with dopamine infusion rates between 10 $\mu g \cdot kg^{-1} \cdot min^{-1}$ and $20 \mu g \cdot kg^{-1} \cdot min^{-1}$, whereas alpha-adrenergic effects of dopamine predominate with doses above $20 \mu g \cdot kg^{-1} \cdot min^{-1}$. High doses of dopamine can inhibit release of insulin, leading to hyperglycemia.

Dopamine is most often used in clinical situations characterized by decreased cardiac output, reduced blood pressure, increased left ventricular end-diastolic pressure, and oliguria. The drug is prepared in a solution of 5 percent dextrose in water. More alkaline intravenous solutions may inactivate dopamine.

Norepinephrine

Norepinephrine, as the endogenous neurotransmitter for adrenoceptive receptors, is responsible for maintaining blood pressure by appropriate

Table 3-2. Pharmacologic Effects and Therapeutic Doses of Catecholamines

Catecholamine	MAP[a]	HR[a]	CO[a]	SVR[a]	RBF[a]	Preparation (mg in 500 ml)	Intravenous Dose ($\mu g \cdot kg^{-1} \cdot min^{-1}$)
Dopamine	+[b]	+	+++[b]	+	+++	400	2–20
Norepinephrine	+++	−[b]	−	+++	−−−[b]	8	0.05–0.2
Epinephrine	+	++[b]	++	++	−−[b]	8	0.05–0.2
Isoproterenol	−	+++	+++	−−	−	2	0.03–0.3
Dobutamine	+	+	+++	±	++	500	2–20

[a] MAP, mean arterial pressure; HR, heart rate; CO, cardiac output; SVR, systemic vascular resitance; RBF, renal blood flow.
[b] +, mild increase; ++, moderate increase; +++, marked increase; −, mild decrease; −−, moderate decrease; −−−, marked decrease.

adjustments in systemic vascular resistance. Vasoconstriction induced by norepinephrine produces increases in systemic vascular resistance reflected by elevations in systolic, diastolic, and mean arterial pressure. Beta-1 agonist effects of norepinephrine on the heart are overshadowed by the alpha-1 agonist effects of this catecholamine on the peripheral vasculature. Cardiac output may be reduced despite the increased blood pressure, reflecting the effect of increased ventricular afterload and baroreceptor-mediated reflex bradycardia. Beta-2 agonist effects of norepinephrine are minimal. Clinically, norepinephrine is seldom used to treat cardiovascular collapse.

Epinephrine

Epinephrine stimulates alpha-1, beta-1, and beta-2 receptors. Low doses of epinephrine stimulate alpha-1 receptors in the skin, mucosa, and hepatorenal vasculature producing vasoconstriction, whereas beta-2 induced vasodilation predominates in skeletal muscles. The net effect is decreased systemic vascular resistance and a preferential distribution of cardiac output to skeletal muscles. Renal blood flow is greatly reduced during infusion of epinephrine, even with an unchanged blood pressure. Stimulation of beta-1 receptors increases heart rate and myocardial contractility, resulting in an increased cardiac output. Since the blood pressure is not greatly elevated, compensatory baroreceptor reflexes are not elicited and the cardiac output is increased. Beta-1 stimulation also increases automaticity of the heart, which mani-

fests as cardiac irritability, most often in the form of ventricular premature contractions.

Of all the catecholamines, epinephrine has the most significant effects on metabolism. For example, beta-adrenergic stimulation from epinephrine increases adipose tissue lipolysis and liver glycogenolysis, whereas alpha-1 stimulation inhibits release of insulin from the pancreas (Table 3-1). Epinephrine release in response to surgical stimulation is a likely explanation for the characteristic hyperglycemia observed in the perioperative period.

Epinephrine may be used as a continuous intravenous infusion to treat reduced myocardial contractility. Subcutaneous epinephrine is also used in combination with local anesthetics to reduce systemic absorption and to provide local hemostasis. In addition, epinephrine is administered during cardiopulmonary resuscitation (see Chapter 34). Finally, epinephrine is indicated in the treatment of life-threatening allergic reactions.

Isoproterenol

Isoproterenol is a synthetic catecholamine with potent stimulant effects on beta-1 and beta-2 receptors and no effect on alpha-1 receptors. Myocardial contractility, heart rate, systolic blood pressure, and cardiac automaticity are increased, whereas systemic vascular resistance and diastolic blood pressure are decreased. The net effect is an increase in cardiac output and occasionally a reduction in mean arterial pressure. Bronchodilation is accompanied by significant cardiovascular effects because isoproterenol does not discriminate between beta-1 and beta-2 receptors (Table 3-1).

Excessive tachycardia and simultaneous diastolic hypotension may reduce coronary blood flow at the time myocardial oxygen requirements are increased by tachycardia. These events, combined with a high incidence of cardiac dysrhythmias and diversion of blood to skeletal muscles, detract from the value of this catecholamine, particularly in patients with coronary artery disease. The major clinical use of isoproterenol is in patients with valvular heart disease associated with pulmonary hypertension. Such patients may benefit from isoproterenol-induced increases in heart rate and reductions in systemic and pulmonary vascular resistance.

Dobutamine

Dobutamine is a synthetic catecholamine with structural characteristics of dopamine and isoproterenol. Removal of the side-chain hydroxyl groups from the isoproterenol portion decreases cardiac dysrhythmogenicity but retains the inotropic properties. Dobutamine acts selectively on beta-1 receptors without significant effects on beta-2 or alpha receptors. Unlike dopamine, this catecholamine does not act indirectly by stimulating endogenous norepinephrine release, nor does it stimulate dopaminergic receptors to increase renal blood flow. The most prominent effect during the infusion of dobutamine (2 μg·kg^{-1}·min^{-1} to 20 μg·kg^{-1}·min^{-1}) is a dose-dependent increase in cardiac output, often with a decrease in systemic vascular resistance. This ability to increase myocardial contractility with minimal chronotropic or alpha stimulation is unique to dobutamine. Dobutamine may be ineffective for those patients who need increased systemic vascular resistance to elevate blood pressure. Drug-induced increases in the rate of atrioventricular conduction of cardiac impulses detracts from the use of dobutamine in patients with atrial fibrillation. Since dobutamine lacks dopaminergic stimulating effects, it is reasonable to consider infusing this catecholamine with dopamine to patients who are hypotensive and oliguric. Dobutamine, like dopamine, can be inactivated when prepared in alkaline intravenous solutions—emphasizing the importance of preparing this drug in a 5-percent dextrose in water solution.

SYMPATHOMIMETICS

Sympathomimetics are synthetic drugs that are used as vasopressors to reverse downward trends in blood pressure that accompany vasodilation produced by spinal or epidural blockade. Likewise, hypotension produced by inhaled anesthetics may be treated with a sympathomimetic to assure maintenance of an adequate perfusion pressure during the time needed to eliminate the excess inhaled drug. Prolonged administration of sympathomimetics to support blood pressure in the presence of hypovolemia is not recommended. Structurally, sympathomimetics resemble catecholamines except that hydroxyl groups are not present on both the 3 and 4 positions of the benzene ring (Fig. 3-5).

Classification

Sympathomimetics are classified according to their selectivity for stimulating alpha- and/or beta-adrenergic receptors (Table 3-3). Knowing the selectivity for either receptor permits selection of a drug specifically to elevate blood pressure by peripheral vasoconstriction, increased myocardial contractility, or a combination of these effects. Most sympathomimetics are mixed, producing both alpha and beta agonist effects. Disadvantages of using sympathomimetics that lack beta-1 effects to maintain blood pressure include intense vasoconstriction and associated blood pressure elevations that evoke baroreceptor reflex-mediated bradycardia that lowers cardiac output.

Sympathomimetics may also be classified as direct- or indirect-acting drugs (Table 3-3). Direct-acting drugs produce effects similar to the sympathetic nervous system neurotransmitter, norepinephrine, such that depletion of norepinephrine or denervation does not reduce the efficacy of these drugs. In contrast, indirect-acting drugs act by evoking the release of endogenous norepinephrine, and their efficacy is reduced by depletion of the neurotransmitter. This classification permits prediction of altered responses to sympathomimetics. For example, antihypertensives that reduce

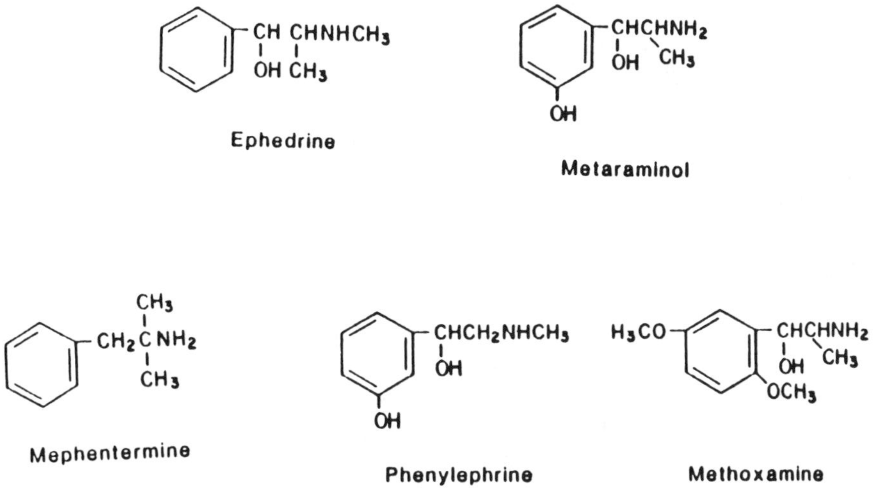

Fig. 3-5. Chemical structure of sympathomimetics.

sympathetic nervous system activity will also decrease the pressor response elicited by indirect-acting sympathomimetics.[4] Conversely, the pressor response elicited by direct-acting drugs may be exaggerated as the receptors are sensitized (denervation hypersensitivity) by a lack of tonic impulses.[4]

Treatment of patients with tricyclic antidepressants or monoamine oxidase inhibitors introduces the potential for adverse drug interactions with sympathomimetics as well as other undesirable responses.

Tricyclic Antidepressants

Tricyclic antidepressants inhibit uptake of previously released norepinephrine back into post-ganglionic sympathetic nerve endings, resulting in increased availability of this neurotransmitter. Therefore, administration of indirect-acting drugs, such as ephedrine, is likely to evoke an exaggerated blood pressure response. Furthermore, administration of pancuronium to halothane-anesthetized dogs who have been pretreated with tricyclic antidepressants is associated with an

Table 3-3. Classification and Therapeutic Doses of Sympathomimetics

Sympathomimetic	Alpha	Beta-1	Beta-2	Direct (D) Indirect (I)	Intravenous Dose for an Adult (mg)
Ephedrine	$++^a$	$+^a$	$+$	I (some D)	10–25
Metaraminol	$++$	$+$	$+$	I (some D)	1.5–5
Mephentermine	$++$	$+$	$+$	I	10–25
Phenylephrine	$+++^a$	0^a	0	D	0.05–0.2
Methoxamine	$+++$	0	0	D	5–10

[a] 0, none; +, mild; + +, moderate; + + +, marked.

elevation of plasma catecholamine concentrations and an increased incidence of cardiac dysrhythmias (Fig. 3-6).[5] Finally, tricyclic antidepressant therapy is associated with anticholinergic effects (dry mouth, central nervous system dysfunction, urinary retention) and, occasionally, with changes in conduction of cardiac impulses that manifest on the electrocardiogram as widening of the QRS complex and prolongation of the PR interval.

Monoamine Oxidase Inhibitors

Monoamine oxidase inhibitors prevent the breakdown of norepinephrine in postganglionic nerve endings and peripheral tissues by monoamine oxidase, resulting in increased availability of this neurotransmitter. Therefore, administration of indirect-acting drugs, such as ephedrine, is likely to evoke an exaggerated blood pressure response. Should treatment of hypotension require administration of sympathomimetics, a useful selection is a reduced dose of direct-acting drugs such as phenylephrine. Administration of even small doses of opioids to patients being treated with monoamine oxidase inhibitors can result in elevations in body temperature, seizures, depression of ventilation, and cardiovascular collapse. In view of these potential adverse perioperative drug interactions and the prolonged effect of monoamine oxidase inhibitors, it is often recommended that this class of drugs be discontinued 14 days to 21 days before elective surgery. Nevertheless, even patients receiving these enzyme inhibitors may be safely anesthetized without waiting for regeneration of new enzyme.[6]

Ephedrine

Ephedrine is an indirect-acting sympathomimetic that exerts its blood pressure effects principally by stimulating the release of norepinephrine. Ephedrine also has some direct-acting effects. Clinically, ephedrine produces responses consistent with alpha- (vasoconstriction) and beta-adrenergic (in-

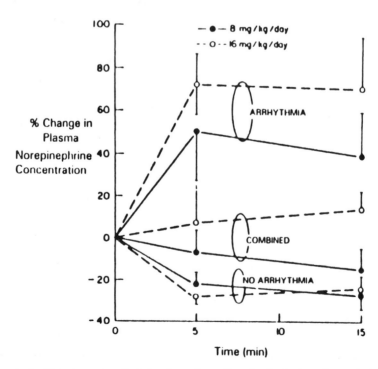

Fig. 3-6. Dogs pretreated with imipramine that developed cardiac dysrhythmias after administration of pancuronium during halothane anesthesia also manifested increased plasma concentrations of norepinephrine. (From Edwards et al.,[5] with permission.)

creased myocardial contractility) stimulation. The systolic and diastolic blood pressure are typically increased and the cardiac output is improved, providing there is adequate venous return to the heart. Increased heart rate is consistent with beta-adrenergic stimulation. Cardiac dysrhythmias have been demonstrated in the dog anesthetized with halothane and treated with ephedrine. Placental blood flow is preserved by ephedrine, making this drug useful for treating anesthetic-induced hypotension in parturients (see Chapter 26).

Cardiovascular stimulating effects of ephedrine diminish with repeated doses. The mechanism of this tachyphylaxis is not known, but depletion of catecholamine stores is a consideration. Alternatively, persistent blockade of alpha receptors, despite return of blood pressure to normal levels, would limit available sites for subsequent doses of ephedrine and thus reduce the blood pressure response evoked compared with prior injections.

Metaraminol

Metaraminol has both indirect and direct actions and overall effects similar to those of norepinephrine. Its vasoconstrictive action is of longer duration than its cardiac stimulating action such that alpha agonist effects predominate. Reflex bradycardia often accompanies drug-induced increases in blood pressure resulting in a decline in cardiac output. It may be useful to think of metaraminol as a potent ephedrine.

Metaraminol depletes and replaces norepinephrine from its storage sites and then acts as a false neurotransmitter. The release of metaraminol rather than norepinephrine in response to an adrenergic stimulus results in less alpha agonist stimulation, since this false neurotransmitter is about one-tenth as potent as the endogenous neurotransmitter. Therefore, continued infusion of metaraminol for longer than 3 hours may have an antihypertensive effect.

Mephentermine

Mephentermine, like ephedrine and metaraminol, acts in part by stimulating the release of catecholamines. In contrast to metaraminol, the cardiac stimulating effects of mephentermine predominate over its peripheral vascular effects. Hence,

cardiac output is increased, but changes in systemic vascular resistance are variable. Cardiac dysrhythmias are less likely to occur with this drug as compared with other sympathomimetics that stimulate alpha- and beta-adrenergic receptors.

Phenylephrine and Methoxamine

Phenylephrine and methoxamine are direct-acting sympathomimetics that increase systemic vascular resistance and blood pressure by selective stimulation of alpha-adrenergic receptors. These drugs are devoid of clinically significant cardiac stimulating effects. The dose of phenylephrine necessary to stimulate alpha-1 receptors is less than that needed to stimulate alpha-2 receptors. As a result, venoconstriction is greater than arterial constriction following administration of phenylephrine. Reflex bradycardia is a predictable response when blood pressure is elevated by phenylephrine and methoxamine.

Choice of phenylephrine or methoxamine to treat hypotension due to volatile anesthetics must consider the possible detrimental cardiac effects of drug-induced vasoconstriction on the anesthetic depressed heart. Hypotension due to spinal or epidural block may be treated with drugs, such as phenylephrine or methoxamine, that elevate blood pressure by increasing systemic vascular resistance. Ephedrine, which increases myocardial contractility, is also a useful drug to treat this form of hypotension.

ANTIHYPERTENSIVES

Antihypertensives are used in the treatment of ambulatory essential hypertension to reduce blood pressure toward normal levels by selectively impairing sympathetic nervous sytem function at the heart and/or peripheral vasculature. Attenuation of sympathetic nervous system activity is reflected by orthostatic hypotension. During anesthesia, exaggerated reductions in blood pressure (as associated with hemorrhage, positive airway pressure, or sudden changes in body position) may reflect an impaired degree of compensatory peripheral vascular vasoconstriction due to inhibitory effects of antihypertensives on sympathetic nervous system activity. The response to sympathomimetics

---

Antihypertensives Used in the Ambulatory Treatment of Essential Hypertension

Central sympatholytics
  Alpha-methyldopa
  Clonidine

Peripheral sympatholytics
  Guanethidine

Peripheral vasodilators
  Hydralazine
  Minoxidil

Alpha-adrenergic antagonists
  Prazosin

Angiotensin converting enzyme inhibitors
  Captopril

Beta-adrenergic antagonists
  Propranolol
  Metoprolol
  Nadolol
  Atenolol
  Timolol

Alpha- and beta-adrenergic antagonists
  Labetalol

---

may be modified by prior treatment with antihypertensives (see the section *Sympathomimetics*). Selective impairment of sympathetic nervous system activity by antihypertensives results in a predominance of parasympathetic nervous system tone, manifesting as bradycardia. Finally, antihypertensives that reduce central nervous system sympathetic activity are associated with sedation and reduced anesthetic requirements (MAC).[4] Despite interference of antihypertensives with normal sympathetic nervous system activity, these drugs should be continued during the perioperative period so as to maintain optimal control of the blood pressure.

Alpha-Methyldopa

The most likely explanation for the antihypertensive effect of alpha-methyldopa is the accumulation of alpha-methylated amines in the central nervous system, resulting in a reduced outflow of sympathetic nervous system impulses. Methyldopa decreases blood pressure by reducing both the cardiac output and systemic vascular resistance. The plasma half-time of this drug in only 1 hour to 2 hours, but its hypotensive effect can last as long as 24 hours, probably because the active metabolite, alpha-methylnorepinephrine, has a long half-time in the brain.

A major side effect of alpha-methyldopa is depression of the central nervous system and drowsiness. In animals, this effect is associated with a dose-dependent 15 percent to 30 percent decrease in MAC.[4] Decreased blood pressure responses following the administration of ephedrine also occurred in these animals. About 20 percent of patients treated with alpha-methyldopa develop a positive Coombs' test, which may result in difficulty in cross-matching whole blood for that patient. As much as 5 percent of patients with a positive Coombs' test secondary to alpha-methyldopa develop hemolytic anemia, necessitating the cessation of treatment with this drug. A rare but important side effect of treatment with alpha-methyldopa is fever with hepatic dysfunction. Patients who are receiving alpha-methyldopa may develop hypertension after administration of propranolol. This hypertensive response presumably reflects the ability of propranolol to block the vasodilating effects of alpha-methylnorepinephrine. As a result, only the potent alpha stimulating effects of this metabolite are apparent. Sudden withdrawal of alpha-methyldopa can cause rebound hypertension, although the incidence of this complication seems to be less than that observed after discontinuation of other centrally acting antihypertensive drugs. Alpha-methyldopa is a logical choice in patients with renal disease because it maintains or increases renal blood flow.

Clonidine

Clonidine is a centrally acting antihypertensive that stimulates alpha-2 receptors in the depressor area of the vasomotor center, leading to a decreased outflow of sympathetic nervous system impulses to the periphery. The net effect of this decreased sympathetic nervous system activity is a reduction in cardiac output, systemic vascular resistance, and blood pressure. Reductions in MAC for injected and inhaled drugs are produced by small doses of clonidine administered preoperatively, presumably reflecting sedative and/or analgesic effects of this drug.[7] Sympathetic nervous system responses evoked by surgical stimulation are attenuated by prior treatment with clonidine. Bradycardia and dry mouth may accompany treatment with clonidine. The duration of action of a single dose of clonidine is 6 hours to 24 hours.

The most important adverse effect of clonidine is rebound hypertension when the drug is discontinued. Indeed, discontinuation of treatment with clonidine has been associated with the development of adverse increases in blood pressure before the induction of anesthesia, as well as in the early postoperative period.[8] The speculated mechanism for this rebound hypertension is an abrupt increase in systemic vascular resistance due to release of catecholamines. Rebound hypertension can usually be controlled or prevented by maintaining clonidine therapy (transdermal clonidine an alternative to oral administration) or substitution of alternative drugs such as hydralazine or alphamethyldopa. Beta antagonists may exaggerate rebound hypertension by blocking beta-2 vasodilating effects of catecholamines and leaving unopposed alpha vasoconstricting actions. Antihypertensive drugs that act independently of central and peripheral nervous system mechanisms (peripheral vasodilators) do not seem to be associated with rebound hypertension following sudden discontinuation of therapy.[8]

Clonidine has been shown to be effective in suppressing the signs and symptoms of withdrawal from opioids. It is speculated that clonidine replaces opioid-mediated inhibition with alpha-2 mediated inhibition of central nervous system sympathetic activity. Clonidine lowers plasma catecholamine concentrations in normal patients but not those with pheochromocytoma. Intravenous or neuraxial administration of clonidine produces analgesia for management of acute or chronic pain.

Guanethidine

Guanethidine lacks significant effects on the central nervous system (MAC is not altered) because its guanidine group prevents easy passage across the blood-brain barrier.[5] This drug acts selectively on the peripheral sympathetic nervous system to depress function of postganglionic sympathetic nerves by inhibiting the presynaptic release of norepinephrine. Resulting reductions in peripheral sympathetic nervous system activity are responsible for a decrease in venous return that leads to a reduction in cardiac output and a subsequent decline in blood pressure. Decreased responsiveness of resistance and capacitance blood vessels to sympathetic nervous system stimulation manifests as orthostatic hypotension.

Hydralazine

Hydralazine probably interferes with calcium transport at the arterial vascular smooth muscle and thus lowers blood pressure by vasodilation. Activity of the baroreceptor reflex remains intact, leading to an increased outflow of sympathetic nervous system activity from the central nervous system. This maintenance of sympathetic nervous system activity prevents orthostatic hypotension but may offset the desired antihypertensive effect of hydralazine by increasing the heart rate. Baroreceptor-mediated reflex stimulation of heart rate can be prevented by combining hydralazine with a beta-adrenergic antagonist. A lupus-erythematosus-like syndrome is likely when the daily dose of hydralazine exceeds 200 mg.

Minoxidil

Minoxidil reduces blood pressure by direct relaxation of arteriolar smooth muscle. As with any peripheral vasodilator, minoxidil is associated with reflex tachycardia, salt retention, and water retention. For these reasons, minoxidil is often administered in combination with a beta-adrenergic antagonist and diuretic. Pulmonary hypertension associated with minoxidil is more likely due to fluid retention than a unique effect of this drug on pulmonary vasculature. Pericardial effusion and cardiac tamponade occur in a small number of patients, especially if renal dysfunction is present.[8] Minoxidil stimulates hair growth and a topical preparation may be used to treat baldness.

Prazosin

Prazosin lowers blood pressure by decreasing systemic vascular resistance due to selective postsynaptic alpha-1 receptor blockade. Absence of drug-induced presynaptic alpha-2 blockade leaves the normal inhibition of norepinephrine release intact. In addition to treating essential hypertension, prazosin may be of value for reducing afterload in patients with cardiac failure. Prazosin is also useful in the preoperative preparation of patients with pheochromocytoma. Fluid retention and orthostatic hypotension are prominent side effects of prazosin therapy.

Labetalol

Labetalol lowers blood pressure by acting as a selective alpha-1 antagonist and nonselective beta-1 and beta-2 receptor antagonist. Bronchospasm is less likely to occur than with other nonselective beta antagonists, but orthostatic hypotension may be prominent.

Captopril

Captopril is an orally effective antihypertensive that acts by competitive inhibition of angiotensin-I converting enzyme. Patient compliance is high with captopril therapy, reflecting minimal side effects compared with drugs acting on the central nervous system.

BETA-ADRENERGIC AGONISTS

Catecholamines are examples of beta-1 agonists used to increase heart rate and myocardial contractility (Table 3-1) (see the section *Catecholamines*). Beta-2 agonists produce relaxation of bronchial, uterine, and vascular smooth muscle, reflecting selective stimulation of beta-2 receptors (Table 3-1). Beta-2 agonists are used to treat bronchial asthma and to stop premature labor.

Drugs selective for beta-2 receptors are less likely than beta-1 agonists to produce adverse cardiac effects such as tachycardia or cardiac dysrhythmias. Nevertheless, reflex tachycardia, presumably due to beta-2 mediated vasodilation and subsequent hypotension, has been observed after administration of these drugs.[9] Another serious hazard of continuous intravenous infusion of a beta-2 agonist as used to stop premature labor is hypokalemia.[10] Hypokalemia most likely reflects

sustained beta-2 stimulation of the sodium pump with transfer of potassium intracellularly. Tachyphylaxis to the effects of beta-2 agonists is attributed to a decreased number or reduced sensitivity of beta receptors (down-regulation) that occurs with chronic stimulation of these receptors.

Drug-induced inhibition of phosphodiesterase enzyme activity results in the accumulation of cAMP, leading to beta agonist effects in the absence of activation of adenylate cyclase (Table 3-1). Aminophylline is an example of a useful drug that produces beta-adrenergic stimulation in part by this mechanism. In addition, aminophylline stimulates the release of norepinephrine. Patients receiving a continuous intravenous infusion of aminophylline to treat bronchial asthma may be at increased risk for developing cardiac dysrhythmias during halothane anesthesia.[11] For this reason, inhaled anesthetics, such as enflurane or isoflurane, which are less likely to evoke cardiac dysrhythmias, may be better choices than halothane when patients treated with aminophylline require surgery.

BETA-ADRENERGIC ANTAGONISTS

Beta antagonists may produce selective beta-1 blockade (decreased heart rate and myocardial contractility) or mixed responses also reflecting drug effects at beta-2 receptors (bronchial and vascular smooth muscle constriction) (Table 3-1). Beta antagonists may also possess membrane stabilizing activity and intrinsic sympathomimetic activity.

Beta antagonists probably decrease blood pressure by reducing cardiac output. Heart rate slowing produced by beta antagonists lasts longer than negative inotropic effects, suggesting a possible subdivision of beta-1 receptors. Beta blockade attenuates baroreceptor-mediated increases in heart rate associated with vasodilator therapy. An important advantage of beta antagonists as used to treat essential hypertension is the absence of orthostatic hypotension. In addition, these drugs do not alter MAC. Fatigue and lethargy, however, are commonly associated with beta antagonist therapy.

In addition to treatment of essential hypertension, beta antagonists are effective in reducing myocardial oxygen requirements by virtue of reductions in heart rate and myocardial contractility. These beta-1 antagonist effects more than offset any adverse effect of an increase in coronary vascular resistance due to concomitant beta-2 receptor blockade. Evidence of reduced myocardial oxygen requirements in patients treated with beta antagonists is relief of angina pectoris. Indeed, beta antagonists may be effective in reducing post-myocardial infarction mortality.

Hazards of beta blockade include excessive myocardial depression and bronchoconstriction. Additive myocardial depression with volatile anesthetics can occur, but this has not proven to be a clinically significant problem. When bronchoconstriction is a likely response, as in patients with bronchial asthma or chronic obstructive airways disease, it is important to select beta antagonists with selective beta-1 blocking effects. Likewise, cardioselective drugs would be logical selections in patients with peripheral vascular disease so as to minimize the occurrence of vasoconstriction that accompanies beta-2 blockade (Table 3-1). Drugs with intrinsic sympathomimetic activity may be logical selections for treatment of patients with depressed left ventricular function or bradycardia. Indeed, beta-adrenergic blockade may produce atrioventricular heart block. Acute discontinuation of beta antagonists can result in excess sympathetic nervous system activity that manifests in 24 hours to 48 hours. Presumably, this enhanced activity reflects an increase in the number or sensitivity of beta receptors (up-regulation) that occurs during chronic therapy. Beta antagonists may accentuate increases in plasma concentrations of potassium associated with infusion of potassium chloride, presumably by interfering with the mechanism necessary for movement of this ion across cell membranes (Fig. 3-7).[12] Warning signs and symptoms of hypoglycemia are blunted by beta-adrenergic blockade, suggesting caution in the use of these drugs in insulin-dependent patients with diabetes mellitus. Cardioselective drugs would be logical selections when diabetes mellitus is present since suppression of insulin secretion is produced by beta-2 blockade (Table 3-1).

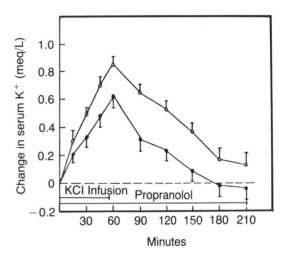

Fig. 3-7. Increases in serum potassium (K^+) concentrations in response to infusion of potassium chloride (KCL) are greater in the presence of propranolol (clear circles) than in its absence (solid circles). Mean ± SE. (From Rosa et al.,[12] with permission.)

Atropine is the initial drug recommended for treatment of signs of excessive beta blockade manifesting as bradycardia or atrioventricular heart block. If signs of excessive beta blockade persist, a specific pharmacologic treatment is administration of a beta agonist such as isoproterenol or dobutamine. However, large doses of these drugs may be required to antagonize excessive beta blockade. Alternatively, calcium chloride administered intravenously antagonizes excessive beta blockade independently of any known effect mediated via beta-adrenergic receptors. As such, conventional doses of calcium chloride (5 $mg \cdot kg^{-1}$ to 10 $mg \cdot kg^{-1}$) are likely to be effective.

It must be recognized that abrupt discontinuation of treatment with beta antagonists can be associated with excessive sympathetic nervous system activity manifesting as hypertension and myocardial ischemia. Therefore, treatment with these drugs should be maintained throughout the perioperative period. Continuous intravenous infusion of esmolol would also be effective in maintaining therapeutic plasma concentrations in adult patients who cannot receive oral medications during the perioperative period.

ANTICHOLINERGICS

Anticholinergics (atropine, scopolamine, glycopyrrolate) prevent the muscarinic effects of acetylcholine by competing for the same receptors as normally occupied by the neurotransmitter. Atropine and scopolamine are tertiary amines and can cross lipid barriers such as the blood-brain barrier and placenta. In contrast, glycopyrrolate acts principally on peripheral cholinergic receptors because its quaternary ammonium structure prevents it from crossing lipid barriers in significant amounts.

Responses produced by anticholinergics include (1) inhibition of salivation (antisialagogue effect), (2) decreased gastric hydrogen ion secretion, (3) increased heart rate, (4) mydriasis, and (5) relaxation of the lower esophageal sphincter. The sensitivity of peripheral cholinergic receptors differs such that low doses of an anticholinergic may be sufficient to inhibit salivation, but large doses are necessary for cardiac of gastrointestinal effects. Furthermore, the magnitude of anticholinergic effects may differ between drugs despite similar doses. For example, scopolamine is a potent antisialagogue, sedative, and amnesic, but has minimal effects on heart rate. Conversely, atropine is a less potent antisialagogue than scopolamine but produces significant cardiac vagolytic effects. As an antisialagogue, glycopyrrolate is more potent and longer lasting than atropine, but the heart rate effects of glycopyrrolate are minimal. Central nervous system toxicity (central anticholinergic syndrome) is more likely to occur after administration of scopolamine than of atropine and is unlikely to develop after glycopyrrolate, since this drug is unable to easily cross the blood-brain barrier.

ANTICHOLINESTERASES

Anticholinesterases are represented by quaternary ammonium (neostigmine, pyridostigmine, and edrophonium) and tertiary amine (physostigmine) drugs. These drugs inhibit the enzyme acetylcholinesterase (true cholinesterase), which is normally responsible for the rapid hydrolysis of acetylcholine after its release from cholinergic nerve endings. Therefore, in the presence of an anticholinesterase, there is accumulation of acetylcholine at nicotinic and muscarinic sites. Quarternary ammonium drugs cannot easily cross the blood-brain barrier such that accumulation of acetylcholine is predominantly at peripheral sites such as the nicotinic neuromuscular junction. Indeed, this is the principle mechanism for pharmacologic reversal of nondepolarizing muscle relaxants (see Chapter 8). Conversely, physostigmine, with its tertiary amine structure, can cross the blood-brain barrier, making this an effective drug for treatment of the central anticholinergic syndrome that manifests as emergence delerium in the recovery room (see Chapter 30).

Organophosphates produce prolonged inhibition of acetylcholinesterase activity. These substances are used as insecticides and are a frequent cause of poisoning (bradycardia, salivation, bronchoconstriction, skeletal muscle weakness) among agricultural workers, emphasizing the potential for their rapid absorption through intact skin. Pralidoxime is a specific antidote for organophosphate poisoning. Medically, organophosphate drugs (echothiophate, isoflurophate) are applied topically to the cornea to produce sustained miosis in the treatment of glaucoma (see Chapter 25). These drugs also inhibit the enzyme activity of plasma cholinesterase (pseudocholinesterase), which introduces the potential for a prolonged response to succinylcholine, as this drug is normally hydrolyzed by plasma cholinesterase.

REFERENCES

1. Lawson NW, Wallfisch HK. Cardiovascular pharmacology: A new look at the pressors. In: Stoelting RK, Barash PG, Gallagher TJ, eds. Advances in Anesthesia. Chicago, Year Book Medical Publishers, 1986;3:195–270.

2. Ram CVS, Kaplan NM. Alpha- and beta-receptor blocking drugs in the treatment of hypertension. In: Harvey WP, et al., eds. Current Problems in Cardiology. Chicago, Year Book Medical Publishers, 1979.

3. Berridge MJ. The molecular basis of communication within the cell. Sci Am 1985;253:(4):142–52.

4. Miller RD, Way WL, Eger EI II. The effects of alpha-methyldopa, reserpine, guanethidine, and iproniazid on minimum alveolar anesthetic requirement (MAC). Anesthesiology 1968;29:1153–8.

5. Edwards RP, Miller RD, Roizen MF, et al. Cardiac

responses to imipramine and pancuronium during anesthesia with halothane or enflurane. Anesthesiology 1979;50:421–5.

6. El-Ganzouri AR, Ivankovich AD, Braverman B, McCarthy R. Monoamine oxidase inhibitors: Should they be discontinued preoperatively? Anesth Analg 1985;64:592–6.

7. Bloor BC, Flacke WE. Reduction in halothane anesthetic requirements by clonidine, an alpha-adrenergic agonist. Anesth Analg 1982;61:741–5.

8. Husserl FE, Messerli FH. Adverse effects of antihypertensive drugs. Drugs 1981;22:188–210.

9. Wheeler AS, Patel KF, Spain J. Pulmonary edema during beta-2 tocolytic therapy. Anesth Analg 1981;60:695–6.

10. Moravec MA, Hurlbert BJ. Hypokalemia associated with terbutaline administration in obstetrical patients. Anesth Analg 1980;59:917–20.

11. Roizen MF, Stevens WC. Multiform ventricular tachycardia due to interaction of aminophylline and halothane. Anesth Analg 1978;57:738–41.

12. Rosa RM, Silva P, Young JB, et al. Adrenergic modulation of extrarenal potassium disposal. N Engl J Med 1980;302:431–4.

Effects of Inhaled Anesthetics on Ventilation and Circulation

Currently used inhaled anesthetics are represented by one gas (nitrous oxide) and three volatile liquids (halothane, enflurane, isoflurane). These anesthetics have important and often differing pharmacologic effects on ventilation and circulation. Data from healthy volunteers breathing equal potent concentrations of these drugs have provided the foundation for establishing comparative differences of inhaled anesthetics on ventilation and circulation in the absence of extraneous influences.[1] It must always be appreciated, however, that surgical patients with other variables (co-existing diseases, drug therapy that influences the function of the autonomic nervous system, preoperative medication, surgical stimulation, altered intravascular fluid volume, extremes of age) can respond differently from healthy volunteers.

VENTILATION

Inhaled anesthetics produce dose-dependent and drug-specific depressant effects on ventilation. Anesthetic-induced depression of ventilation most likely reflects direct depressant effects of these drugs on the medullary ventilatory center and perhaps peripheral effects on intercostal muscle function. The incidence of postoperative pulmonary complications is not different in patients anesthetized with halothane, enflurane, or isoflurane.

Pattern of Breathing

Inhaled anesthetics, except for isoflurane, produce dose-dependent increases in the rate of breathing (Fig. 4-1).[2] Isoflurane increases the rate of breathing similar to other inhaled anesthetics up to about 1 MAC, and above this dose the breathing frequency does not increase further. Nitrous oxide increases the rate of breathing more than other inhaled anesthetics at concentrations above 1 MAC. The effect of inhaled anesthetics on breathing frequency most likely reflects central nervous system stimulation and not, with the possible exception of nitrous oxide, stimulation of pulmonary stretch receptors.

Tidal volume is decreased in association with anesthetic-induced increases in the rate of breathing. The increase in rate of breathing is insufficient to offset the reduction in tidal volume, leading to a decline in minute ventilation and an elevation in $PaCO_2$ (Fig. 4-2)[1] (see the section *Arterial Partial Pressure of Carbon Dioxide*). Overall, the pattern of breathing during general anesthesia is characterized as rapid, shallow, regular, and rhythmic in contrast to the awake pattern of intermittent deep breaths separated by varying intervals.

Arterial Partial Pressure of Carbon Dioxide

The resting $PaCO_2$ is the most frequently used index of the dose-dependent depression of ventilation produced by inhaled anesthetics. In healthy

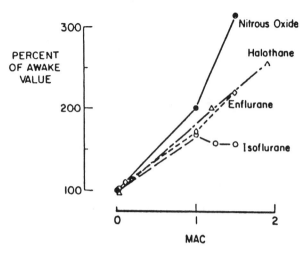

Fig. 4-1. Inhaled anesthetics produce similar increases in the rate of breathing (percent of awake value) up to doses of about 1 MAC. Increasing the dose above 1 MAC does not further increase the rate of breathing during inhalation of isoflurane. (From Eger,[2] with permission.)

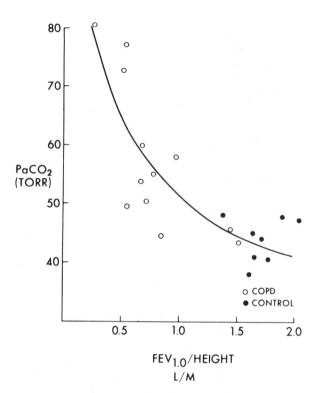

Fig. 4-3. The effects of halothane (1 percent alveolar concentration) on the $PaCO_2$ (torr, mmHg) were measured during spontaneous ventilation in patients with chronic obstructive airways disease and in normal patients of similar age. During halothane anesthesia, the $PaCO_2$ was increased more (depression of ventilation was greater) in patients with co-existing pulmonary disease compared with normal patients. The magnitude of the elevation of $PaCO_2$ was best related to preoperative measurements of the forced exhaled volume in 1 second (FEV_1) expressed in terms of body height. (From Pietak et al.,[3] with permission.)

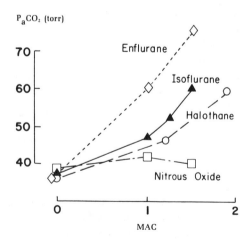

Fig. 4-2. Increasing MAC levels of enflurane, isoflurane, and halothane produce dose-dependent elevations in the $PaCO_2$ when administered to healthy volunteers. Nitrous oxide was given in a pressure chamber and did not increase the $PaCO_2$. (From Eger,[1] with permission.)

volunteers breathing equally potent concentrations of volatile anesthetics, the $PaCO_2$ is increased most by enflurane and less by isoflurane and halothane (Fig. 4-2).[1] The presence of chronic obstructive airways disease may accentuate the magnitude of increase in $PaCO_2$ produced by volatile anesthetics such as halothane (Fig. 4-3).[3] Nitrous oxide administered to volunteers in a hyperbaric chamber does not alter $PaCO_2$ from awake levels. Indeed, substitution of nitrous oxide for an equivalent

Table 4-1. Recovery from Drug-Induced Ventilatory Depression with Time

| | PaCO$_2$ | |
Enflurane	1 Hour of Administration	5 Hours of Administration
1 MAC	61 mmHg	46 mmHg
2 MAC	Apnea	67 mmHg

(Data from Calverley et al.[4])

portion of the volatile anesthetic results in less elevation of the PaCO$_2$ than that produced by the volatile anesthetic alone. Likewise, the addition of nitrous oxide without changing the inhaled concentration of volatile anesthetic does not further increase the PaCO$_2$, despite the greater depth of anesthesia in the presence of both inhaled drugs. The beneficial effect of nitrous oxide on limiting the increase in PaCO$_2$ is seen with all three volatile anesthetics, but the greatest impact is present when nitrous oxide is used to replace an equivalent amount of enflurane.

In addition to nitrous oxide, surgical stimulation and duration of administration may influence the magnitude of increase in PaCO$_2$ associated with the inhalation of volatile anesthetics. For example, surgical stimulation increases the tidal volume and breathing rate such that minute ventilation increases about 40 percent.[1] However, the PaCO$_2$ declines only about 5 mmHg (10 percent) in response to surgical stimulation.[1] This discrepancy is presumed to reflect increased production of carbon dioxide by activation of the sympathetic nervous system in response to surgical stimulation. This increased production of carbon dioxide prevents the increase in ventilation from reducing the PaCO$_2$ by the same magnitude. Finally, the magnitude of PaCO$_2$ elevation produced by the same dose of volatile anesthetic is less after 5 hours to 6 hours of administration than after 1 hour to 3 hours of administration (Table 4-1).[4] The reason for this apparent lessening of depression of ventilation with time is not known.

Assisted ventilation of the lungs is not greatly effective in lowering the PaCO$_2$ since the apneic threshold (maximum PaCO$_2$ that does not initiate spontaneous ventilation) is only about 5 mmHg below the resting PaCO$_2$, regardless of the level of the resting PaCO$_2$. For example, patients inhaling a volatile anesthetic at a dose sufficient to elevate the PaCO$_2$ to 50 mmHg would likely become apneic when assisted ventilation of the lungs lowered the PaCO$_2$ to about 45 mmHg. For this reason, assisted ventilation of the lungs is not a highly effective method to reduce the PaCO$_2$ during general anesthesia. Controlled ventilation of the lungs is the most predictable method for preventing elevations in the PaCO$_2$ during inhalation of volatile anesthetics.

Ventilatory Response to Carbon Dioxide

Plotting the volume of ventilation at increasing levels of PaCO$_2$ (carbon dioxide response curve) is a sensitive method for quantitating the effects of drugs on ventilation (Fig. 4-4). In awake humans, inhalation of carbon dioxide increases minute ventilation 1 L·min^{-1} to 3 L·min^{-1} for every mmHg increase in PaCO$_2$. Inhaled anesthetics including nitrous oxide produce dose-dependent depression of the slope of the carbon dioxide response curve. In addition, the position of the carbon dioxide response curve is shifted to the right as compared with the awake curve. A decreased slope reflects reduced sensitivity to the ventilatory stimulant effects of carbon dioxide, whereas rightward displacement depicts an attenuated responsiveness to carbon dioxide.

The depression of the ventilatory response to carbon dioxide implies that the drive to overcome resistance to breathing (upper airway obstruction, kinked endotracheal tube, airway secretions) could be reduced in the presence of these drugs. Yet the slope and position of the carbon dioxide response curve during inhalation of volatile anesthetics returns toward normal (like the PaCO$_2$) after 5 hours to 6 hours of administration of these drugs.

Substitution of nitrous oxide for a portion of the volatile anesthetic (while maintaining the same total dose of anesthetic) results in a return of the slope and position of the carbon dioxide response curve toward the awake level. This effect of nitrous oxide is present with all three volatile anesthetics, but the impact is most apparent when nitrous

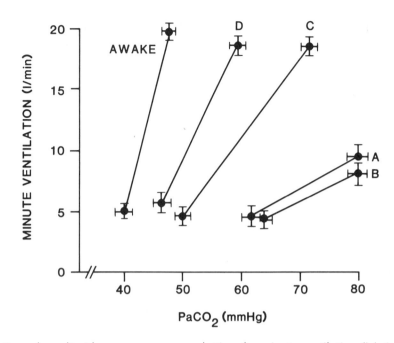

Fig. 4-4. Schematic carbon dioxide response curves plotting the minute ventilation (L/min) versus PaCO$_2$ (mmHg). In the awake state minute ventilation increases 1 L·min^{-1} to 3 L·min^{-1} for every mmHg increase in PaCO$_2$ (curve AWAKE). The carbon dioxide response curve is dramatically shifted to the right and the slope decreased during the first 2 hours to 3 hours of inhalation of 1.1 MAC concentrations of volatile anesthetics (curve A). Addition of 70 percent nitrous oxide to 1.1 MAC concentrations of volatile anesthetics does not significantly alter the position or slope of the carbon dioxide response curve despite the increased anesthetic depth produced by the drug combination (curve B). The combination of 70 percent nitrous oxide with sufficient concentrations of volatile anesthetics to result in a 1.1 MAC concentration produces less depression of ventilation than that seen with a 1.1 MAC concentration of volatile anesthetics alone (curve C). Recovery from the ventilatory depressant effects produced by 1.1 MAC concentrations of volatile anesthetics occurs after 5 hours to 6 hours of administration (curve D).

oxide is substituted for an equivalent amount of enflurane.

Ventilatory Response to Arterial Hypoxemia

Reductions in the PaO$_2$ below 60 mmHg normally produce increases in minute ventilation. This response in humans is mediated by peripheral chemoreceptors known as the carotid bodies. Subanesthetic concentrations (0.1 MAC) of inhaled anesthetics greatly attenuate, and anesthetic concentrations (1 MAC) abolish the ventilatory response to arterial hypoxemia (Table 4-2).[5] Conversely, subanesthetic concentrations of inhaled anesthetics do not depress the ventilatory response

to carbon dioxide to the same degree (Table 4-2).[5] Inhaled anesthetics also attenuate the usual synergistic effect of arterial hypoxemia and hypercapnia on stimulation of ventilation. The depression of hypoxic responsiveness by subanesthetic concentrations of inhaled drugs suggests that patients could manifest a diminished ventilatory response to arterial hypoxemia in the recovery room (see Chapter 30).

Bronchodilation

Volatile anesthetics administered at 1 MAC concentrations produce similar attenuation of antigen-induced bronchospasm in dogs (Fig. 4-5).[6] Despite

Table 4-2. Ventilatory Responses to Arterial Hypoxemia or Hypercapnia during Administration of Halothane to Humans

| Halothane Concentration (MAC) | Percent of Awake Response | |
	Arterial Hypoxemia	Hypercapnia
0.1	31	100
1.1	0	36
2.0	0	17

(Data from Knill and Gelb.[5])

these observations, there is lack of evidence that bronchodilating effects of volatile anesthetics are an effective method for treating status asthmaticus that is unresponsive to more conventional treatments. The relaxant effect of volatile anesthetics on bronchial smooth muscle most likely reflects anesthetic-induced reductions in afferent nerve traffic or central medullary depression of bronchoconstriction reflexes. In addition, volatile anesthetics may produce bronchial smooth muscle relaxation by direct effects. Indeed, it has been suggested that halothane exerts beta agonist effects on bronchial smooth muscle leading to bronchodilation.

Hypoxic Pulmonary Vasoconstriction

Hypoxic pulmonary vasoconstriction is the reflex constriction of pulmonary arterioles in areas of atelectasis in attempts to reduce or prevent perfusion of unventilated alveoli. This reflex vasoconstriction is protective and its inhibition by inhaled anesthetics could adversely affect the PaO_2. Many drugs, including inhaled anesthetics, inhibit hypoxic pulmonary vasoconstriction. Nevertheless, halothane and isoflurane do not further impair arterial oxygenation in anesthetized patients during one lung ventilation, suggesting that these inhaled anesthetics do not inhibit hypoxic pulmonary vasoconstriction (see Fig. 20-5). Based on available data, it would seem premature to select one inhaled anesthetic over another based on presumed effects on hypoxic pulmonary vasoconstriction.

Respiratory Muscle Function

Optimal respiratory muscle function occurs when descent of the diaphragm is coupled with expansion of the rib cage produced by contraction of the intercostal muscles. Halothane produces preferential suppression of intercostal muscle function with relative sparing of the diaphragm.[7] Depression of intercostal muscle function interferes with rib cage expansion in response to chemical stimuli such as arterial hypoxemia or hypercapnia. Furthermore, depression of intercostal muscle function means that stabilization of the rib cage is reduced during spontaneous ventilation such that descent of the diaphragm tends to cause the chest to collapse inward contributing to reductions in lung volumes, particularly the functional residual capacity. It is concluded that, in addition to depression of the medullary ventilatory center, halothane produces depression of ventilation by virtue of interfering with normal intercostal muscle function. The effects of other inhaled anesthetics on intercostal muscle function have not been reported.

CIRCULATION

Inhaled anesthetics produce dose-dependent and drug-specific effects on the circulation.[1] Data obtained from healthy volunteers during controlled ventilation of the lungs to maintain normocarbia permits isolation of circulatory changes due solely to the inhaled anesthetic. Again, surgical patients characterized by other variables that influence circulatory responses can respond differently from healthy volunteers.

Arterial Blood Pressure

Dose-dependent reductions of arterial blood pressure are produced by halothane, enflurane, and isoflurane; whereas nitrous oxide alone usually does not alter the blood pressure (Fig. 4-6).[1] Decreases in blood pressure are similar for isoflurane and enflurane and greater than that produced by halothane. Decreases in myocardial contractility and cardiac output are primarily responsible for

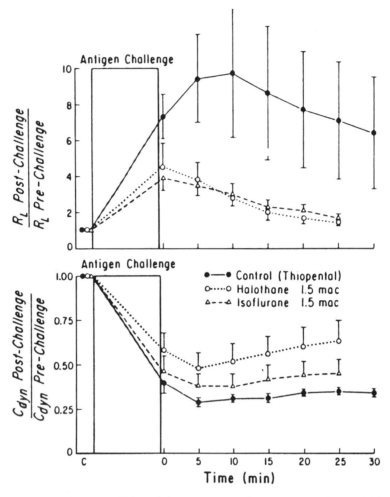

Fig. 4-5. Increases in airway resistance (R_L) and decreases in pulmonary compliance (Cdyn) following Ascaris antigen challenge were measured during thiopental, halothane, and isoflurane anesthesia in dogs. The horizontal axis shows elapsed time from the conclusion of antigen administration. Halothane and isoflurane were equally effective in attenuating the antigen-induced increases in R_L as compared with thiopental. Conversely, halothane was somewhat more effective than isoflurane in minimizing concomitant decreases in Cdyn. (From Hirshman et al.,[6] with permission.)

reductions in blood pressure produced by inhalation of halothane and enflurane. Conversely, isoflurane-induced reductions in blood pressure are due principally to peripheral vasodilation and associated reductions in systemic vascular resistance. Surgical stimulation and/or substitution of nitrous oxide for an equivalent portion of the volatile anesthetic results in less blood pressure decrease at the same anesthetic dose (Fig. 4-7).

Heart Rate

Heart rate is unchanged by halothane and only minimally increased by nitrous oxide (Fig. 4-8).[1] Isoflurane increases heart rate 20 percent above awake levels (Fig. 4-8).[1] Isoflurane-induced heart rate increases are more likely to occur in young than elderly patients and may be accentuated by the presence of other drugs (atropine, meperidine,

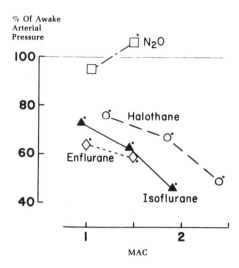

Fig. 4-6. Isoflurane, halothane, and enflurane, but not nitrous oxide, administered to healthy volunteers decreases arterial blood pressure from the awake value in a dose-dependent manner. Asterisks indicate significant changes from awake values. (From Eger,[1] with permission.)

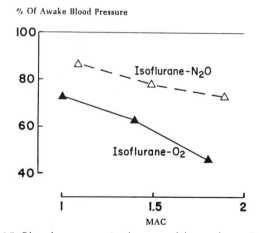

Fig. 4-7. Blood pressure is depressed less when nitrous oxide is substituted for a portion of the isoflurane dose but keeping the total MAC concentration the same as with isoflurane alone. (From Eger,[1] with permission.)

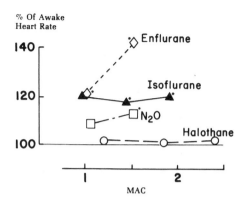

Fig. 4-8. Halothane and nitrous oxide produce minimal to no change in heart rate when administered to healthy volunteers. Heart rate is increased about 20 percent by 1 MAC and 2 MAC isoflurane. Enflurane produces a dose-dependent increase in heart rate. Asterisks indicate significant changes from awake values. (From Eger,[1] with permission.)

pancuronium) that independently increase heart rate. Furthermore, inclusion of morphine in the preoperative medication or intravenous administration of fentanyl during surgery prevents increases in heart rate associated with inhalation of volatile anesthetics including isoflurane (Fig. 4-9)[8] (see Chapter 10). Enflurane is the only anesthetic that produces dose-dependent increases in heart rate in volunteers (Fig. 4-8).[1] In surgical patients, however, enflurane-induced heart rate changes have not been prominent (Fig. 4-9).[8]

Anesthetic-induced reductions in blood pressure would tend to increase heart rate via stimulation of the carotid sinus baroreceptors. The presence of this reflex response is suggested by the increased heart rate that accompanies isoflurane and enflurane-induced reductions in blood pressure. By contrast, halothane inhibits the baroreceptor reflex response, and heart rate usually remains unchanged despite halothane-induced reductions in blood pressure.

Cardiac Output

Volatile anesthetics produce dose-dependent reductions in cardiac output (Fig. 4-10).[1] Isoflurane produces the least depression, and at a 1 MAC concentration of this drug the cardiac output is

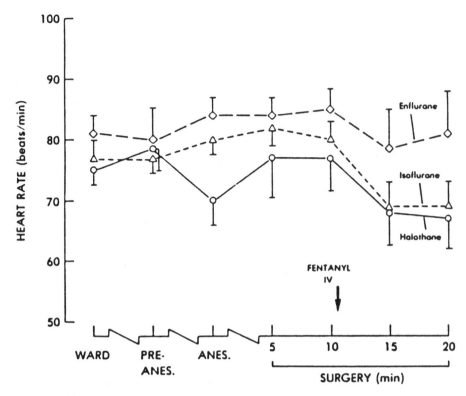

Fig. 4-9. Heart rate did not change significantly from awake levels (ward and pre-anes) following induction of anesthesia (thiopental-succinylcholine) or inhalation of volatile anesthetics (surgery) at doses of about 0.9 MAC plus 60 percent nitrous oxide. Heart rate declined when fentanyl was administered intravenously. (From Cahalan et al.,[8] with permission.)

not reduced below awake values. The depression of cardiac output produced by halothane and enflurane parallels the reductions in blood pressure produced by these drugs. In contrast to volatile anesthetics, nitrous oxide is associated with mild increases in cardiac output, presumably reflecting weak sympathomimetic effects of this drug.[1]

Stroke Volume

Halothane, enflurane, and isoflurane produce dose-dependent reductions in calculated stroke volume (cardiac output divided by heart rate), with the greatest decreases occurring during inhalation of enflurane (Fig. 4-11).[1] Stroke volume is not changed by nitrous oxide. Reductions in stroke volume are consistent with decreased myocardial contractility manifesting as a lowered cardiac out-

put. It is also possible that cardiac output would not be as well maintained during inhalation of isoflurane should increases in heart rate not accompany administration of this drug (see the section *Heart Rate*). Increased heart rate during inhalation of isoflurane offsets the decreased stroke volume and cardiac output is unchanged. Increased heart rate associated with inhalation of enflurane is insufficient to offset the reduction in stroke volume and cardiac output decreases.

Myocardial Contractility

Inhaled anesthetics studied in vitro (isolated papillary muscle preparations) produce dose-dependent direct myocardial depression. Depression produced by nitrous oxide, however, is less than that produced by comparable concentrations of volatile anesthetics. Depression of myocardial con-

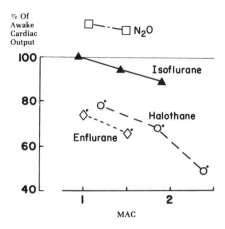

Fig. 4-10. Cardiac output during inhalation of nitrous oxide is increased above awake levels while 1 MAC isoflurane produces no change and higher concentrations result in only small decreases. Conversely, halothane and enflurane produce dose-dependent reductions in cardiac output. Asterisks indicate significant changes from awake values. (From Eger,[1] with permission.)

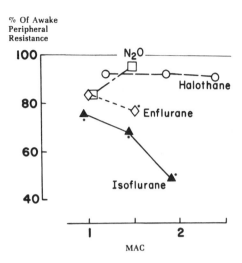

Fig. 4-12. Isoflurane, and to a lesser degree, enflurane, produce dose-dependent decreases in calculated systemic (peripheral) vascular resistance when administered to healthy volunteers. Halothane and nitrous oxide do not alter systemic vascular resistance. Asterisks indicate significant changes from awake values. (From Eger,[1] with permission.)

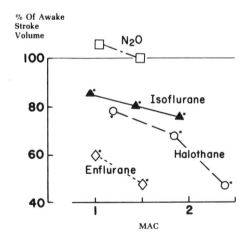

Fig. 4-11. Volatile anesthetics, but not nitrous oxide, administered to healthy volunteers result in dose-dependent decreases in stroke volume with the greatest reductions produced by enflurane. Asterisks indicate significant changes from awake values. (From Eger,[1] with permission.)

tractility is greater in papillary muscles taken from animals in congestive heart failure as compared with measurements in muscles taken from normal animals. Therefore, patients with impaired myocardial contractility due to congestive heart failure might be particularly vulnerable to the direct myocardial depressant effects of inhaled anesthetics. Nevertheless, cardiac depression is not consistently seen in vivo, presumably because compensatory homeostatic mechanisms, particularly autonomic nervous system activity, can obscure these direct depressant effects.

Systemic Vascular Resistance

Isoflurane and, to a lesser extent, enflurane reduce calculated systemic vascular resistance (mean arterial pressure minus right arterial pressure divided by cardiac output), but no significant change is produced by halothane or nitrous oxide (Fig. 4-12).[1] Decreases in calculated systemic vascular resistance associated with inhalation of isoflurane are predictable considering the decrease in blood pressure and unchanged cardiac output associated with administration of this drug. Conversely, re-

ductions in blood pressure associated with halothane administration parallels the decrease in cardiac output and the calculated systemic vascular
resistance is unchanged. This does not mean that
halothane lacks vasodilating effects on specific
organ systems. Indeed, the prominence of superficial cutaneous veins during inhalation of halothane and other volatile drugs reflects venodilation. Anesthetic-induced increases in skin blood
flow at the onset of anesthesia most likely reflect
central inhibitory actions of these drugs on tem-
perature-regulating mechanisms. All volatile anesthetics produce cerebral vasodilation and increase cerebral blood flow (halothane the most
and isoflurane the least) regardless of their overall
effects on calculated systemic vascular resistance.
Isoflurane is unique in its ability to produce twofold to threefold increases in skeletal muscle blood
flow that contribute to reductions in systemic vascular resistance associated with administration of
this drug. Muscle blood flow is not altered by
nitrous oxide and is diminished by halothane,
reflecting decreased perfusion pressure rather
than vasoconstriction.

The magnitude of reduction in systemic vascular
resistance produced by isoflurane is less when
nitrous oxide is substituted for an equivalent
amount of isoflurane. The lesser reduction in
systemic vascular resistance is consistent with the
attenuation of decreases in blood pressure produced by isoflurane when administered with nitrous oxide (Fig. 4-7).[1]

Absence of changes in calculated systemic vascular resistance during the inhalation of halothane
emphasizes that depth of halothane anesthesia
parallels cardiac depression as reflected by reductions in blood pressure. Conversely, reductions in
blood pressure during administration of enflurane
or isoflurane can occur at light levels of anesthesia,
reflecting decreases in systemic vascular resistance
rather than myocardial depression.

Coronary Vascular Resistance

Isoflurane, but not halothane or enflurane, selectively dilates coronary arterioles in animal models.[9]
Theoretically, isoflurane-induced coronary arteriole vasodilation could result in diversion of blood
flow from ischemic areas of myocardium (arter-

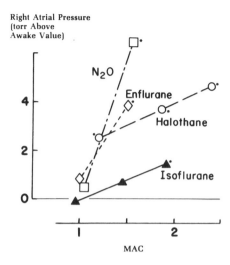

Fig. 4-13. Nitrous oxide, enflurane and halothane administered to healthy volunteers produce dose-dependent
increases in right atrial pressures. Right atrial pressures
are minimally changed by isoflurane. Asterisks indicate
significant changes from awake values. (From Eger,[1]
with permission.)

ioles already maximally dilated) to areas with normally responsive vessels (i.e., coronary artery steal
syndrome). Nevertheless, most patients do not
develop myocardial ischemia during administration of volatile anesthetics, including isoflurane,
emphasizing the importance of avoiding drug-
induced events that adversely alter myocardial
oxygen delivery (hypotension) or myocardial oxygen requirements (tachycardia) (see Chapter 19).
Autoregulation of coronary blood flow seems to
be maintained during administration of inhaled
anesthetics.

Right Atrial Pressure

Right atrial pressure is increased in a dose-dependent manner by inhaled anesthetics (Fig. 4-13).[1]
Myocardial depression produced by volatile anesthetics would result in elevations of right atrial
pressures. Despite evidence of similar depression
of myocardial contractility produced in vitro by
halothane, enflurane, and isoflurane increases in
right atrial pressures are least during inhalation
of isoflurane, presumably reflecting peripheral
vasodilating effects of this drug. Elevated right

atrial pressures during inhalation of nitrous oxide most likely reflects increased pulmonary vascular resistance due to sympathomimetic effects of this drug.[1]

Mechanism of Circulatory Effects

No single or predominant mechanism explains circulatory effects produced by inhaled anesthetics. Proposed mechanisms include

1. Direct myocardial depression
2. Inhibition of sympathetic nervous system outflow from the central nervous system
3. Depression of transmission of impulses through autonomic ganglia
4. Impairment of baroreceptor reflex activity
5. Decreased formation of cAMP
6. Increased formation of cGMP
7. Decreased release of catecholamines from the adrenal medulla
8. Inhibition of calcium reuptake by myocardial sarcoplasmic reticulum
9. Decreased influx of calcium through slow channels.

Plasma catecholamine concentrations usually do not increase during administration of volatile anesthetics as evidenced by the fact that these drugs do not activate the sympathetic nervous system.

Isoflurane is possibly unique among volatile anesthetics in possessing mild beta agonist properties. This property may oppose direct depressant effects of isoflurane on the heart and is consistent with maintenance of cardiac output, increased heart rate, elevated skeletal muscle blood flow, dilation of coronary arterioles, and decreased systemic vascular resistance associated with administration of this drug. Furthermore, isoflurane interferes with calcium influx less and is less likely than enflurane or halothane to depress baroreceptor reflex responses.[10] Another possible explanation for the lesser impact of isoflurane on myocardial contractility may be a greater anesthetic potency of isoflurane relative to halothane and enflurane. The implication is that isoflurane may more readily depress the brain and thus, at a given MAC value, appear to spare the heart. Indeed, in animals, the lesser myocardial depression associated with inhalation of isoflurane manifests as a greater margin of safety between the dose that produces anesthesia and that which produces cardiovascular collapse (Table 4-3).[11]

Nitrous oxide alone or when added to unchanged concentrations of volatile anesthetics produce signs of mild sympathomimetic stimulation characterized by elevations in circulating levels of catecholamines, mydriasis, and increased systemic and pulmonary vascular resistance. Animal studies suggest that increases in systemic vascular resistance result from activation of the sympathetic nervous system due to the actions of nitrous oxide on suprapontine areas of the brain. Sympathomimetic effects of nitrous oxide are most evident when this drug is added to halothane, intermediate with isoflurane and minimal with enflurane. Conceivably, sympathetic nervous system stimulation produced by nitrous oxide alone or in combination with volatile drugs is responsible for the minimal to absent cardiac depression associated with inhalation of this drug.

Cardiac Rhythm

Halothane reduces the amount of circulating epinephrine required to elicit ventricular premature contractions. This anesthetic-induced sensitization of the myocardium to the effects of epinephrine is less with enflurane and least with isoflurane (Fig. 4-14).[12] Enflurane is intermediate in dysrhythmogenic potential, but the flat nature of the dose response curve makes it impossible to predict the epinephrine dose likely to produce ventricular

Table 4-3. Anesthetic Indices

Drug	Cardiac Anesthetic Index[a]
Isoflurane	5.7
Enflurane	3.3
Halothane	3.0
Halothane Nitrous Oxide (50%)	3.7

[a] Concentration of anesthetic in heart that produces cardiac failure: concentration of anesthetic in heart at establishment of anesthesia.
(Data from Wolfson et al.[11])

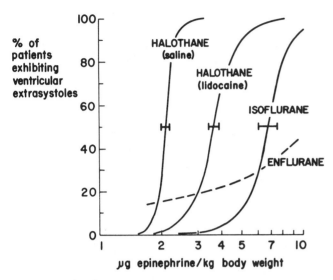

Fig. 4-14. The dose (ED_{50}) of submucosal epinephrine necessary to produce ventricular premature contractions (ventricular extrasystoles) was determined in adult normocapnic patients anesthetized with 1.25 MAC halothane, isoflurane or enflurane. The results of the statistical analysis suggest that the halothane and isoflurane curves (but not the enflurane curve) are parallel and that the ED_{50}s are significantly different from each other ($P < 0.01$). For example, the ED_{50} for halothane was 2.1 $\mu g \cdot kg^{-1}$ versus 6.7 $\mu g \cdot kg^{-1}$ for isoflurane. (From Johnston et al.,[12] with permission.)

dysrhythmias (Fig. 4-14).[12] Nevertheless, the incidence of cardiac dysrhythmias during inhalation of enflurane is low.

The mechanism for the difference between volatile anesthetics and sensitization of the myocardium to catecholamines may reflect differences in the effects of these drugs on transmission of cardiac impulses. For example, halothane, enflurane, and isoflurane slow transmission of cardiac impulses through the atrioventricular node, but only halothane slows conduction through the His-Purkinje system. Re-entry and appearance of ventricular premature contractions are more likely in the presence of halothane-induced prolongation of His-Purkinje conduction times. Furthermore, the ability of alpha-1 receptor blockade with prazosin to increase the dysrhythmogenic dose of epinephrine more than beta receptor blockade

suggests that stimulation of alpha-1 receptors in the heart is important for halothane-induced sensitization.[13] In animals, enhancement of the dysrhythmogenic potential of epinephrine is independent of the dose of halothane between alveolar concentrations of 0.5 percent and 2 percent. If true in patients, it is likely that therapeutic interventions other than decreasing the inhaled concentrations of halothane will be required to promptly treat cardiac dysrhythmias caused by epinephrine.

Junctional rhythm leading to reductions in blood pressure is common during inhalation of halothane. The appearance of this cardiac rhythm disturbance most likely reflects suppression of sinus node activity by halothane.

Pulmonary Vasculature

The effect of volatile anesthetics on the pulmonary vasculature in the absence of any underlying pulmonary vascular abnormality is small. Conversely, nitrous oxide can increase pulmonary vascular resistance particularly when administered to patients with co-existing pulmonary hypertension.[14]

Spontaneous Ventilation

Spontaneous ventilation during inhalation of volatile anesthetics leads to the accumulation of carbon dioxide. Accumulation of carbon dioxide may stimulate the sympathetic nervous system and produce peripheral vasodilation, thus altering circulatory effects produced by volatile anesthetics during spontaneous ventilation as compared with measurements obtained during controlled ventilation of the lungs and normocarbia. For example, heart rate and cardiac output are greater (sympathetic nervous system stimulation) and the systemic vascular resistance decreased more (peripheral vasodilation) during spontaneous inhalation of volatile anesthetics.[1] Despite these changes, the blood pressure is not altered from that observed during controlled ventilation of the lungs. In addition to affecting the circulation by allowing the accumulation of carbon dioxide, spontaneous ventilation of the lungs favors venous return to the heart.

Surgical Stimulation

Surgical stimulation modifies the circulatory effects produced by inhaled anesthetics. Indeed, sympathetic nervous system stimulation produced by the surgical incision often results in increased blood pressure and heart rate. Volatile anesthetics oppose this response in a dose-dependent manner. For example, 1.47 MAC halothane or 1.63 MAC enflurane prevents blood pressure and heart rate responses evoked by surgical skin incision in 50 percent of patients.[15]

Duration of Administration

Inhalation of volatile anesthetics for 5 hours to 6 hours is associated with an increased heart rate, cardiac output, right atrial pressure, and decreased systemic vascular resistance compared with similar measurements after 1 hour of administration. Despite the increased cardiac output, blood pressure is unchanged with time reflecting decreases in systemic vascular resistance. This recovery from depressant effects of volatile anesthetics with time is most apparent during inhalation of halothane, intermediate with enflurane, and minimal with isoflurane. Prior administration of propranolol prevents these time-related changes, suggesting increased sympathetic nervous system activity as the mechanism.

Co-Existing Diseases

Co-existing diseases, particularly of the heart, may influence the significance of circulatory effects produced by inhaled anesthetics. For example, drug-induced reductions in myocardial contractility are additive with co-existing decreases in contractility associated with congestive heart failure. In patients with coronary artery disease, inhalation of nitrous oxide produces evidence of myocardial depression that does not occur in patients without heart disease. Patients with stenotic lesions of the aortic or mitral valves tolerate poorly changes in blood pressure and systemic vascular resistance produced by inhaled anesthetics (see Chapter 19). Anemia does not predictably alter anesthetic-induced circulatory effects.

Prior Drug Therapy

Prior drug therapy that alters sympathetic nervous system activity (antihypertensives, beta-adrenergic antagonists) may exaggerate the magnitude of circulatory effects produced by inhaled anesthetics. For example, the magnitude of cardiac depression produced by enflurane, but not isoflurane, seems to be accentuated by concomitant drug therapy with beta-adrenergic antagonists such as propranolol. Circulatory changes during inhalation of halothane in the presence of beta-adrenergic blockade are intermediate between isoflurane and enflurane. Calcium entry blockers decrease myocardial contractility and thus render the heart more vulnerable to direct depressant effects of inhaled anesthetics. In animals, depressant effects of verapamil on cardiac output are greater during administration of enflurane than isoflurane. Despite these differences, clinical experience has not suggested that a specific volatile anesthetic is indicated for administration to patients being treated with drugs that act on the heart or depress the sympathetic nervous system. Since additive depression may occur with these drugs, however, it may be necessary to decrease the dose of volatile anesthetics, especially when enflurane is being administered. Discontinuation of previously established efficacious drug therapy is not recommended as this practice may provoke an abrupt return of drug-suppressed symptoms such as hypertension or myocardial ischemia.

REFERENCES

1. Eger EI II. Isoflurane (Forane). A compendium and reference. Madison, WI, Anaquest, a division of BOC, Inc. 1986:1–160.
2. Eger EI II. Respiratory effects of nitrous oxide. In: Nitrous Oxide. New York. Elsevier, 1985:109–23.
3. Pietak S, Weenig CS, Hickey RF, Fairley HB. Anesthetic effects of ventilation in patients with chronic obstructive pulmonary disease. Anesthesiology 1975;42:160–6.
4. Calverley RK, Smith NT, Jones CW, Prys-Roberts C, Eger EI II. Ventilatory and cardiovascular effects of enflurane anesthesia during spontaneous ventilation in man. Anesth Analg 1978;57:610–8.
5. Knill RL, Gelb AW. Ventilatory responses to hypoxia and hypercapnia during halothane sedation and anesthesia in man. Anesthesiology 1978;49:244–51.

6. Hirshman CA, Edelstein G, Peetz S, Wayne R, Downes H. Mechanism of action of inhalational anesthesia on airways. Anesthesiology 1982;56:107–11.

7. Tusiewicz K, Bryan AC, Froese AB. Contributions of changing rib cage-diaphragm interactions to the ventilatory depression of halothane anesthesia. Anesthesiology 1977;47:327–37.

8. Cahalan MK, Lurz FW, Eger EI II, Schwartz LA, Beaupre PN, Smith JS. Narcotics decrease heart rate during inhalation anesthesia. Anesth Analg 1987;66:166–70.

9. Sill JC, Bove AA, Nugent M, Blaise GA, Dewey JD, Grabau C. Effects of isoflurane on coronary arterioles in the intact dog. Anesthesiology 1987;66:273–9.

10. Hilgenberg JC, McCammon RL, Stoelting RK. Pulmonary and systemic vascular responses to nitrous oxide in patients with mitral stenosis and pulmonary hypertension. Anesth Analg 1980;59:323–6.

11. Wolfson B, Hetrick WD, Lake CL, Siker ES. Anesthetic indices—further data. Anesthesiology 1978;48:187–90.

12. Johnston RR, Eger EI II, Wilson C. A comparative interaction of epinephrine with enflurane, isoflurane and halothane in man. Anesth Analg 1976;55:709–12.

13. Maze M, Smith CM. Identification of receptor mechanism mediating epinephrine induced arrhythmias during halothane anesthesia in the dog. Anesthesiology 1983;59:322–6.

14. Schulte-Sasse U, Hess W, Tarnow J. Pulmonary vascular responses to nitrous oxide in patients with normal and high pulmonary vascular resistance. Anesthesiology 1982;57:9–13.

15. Roizen MF, Horrigan RW, Frazer BM. Anesthetic doses blocking adrenergic (stress) and cardiovascular responses to incision—MAC BAR. Anesthesiology 1981;54:390–8.

Chapter 5

Metabolism and Toxicity of Inhaled Anesthetics

For many years, inhaled anesthetics were considered to be chemically inert and thus resistant to even minimal metabolism (biotransformation). It is now recognized that inhaled anesthetics can undergo varying degrees of metabolism in the liver and to a lesser extent in the lungs, kidneys, and gastrointestinal tract (Tables 5-1 and 5-2).[1-4] The significance of this metabolism can relate to toxic effects of metabolism on the liver, kidneys, and reproductive organs (see the section *Organ Toxicity Due to Anesthetic Metabolism*). In addition to organ toxicity, the magnitude of metabolism of methoxyflurane and halothane may be sufficient to influence the rate of elimination of these drugs from the blood—a process normally attributed solely to ventilation of the lungs[1,5] (see Chapter 30). Metabolism does not influence the rate of induction of anesthesia or the inhaled concentrations of anesthetics necessary for the maintenance of anesthesia because the inhaled anesthetics are administered in great excess of the amount metabolized.

DETERMINANTS OF METABOLISM

Metabolism of inhaled anesthetics is dependent on the activity of cytochrome P-450 enzymes located in the endoplasmic reticulum of hepatocytes. These enzymes mediate both oxidative and reductive metabolism of inhaled anesthetics. Cytochrome P-450 enzymes are susceptible to induction by many drugs including the inhaled anesthetics. With the prevalence of polypharmacy, enzyme induction may be a common occurrence in patients undergoing surgery. Indeed, anesthetic-induced hepatotoxicity and nephrotoxicity are often attributed to increased production of toxic metabolites as a reflection of enzyme induction. Nevertheless, a study of surgical patients in whom enzymes were induced failed to show an increased incidence of toxic effects.[6] Finally, genetic factors appear to be the most important determinant of drug metabolizing enzyme activity.

Chemical structure is important in determining the susceptibility of anesthetic molecules to metabolism. The ether bond (carbon-oxygen-carbon) and carbon-halogen bond are the sites most likely to undergo oxidative metabolism mediated by cytochrome P-450 enzymes. Two halogen atoms on a terminal carbon atom represent the optimal condition for dehalogenation, whereas a terminal carbon atom with three fluorine atoms (trifluorocarbon molecule) is stable and resistant to oxidative metabolism. Oxidation of the ether bond is less likely when hydrogen atoms on the carbons surrounding the oxygen atom of this bond are replaced with halogen atoms. Reductive (anaerobic) metabolism of inhaled anesthetics is rare, occurring to a significant degree only with halothane.

Table 5-1. Estimates of the Magnitude of Metabolism of Inhaled Anesthetics

Anesthetic	Percent of Absorbed Anesthetic Recovered as Metabolites[2-4]	Percent Metabolized Based on Total Uptake Minus Total Recovered in Exhaled Gases[1]
Nitrous Oxide	0.004	
Isoflurane	0.17	0[a]
Enflurane	2.4	8.5
Halothane	20	46.1
Methoxyflurane	50	75.3

[a] Metabolism of isoflurane was assumed to be zero for this calculation.[1]

Hydrolysis of inhaled anesthetics does not occur because these drugs do not contain ester bonds.

EXTENT OF METABOLISM

Estimates of the total amount of inhaled anesthetic that is metabolized have traditionally been based on the recovery of metabolites in the urine (Table 5-1).[1-4] This approach may underestimate the true extent of metabolism as it is unlikely that all metabolites can be accounted for or recovered.[1] For example, estimates of metabolism based on organic fluoride excretion in urine must compensate for loss to bone by multiplying urinary excretion by a correction factor which at best is an approximation. The problem of incomplete recovery of metabolites can be circumvented by esti-

mating metabolism as the difference between the total anesthetic recovered in exhaled gases after anesthetic administration is discontinued compared with the total taken up during administration.[1] Applying this technique, estimates of the extent of metabolism of inhaled anesthetics are 1.5 times to 3 times greater than estimates determined by recovery of metabolites (Table 5-1).[1-4]

Alveolar concentrations of an inhaled anesthetic may be an important determinant of the fraction of anesthetic metabolized. For example, high concentrations (1 MAC) saturate hepatic enzymes, reducing the fraction of inhaled anesthetic that is metabolized on passage through the liver (Fig. 5-1).[4] Conversely, subanesthetic concentrations (0.1 MAC or less) undergo extensive metabolism on passage through the liver (Fig. 5-1).[4] Inhaled an-

Table 5-2. Comparative Serum Fluoride Concentrations in Nonobese Patients

Anesthetic	Peak Fluoride Concentration ($\mu M \cdot L^{-1}$)	Time to Peak Fluoride Concentration after Anesthesia (hr)	Dose[a] (MAC hr)
Halothane	No Change		4.7
Isoflurane	4.4	6	4.1
Enflurane	22.2	4	2.7
Methoxyflurane	61	48	2.5

[a] MAC hr is calculated as the MAC concentration × duration of administration in hours. Administration of a 1 MAC concentration for 2.5 hours is a 2.5 MAC hr dose.

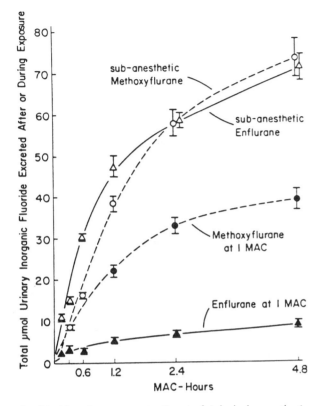

Fig. 5-1. Alveolar concentrations of inhaled anesthetics are important determinants of the fraction of anesthetic metabolized. Mean ± SE. (From White et al.,[4] with permission.)

esthetics, such as nitrous oxide, isoflurane, and enflurane, that are poorly soluble in blood and tissue lipids tend to be rapidly eliminated by ventilation of the lungs at the conclusion of their administration. As a result, less drug is available to recirculate through the liver at low concentrations conducive to metabolism, and the magnitude of metabolism of these drugs is likely to be minimal (Table 5-1).[1–4] Halothane and methoxyflurane are more soluble in blood and tissue lipids providing a reservoir to maintain subanesthetic concentrations in the blood for prolonged periods following their discontinuation. Indeed, the magnitude of metabolism of halothane and methoxyflurane is large compared to less lipid soluble inhaled anesthetics (Table 5-1).[1–4]

Despite the speculated importance of blood and lipid solubility in maintaining plasma and alveolar concentrations of inhaled anesthetics, there is evidence that alveolar partial pressures of methoxyflurane (high lipid solubility) and enflurane (low lipid solubility) decrease at nearly the same rate (see Fig. 2-5).[5] Therefore, a slow decline in partial pressure and resultant recirculation through the liver at concentrations conducive to metabolism is not the cause of increased metabolism of methoxyflurane. Rather, methoxyflurane (and to a lesser extent halothane) is metabolized so rapidly that the decline in its alveolar partial pressure is accelerated resulting in a rate of decrease similar to the less lipid soluble anesthetic, enflurane (see Fig. 2-5).[5]

Disease states, such as cirrhosis of the liver or congestive heart failure, may decrease the magnitude of metabolism of inhaled anesthetics by reducing hepatic blood flow and the subsequent delivery of these drugs to hepatic enzymes for metabolism. Cirrhosis of the liver may also reduce enzyme activity due to loss of hepatic parenchyma. Finally, morbid obesity, for unknown reasons, is associated with increased defluorination of volatile anesthetics (Fig. 5-2).[7]

HALOTHANE METABOLISM

Halothane undergoes significant metabolism in humans with an estimated 20 percent to 46 percent of the absorbed drug undergoing metabolism (Table 5-1).[1–4] Based on the higher estimate of halothane metabolism, it is concluded that elimination of this drug after discontinuation of its administration is equally via ventilation of the lungs and metabolism.[1]

Oxidative and reductive pathways for metabolism are present, but halothane preferentially undergoes oxidative metabolism. This is fortunate since oxidative metabolites are not likely to be toxic, but metabolites formed during reductive metabolism of halothane may produce hepatotoxicity (see the section *Halothane-Associated Hepatic Dysfunction*).

Oxidative Metabolism

The major metabolite of oxidative metabolism of halothane is trifluoroacetic acid, which is excreted in the urine. Trifluoroacetic acid has no known

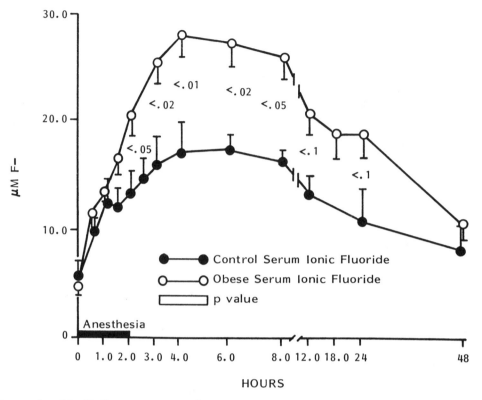

Fig. 5-2. Serum fluoride (F^{-1}) concentrations during and following 2 hours of enflurane administration to obese (127 kg) and nonobese (67 kg) patients. Mean ± SE. (From Bentley et al.,[7] with permission.)

adverse effects, perhaps reflecting the highly ionized characteristic of this metabolite, which limits its ability to cross lipid membranes and gain access to intracellular structures. Other oxidative metabolites that appear in the urine are chloride and bromide. Based on measurements in patients, serum bromide concentrations will increase approximately 0.5 $mEq \cdot L^{-1} \cdot MAC\, hr^{-1}$ of halothane administration (Fig. 5-3).[8] Since signs of bromide toxicity (somnolence, mental confusion) do not occur until serum bromide concentrations exceed 6 $mEq \cdot L^{-1}$, the likelihood of symptoms due to accumulation of bromide from metabolism of halothane is remote. Trifluoroethanol and trifluoroacetaldehyde, although it is theoretically possible, have not been detected as a result of the metabolism of halothane.

Reductive Metabolism

Reductive metabolism of halothane is most likely to occur in the presence of inadequate oxygen delivery to hepatocytes and stimulation of hepatic microsomal enzyme activity by drugs (phenobarbital) or exposure to chemicals (polychlorobiphenyls). Metabolism of halothane by reductive pathways results in the formation of reactive intermediary metabolites and fluoride. The presumed significance of formation of reactive intermediary metabolites is their potential to produce liver damage either by direct effects on hepatocytes or initiation of an immune-mediated hypersensitivity (allergic) reaction (see the section *Halothane-Associated Hepatic Dysfunction*). Acceptance of an hepatotoxic role of reductive intermediary metabo-

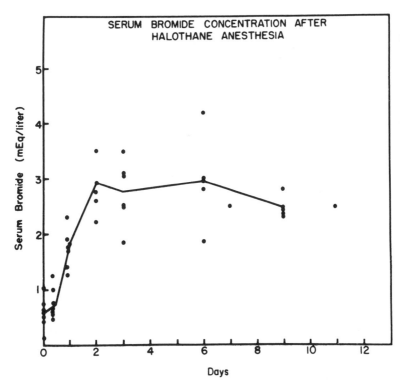

Fig. 5-3. Serum bromide concentrations were measured in seven healthy male volunteers following a prolonged exposure (about 7 hours) to halothane. Mean serum bromide concentration was 2.9 mEq·L^{-1} on the second day after anesthesia. Nine days after anesthesia, serum bromide was still elevated to 2.5 mEq·L^{-1}. Individual values peaked on the second day to sixth day with the highest concentration being 4.2 mEq·L^{-1}. (From Johnstone et al.,[8] with permission.)

lites of halothane, however, is challenged by occurrence of similar hepatic damage in the hypoxic rat model after administration of other anesthetics that either do not undergo significant metabolism or undergo metabolism by pathways other than reductive routes (Fig. 5-4).[9,10]

An increase in the serum concentration of fluoride after the administration of halothane implies that reductive metabolism and the formation of potentially hepatotoxic reactive intermediary metabolites has occurred. Serum fluoride concentrations increase after the administration of halothane to obese but not to nonobese patients. Evidence of liver dysfunction, however, based on measurements of serum glutamic transaminase concentrations in these obese patients does not occur. Like-

wise, peak serum fluoride concentrations (about 10 µM·L^{-1}) are far below the 50 µM·L^{-1} concentration likely to be associated with renal dysfunction (see the section *Fluoride-Induced Nephrotoxicity*).

ENFLURANE METABOLISM

Enflurane undergoes minimal oxidative metabolism in humans with an estimated 2.4 percent to 8.5 percent of the absorbed drug undergoing metabolism (Table 5-1).[1-4] This degree of metabolism is not sufficient to influence elimination of this drug after discontinuation of its administration. Therefore, elimination of enflurane is primarily by ventilation of the lungs.[1]

The most important metabolite of enflurane

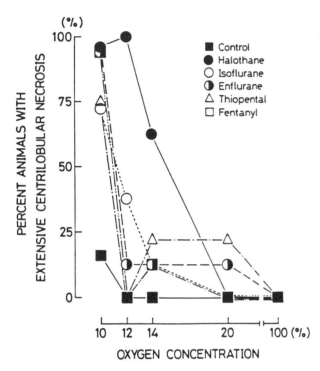

Fig. 5-4. Extensive centrilobular necrosis is present in the hypoxic rat model following administration of inhaled or injected drugs when the inhaled concentration of oxygen is 10 percent. (From Shingu et al.,[10] with permission.)

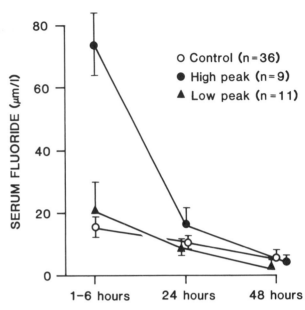

Fig. 5-5. Serum fluoride concentrations were measured in 36 control patients taking no drugs and 20 patients treated with 300 mg of isoniazid daily for periods of up to 1 year. Anesthesia was maintained in all patients using enflurane with or without nitrous oxide. Nine isoniazid-treated patients (high dose peak) had serum fluoride concentrations significantly higher ($P < 0.001$) than either the 11 other isoniazid-treated patients (low peaks) or the control patients. These high peak serum fluoride concentrations occurred 1 hour to 6 hours after anesthesia. It is speculated that isoniazid resulted in enzyme induction and accelerated defluorination in these nine patients, presumably reflecting a genetically determined ability for rapid acetylation. (Data from Mazze et al.[11])

metabolism is fluoride, which originates from the terminal carbon atom (Table 5-2).[1–4] Oxidation of the ether bond and release of additional fluorine atoms does not occur, reflecting the stability imparted to this bond by the surrounding halogens. In addition to this chemical stability, the low blood and lipid solubility of enflurane facilitates its removal by ventilation of the lungs before significant hepatic metabolism can occur.

Enzyme induction with phenobarbital does not increase the defluorination of enflurane. Conversely, defluorination of enflurane is increased in patients being treated chronically with isoniazid (Fig. 5-5).[11] Likewise, in vitro incubations of hepatic microsomes from rats pretreated with ethanol reveals increased defluorination of enflurane when compared with untreated rats. Excessive serum concentrations of fluoride from the metabolism of enflurane could result in renal dysfunc-

tion (see the section *Fluoride-Induced Nephrotoxicity*). Finally, serum fluoride concentrations are greater after administration of enflurane to obese as compared with nonobese patients (Fig. 5-2).[7] The incidence of renal dysfunction, however, has not been reported to be increased in obese patients after administration of enflurane.

ISOFLURANE METABOLISM

Isoflurane undergoes insignificant oxidative metabolism in humans with an estimated 0.17 percent of the absorbed drug undergoing metabolism

(Table 5-1).[1-4] Clearly, ventilation of the lungs is primarily responsible for elimination of isoflurane after discontinuation of its administration.[1]

Chemical stability of isoflurane is assured by the trifluorocarbon molecule and the presence of halogen atoms on three sides of the ether bond. Likewise, the low blood and lipid solubility of isoflurane favors its rapid elimination by ventilation of the lungs before significant metabolism can occur.

The primary pathway of isoflurane metabolism most likely begins with the oxidation of the ethyl alpha carbon atom, ultimately resulting in the formation of difluoromethanol and trifluoroacetic acid. Difluoromethanol is unstable, leading to the production of formic acid and the release of fluoride.

The resistance of isoflurane to metabolism is evidenced by the minimal increase in serum fluoride concentrations that accompany prolonged administration of this anesthetic (Table 5-2).[1-4] Enzyme induction with drugs, including isoniazid, does not significantly increase the metabolism of isoflurane to fluoride. The insignificant metabolism of isoflurane makes hepatic or renal toxicity after the administration of this drug unlikely.

METHOXYFLURANE METABOLISM

Methoxyflurane undergoes substantial oxidative metabolism in humans with an estimated 50 percent to 75 percent of the absorbed drug undergoing metabolism (Table 5-1).[1-4] Based on these estimates of metabolism, it is concluded that elimination of this drug after discontinuation of its administration is more dependent on metabolism than on ventilation of the lungs.[1]

Methoxyflurane can be dehalogenated at the dichloromethyl carbon atom or at the ether bond. The most significant metabolite of methoxyflurane is fluoride (Table 5-2).[1-4] Other metabolites are oxalic acid, dichloroacetic acid, and probably methoxydifluoroacetic acid. Methoxydifluoroacetic acid is labile and would be expected to break down in the acid environment of the kidneys to release oxalic acid and fluoride. Metabolism of methoxyflurane is increased by enzyme induction. As with enflurane, the serum fluoride concentrations are greater after administration of methoxyflurane to obese compared with nonobese patients. Serum fluoride concentrations are lower in pediatric patients compared with adults receiving methoxyflurane, presumably due to avid uptake of fluoride by metabolically active bone.

NITROUS OXIDE METABOLISM

Nitrous oxide undergoes almost imperceptible reductive metabolism (an estimated 0.004 percent of an absorbed dose) to nitrogen in the gastrointestinal tract (Table 5-1).[1-4] Anaerobic bacteria, such as *Pseudomonas*, are responsible for this reductive metabolism. The potential toxic effects, if any, of nitrous oxide metabolism remain undocumented. There is no evidence that nitrous oxide undergoes oxidative metabolism.

ORGAN TOXICITY DUE TO ANESTHETIC METABOLISM

Organ toxicity due to toxic metabolites of inhaled anesthetics may manifest postoperatively as halothane-associated hepatic dysfunction or fluoride-induced nephrotoxicity. In addition, adverse responses may occur in personnel who are chronically exposed to trace concentrations of inhaled anesthetics present in the operating room atmosphere.

Halothane-Associated Hepatic Dysfunction

The mechanism responsible for halothane-associated hepatic dysfunction is unknown. The most frequently invoked theories include metabolism of halothane to an hepatotoxic reactive intermediary metabolite or the occurrence of an allergic reaction. With respect to toxic metabolites, it is speculated that products of reductive metabolism can bind irreversibly (covalently) to intracellular constituents of hepatocytes and cause their destruction (i.e., an autoimmune hepatic necrosis) in susceptible patients.[12] Indeed, lymphocytes from patients with halothane hepatitis and their families are more sensitive to a standard test of toxicity, emphasizing the possible presence of a familial factor that predisposes these individuals to halothane-associated hepatic dysfunction.[13] Conversely, evidence of an allergic reaction as the cause of liver damage produced by halothane is the rarity of the response, the occurrence of eosinophilia, and accelerated liver dysfunction after a second or repeat exposure to halothane. It is possible that halothane or one of its metabolites alters the antigenicity of liver cell constituents, leading to the production of antibodies that initiate an allergic reaction with the liver as a target organ. Indeed, genetic factors could be important in determining the likelihood that patients will form antibodies or use reductive pathways of metabolism for halothane.

Hypoxia alone has been shown to produce a mild degree of hepatic dysfunction after administration of nitrous oxide, halothane, enflurane, or isoflurane (Fig. 5-4).[9,10] These observations suggest liver damage previously attributed to reductive metabolism of halothane may have been caused by arterial hypoxemia. Indeed, it has been proposed that halothane-associated hepatic dysfunction is two entities.[14] One entity is a mild and transient form of hepatic dysfunction unrelated to the anesthetic but rather reflects unrecognized hepatocyte hypoxia during or after anesthesia. This unrecognized hypoxia may directly damage hepatocytes and/or favor the production of reductive metabolites that are toxic to the liver. Perhaps, reductions in hepatic blood flow during anesthesia and surgery contribute to inadequate delivery of oxygen to hepatocytes, regardless of the drug used for anesthesia. The other, rarer but fulminant variety of halothane-associated hepatic dysfunction is speculated to be due to an allergic reaction.

Diagnosis of liver dysfunction due to halothane depends on the elimination of other possible causes (hepatocyte hypoxia, hypotension, sepsis, viral infections, cholestasis, bilirubin overload, nonanesthetic hepatotoxic drugs, co-existing liver disease) as likely explanations. Undoubtedly, halothane has been wrongfully incriminated in the past as a cause for hepatic dysfunction when more detailed investigations would have exonerated the anesthetic. Nevertheless, most cases of alleged halothane-associated hepatic dysfunction have occurred in middle-aged obese women, especially with repeat administration of halothane within 4 weeks of a previous halothane anesthetic. An unexplained postoperative fever is often present. Laboratory measurements in these patients suggest hepatocellular damage (markedly elevated serum transaminase enzyme concentrations) and eosinophilia may be present. Finally, pediatric patients seem less likely than adults to experience halothane-associated hepatic dysfunction even with reexposure to the drug at short intervals.

Fluoride-Induced Nephrotoxicity

Metabolism of methoxyflurane, and to a lesser extent enflurane, to fluoride may result in nephrotoxicity. Fluoride-induced nephrotoxicity is characterized by an inability to concentrate urine. The resulting polyuria leads to dehydration with hypernatremia and increased serum osmolarity. Inability to concentrate urine may reflect fluoride-induced inhibition of adenylate cyclase activity necessary for the normal action of antidiuretic hormone on distal convoluted renal tubules. Alternatively, fluoride may produce intrarenal vasodilation with increased medullary blood flow, which interferes with the countercurrent mechanism in the kidneys necessary for optimal concentration of urine.

Detectable renal dysfunction is likely when the administered dose of methoxyflurane results in serum fluoride concentrations that exceed 50 $\mu M \cdot L^{-1}$.[15] This level of fluoride elevation is likely when the duration of methoxyflurane administration to adult patients exceeds 2.5 MAC hours (Table 5-2).[1-4] The nephrotoxic potential of methoxyflurane has led to the almost total abandonment of the use of this drug to produce general anesthesia.

Metabolism of enflurane to fluoride, although much less than with methoxyflurane, is potentially great enough to produce transient decreases in urine concentrating ability, particularly after prolonged administration (1 MAC for 9.6 hours).[13] Nevertheless, short administration (1 MAC for 2.7 hours) does not reveal a difference between enflurane or halothane with respect to urine concentrating ability. Indeed, the likelihood of fluoride-induced nephrotoxicity due to metabolism of enflurane seems remote since serum concentrations of fluoride after clinical use of this drug are about one-half the speculated toxic level of 50 $\mu M \cdot L^{-1}$ (Table 5-2).[1-4] Nevertheless, the administration of enflurane to patients with known renal disease or undergoing operations likely to be associated with renal dysfunction is controversial. This controversy is based on the realization that elimination of fluoride depends on glomerular filtration rate. Therefore, it is likely that patients with decreased glomerular filtration rates will maintain elevated circulating levels of fluoride for longer periods of time than normal patients. Fluoride-induced nephrotoxicity depends on the duration of the exposure of the renal tubules to fluoride, as well as on the absolute increase of the serum fluoride concentration. As a result, it is possible that patients with decreased glomerular filtration rates are at an increased risk in the presence of fluoride concentrations usually considered to be nontoxic (i.e., below 50 $\mu M \cdot L^{-1}$). Nevertheless, there is no detectable reduction in renal function in patients with chronic renal disease who undergo elective operations and receive enflurane or halothane.[16]

Trace Concentrations of Inhaled Anesthetics

Approximately 225,000 operating room personnel are chronically exposed to trace concentrations of inhaled anesthetics. This is of concern since the mutagenicity, teratogenicity, and carcinogenicity of chemicals (including anesthetics) probably results from direct alteration of chromosomal proteins (DNA) by these substances. Reactive intermediary metabolites, and not the relatively stable parent molecule, are most likely to attack (adduct to) chromosomal proteins. Depending on the point in life at which adduction occurs, the result may be fetal death and spontaneous abortion, a birth defect, or cancer.

Synthesis of chromosomal protein may be inhibited by nitrous oxide-induced inactivation of the vitamin B_{12} dependent enzymes methionine synthetase and thymidylate synthetase (Fig. 5-6).[17] Nitrous oxide produces this inactivation by irreversibly oxidizing the cobalt atom of vitamin B_{12}. Animals seem more sensitive to this effect of nitrous oxide than humans. For example, patients inhaling 60 percent to 70 percent nitrous oxide for 4 hours do not show evidence of enzyme inhibition.[18] Nevertheless, anemia and polyneuropathy resembling pernicious anemia and bone marrow depression that can accompany prolonged exposure to nitrous oxide are consistent with drug-induced inactivation of these enzymes. Unlike ni-

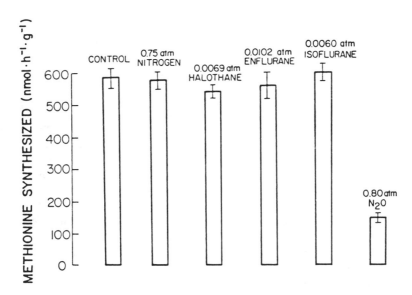

Fig. 5-6. Synthesis of methionine synthetase was reduced in the livers of mice exposed to nitrous oxide for 4 hours. Volatile anesthetics did not alter methionine synthetase activity. Mean ± SE. (From Koblin et al.,[17] with permission.)

trous oxide, volatile anesthetics do not inhibit methionine synthetase (Fig. 5-6).[17]

Mutagenicity

The Ames test is the most widely used in vitro test for determination of the mutagenic and carcinogenic potential of chemicals. Nitrous oxide, halothane, enflurane, and isoflurane give negative Ames test results, suggesting that the mutagenic and thus carcinogenic potential of these inhaled anesthetics are low if not nonexistent. Nevertheless, potential metabolites of halothane may give a positive Ames test. In addition, inhaled anesthetics containing vinyl groups (divinyl ether, fluroxene) give a positive Ames test. Therefore, these drugs and any new drugs with a vinyl moiety should be considered potential carcinogens.

Teratogenicity

Female operating room personnel have an increased incidence of spontaneous abortion (1.3 times to 2 times) compared with matched controls not working in the operating rooms.[19] Less well documented than the increased incidence of spontaneous abortion is an increased incidence of minor and major congenital malformations in the offspring of these anesthetic-exposed females. Even less well documented is an increased incidence of spontaneous abortion among spouses of anesthetic-exposed males. Furthermore, the role of stress or exposure to radiation have not been adequately evaluated as explanations for the increased incidence of spontaneous abortion among females working in operating rooms.

The cause of the increased incidence of spontaneous abortion or other adverse responses observed in operating room personnel is not known, but chronic exposure to trace concentrations of inhaled anesthetics, particularly nitrous oxide, has received much attention. Indeed, the rationale for scavenging systems is to reduce the trace concentrations of anesthetic gases in the operating room atmosphere and, it is hoped, reduce any toxic effects associated with chronic exposure to these gases (see Chapter 11). Nevertheless, data to support beneficial effects of scavenging are not available. Furthermore, animal studies employing intermittent exposure to trace concentrations of

nitrous oxide, halothane, enflurane, and isoflurane have not revealed harmful reproductive effects.[20]

Carcinogenicity

No study has demonstrated the existence of a cause and effect relationship between inhaled anesthetics and cancer. Nevertheless, there is an increase in cancer among female, but not male, operating room personnel. Additional data are needed before it can be concluded, however, that the incidence of cancer is truly increased in females chronically exposed to trace concentrations of anesthetics. As with spontaneous abortion, the possible role of stress and exposure to radiation associated with working in operating rooms will also have to be considered.

Gonadal Toxicity

Inhaled anesthetics and their metabolites may be directly toxic to the testes. Evidence for this toxicity is from animals who manifest injury to the seminiferous tubules and damage to spermatogenic cells after prolonged exposure to nitrous oxide.

RESISTANCE TO INFECTION

Inhaled anesthetics, particularly nitrous oxide, produce dose-dependent inhibition of mobilization of polymorphonuclear leukocytes and subsequent migration for phagocytosis that is necessary for the inflammatory response to infection. Nevertheless, the effects produced by these drugs are probably clinically insignificant, considering the usual duration of anesthesia and the dose used. Therefore, a decrease in the resistance to infection in the postoperative period due to persistent effects of inhaled anesthetics seems remote. Rather, the occurrence of postoperative infections seems more likely to be related to surgical trauma and associated release of cortisol and catecholamines that are known to inhibit phagocytosis.

Inhaled anesthetics do not have a bacteriostatic effect at clinically useful concentrations. Low concentrations (0.2 MAC) of volatile anesthetics inhibit replication of measles virus by 50 percent, whereas 0.5 MAC to 1 MAC greatly inhibits replication. Furthermore, volatile anesthetics have been shown to reduce mortality in mice receiving intranasal influenza virus during anesthesia.[21] These data suggest that if volatile anesthetics inhibit the body's immune defenses against infection, they may also directly inhibit growth of the infecting organism.

REFERENCES

1. Carpenter RL, Eger EI II, Johnson BH, Unadkat JD, Sheiner LB. The extent of metabolism of inhaled anesthetics in humans. Anesthesiology 1986;65:201–5.
2. Blitt CD, Gandolfi AJ, Soltis JJ, Brown BR. Extrahepatic biotransformation of halothane and enflurane. Anesth Analg 1981;60:129–32.
3. Hong K, Trudell JR, O'Neil JR, Cohen EN. Metabolism of nitrous oxide by human and rat intestinal contents. Anesthesiology 1980;52:16–9.
4. White AE, Stevens WC, Eger EI II, Mazze RI, Hitt BA. Enflurane and methoxyflurane metabolism at anesthetic and subanesthetic concentrations. Anesth Analg 1979;58:221–4.
5. Carpenter RL, Eger EI II, Johnson BH, Unadkat JD, Sheiner LB. Pharmacokinetics of inhaled anesthetics in humans: Measurements during and after the simultaneous administration of enflurane, halothane, isoflurane, methoxyflurane and nitrous oxide. Anesth Analg 1986;65:575–82.
6. Greene NM. Halothane anesthesia and hepatitis in a high risk population. N Engl J Med 1973;289:304–7.
7. Bentley JB, Vaughan RW, Miller MS, Calkins JM, Gandolfi AJ. Serum inorganic fluoride levels in obese patients during and after enflurane anesthesia. Anesth Analg 1979;58:409–12.
8. Johnstone RE, Kennell EM, Behar MG, Brummund W, Ebersole RC, Shaw LM. Increased serum bromide concentration after halothane anesthesia in man. Anesthesiology 1975;42:598–601.
9. Fassoulaki A, Eger EI II, Johnson BH, et al. Nitrous oxide, too, is hepatotoxic in rats. Anesth Analg 1984;63:1076–80.
10. Shingu K, Eger EI II, Johnson BH, VanDyke RA, Lurz FW, Cheng A. Effect of oxygen concentration, hyperthermia, and choice of vendor on anesthetic-induced hepatic injury in rats. Anesth Analg 1983;62:146–50.
11. Mazze RI, Woodruff RE, Heerdt ME. Isoniazid-induced enflurane defluorination in humans. Anesthesiology 1982;57:5–8.
12. Brown BR. Halothane hepatitis revisited. N Engl J Med 1985;313:1347–8.
13. Farrell G, Prendergast D, Murray M. Halothane hepatitis: Detection of a constitutional factor. N Engl J Med 1985;313:1310–4.
14. Pohl LR, Gillette JR. A perspective on halothane-induced hepatotoxicity (editorial). Anesth Analg 1982;61:809–11.
15. Cousins MJ, Greenstein LR, Hitt BA, Mazze RI. Metabolism and renal effects of enflurane in man. Anesthesiology 1976;44:44–53.
16. Mazze RI, Sievenpiper TS, Stevenson J. Renal effects of enflurane and halothane in patients with abnormal renal function. Anesthesiology 1984;60:161–3.
17. Koblin DD, Watson JE, Deady JE, Stokstad ELR, Eger EI II. Inactivation of methionine synthetase by nitrous oxide in mice. Anesthesiology 1981;54:318–24.
18. Nunn JF, Sharer NM, Bottiglieri T, Rossiter J. Effect of short-term administration of nitrous oxide on plasma concentrations of methionine, tryptophan, phenylalanine and S-adenosyl methionine in man. Br J Anaesth 1986;58:1–10.
19. American Society of Anesthesiologists. Report of an ad hoc committee on the effect of trace anesthetics on the health of operating room personnel. Occupational disease among operating room personnel. A national study. Anesthesiology 1974;41:321–40.
20. Mazze RI, Fujinaga M, Rice SA, Harris SB, Baden JM. Reproductive and teratogenic effects of nitrous oxide, halothane, isoflurane, and enflurane in Sprague-Dawley rats. Anesthesiology 1986;64:339–44.
21. Knight PR, Bedows E, Nahrwold ML, Maassab HF, Smitka CW, Busch MT. Alterations in influenza virus pulmonary pathology induced by diethyl ether, halothane, enflurane and pentobarbital in mice. Anesthesiology 1983;58:209–15.

Chapter 6

Intravenous Anesthetics

Drugs classified as intravenous anesthetics are most often used to produce induction of anesthesia. Usually, combined with inhaled anesthetics, these drugs may also be used for maintenance of anesthesia, either by intermittent bolus or constant intravenous infusion. Examples of intravenous anesthetics are barbiturates, benzodiazepines, opioids, and miscellaneous drugs such as ketamine, etomidate, and propofol.

BARBITURATES

Historically, barbiturates have been classified as long-acting, intermediate-acting, short-acting, and ultrashort-acting. This classification is no longer recommended as it incorrectly implies the action of these drugs ends predictably after specified time intervals. This is not true as drug effects persist for several hours even after administration of thiopental, thiamylal, or methohexital (ultrashort-acting barbiturates) for induction of anesthesia. Thiopental is the most commonly used barbiturate and the drug against which all other drugs used for induction of anesthesia are compared.

General Pharmacology

Structure Activity Relationships

Barbiturates result from substitution at the number 2 and number 5 carbon atoms of barbituric acid (Fig. 6-1). Oxybarbiturates retain an oxygen atom on the number 5 carbon, whereas replacement of this atom with a sulfur atom results in more lipid soluble thiobarbiturates. Increased lipid solubility contributes to a more rapid onset and shorter duration of action. For example, thiopental and thiamylal have a more rapid onset and shorter duration of action than their less lipid soluble oxybarbiturate analogs, pentobarbital and secobarbital. Addition of a methyl group to the nitrogen atom of the barbituric acid ring results in a short duration of action as produced by methohexital.

Mechanism of Action

Barbiturates probably have numerous sites of action in the central nervous system. For example, these drugs depress polysynaptic responses perhaps by decreasing release of neurotransmitters such as acetylcholine. Barbiturates may decrease the rate of dissociation of the inhibitory neurotransmitter gamma-aminobutyric acid (GABA) from ion channels, resulting in hyperpolarization and inhibition of postsynaptic neurons. Transmission of impulses through sympathetic nervous system ganglia is depressed by concentrations of barbiturates that have no detectable effect on nerve conduction. Barbiturates seem uniquely capable of depressing the reticular activating system, which functions to maintain wakefulness. There is no

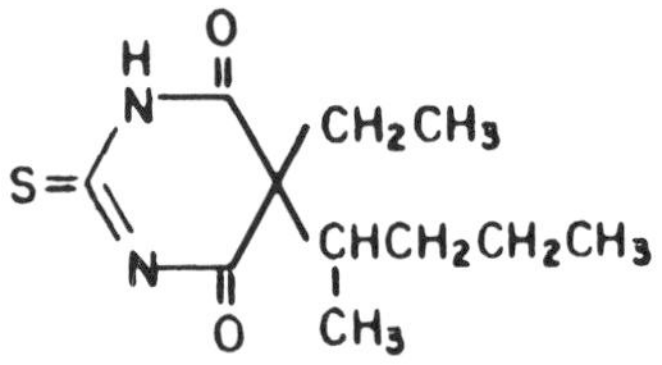

Fig. 6-1. Chemical structures of barbiturates administered intravenously most often for induction of anesthesia.

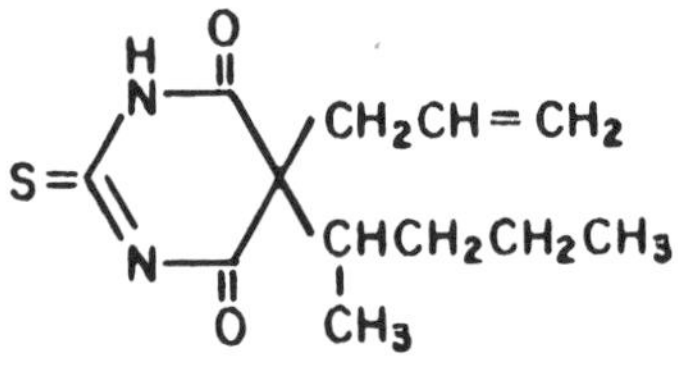

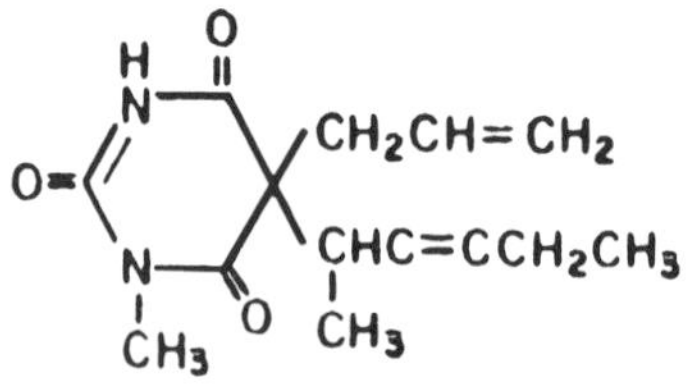

specific pharmacologic antagonist for barbiturate effects on the central nervous system.

Cardiovascular System

Administration of barbiturates to produce induction of anesthesia typically produces modest reductions in blood pressure (10 mmHg to 20 mmHg) that are transient due to compensatory baroreceptor mediated increases in heart rate (Fig. 6-2).[1] This blood pressure reduction is principally due to peripheral vasodilation, reflecting barbiturate induced depression of the medullary vasomotor center and decreased sympathetic nervous system outflow from the central nervous system. Resulting dilation of peripheral capacitance vessels leads to pooling of blood, decreased venous return, and the potential for decreases in cardiac output and blood pressure. Indeed, hypovolemic patients, who are less able to compensate for peripheral vasodilating effects, are likely to experience exaggerated reductions in blood pressure when barbiturates are injected rapidly intravenously for the induction of anesthesia. Patients treated with beta antagonists or centrally-acting antihypertensives that inhibit compensatory baroreceptor reflex responses could also be at increased risk to experience exaggerated decreases in blood pressure after intravenous administration of barbiturates. Negative inotropic effects of barbiturates, which are readily demonstrated using isolated heart preparations, are obscured in vivo by baroreceptor mediated reflex responses.

Ventilation

Barbiturates depress medullary ventilatory centers as reflected by decreased responsiveness to ventilatory stimulant effects of carbon dioxide. Induction of anesthesia with barbiturates is likely to produce transient apnea requiring temporary controlled ventilation of the lungs. Apnea is particularly likely to occur when depressant drugs have been included in the preoperative medication. Resumption of spontaneous breathing after induction doses of barbiturates is characterized by a slow rate of breathing and a reduced tidal volume. Laryngeal reflexes and cough reflexes are not greatly depressed by induction doses of barbiturates. Indeed, stimulation of the upper airway or trachea (secretions, laryngoscopy, intubation of the trachea) in the presence of inadequate depression of airway reflexes by barbiturates may result in laryngospasm or bronchospasm. This response

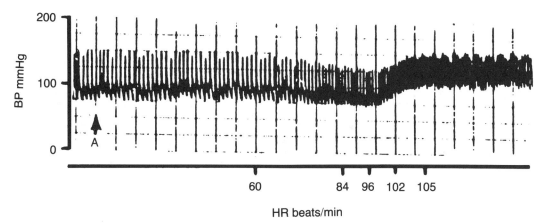

Fig. 6-2. In normovolemic patients the intravenous administration of thiopental (A) is followed by a modest decline in blood pressure which is subsequently offset by a compensatory increase in heart rate (HR). (From Filner and Karliner,[1] with permission.)

should not be interpreted as unique to barbiturates but rather as an example of an adverse response to stimulation in the presence of inadequate drug-induced suppression of airway reflexes.

Central Nervous System

Barbiturates are potent cerebral vasoconstrictors producing predictable reductions in cerebral blood flow, cerebral blood volume, and intracranial pressure. Cerebral metabolic oxygen requirements ($CMRO_2$) are reduced maximally when the electroencephalogram (EEG) is rendered isoelectric. The ability of barbiturates to decrease intracranial pressure and $CMRO_2$ makes these drugs useful selections in the management of anesthesia for patients with space occupying intracranial lesions (see Chapter 24). An exception to the generalization that barbiturates reduce electrical activity on the EEG is methohexital, which activates epileptic foci, making their identification easier during surgery designed to ablate these sites. Barbiturates may provide protection of the brain from adverse effects produced by regional cerebral ischemia but not global cerebral ischemia, which is likely to accompany cardiac arrest (see Chapter 34).

Pharmacokinetics

Maximal brain uptake of barbiturates occurs wthin 30 seconds after their intravenous administration, accounting for the rapid induction of anesthesia (one to two circulation times) produced by these drugs. Prompt awakening following intravenous administration of thiopental, thiamylal, and methohexital reflects redistribution of these drugs from the brain to inactive tissues, especially skeletal muscles and fat. Ultimately, however, elimination of barbiturates from the body depends almost entirely on metabolism because less than 1 percent of these drugs are cleared unchanged by the kidneys. Large or repeated doses of lipid soluble barbiturates may saturate inactive tissue sites, resulting in prolonged effects of these usually short-acting drugs. The elimination half-time of methohexital is less than thiopental, reflecting the greater hepatic metabolism of methohexital (Table 6-1).[2] These characteristics of methohexital should result in more rapid awakening than after administration of thiopental, especially if repeated doses of barbiturates are injected. For this reason methohexital is sometimes recommended for outpa-

Table 6-1. Pharmacokinetics of Barbiturates

	Thiopental	Methohexital
Elimination half-time (hours)	11.6	3.9[a]
Clearance (ml·kg^{-1}·min^{-1})	3.4	10.9[a]
Volume of distribution (L·kg^{-1})	2.5	2.2

[a] Significantly different from thiopental.
(Data from Hudson et al.[2])

tient procedures when rapid awakening is especially important.

Clinical Uses

Barbiturates are used most often for induction of anesthesia and occasionally to aid in the maintenance of anesthesia in combination with other inhaled drugs. When used for induction of anesthesia, thiopental or thiamylal 3 mg·kg^{-1} to 5 mg·kg^{-1} or methohexital 1 mg·kg^{-1} to 1.5 mg·kg^{-1} is injected rapidly intravenously followed by succinylcholine or nondepolarizing muscle relaxants to produce skeletal muscle paralysis and facilitate subsequent intubation of the trachea. This approach is referred to as *rapid sequence* induction of anesthesia. An important advantage of rapid sequence induction of anesthesia is early endotracheal intubation to provide protection against inhalation of gastric fluid. Although rapid sequence induction of anesthesia is pleasant for the patient, it has associated hazards. For example, if the trachea cannot be immediately intubated, the paralyzed patient will be totally dependent on the anesthesiologist for adequate ventilation of the lungs. The need for prolonged manual ventilation of the lungs may increase the likelihood of inflating the patient's stomach with gas and associated hazards of regurgitation and aspiration.

An alternative approach to rapid sequence induction of anesthesia is administration of small doses of barbiturates (thiopental 0.5 mg·kg^{-1} to 1 mg·kg^{-1}) followed by application of the anesthesia mask to the patient's face and delivery of inhaled anesthetics to complete the induction of anesthesia. The low dose of barbiturate improves patient acceptance of the anesthesia mask and the pungent volatile anesthetics, especially enflurane and isoflurane. This slow induction of anesthesia is not a likely selection for patients with a history of recent food ingestion who are considered to be at risk for aspiration of gastric contents.

After induction of anesthesia, maintenance is with inhaled or injected drugs (opioids, benzodiazepines). For short surgical procedures not requiring skeletal muscle relaxation (dilation and curettage or breast biopsy) repeated injections of small doses of barbiturates combined with nitrous oxide may be used for maintenance of anesthesia.

Signs of light anesthesia (hypertension, tachycardia, diaphoresis, skeletal muscle movement) are used as indications for the need to administer additional doses of barbiturate.

Venous thrombosis following intravenous administration of barbiturates for induction of anesthesia presumably reflects deposition of barbiturate crystals (pH of blood too low to keep alkaline barbiturates in solution—thiopental pH 10.5) in veins. Accidental intra-arterial injection of barbiturates results in excruciating pain and intense vasoconstriction, often leading to gangrene despite aggressive therapy, including sympathetic nervous system blockade (stellate ganglion block) of the involved extremity. It is likely that barbiturate crystal formation results in occlusion of more distal small diameter arteries and arterioles. Barbiturate crystal formation in veins is less hazardous because of the ever increasing diameter of veins. Accidental subcutaneous injection (extravasation) of barbiturates results in local tissue irritation, emphasizing the importance of using dilute concentrations (thiopental and thiamylal 2.5 percent, methohexital 1.0 percent) of barbiturates. If extravasation occurs some recommend local injection of 5 ml to 10 ml to 0.5 percent lidocaine in an attempt to dilute the barbiturate concentration. Life-threatening allergic reactions are a rare (estimated 1 in 30,000 patients) risk of induction of anesthesia with barbiturates.

BENZODIAZEPINES

Benzodiazepines commonly used in the perioperative period include diazepam, lorazepam, and midazolam (Fig. 6-3). In addition to their hypnotic effects, favorable pharmacologic characteristics of benzodiazepines include (1) production of amnesia, (2) minimal depression of circulation, and (3) specific sites of action as anticonvulsants.

General Pharmacology

The hypnotic effect of benzodiazepines is likely to be related to GABA accumulation and occupation of specific receptors.[3] Benzodiazepines facilitate inhibitory actions of GABA on nerve conduction by acting on receptors that occur almost exclusively on postsynaptic nerve endings in the central ner-

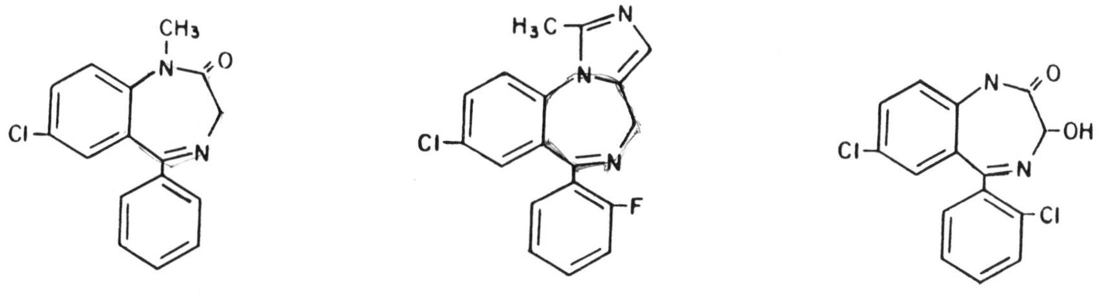

Fig. 6-3. Chemical structures of benzodiazepines commonly administered in the perioperative period.

vous system, especially the cerebral cortex.[4] Consistent with its greater potency, midazolam has an affinity for these receptors that is approximately twice that of diazepam.[5] Central nervous system effects of benzodiazepines are antagonized by a specific antagonist (flumazenil). Anticholinesterases, such as physostigmine, are both nonspecific and inconsistent antagonists of benzodiazepine effects. The incidence and magnitude of depression of ventilation and production of hypotension produced by benzodiazepines seem to be less than that associated with barbiturates as used for induction of anesthesia. Benzodiazepines, like barbiturates, reduce cerebral blood flow and $CMRO_2$.

Pharmacokinetics

Benzodiazepines are highly lipid-soluble drugs resulting in rapid entrance into the central nervous system followed by redistribution to inactive tissue sites. Diazepam undergoes hepatic metabolism to active metabolites (desmethyldiazepam and oxazepam) that may contribute to prolonged effects of this drug. In contrast, metabolites of midazolam seem to possess little or no pharmacologic activity. The elimination half-time of diazepam greatly exceeds that of midazolam, emphasizing the likely prolonged central nervous system effects of diazepam compared with midazolam (Table 6-2).

Clinical Uses

Benzodiazepines are used for (1) preoperative medication, (2) intravenous sedation, (3) induction of anesthesia, (4) maintenance of anesthesia, and (5) suppression of seizure activity. Amnesic, calming, and sedative effects of benzodiazepines are the basis for the use of these drugs in preoperative medication (see Chapter 10). Diazepam (5 mg to 10 mg) or midazolam (1 mg to 2.5 mg) administered intravenously are useful for sedation during regional anesthesia. Midazolam produces a more rapid onset and greater degree of amnesia than

Table 6-2. Pharmacokinetics of Benzodiazepines

	Elimination Half-time (hours)	Clearance ($ml \cdot kg^{-1} \cdot min^{-1}$)	Volume of Distribution ($L \cdot kg^{-1}$)
Diazepam	21–37	0.2–0.5	1–1.5
Midazolam	1–4	6–8	1–1.5
Lorazepam	10–20	0.7–1	0.8–1.3

diazepam when administered for intravenous sedation. Induction of anesthesia can be produced by the intravenous administration of diazepam (0.2 mg·kg^{-1} to 0.3 mg·kg^{-1}) or midazolam (0.1 mg·kg^{-1} to 0.2 mg·kg^{-1}). Induction of anesthesia is more rapid after administration of midazolam (about 80 seconds) than it is after that of diazepam but it is still slower than after administration of barbiturates (about 30 seconds).[6] Prior administration of opioids, as in the preoperative medication or intravenously immediately before injection of benzodiazepines, may facilitate the speed of induction of anesthesia produced by these drugs. Despite the possible production of lesser circulatory effects, it is unlikely that benzodiazepines offer any advantages over barbiturates as used for rapid sequence induction of anesthesia. Delayed awakening is a potential disadvantage of administering benzodiazepines for the induction of anesthesia. The efficacy of benzodiazepines as anticonvulsants, especially diazepam, is consistent with the ability of these drugs to enhance the inhibitory effects of GABA, especially in the limbic system. Indeed, diazepam, 0.1 mg·kg^{-1}, administered intravenously, is effective in abolishing seizure activity produced by local anesthetics, alcohol withdrawal, and status epilepticus.

Pain during intravenous injection of diazepam and subsequent thrombophlebitis reflect the poor water solubility of this benzodiazepine. It is the organic solvent, propylene glycol, required to dissolve diazepam that is most likely responsible for venoirritation, as well as unpredictable absorption after intramuscular injection. Midazolam is water soluble, obviating the need for an organic solvent and reducing the likelihood of exaggerated pain or erratic absorption after intramuscular injection or venoirritation during or following intravenous administration. Exposure of midazolam to blood pH causes a change in structure converting this drug to a highly lipid soluble substance capable of crossing the blood-brain barrier to gain access to the central nervous system. The slow onset and prolonged duration of action of lorazepam limits its usefulness for preoperative medication or induction of anesthesia, especially when rapid awakening at the end of surgery is desirable.

OPIOIDS

Opioids include all exogenous substances that bind specifically to opioid receptors and produce at least some agonist responses. Although several opioids are available, those most often used in the perioperative period are morphine and meperidine for preoperative medication and fentanyl, sufentanil, and alfentanil for induction of anesthesia and/or maintenance of anesthesia (Fig. 6-4). All opioids have a role in production of analgesia either before or after surgery. Morphine is the opioid to which all other opioids are compared.

General Pharmacology

Mechanism of Action

Opioids act as agonists at opioid receptors in the central nervous system and other tissues (Table 6-3). Analgesia is mediated through a complex interaction of mu, delta, and kappa receptors. Supraspinally, mu receptors are more important, whereas delta and kappa receptors are involved at the spinal level.[7] These same opioid receptors are normally activated by endogenous ligands known as endorphins. The affinity of most opioid agonists for receptors parallels their analgesic potency. Binding of opioids to specific receptors results in inhibition of adenylate cyclase activity, as well as interference with calcium ion transport and release of neurotransmitters including acetylcholine, norepinephrine, and substance P.

Table 6-3. Opioid Receptors and Response to Stimulation

Receptor	Response Evoked by Agonists
Mu-1	Supraspinal analgesia
Mu-2	Depression of ventilation
	Most cardiovascular effects
	Physical dependence
	Euphoria
Delta	Modulation of mu receptor activity
Kappa	Spinal analgesia
	Sedation
	Miosis
Sigma	Dysphoria
	Hypertonia

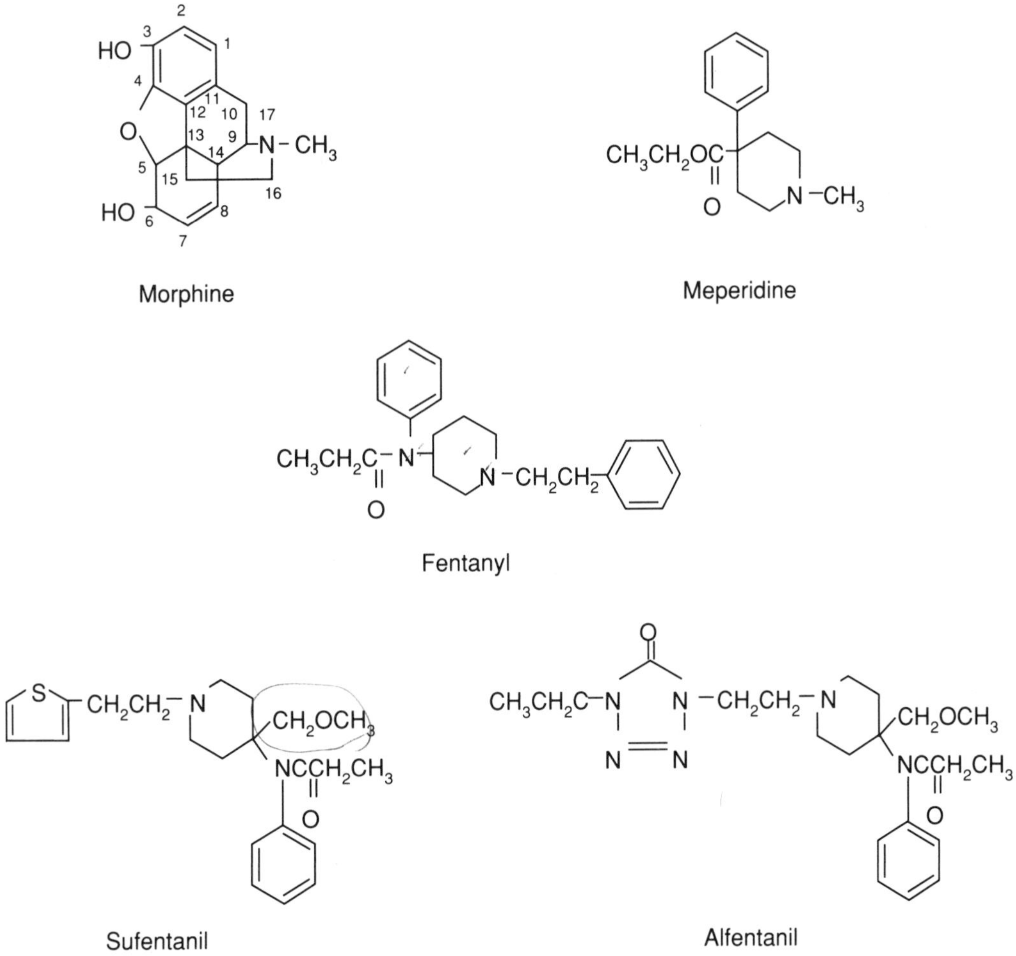

Fig. 6-4. Chemical structures of opioid agonists commonly administered in the perioperative period.

Cardiovascular Effects

Administration of even large doses of opioids to supine normovolemic patients is unlikely to cause significant changes in myocardial contractility (exception meperidine) or reductions in blood pressure. Orthostatic hypotension may be prominent when patients change from the supine position or hypovolemia is present, reflecting the ability of opioids to reduce sympathetic nervous system tone to peripheral veins. Morphine, but not fentanyl, sufentanil, or alfentanil, can evoke release of histamine, especially when high doses are administered (Fig. 6-5).[8] Bradycardia often accompanies opioid administration (exception meperidine), pre-

sumably reflecting stimulation of the vagal nucleus in the medulla. Heart rate slowing is particularly prominent after the administration of sufentanil. Opioids do not sensitize the heart to cardiac dysrhythmic effects of catecholamines.

Ventilation

Opioids produce rapid and sustained dose-dependent depression of ventilation characterized by elevations in the resting $PaCO_2$ and decreased responsiveness to the ventilatory stimulant effects of carbon dioxide (CO_2 response curve shifted to the right). Depression of ventilation reflects effects of opioids on medullary ventilatory centers, which may include decreased release of the neurotrans-

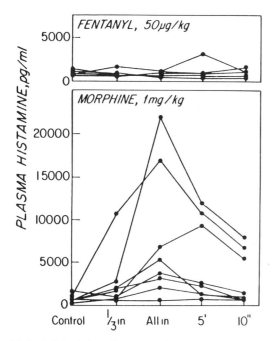

Fig. 6-5. Individual data for arterial concentrations of histamine before and after intravenous administration of large doses of fentanyl or morphine. (From Rosow et al.,[8] with permission.)

mitter, acetylcholine. Frequency of breathing is decreased while tidal volume is often increased as an incomplete compensatory response. Death due to opioids is almost invariably the result of depression of ventilation. Hypoventilation and arterial hypoxemia can also result from opioid-induced spasm of thoracoabdominal muscles (see the section *Skeletal and Smooth Muscle*).[9]

Central Nervous System

Opioids even in high doses do not reliably produce unconsciousness, especially in young patients, emphasizing that these drugs cannot be considered true anesthetics. In the absence of hypoventilation, opioids act as cerebral vasoconstrictors producing reductions in cerebral blood flow and intracranial pressure. Miosis is a central nervous system effect of opioids. Stimulation of the chemoreceptor trigger zone by opioids may cause nausea and vomiting.

Skeletal and Smooth Muscle

High doses of opioids may cause spasm of the thoracoabdominal muscles ("stiff-chest" syndrome) resulting in hypoventilation.[9] This skeletal muscle rigidity commonly occurs during induction of anesthesia, interfering with positive pressure ventilation of the lungs before tracheal intubation. Opioid-induced skeletal muscle rigidity can be terminated by administration of a muscle relaxant or an opioid antagonist such as naloxone. Opioids can cause spasm of biliary smooth muscle, resulting in increases in intrabiliary pressure that produce epigastric distress or mimic the presence of a common duct stone during performance of intravenous cholangiography. This effect on biliary smooth muscle detracts from the use of opioids in patients undergoing cholecystectomies. Opioid-induced enhancement of bladder sphincter tone may make spontaneous urination difficult.

Pharmacokinetics

Clearance of opioids is principally by hepatic metabolism, but large differences in lipid solubility account for greatly different elimination half-times between these drugs (Table 6-4). Typically, metabolites of opioids possess greatly reduced pharmacologic activity.

A single dose of fentanyl administered intravenously has a more rapid onset and shorter duration of action than morphine. This reflects fentanyl's greater lipid solubility that facilitates entrance into the central nervous system followed by prompt redistribution to inactive tissue sites, such as skeletal muscles and fat. High doses of fentanyl or continuous infusions of fentanyl lead to progressive saturation of these inactive tissue sites. As a result, plasma concentrations of fentanyl do not decline promptly, and pharmacologic effects, including depression of ventilation, are prolonged. Indeed, persistent or recurrent depression of ventilation owing to lingering effects of fentanyl (presumably other opioids too) is a potential postoperative problem[10] (see Chapter 30).

Sufentanil and alfentanil are synthetic derivatives of fentanyl. A greater affinity for opioid receptors accounts for the increased potency of

Table 6-4. Pharmacokinetics of Opioids

	Equivalent Potency	Elimination Half-time (minutes)	Clearance $(ml \cdot kg^{-1} \cdot min^{-1})$	Volume of Distribution $(L \cdot kg^{-1})$
Morphine	1	114	14.7	3.2
Meperidine	$\frac{1}{10}$ as morphine	180–264	15.1	3.8
Fentanyl	75 to 125 times morphine	185–219	11.6	4.1
Sufentanil	5 to 10 times fentanyl	148–164	12.7	1.7
Alfentanil	$\frac{1}{5}$ to $\frac{1}{10}$ as fentanyl	70–98	6.4	0.86

sufentanil (Table 6-4). Like fentanyl, the high lipid solubility of sufentanil contributes to its prompt onset and subsequent redistribution to inactive tissue sites, as well as to the potential for cumulative effects. Alfentanil has the most rapid onset of all the listed opioids reflecting its high degree of nonionization at physiologic pH. This facilitates the passage of alfentanil into the central nervous system and more than offsets the impact of its lower lipid solubility. Unlike other opioids, continuous infusions of alfentanil do not seem to produce cumulative drug effects, and postoperative awakening is prompt (rapid dissociation from opioid receptors) with minimal lingering side effects such as depression of ventilation.[11]

Clinical Uses

Clinical uses of opioids are numerous including (1) provision of analgesia before or after surgery, (2) induction of anesthesia and maintenance of anesthesia especially in patients with severe cardiac dysfunction, (3) inhibition of reflex sympathetic nervous system activity, and (4) supplementation of inhaled anesthetics being used for maintenance of anesthesia.

Postoperative pain relief for prolonged periods (12 hours to 24 hours) may be produced by injection of low doses of opioids (most often morphine) into the subarachnoid or epidural space. Pain relief provided in this manner reflects attachment of opioids to specific receptors in the dorsal horn of the spinal cord in the substantia gelatinosa. Delayed depression of ventilation (6 hours or more after injection) most likely reflects cephalad spread of opioids to medullary ventilatory centers in the area of the fourth ventricle.

High doses of fentanyl (50 $\mu g \cdot kg^{-1}$ to 150 $\mu g \cdot kg^{-1}$) or equivalent doses of sufentanil may be used as the sole anesthetic in patients who would not tolerate even modest direct cardiac depression produced by inhaled anesthetics. More often, however, opioids are administered in lower doses during maintenance of anesthesia as intermittent injections or as continuous infusions to supplement inhaled anesthetics. Alfentanil may be particularly useful for both, producing induction of anesthesia (150 $\mu g \cdot kg^{-1}$ to 300 $\mu g \cdot kg^{-1}$ produces unconsciousness in about 45 seconds) and providing for anesthetic maintenance (continuous infusions of 25 $\mu g \cdot kg^{-1}$ to 150 $\mu g \cdot kg^{-1}$) in combination with inhaled anesthetics.[7] Small doses of opioids (fentanyl 1 $\mu g \cdot kg^{-1}$ to 2 $\mu g \cdot kg^{-1}$ or equivalent doses of sufentanil or alfentanil) administered intravenously 1 minute to 3 minutes before induction of anesthesia may attenuate blood pressure and heart rate responses evoked by direct laryngoscopy and intubation of the trachea. Conversely, opioids are frequently not useful when administered after noxious stimulation has evoked hypertension. Intraoperative tachycardia, however, may respond to small intravenous injections of opioids.

Residual effects of opioids may be antagonized by a specific opioid antagonist, naloxone. Naloxone, however, is a nonselective antagonist, reversing desirable effects (analgesia), as well as undesirable effects (depression of ventilation). Large doses of naloxone (3 $\mu g \cdot kg^{-1}$ to 5 $\mu g \cdot kg^{-1}$) may result in abrupt awakening associated with intense pain and activation of the sympathetic nervous system manifesting as hypertension, tachycardia, and cardiac dysrhythmias. Intermittent administration of small doses of naloxone ($0.1\ \mu g \cdot kg^{-1}$ to $0.3\ \mu g \cdot kg^{-1}$) is more likely to reverse unacceptable degrees of depression of ventilation while leaving intact a sufficient amount of analgesia to maintain patient comfort. Unfortunately, the duration of action of naloxone is brief (about 30 minutes), and previously antagonized undesirable effects of opioids are likely to recur unless supplemental doses of the antagonist are administered.

Agonist-Antagonist Opioids

Opioids classified as agonist-antagonists include pentazocine, butorphanol, nalbuphine, and buprenorphine. These drugs are often strong kappa and weak mu receptor agonists. In contrast to pure agonists, the agonist-antagonists have limited analgesic properties (ceiling effect after which increasing doses do not produce additional analgesia) and are thus unlikely to be used alone or in combination with other anesthetics for induction or maintenance of anesthesia. The antagonist properties of these drugs, however, have been used to an advantage to provide postoperative analgesia with the hope that associated depression of ventilation will be minimal.

KETAMINE

Ketamine is a phencyclidine derivative that produces dissociative anesthesia characterized by EEG evidence of dissociation between the thalamus and limbic system. Induction of anesthesia is achieved in less than 60 seconds after intravenous administration of ketamine ($1\ mg \cdot kg^{-1}$ to $2\ mg \cdot kg^{-1}$) and within 2 minutes to 4 minutes after intramuscular injection ($5\ mg \cdot kg^{-1}$ to $10\ mg \cdot kg^{-1}$). Patients appear to be in cataleptic states in which the eyes remain open with a slow nystagmic gaze. Amnesia is present and analgesia is intense. Varying degrees of hypertonus and purposeful skeletal muscle movements can occur. Skeletal muscle tone helps maintain a patent upper airway, but the presence of protective upper airway reflexes should vomiting or regurgitation occur cannot be assumed.

Cardiovascular stimulation due principally to direct stimulation of sympathetic nervous system outflow from the central nervous system by ketamine is useful for induction of anesthesia and even maintenance of anesthesia in patients who are hypovolemic. These cardiac stimulant effects may be absent in the presence of catecholamine depletion.[12] Furthermore, ketamine-induced cardiac stimulation may adversely increase myocardial oxygen requirements in patients with coronary artery disease. Airway secretions are increased by ketamine, emphasizing the value of including anticholinergics in the preoperative medication when the use of this drug is planned. Reductions in airway resistance produced by sympathetic nervous system stimulation may be beneficial in patients with bronchial asthma. Ketamine is a potent cerebral vasodilator and predictably increases intracranial pressure in patients with space occupying intracranial lesions.

Ketamine is highly lipid soluble and undergoes extensive hepatic metabolism. Redistribution to inactive tissue sites, as with barbiturates, is important in early awakening after administration of ketamine. Elimination half-time is 1 hour to 2 hours. Repeated anesthetics with ketamine, as is popular for burn dressing changes, may be associated with the development of tolerance, as manifested by progressive increases in dose requirements with each successive anesthetic.

Emergence from ketamine may be associated with unpleasant visual, auditory, and proprioceptive illusions that may progress to delirium. The incidence of emergence delirium may approach 30 percent, causing many anesthesiologists to avoid the use of this drug. Administration of benzodiazepines, either preoperatively or after the induction of anesthesia, can reduce the incidence of emergence reactions associated with ketamine.

ETOMIDATE

Etomidate is a carboxylated imidazole derivative that produces rapid induction of anesthesia (usually less than 30 seconds) followed by awakening that is more prompt than after administration of barbiturates. Rapid awakening reflects nearly complete hydrolysis of etomidate to pharmacologically inactive metabolites. Etomidate is useful for induction of anesthesia in outpatients where prompt awakening is desirable. Cardiovascular stability is characteristic of patients receiving etomidate, suggesting that this drug may be useful in patients with limited cardiac reserve. Blood pressure declines are modest and reflect principally decreases in systemic vascular resistance. These blood pressure changes would likely be exaggerated in the presence of hypovolemia. Etomidate reduces cerebral blood flow, $CMRO_2$, and intracranial pressure and, like methohexital, activates seizure foci.

Disadvantages of etomidate include pain during intravenous injection, involuntary skeletal muscle movements, and an increased incidence of postoperative nausea and vomiting. More important, etomidate suppresses adrenocortical function for up to 8 hours after an induction dose.[13] During this time, the adrenal cortex is not responsive to adrenocorticotrophic hormone. This suppression may be desirable for stress-free anesthesia or undesirable if it prevents useful protective responses against stresses that accompany the perioperative period.

PROPOFOL

Propofol is a lipid-soluble-substituted isopropylphenol that produces rapid induction of anesthesia (usually less than 30 seconds after administration of 1.5 mg·kg^{-1} to 3 mg·kg^{-1}) followed by awakening in 4 minutes to 8 minutes. Continous intravenous infusion of propofol plus inhalation of nitrous oxide may be acceptable for maintenance of anesthesia in selected operations. In contrast to barbiturates, awakening is associated with minimal residual sedative effects, making this drug useful for brief operations. Hepatic metabolism to inactive metabolites is rapid, but redistribution to inactive tissue sites also plays an important role in early awakening. Depressant effects on circulation and ventilation resemble, but may exceed, those produced by barbiturates. The incidence of nausea and vomiting following administration of propofol is low.

REFERENCES

1. Filner BF, Karliner JS. Alterations of normal left ventricular performance by general anesthesia. Anesthesiology 1976;45:610–20.
2. Hudson RJ, Stanski DR, Burch PG. Pharmacokinetics of methohexital and thiopental in surgical patients. Anesthesiology 1983;59:215–9.
3. Richter JJ. Current theories about the mechanism of benzodiazepines and neuroleptic drugs. Anesthesiology 1981;54:66–72.
4. Reves JG, Fragen RJ, Vinik HR, Greenblatt DJ. Midazolam: Pharmacology and uses. Anesthesiology 1985;62:310–24.
5. Fleischer JE, Milde JH, Moyer TP, Michenfelder JD. Cerebral effects of high-dose midazolam and subsequent reversal with RO 15-1788 dogs. Anesthesiology 1988;68:234–42.
6. Sarnquist FH, Mathers WD, Brock-Utne J, Carr B, Canup C, Brown CR. A bioassay of a water-soluble-benzodiazepine against sodium thiopental. Anesthesiology 1980;52:149–53.
7. Pasternak GW. Multiple morphine and enkephalin receptors and the relief of pain. JAMA 1988;259:1362–7.
8. Rosow CE, Moss J, Philbin DM, Savarese JJ. Histamine release during morphine and fentanyl anesthesia. Anesthesiology 1982;56:93–6.
9. Benthuysen JL, Smith NT, Sanford TJ, Head N, Dec-Silver H. Physiology of alfentanil-induced rigidity. Anesthesiology 1986;64:440–6.
10. Becker LD, Paulson BA, Miller RD, Severinghaus JW, Eger EI II. Biphasic respiratory depression after fentanyl-droperidol or fentanyl alone used to supplement nitrous oxide anesthesia. Anesthesiology 1976;44:291–6.
11. Nauta J, deLange S, Koopman D, Spierdijk J, vanKleff J, Stanley TH. Anesthetic induction with alfentanil: A new short-acting narcotic analgesic. Anesth Analg 1982;61:267–72.
12. Weiskopf RB, Bogetz MS, Roizen MF, Reid IA. Cardiovascular and metabolic sequelae of inducing anesthesia with ketamine or thiopental in hypovolemic swine. Anesthesiology 1984;60:214–9.
13. Wagner RL, White PF, Kan PB, Rosenthal MH, Feldman D. Inhibition of adrenal steroidogenesis by the anesthetic etomidate. N Engl J Med 1984; 310:1415–21.

Local Anesthetics

Local anesthetics, when placed in proximity to nerve membranes, produce reversible conduction blockade of nerve impulses. Progressive increases in the concentrations of local anesthetics results in interruption of transmission of autonomic, somatosensory, and somatomotor impulses producing autonomic nervous system blockade, sensory anesthesia, and skeletal muscle paralysis in the areas innervated by the affected nerves. Subsequent recovery from the effects of local anesthetics is spontaneous and complete without evidence of damage to nerve fibers.

HISTORY

Since prehistoric times, the natives of Peru have chewed the leaves of the indigenous plant, erythroxylon coca, the source of cocaine, to obtain a feeling of well-being and reduced fatigue. Cocaine was introduced into clinical medicine by Köller in 1884 as a topical anesthetic for the cornea. The ability of cocaine to produce psychologic dependence and its irritant properties when placed topically or around nerves led to a search for a better local anesthetic. The first synthetic local anesthetic was introduced by Einhorn in 1905. Lidocaine, synthesized in 1943 by Lofgren, is the present-day, prototype local anesthetic to which all other such drugs are compared.

GENERAL PHARMACOLOGY

Structure Activity Relationships

Local anesthetics consist of a lipophilic (unsaturated benzene ring) and hydrophilic (tertiary amine) portion separated by a hydrocarbon connecting chain. Linkage of the hydrocarbon chain to the lipophilic portion is by an ester (–CO–) or amide (–HNC–) bond. The nature of this bond is the basis for classifying local anesthetics as esters or amides (Fig. 7-1). Important differences between ester and amide local anesthetics relate to the site of metabolism and the potential to produce allergic reactions.

Mechanism of Action

Local anesthetics produce conduction blockade of nerve impulses by preventing increases in permeability of nerve membranes to sodium ions. Failure of permeability to sodium ions to increase slows the rate of depolarization such that threshold potential is not reached and an action potential is not propagated (Fig. 7-2). Local anesthetics do not alter the resting transmembrane potential or threshold potential.

It is likely that local anesthetics stabilize and maintain sodium channels in the inactivated closed states by binding to specific receptors located in the inner portion of sodium channels.[1] Local an-

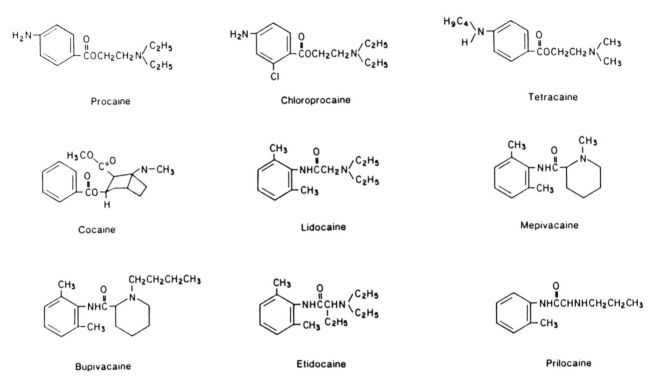

Fig. 7-1. Chemical structures of ester (procaine, chloroprocaine, tetracaine, cocaine) and amide (lidocaine, mepivacaine, bupivacaine, etidocaine, prilocaine) local anesthetics.

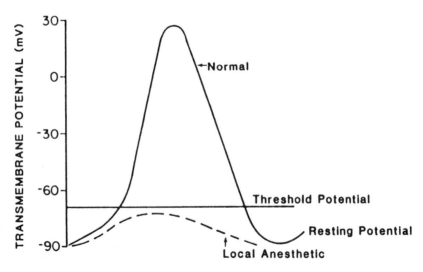

Fig. 7-2. Local anesthetics slow the rate of depolarization of the nerve action potential such that threshold potential is not reached. As a result, an action potential cannot be propagated in the presence of local anesthetics and conduction blockade occurs.

esthetics may also prevent changes in sodium permeability by obstructing sodium channels near their external openings.

Frequency-Dependent Blockade

Frequency-dependent blockade reflects recovery from local anesthetic-induced conduction blockade between action potentials and development of additional conduction blockade each time sodium channels open during an action potential. This emphasizes that local anesthetics gain access to receptors only when sodium channels are in activated-open states (not in the inactivated-closed and rested-closed states). For this reason, selective conduction blockade of nerve fibers by local anesthetics may be related to the nerve's characteristic frequencies of activity.

Classification of Nerves

Nerves can be classified according to fiber diameter, presence or absence of myelin, and function (Table 7-1). In essence, a smaller diameter nerve is more susceptible to blockade than is a larger diameter nerve, a myelinated nerve is more susceptible to blockade than is a nonmyelinated nerve, and an active nerve is more susceptible to blockade than is an inactive nerve. A combination of these factors will ultimately determine whether a given nerve can be blocked by a certain concentration of local anesthetic.

As previously indicated, ability of local anesthetics to block nerve conduction is indirectly related to the diameter of the nerve fiber. For example, the minimum concentration of local anesthetic (Cm, which is analogous to the minimum alveolar concentration [MAC] for inhaled anesthetics) required to block nerve conduction is greater in large diameter nerve fibers. The Cm of motor fibers is about twice that for sensory fibers, emphasizing that sensory anesthesia may not be accompanied by skeletal muscle paralysis. Further evidence of differential conduction blockade is selective blockade of preganglionic sympathetic nervous system type B fibers with low concentrations of local anesthetics that do not interrupt conduction in type A fibers.

Peripheral nerves are made up of myelinated type A and type B fibers and unmyelinated type C fibers. There is a minimal length of myelinated nerve fiber that must be exposed to an adequate concentration of local anesthetic for conduction blockade of nerve impulses to occur. For example, if only one node of Ranvier is blocked (i.e., site of changes in sodium permeability), nerve impulses can bypass this node and conduction blockade does not occur. Conduction blockade is predictably present if at least three successive nodes of Ranvier are exposed to adequate concentrations of local anesthetics. Both types of pain-conducting fibers (myelinated type A delta and nonmyelinated type C fibers) are blocked by similar concentrations of local anesthetics despite differences in diameters of these fibers. Preganglionic type B fibers are more readily blocked by local anesthetics than any fiber even though these fibers are larger in diameter than type C fibers. Presumably, the presence of myelin and its rather small diameter make these fibers especially susceptible to blockade by local anesthetics.

Table 7-1. Classification of Nerves

Fiber Type	Diameter (μ)	Myelin	Sensitivity to Block	Function
Type A				
Alpha	12–20	Yes	+	Proprioception, motor
Beta	5–12	Yes	+ +	Proprioception, motor
Gamma	3–6	Yes	+ +	Muscle tone
Delta	2–5	Yes	+ + +	Pain, temperature, touch
Type B	< 3	Yes	+ + + +	Preganglionic autonomic
Type C	0.3–1.2	No	+ + +	Pain and postganglionic autonomic

Symbols: + + + + extremely sensitive; + + + very sensitive; + + moderately sensitive; + slightly sensitive.

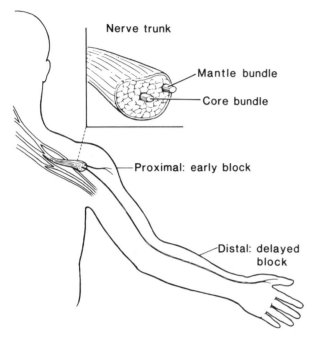

Fig. 7-3. Local anesthetics deposited around a peripheral nerve diffuse along a concentration gradient to block nerve fibers on the outer surface (mantle) before more centrally located (core) fibers. This accounts for early manifestations of anesthesia in more proximal areas of the extremity.

Location of a Nerve in the Nerve Bundle

When local anesthetics are deposited around a peripheral nerve, they diffuse from the outer surface (mantle) toward the center (core) of the nerve along a concentration gradient (Fig. 7-3).[2] As a result, nerve fibers located in the mantle of the mixed nerve are blocked first. These mantle fibers are often distributed to more proximal anatomic structures in contrast to distal structures innervated by nerve fibers near the core of the nerve. This explains the initial development of analgesia proximally with subsequent distal spread as local anesthetics diffuse to reach more central core nerve fibers. Skeletal muscle paralysis may precede the onset of sensory blockade if motor nerve fibers are distributed peripheral to sensory fibers in the mixed peripheral nerve. Indeed, the sequence of onset and recovery from blockade of sympathetic, sensory, and motor nerve fibers in a mixed peripheral nerve probably depends as much

on the anatomic location of the nerve fibers within the mixed nerve as on their sensitivity to local anesthetics.

PHARMACOKINETICS

The pKa of local anesthetics is such that less than one-half the total local anesthetic exists is a lipid-soluble nonionized form at physiologic pH (Table 7-2). This is important because the nonionized form of local anesthetics are necessary to cross the lipophilic nerve sheath to gain access to sodium channels on the nerve membrane. This is consistent with the observation that local tissue acidosis as produced by infection is associated with poor quality local anesthesia, presumably reflecting an increased ionized drug fraction that limits the amount of drug available to act on sodium channels.

Lipid solubility is a primary determinant of local anesthetic potency. Peak plasma concentrations of local anesthetics after their absorption from tissue injection sites is ultimately determined by the rate of tissue distribution and rate of clearance of the drug. Clearance of local anesthetics represent hydrolysis of ester drugs, whereas amide local anesthetics undergo metabolism by hepatic microsomal enzymes. The rate of metabolism influences systemic toxicity. For example, rapid metabolism prevents accumulation of local anesthetics in the plasma and systemic toxicity is unlikely (see the section *Systemic Toxicity*). In this regard, ester local anesthetics (hydrolysis of chloroprocaine more rapid than tetracaine) may be less likely to produce sustained plasma concentrations and resultant systemic toxicity than more slowly metabolized amide local anesthetics (lidocaine metabolized more rapidly than bupivacaine). Patients with atypical plasma cholinesterase enzyme may be at increased risk for developing excessive plasma concentrations of ester local anesthetics due to absent or limited plasma hydrolysis. Hepatic metabolism of lidocaine is extensive such that clearance of this local anesthetic from the plasma parallels hepatic blood flow. Hepatic disease or reductions in hepatic blood flow as occur during congestive heart failure or general anesthesia can reduce the rate of metabolism of lidocaine. Metabolites of lido-

Table 7-2. Comparative Pharmacology of Local Anesthetics

Classification	Potency	Onset	Duration After Infiltration (Minutes)	Maximum Single Dose for Infiltration (Adult, mg[a])	Toxic Plasma Concentration ($\mu g \cdot ml^{-1}$)	pKa	Nonionized %	
							pH 7.2	pH 7.4
Esters								
Procaine	1[b]	Slow	45–60	500		8.9	2	3
Chloroprocaine	4	Rapid	30–45	600		8.7	3	5
Tetracaine	16	Slow	60–180	100 (Topical)		8.5	5	7
Amides								
Lidocaine	1[c]	Rapid	60–120	300	5	7.9	17	25
Mepivacaine	1	Slow	90–180	300	5	7.6	28	39
Bupivacaine	4	Slow	240–480	175	About 1.5	8.1	11	15
Etidocaine	4	Slow	240–480	300	About 2	7.7	24	33
Prilocaine	1	Slow	60–120	400	5	7.9	17	24

[a] Increased if solution contains epinephrine.
[b] Standard of comparison for esters.
[c] Standard of comparison for amides.

caine, like the parent compound, possess cardiac antidysrhythmic effects (Fig. 7-4). Poor water solubility of local anesthetics limits renal excretion of unchanged drug to usually less than 5 percent of the injected dose.

Vasoconstrictors

Addition of epinephrine (1:200,000, 5 $\mu g \cdot ml^{-1}$) or phenylephrine (1:20,000) to local anesthetic solutions produces local vasoconstriction, which

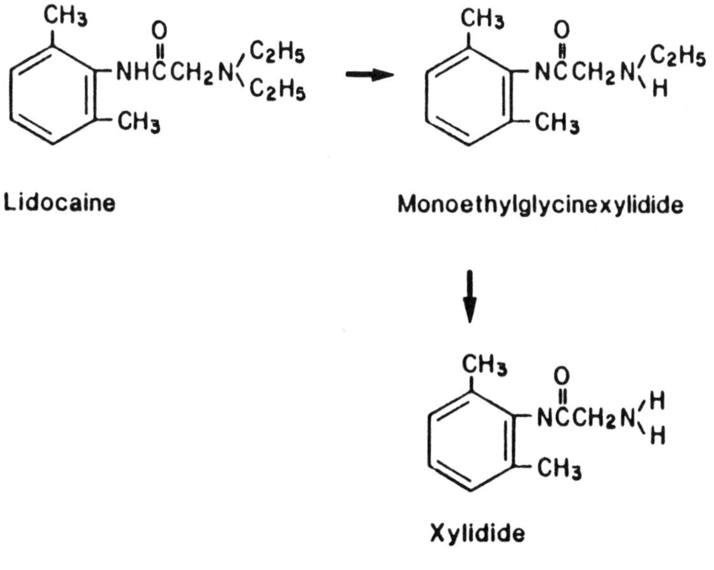

Fig. 7-4. Metabolism of lidocaine results in metabolites with cardiac antidysrhythmic properties.

limits systemic absorption and prolongs the duration of action of local anesthetics by keeping them in contact with nerve fibers. For example, addition of epinephrine prolongs the duration of lidocaine conduction blockade by about 50 percent and reduces systemic absorption by about 30 percent.[3] The impact of epinephrine, however, in prolonging the duration of action and reducing systemic absorption of bupivacaine and etidocaine is less, presumably because the high lipid solubility of these drugs causes them to avidly bind to tissues. Decreased systemic absorption of local anesthetics produced by epinephrine increases the likelihood that the rate of metabolism will match absorption, thus reducing the possibility of systemic toxicity. The addition of epinephrine to local anesthetic solutions has little if any effect on the rate of onset of local anesthesia. Systemic absorption of epinephrine may contribute to cardiac dysrhythmias in the presence of volatile anesthetics or accentuate hypertension in vulnerable patients.

SIDE EFFECTS

Systemic toxicity, neurotoxicity, and allergic reactions represent rare but important side effects associated with use of local anesthetics.

Systemic Toxicity

Systemic toxicity of local anesthetics is due to excess plasma concentrations of these drugs, most often due to accidental intravascular injection of local anesthetic solutions during performance of nerve blocks. Less often, excess plasma concentrations of local anesthetics result from absorption of local anesthetics from tissue injection sites. The magnitude of this systemic absorption depends on the (1) dose injected, (2) vascularity of the injection site, and (3) inclusion of a vasoconstrictor in the local anesthetic solutions. Establishment of maximal acceptable doses for use during performance of regional blocks is an attempt to limit plasma concentrations that result from systemic absorption of injected local anesthetics (Table 7-2). Systemic absorption of local anesthetics is greatest after injection for intercostal nerve blocks and caudal blocks, intermediate following epidural blocks, and least after brachial plexus blocks (Fig. 7-5).[4]

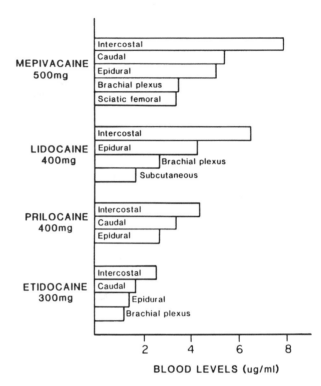

Fig. 7-5. Peak plasma concentrations of local anesthetics resulting during performance of various types of regional anesthetic procedures. (From Covino and Vassallo,[4] with permission.)

Systemic toxicity of local anesthetics manifests most prominently as changes in the central nervous system and cardiovascular system.

Central Nervous System

Increasing plasma concentrations of local anesthetics are associated initially with restlessness, vertigo, tinnitus, and slurred speech culminating in tonic-clonic seizures. Seizures can be followed by central nervous system depression (apnea) and death. The onset of seizures may reflect selective depression of inhibitory cortical neurons by local anesthetics leaving excitatory pathways unopposed.

Seizures

Treatment of local anesthetic induced seizures includes administration of (1) drugs to stop seizures and (2) supplemental oxygen, as arterial hypoxemia and metabolic acidosis can occur rapidly.[5] Hyperventilation of the lungs reduces delivery of additional local anesthetic to the brain, whereas associated respiratory alkalosis and hypokalemia results in hyperpolarization of nerve membranes and decreased local anesthetic effects. Diazepam administered intravenously in doses of 0.1 mg·kg^{-1} is effective in stopping local anesthetic-induced seizures, most likely by specific effects on the limbic system. Alternatively, small intravenous doses of thiopental, 0.5 mg·kg^{-1} to 2 mg·kg^{-1} stop seizures (and have a shorter duration of action than does diazepam), but their site of action in the central nervous system is nonspecific. Paralyzing doses of rapid acting muscle relaxants stop peripheral but not central nervous system manifestations of seizure activity. Muscle relaxants followed by intubation of the trachea are indicated when benzodiazepines or barbiturates are not promptly effective in stopping seizure activity. Placement of a cuffed tracheal tube reduces the likelihood of pulmonary aspiration of gastric contents and facilitates delivery of oxygen to the lungs.

Cardiovascular System

The cardiovascular system is more resistant to toxic effects of local anesthetics than is the central nervous system. Nevertheless, high plasma concentrations of local anesthetics can produce profound hypotension due to relaxation of arteriolar vascular smooth muscle and direct myocardial depression. Part of the cardiac toxicity reflects the ability of local anesthetics to block cardiac sodium channels. As a result, cardiac automaticity and conduction of cardiac impulses is impaired, manifesting on the electrocardiogram as prolongation of the P–R interval and widening of the QRS complex. Local anesthetics differ in their ability to produce cardiotoxicity. For example, the ratio between cardiovascular/central nervous system toxicity is 4 with lidocaine and 2 with bupivacaine. Thus, bupivacaine has a greater tendency to produce cardiotoxicity than does lidocaine.

Selective Cardiac Toxicity

Accidental intravenous injection of bupivacaine may result in precipitous hypotension, cardiac dysrhythmias (including ventricular tachycardia

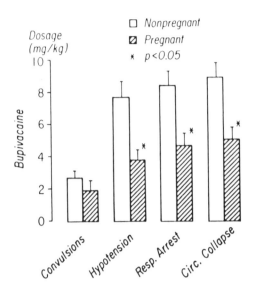

Fig. 7-6. The dose of bupivacaine (mean ± SE) required to produce toxic effects is less in pregnant than in nonpregnant ewes. (From Morishima et al.,[7] with permission.)

and fibrillation), and atrioventricular heart block.[6] Pregnancy may increase sensitivity to cardiotoxic effects of bupivacaine (Fig. 7-6).[7] Presumably, dissociation of highly lipid soluble bupivacaine from cardiac sodium channels is slow (i.e., fast in, slow out local anesthetic) accounting for its exaggerated and persistent depressant effects on cardiac function. In contrast, less lipid soluble lidocaine leaves sodium channels rapidly (i.e., fast in, fast out local anesthetic) and cardiac toxicity is low. In an effort to minimize the potential for cardiotoxicity should accidental intravascular injection occur, the maximum recommended concentrations of bupivacaine to be used for epidural block in obstetrical anesthesia are 0.5 percent.

Methemoglobinemia

Prilocaine administered in large doses (greater than 8 mg·kg^{-1}) may result in accumulation of the metabolite, ortho-toluidine, an oxidizing compound capable of converting hemoglobin to methemoglobin. When sufficient methemoglobin is present, patients may appear cyanotic and the blood chocolate-colored. Methemoglobinemia is readily reversed by the intravenous administration of methylene blue. Nevertheless, the unique ability of prilocaine to cause dose-related methemoglobinemia limits the clinical usefulness of this local anesthetic.

Neurotoxicity

Local anesthetics are not neurotoxic when administered at recommended concentrations, except for chloroprocaine, which is not recommended for intravenous regional anesthesia or spinal block because of potential irritant effects. For example, accidental injection of large volumes of chloroprocaine into the subarachnoid space during the intended performance of an epidural block may result in prolonged to even permanent neurologic damage.[8] It is possible that these neurotoxic effects are due to a low pH (3.0) and sodium bisulfite, an antioxidant in chloroprocaine and thus not a unique effect of the local anesthetic.[9]

Allergic Reactions

Allergic reactions to local anesthetics are rare despite the frequent use of these drugs. Indeed, it is estimated that less than 1 percent of all adverse reactions to local anesthetics are due to allergic mechanisms. This emphasizes that the vast majority of adverse responses that are often attributed to allergic reactions are in fact manifestations of systemic toxicity due to excessive plasma concentrations of the drug.

Ester local anesthetics that produce metabolites related to para-aminobenzoic acid are more likely to evoke allergic reactions than are amide local anesthetics, which are not metabolized to para-aminobenzoic acid. Allergic reactions following use of local anesthetics may be due to methylparaben or similar substances used as preservatives in commercial preparations of ester and amide local anesthetics. These preservatives resemble para-aminobenzoic acid and may be responsible for stimulation of antibody production and subsequent allergic reactions independent of the local anesthetic. Cross-sensitivity does not exist between classes of local anesthetics. Therefore, patients known to be allergic to ester local anesthetics could receive amide local anesthetics. This recommendation, however, assumes that the local anesthetic

and not preservatives, which may be common to both classes of drugs, was responsible for evoking the initial allergic reaction.

Documentation of allergy to local anesthetics is based on clinical history (occurrence of rash, laryngeal edema, hypotension, bronchospasm) and perhaps use of intradermal testing with preservative-free solutions. Hypotension associated with syncope, tachycardia, or bradycardia when epinephrine-containing local anesthetic solutions are used is more suggestive of an accidental intravascular injection or a psychogenic-vagally mediated reaction than an allergic reaction.

CLINICAL USES

Local anesthetics are used most often to produce regional anesthesia. Occasional unique uses of lidocaine include its intravenous administration to (1) prevent or treat cardiac ventricular dysrhythmias, (2) attenuate pressor responses associated with intubation of the trachea, (3) prevent or treat increases in intracranial pressure as are often associated with intubation of the trachea, and (4) minimize coughing during intubation or extubation of the trachea.

Regional anesthesia is classified according to the site of the local anesthetic placement as (1) topical or surface anesthesia, (2) local or subcutaneous infiltration, (3) intravenous block, and (4) nerve block (Table 7-3). Nerve block is produced by injection of local anesthetics into the epidural or subarachnoid spaces or near specific nerves (peripheral nerve block) to selectively produce anesthesia in areas innervated by the affected nerves (see Chapters 13 and 14).

Topical Anesthesia

Local anesthetics are used to produce topical anesthesia by placement on mucous membranes of areas such as the nose, mouth, or tracheobronchial tree. For example, lidocaine is commonly applied topically on the pharynx and trachea before intubation of the trachea. Tetracaine is an effective topical anesthetic and is commonly used to provide topical anesthesia for bronchoscopy. Cocaine has the unique advantage of producing topical anes-

Table 7-3. Uses of Local Anesthetics to Produce Regional Anesthesia

	Topical Anesthesia	Local Infiltration	Intravenous Block	Peripheral Nerve Block	Epidural Block	Subarachnoid Block
Procaine	No	Yes	No	Yes	No	Yes
Chloroprocaine	No	Yes	No	Yes	Yes	No
Tetracaine	Yes	No	No	No	No	Yes
Lidocaine	Yes	Yes	Yes	Yes	Yes	Yes
Mepivacaine	No	Yes	No	Yes	Yes	No
Bupivacaine	No	Yes	Yes	Yes	Yes	Yes
Etidocaine	No	Yes	No	Yes	Yes	No
Prilocaine	No	Yes	Yes	Yes	Yes	No

thesia and vasoconstriction (prevents uptake of norepinephrine back into postganglionic adrenergic nerve endings). Vasoconstriction produced in the area where cocaine is applied is useful in decreasing the likelihood of nasal hemorrhage due to nasotracheal intubation. Procaine and chloroprocaine penetrate mucous membranes poorly and are not effective topical anesthetics.

Local Infiltration

Local infiltration of local anesthetics is designed to produce sensory anesthesia in the injected area without any attempt to block specific nerves. For example, lidocaine is commonly injected into the area chosen for placement of an intravenous catheter.

REFERENCES

1. Hille B. Local anesthetics: Hydrophilic and hydrophobic pathways for the drug receptor interaction. J Gen Physiol 1977;69:497–515.
2. Winnie AP, Tay C-H, Patel KP, Ramamurthy S, Durranie Z. Pharmacokinetics of local anesthetics during plexus blocks. Anesth Analg 1977;56:852–61.
3. Scott DB, Jebson PJR, Braid B, Ortengren B, Fisch P. Factors affecting plasma levels of lignocaine and prilocaine. Br J Anaesth 1972;44:1040–9.
4. Covino BG, Vassallo HG. Local Anesthetics: Mechanisms of Action in Clinical Use. Orlando, FL, Grune & Stratton, 1976.
5. Moore DC, Crawford RD, Scurlock JE. Severe hypoxia and acidosis following local anesthetic-induced convulsions. Anesthesiology 1980;53:259–60.
6. Albright GA. Cardiac arrest following regional anesthesia with etidocaine or bupivacaine. Anesthesiology 1979;51:285–7.
7. Morishima HO, Pederson H, Finster M, et al. Bupivacaine toxicity in pregnant and nonpregnant ewes. Anesthesiology 1985;63:134–9.
8. Ravindran RS, Bond VK, Tasch MD, Gupta CD, Luerssen TG. Prolonged neural blockade following regional analgesia with 2-chloroprocaine. Anesth Analg 1980;59:447–51.
9. Wang BC, Hillman DE, Spielholz NI, Turndorf H. Chronic neurological deficits and Nesacaine-CE: An effect of the anesthetic 2-chloroprocaine, or the antioxidant, sodium bisulfite. Anesth Analg 1984; 63:445–7.

Chapter 8

Muscle Relaxants

Muscle relaxants are drugs that interrupt transmission of nerve impulses at the neuromuscular junction. As such, these drugs are more accurately described as neuromuscular blockers. Nevertheless, the designation as muscle relaxants remains a commonly used and accepted term. Skeletal muscle relaxation or paralysis can also be achieved by high doses of volatile anesthetics or regional anesthesia. Muscle relaxants used clinically are classified as depolarizing or nondepolarizing.

The principal uses of muscle relaxants are to provide skeletal muscle relaxation to facilitate intubation of the treachea and to provide optimal surgical working conditions. Muscle relaxants are also administered in the intensive care setting to facilitate mechanical ventilation of the lungs. It is essential to recognize that muscle relaxants lack anesthetic or analgesic effects and must not be used to render an inadequately anesthetized patient immobile. Ventilation of the lungs must be mechanically provided whenever significant skeletal muscle weakness is produced by these drugs. Clinically, intraoperative evaluation of neuromuscular blockade is typically provided by visually monitoring the mechanical response (twitch response) produced by an electrical stimulus delivered from a peripheral nerve stimulator (see the section *Monitoring Effects of Muscle Relaxants*).

Choice of muscle relaxant is influenced by the speed of onset, duration of action, route of elimination, and associated side effects (most often circulatory). A rapid onset and brief duration of skeletal muscle paralysis, as provided by succinylcholine, is useful when intubation of the trachea is the reason for administering a muscle relaxant. When longer periods of neuromuscular blockade are needed, succinylcholine can be administered as a continuous intravenous infusion or nondepolarizing muscle relaxants are selected. When rapid onset of skeletal muscle paralysis is not necessary, it is acceptable to produce skeletal muscle paralysis by administration of nondepolarizing muscle relaxants to facilitate intubation of the trachea.

NEUROMUSCULAR JUNCTION

The neuromuscular junction consists of a prejunctional motor nerve ending separated from a highly folded postjunctional membrane of the skeletal muscle by a synaptic cleft (Fig. 8-1).[1] Neuromuscular transmission is initiated by arrival of an impulse at the motor nerve terminal with an associated influx of calcium and a resultant release of the neurotransmitter, acetylcholine. Acetylcholine binds to nicotinic cholinergic receptors on postjunctional membranes, causing a change in membrane permeability to ions, principally potassium and sodium. This change in permeability and movement of ions causes a decline in the trans-

---

Classification of Muscle Relaxants

Depolarizers
  Succinylcholine
  Decamethonium
Nondepolarizers
  Long-acting
    d-Tubocurarine
    Metocurine
    Gallamine
    Pancuronium
    Pipecuronium
    Doxacurium
  Intermediate-acting
    Atracurium
    Vecuronium
    Mivacurium

---

membrane potential from about -90 mV to -45 mV (threshold potential) at which point a propagated action potential spreads over the surfaces of skeletal muscle fibers leading to muscular contraction. Acetylcholine is rapidly hydrolyzed (within 15 msec) by the enzyme acetylcholinesterase (true cholinesterase), thus restoring membrane permeability (repolarization) and preventing sustained depolarization. Acetylcholinesterase is primarily located in the folds of the endplate region, placing it in close proximity to the site of action of acetylcholine.

Nicotinic Cholinergic Receptors

Nicotinic cholinergic receptors are situated on both the prejunctional and postjunctional membranes. Prejunctional receptors influence the release of acetylcholine. Postjunctional receptors are confined to the area of the endplate precisely opposite prejunctional receptors, and extrajunctional receptors are present throughout skeletal muscle. Postjunctional receptors are the most important sites of action of muscle relaxants. Extrajunctional receptor synthesis is normally suppressed by neural activity. Denervation or trauma to skeletal muscle (burn injury) is associated with a rapid proliferation of extrajunctional receptors.

Postjunctional Receptors

Postjunctional receptors are glycoproteins consisting of five subunits designated as alpha (two subunits), beta, gamma, and delta (Fig. 8-2).[2] The subunits of the receptor are arranged such that a channel is formed that allows the flow of ions along a concentration gradient across cell membranes. This flow of ions is the basis of normal neuromuscular transmission.

The two alpha subunits are the binding sites for acetylcholine and are the sites occupied by muscle relaxants. For example, occupation of one or both alpha subunits by a nondepolarizing muscle relaxant causes the channel to remain closed, and ion flow to produce depolarization cannot occur. Succinylcholine attaches to alpha sites and causes the channel to remain open (mimics acetylcholine), resulting in prolonged depolarization. Large molecules can also act to plug the channel and in this way prevent the normal flow of ions. This is probably what happens when large overdoses of nondepolarizing muscle relaxants are administered. Unfortunately, this type of neuromuscular blockade cannot be readily reversed by anticholinesterases. Finally, the lipid environment around cholinergic receptors can be altered by drugs such as inhaled anesthetics (especially enflurane), thus changing the channel properties.

STRUCTURE ACTIVITY RELATIONSHIPS

Muscle relaxants resemble the structure of acetylcholine (Fig. 8-3). For example, succinylcholine consists of two molecules of acetylcholine linked by methyl groups. Nondepolarizing muscle relaxants are bulky, rigid molecules that contain portions similar to acetylcholine. Acetylcholine and all muscle relaxants contain at least one positively charged quaternary ammonium group. This is important for attraction to the negatively charged cholinergic receptor.

DEPOLARIZING MUSCLE RELAXANTS

Succinylcholine is the only depolarizing muscle relaxant used clinically (Table 8-1). Typically, doses of 0.6 mg·kg^{-1} to 2.0 mg·kg^{-1} are admin-

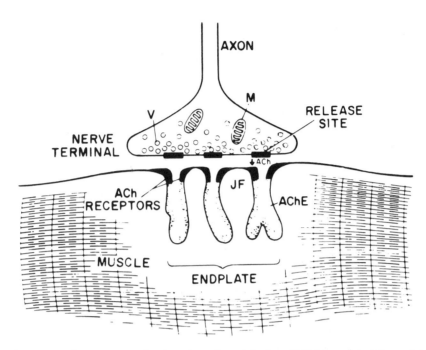

Fig. 8-1. Schematic depiction of neuromuscular junction. Acetylcholine (ACh) is present in vesicles (V) of the axon for release in response to nerve impulses. ACh diffuses across the synaptic cleft to attach to receptors that are concentrated on the junctional folds (JF) of the skeletal muscle endplate. Acetylcholinesterase (AChE) is present in the JF to facilitate rapid hydrolysis of ACh. (From Drachman,[1] with permission.)

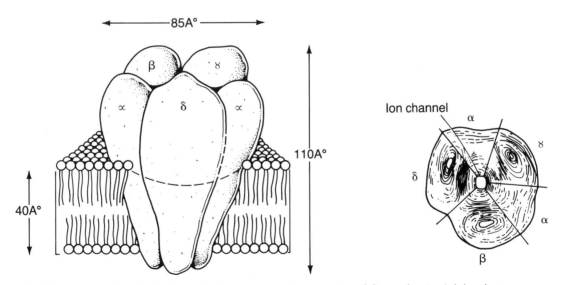

Fig. 8-2. The postjunctional nicotinic cholinergic receptor consists of five subunits (alpha, beta, gamma, delta) arranged to form an ion channel (From Taylor,[2] with permission.)

Table 8-1. Comparison of a Typical Depolarizing (Succinylcholine) and Long-Acting Nondepolarizing (Pancuronium) Muscle Relaxant

	Succinylcholine		Pancuronium
	Phase I	Phase II	
Administration of pancuronium	Antagonize	Augment	Augment
Administration of succinylcholine	Augment	Augment	Antagonize
Administration of neostigmine	Augment	Antagonize	Antagonize
Fasiculations	Yes		None
Response to single twitch	Decreased	Decreased	Decreased
Train-of-four ratio	0.7	0.3	0.3
Response to tetanic stimulation	Sustained	Unsustained	Unsustained
Post-tetanic facilitation	No	Yes	Yes

istered, producing a rapid onset of skeletal muscle paralysis (0.5 minute to 1 minute) that lasts 5 minutes to 10 minutes. These characteristics make succinylcholine useful for providing rapid skeletal muscle paralysis to facilitate intubation of the trachea during induction of anesthesia.

Characteristics of Blockade

Succinylcholine mimics the action of acetylcholine, producing depolarization of the postjunctional membrane. Compared with acetylcholine, the hydrolysis of succinylcholine is slow, resulting in sustained depolarization. Skeletal muscle paralysis occurs because a depolarized postjunctional membrane cannot respond to subsequent release of acetylcholine (hence the designation *depolarizing neuromuscular blockade*). Depolarizing neuromuscular blockade is also referred to as phase I blockade. Phase II blockade is present when the postjunctional membrane has become repolarized but still does not respond normally to acetylcholine (i.e., desensitization neuromuscular blockade). The mechanism of phase II blockade is unknown but may reflect development of a nonexcitable area around the endplate, which becomes repolarized but prevents spread of impulses initiated by the action of acetylcholine. Phase II blockade predominates when the dose of succinylcholine exceeds 2 mg·kg^{-1} to 4 mg·kg^{-1}, and characteristics of this neuromuscular blockade resemble that produced by nondepolarizing muscle relaxants.[3]

The sustained depolarization produced by initial administration of succinylcholine is initially manifested by transient generalized skeletal muscle contractions known as fasiculations. Furthermore, sustained opening of ion channels produced by succinylcholine is associated with leakage of potassium from the interior of cells sufficient to elevate plasma concentrations of potassium an average of 0.5 mEq·L^{-1}.

Metabolism

Hydrolysis of succinylcholine to inactive metabolites is by plasma cholinesterase (pseudocholinesterase) produced in the liver (Fig. 8-4). Plasma cholinesterase has an enormous capacity to hydrolyze succinylcholine at a rapid rate such that only a small fraction of the original intravenous dose reaches the neuromuscular junction. Because plasma cholinesterase is not present at the neuromuscular junction, neuromuscular blockade produced by succinylcholine is terminated by its diffusion away from the neuromuscular junction into extracellular fluid. Therefore, plasma cholinesterase influences the duration of action of succinylcholine by controlling the amount of muscle relaxant that is hydrolyzed before reaching the neuromuscular junction. Liver disease must be severe before reductions in synthesis of plasma cholinesterase enzyme are sufficient to prolong the effects of succinylcholine. Potent anticholinesterases, as used in insecticides and treatment of myasthenia gravis, and certain chemotherapeutic drugs (nitrogen mustard, cyclophosphamide) may

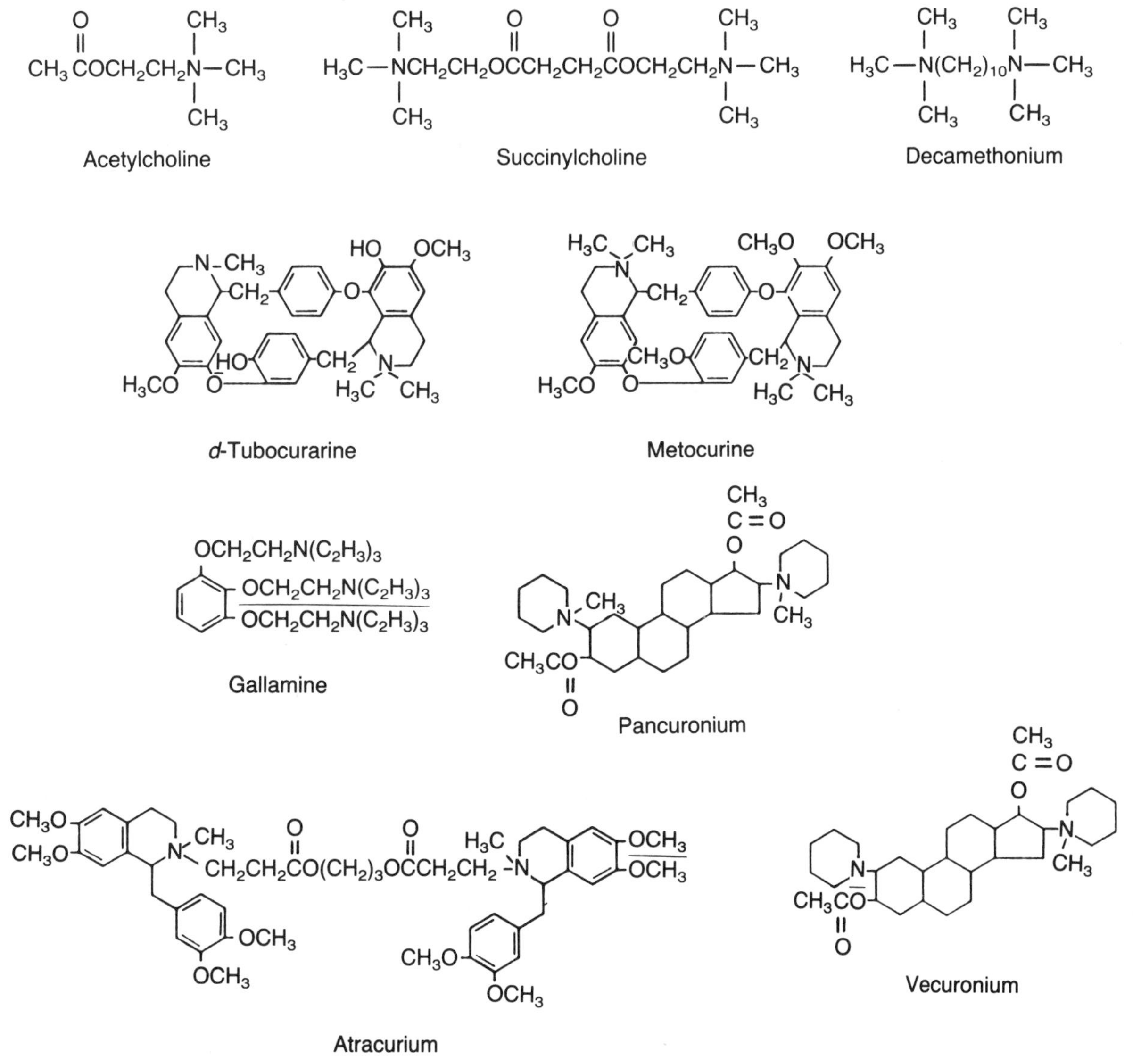

Fig. 8-3. Chemical structure of acetylcholine and muscle relaxants.

so reduce plasma cholinesterase activity that prolonged skeletal muscle paralysis follows administration of succinylcholine.

Atypical Plasma Cholinesterase

Atypical plasma cholinesterase enzyme lacks the ability to hydrolyze ester bonds in drugs such as succinylcholine. The presence of this atypical enzyme is often recognized only after an otherwise healthy patient experiences prolonged skeletal muscle paralysis (greater than 1 hour) after administration of a conventional dose of succinylcholine. Subsequent determination of the dibucaine number permits diagnosis of the presence of atypical plasma cholinesterase. Dibucaine is an amide local anesthetic that inhibits normal plasma cholin-

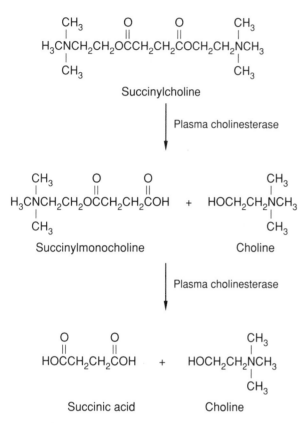

Fig. 8-4. The brief duration of action of succinylcholine is principally due to its rapid hydrolysis in the plasma by cholinesterase enzyme to inactive metabolites (succinylcholine has 1/20 to 1/80 the activity of succinylcholine at the neuromuscular junction).

esterase activity by about 80 percent, whereas activity of atypical enzyme is inhibited by only about 20 percent (Table 8-2). It is important to recognize that the dibucaine number reflects the quality of plasma cholinesterase enzyme (i.e., ability to metabolize succinylcholine) and not the quantity of enzyme that is circulating in the plasma. For example, reductions in plasma cholinesterase activity due to liver disease or anticholinesterases are associated with a normal dibucaine number.

Adverse Side Effects

Adverse side effects following administration of succinylcholine are numerous and may limit or contraindicate the use of this muscle relaxant in certain patients.

Adverse Side Effects of Succinylcholine

Cardiac dysrhythmias
    Sinus bradycardia
    Junctional rhythm
    Sinus arrest
Hyperkalemia
Myalgia
Myoglobinuria
Increased intraocular pressure
Increased intragastric pressure
Increased intracranial pressure
Trismus

Cardiac Dysrhythmias

Sinus bradycardia, junctional rhythm, and even sinus arrest may follow the administration of succinylcholine These responses reflect the action of succinylcholine at cardiac postganglionic muscarinic receptors where this drug mimics the normal effects of acetylcholine (Table 8-3). Cardiac dysrhythmias are most likely to occur when a second intravenous dose of succinylcholine is administered about 5 minutes after the first dose. Intravenous administration of atropine or subparalyzing doses of nondepolarizing muscle relaxants (pretreatment) 1 minute to 3 minutes before succinylcholine reduces the likelihood of these cardiac responses. Atropine administered intramuscularly with the preoperative medication does not reliably protect against succinylcholine-induced heart rate slowing. The effects of succinylcholine at autonomic nervous system ganglia also mimic the actions of the neurotransmitter, acetylcholine, which may manifest as ganglionic stimulation with associated elevations in blood pressure and heart rate (Table 8-3).

Hyperkalemia

Hyperkalemia sufficient to cause cardiac arrest may follow administration of succinylcholine to patients with denervation such as caused by spinal cord injury or skeletal muscle injury as associated with third-degree burns.[4] Vulnerability to hyper-

Table 8-2. Variants of Plasma Cholinesterase Enzyme

	Approximate Duration of Succinylcholine-induced Neuromuscular Blockade	Dibucaine Number (% Inhibition of Enzyme Activity)	Incidence
Homozygous	5–10 minutes	80	
Heterozygous	20 minutes	40–60	1 in 480
Homozygous atypical	60–180 minutes	20	1 in 3200

kalemia may reflect proliferation of extrajunctional receptors, thus providing more sites for potassium to leak outward across cell membranes during depolarization. Although the potential for excessive potassium release may develop within 2 days of injury and persist for up to 2 years or more, the more common vulnerable period is 7 days to 6 months after injury. Pretreatment with nondepolarizing muscle relaxants minimally influences the magnitude of potassium release evoked by succinylcholine and cannot be relied on as a safeguard. Patients with renal failure are not susceptible to exaggerated release of potassium, and succinylcholine can be safely administered to these patients, assuming they are normokalemic.[5]

Myalgia

Postoperative skeletal muscle myalgia manifesting particularly in the muscles of the neck, back, and abdomen may follow administration of succinylcholine. Young adults undergoing minor surgical procedures that permit early ambulation seem most likely to complain of myalgia. It is speculated that unsynchronized contractions of skeletal muscle fibers associated with generalized depolarization lead to myalgia. Indeed, prevention of fasiculations by prior administration of subparalyzing doses of nondepolarizing muscle relaxants prevents or attenuates the incidence of myalgia (see Chapter 29). Further evidence of skeletal muscle damage is the appearance of myoglobinuria in some patients, especially pediatric patients during halothane anesthesia, after administration of succinylcholine.

Increased Intraocular Pressure

Succinylcholine causes a transient increase in intraocular pressure that is maximal 2 minutes to 4 minutes after injection of the drug (see Chapter 25). The mechanism for this effect has not been

Table 8-3. Autonomic Effects of Muscle Relaxants

Drug	Histamine Release	Autonomic Ganglia	Muscarinic Receptors
Succinylcholine	Slight	Modest stimulation	Modest stimulation
d-Tubocurarine	Moderate	Moderate blockade[a]	None
Metocurine	Slight	Slight blockade	None
Gallamine	None	None	Strong blockade
Pancuronium	None	None	Modest blockade
Pipecuronium	None	None	None
Doxacurium	None	None	None
Vecuronium	None	None	None
Atracurium	Slight[a]	None	None
Mivacurium	Slight[a]	None	None

[a] Occurs only with higher doses.

clearly defined but may involve contraction of myofibrils or transient dilation of choroidal blood vessels. For these reasons, succinylcholine may theoretically contribute to extrusion of intraocular contents in patients with open eye injuries, although this fear has not been realized with widespread clinical use.[6]

Increased Intragastric Pressure

Succinylcholine produces unpredictable elevations in intragastric pressure. When intragastric pressure does increase, it seems to be related to the intensity of fasiculations, emphasizing the potential value of preventing this skeletal muscle activity by prior administration of subparalyzing doses of nondepolarizing muscle relaxants. Presumably, these increased intragastric pressures may facilitate passage of gastric fluid and contents into the esophagus and pharynx with the subsequent risk of pulmonary aspiration.

Increased Intracranial Pressure

Succinylcholine produces modest and transient increases in intracranial pressure that are attenuated or prevented by prior administration of subparalyzing doses of nondepolarizing muscle relaxants. The clinical importance of these increases in intracranial pressure has not been ascertained.

Trismus

Varying degrees of increased tension in the masseter muscles may accompany administration of succinylcholine, especially in pediatric patients. In extreme cases, this response may manifest as trismus, leading to difficulty in opening the mouth for direct laryngoscopy and intubation of the trachea. Patients who develop trismus should be considered susceptible to malignant hyperthermia (see Chapter 27).

NONDEPOLARIZING MUSCLE RELAXANTS

Nondeolarizing muscle relaxants can be subdivided into long- and intermediate-acting. Long-acting nondepolarizing muscle relaxants administered in equivalent doses produce skeletal muscle paralysis in 3 minutes to 5 minutes that lasts 60 minutes to 90 minutes (Table 8-4). These drugs are used most often to produce surgical muscle relaxation during maintenance of anesthesia.

Atracurium and vecuronium are intermediate-acting nondepolarizing muscle relaxants that serve as useful alternatives to succinylcholine and long-acting nondepolarizing muscle relaxants, especially when intubation of the trachea and/or skeletal muscle relaxation are needed for short operations. Compared with long-acting nondepolarizing muscle relaxants, these drugs (1) have a similar rate of onset of neuromuscular blockade, (2) have about one-third to one-half the duration of action (hence the designation intermediate-acting), (3) are relatively independent (especially atracurium) of renal function for clearance from the plasma, and (4) evoke minimal (especially vecuronium) circulatory effects (Table 8-5). Drugs and events that alter responses produced by long-acting nondepolarizing muscle relaxants produce similar directional changes after administration of intermediate-acting muscle relaxants.

Characteristics of Blockade

Nondepolarizing muscle relaxants compete with acetylcholine for alpha subunits and prevent changes in permeability of the postjunctional membranes. As a result, depolarization cannot occur (hence, the designation nondepolarizing neuromuscular blockade) and skeletal muscle paralysis develops (Table 8-1). Skeletal muscle fasiculations do not accompany the onset of nondepolarizing neuromuscular blockade.

Pharmacokinetics

Nondepolarizing muscle relaxants are highly ionized at physiologic pH and possess limited lipid solubility. As a result, the volume of distribution of these muscle relaxants is small, being limited principally to the extracellular fluid. In addition, these muscle relaxants cannot easily cross lipid membrane barriers, such as the blood-brain barrier, renal tubular epithelium, gastrointestinal epithelium, or placenta. Therefore, these muscle relaxants do not produce central nervous system effects, renal tubular reabsorption is minimal, oral administration is not effective, and maternal administration does not affect the fetus.

Table 8-4. Comparative Pharmacology of Nondepolarizing Muscle Relaxants

	d-Tubo-curarine	Metocurine	Gallamine	Pancuronium	Pipecuronium	Doxacurium
ED_{95} (mg·kg^{-1})	0.51	0.28	1.0[a]	0.07	0.07	0.25–0.40
Onset to maximum twitch depression (minutes)	3–5	3–5	3–5	3–5	3–5	4–6
Recovery to control twitch height (minutes)	60–90	60–90	60–90	60–90	50–80	60–80
Renal excretion (percent unchanged)	45	43	95	80	70	70 (probable)
Biliary excretion (percent unchanged)	10–40	2	0	5–10	20	[b]
Hepatic degradation (percent)	Insignificant	Insignificant	Insignificant	10	10	[b]

[a] Estimate
[b] Unknown.

Long-Acting Muscle Relaxants

The rate of disappearance of long-acting nondepolarizing muscle relaxants from the plasma is characterized by an initial rapid decline followed by a slower decline (Fig. 8-5).[7] Distribution of drug to tissues is the major cause of the initial rapid decrease in the plasma concentrations, and the slower decline is due to hepatic and renal clearance mechanisms (Table 8-4). Although the major route of excretion of pancuronium is via the kidney, it is also metabolized to 3- and 17-hydroxymetabolites that possess limited muscle relaxant properties. The route of excretion for muscle relaxant that cannot be accounted for by known clearance mechanisms may reflect storage in mucopolysaccharides of connective tissues for prolonged periods of time.

Renal disease can greatly affect the pharmacokinetics of all long-acting nondepolarizing muscle relaxants. The rate at which the plasma concen-

Table 8-5. Comparative Pharmacology of Intermediate-Acting Muscle Relaxants

	Atracurium	Vecuronium	Mivacurium
ED_{95} (mg·kg^{-1})	0.15–0.30	0.04–0.07	0.08
Onset of maximal twitch depression (minutes)	3–5	3–5	2.5–4
Recovery to 25 percent of control twitch height (minutes)	20–35	20–35	12–20
Dose for continuous infusion (µg·kg^{-1}·min^{-1})	6–8	1	1
Active metabolites	No	Slight	Unlikely
Degradation dependent on			
Body temperature	Yes	Yes	[a]
Blood pH	Yes	No	[a]
Renal function	No	Slight	No
Hepatic function	No?	Yes	[a]
Circulatory effects	Slight	No	Slight

[a] Unknown.

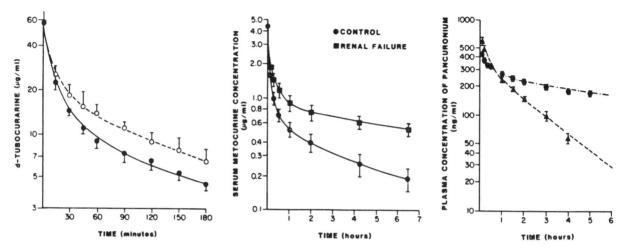

Fig. 8-5. The rate at which the plasma concentrations of pancuronium decrease is more influenced by renal failure than is the rate of decline in the plasma concentrations of d-tubocurarine or metocurine. (From Stoelting,[7] with permission.)

trations of pancuronium decrease is more influenced by renal failure than is the rate of decline in plasma concentrations of d-turbocurarine or metocurine (Fig. 8-5).[7] The new long-acting muscle relaxants, doxacurium, and pipecuronium are highly dependent on the kidneys for their elimination. Patients with biliary obstruction and cirrhosis of the liver manifest reduced plasma clearance and prolonged elimination half-times of pancuronium; doxacurium and pipecuronium have not been tested in these patients.

Intermediate-Acting Muscle Relaxants

Atracurium undergoes extensive metabolism (Hofmann elimination and ester hydrolysis) accounting for its independence from the kidneys for its clearance. Hofmann elimination is a pH and temperature dependent breakdown that occurs spontaneously. Ester hydrolysis uses different enzymes from plasma cholinesterase, and patients with atypical cholinesterase enzyme will not experience prolonged responses after administration of atracurium. The principal metabolite of atracurium is laudanosine, which is inactive at the neuromuscular junction but in high concentrations may act as a central nervous system stimulant. Doses of atracurium administered during surgery result in low plasma concentrations of laudanosine (less

than 1 $\mu g \cdot ml^{-1}$) that are unlikely to produce central nervous system effects. Continuous infusions of atracurium for several days to patients in the intensive care unit may result in plasma concentrations of laudanosine as high as 5 $\mu g \cdot ml^{-1}$ to 6 $\mu g \cdot ml^{-1}$; whether these levels are sufficient to cause seizures in some patients remains to be determined.

Vecuronium is a monoquaternary analog of pancuronium that unlike its analog lacks vagolytic effects or substantial dependence on renal function for its clearance from the plasma. Metabolism is by deacetylation in the liver to metabolites that have reduced blocking properties at the neuromuscular junction. In addition, both unchanged vecuronium and its metabolites (up to 60 percent of an injected dose) are excreted predominantly in the bile.

Mivacurium is primarily metabolized by plasma cholinesterase and apparently is minimally dependent on the kidneys or liver for its elimination.[8] Metabolites of mivacurium are pharmacologically inactive. Dependence of mivacurium on hydrolysis by plasma cholinesterase might result in a longer duration of action should this drug be administered to patients with atypical cholinesterase. Despite the ability of anticholinesterase drugs to inhibit activity of both plasma and true cholinesterase, it appears that antagonism of mivacurium induced neuromuscular blockade with drugs such as neostigmine is rapid.

The rapid clearance of intermediate-acting drugs from the plasma allows adjustment of the dose to parallel loss of drug. As a result, continuous intravenous infusions of atracurium or vecuronium enhance the likelihood of maintaining an optimal and unchanging degree of neuromuscular blockade.

Cardiovascular Effects

Nondepolarizing muscle relaxants may exert cardiovascular effects by virtue of (1) drug-induced histamine release, (2) effects at cardiac postganglionic muscarinic receptors, or (3) effects on nicotinic receptors at autonomic ganglia (Table 8-3). d-Tubocurarine, and to a lesser extent, metocurine, atracurium, and mivacurium produce reductions in blood pressure principally as a result of the release of histamine. In contrast, pancuronium produces modest (10 percent to 15 percent) increases in heart rate and blood pressure. These cardiovascular effects are due principally to selective cardiac vagal blockade (atropine-like effect) and to a lesser extent activation of the sympathetic nervous system. Cardiovascular effects likely to be evoked by muscle relaxants are often considered in selection of these drugs. For example, in hypovolemic patients, blood pressure decreases produced by histamine release after administration of d-tubocurarine could be exaggerated, whereas in these same patients modest increases in heart rate and blood pressure produced by pancuronium would be desirable. Vecuronium, doxacurium, and pipecuronium produce little or no cardiovascular effects.

Causes of Altered Responses to Nondepolarizing Muscle Relaxants

Drugs administered in the perioperative period (volatile anesthetics, aminoglycoside antibiotics, magnesium, local anesthetics, cardiac antidysrhythmics, calcium entry blockers) may enhance effects of nondepolarizing muscle relaxants. Hypothermia prolongs neuromuscular blockade produced by muscle relaxants, especially atracurium and vecuronium. Reductions in pH may prolong

the action of nondepolarizing muscle relaxants, especially atracurium, by inhibiting Hofmann elimination. Hypokalemia, as produced by chronic treatment with diuretics, may be associated with enhanced effects of muscle relaxants. Nevertheless, the changes produced by chronic hypokalemia at the neuromuscular junction are complex and often unpredictable. Burn injury that is accompanied by a proliferation of extrajunctional cholinergic receptors results in resistance to the effects of nondepolarizing muscle relaxants. This is a pharmacodynamic change, as the plasma concentrations of muscle relaxants required to produce the same degree of neuromuscular blockade are greater in burn than in normal patients. Allergic reactions rarely accompany administration of muscle relaxants. When allergy is present, cross-sensitivity is likely to exist between all drugs including succinylcholine.

Volatile Anesthetics

Volatile anesthetics produce dose-dependent and drug specific (greatest with isoflurane and enflurane) enhancement of the magnitude and duration of neuromuscular blockade produced by nondepolarizing muscle relaxants (Fig. 8-6).[9] This enhancement is partly due to anesthetic-induced depression of the central nervous system, which reduces the tone of skeletal muscles. In addition, volatile anesthetics may alter the sensitivity of postjunctional membranes to depolarization. Release of acetylcholine from the motor nerve ending or configuration of the cholinergic receptor is not altered by volatile anesthetics.

Aminoglycoside Antibiotics and Magnesium

Enhancement of neuromuscular blockade by certain antibiotics and magnesium, as is used in the treatment of toxemia of pregnancy, reflects complex changes at prejunctional (decreased release of acetylcholine) and postjunctional (stabilization) membranes. Inhibition of the prejunctional release of acetylcholine may reflect competition of these drugs with calcium. Indeed, calcium has been used to reverse antibiotic-enhanced neuromuscular blockade. Nevertheless, the response to calcium is unpredictable, and the usual recommendation is to mechanically support ventilation of the lungs

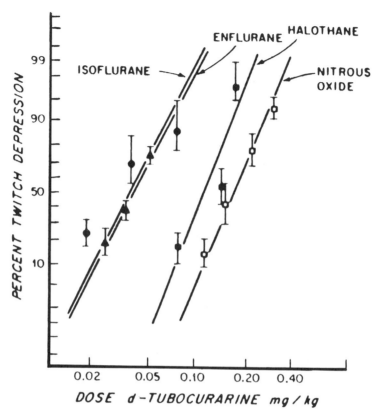

Fig. 8-6. Volatile anesthetics cause dose-dependent and drug-specific enhancement of neuromuscular blockade produced by long-acting nondepolarizing muscle relaxants. (From Ali and Savarese,[9] with permission.)

until the blockade dissipates spontaneously. Antibiotics that do not enhance neuromuscular blockade include the penicillins and cephalosporins.

Local Anesthetics and Cardiac Antidysrhythmics

Lidocaine and quinidine, as administered intravenously to treat cardiac dysrhythmias, may augment co-existing neuromuscular blockade. This potential drug interaction should be considered when administering these drugs to patients recovering from general anesthesia that includes use of nondepolarizing muscle relaxants. Depending on the dose, local anesthetics and cardiac antidysrhythmics interfere with the prejunctional release of acetylcholine, stabilize postjunctional membranes, and directly depress skeletal muscle fibers.

Verapamil potentiates the effects of depolarizing and nondepolarizing muscle relaxants.

PRIMING PRINCIPLE

The priming principle is the administration of a subparalyzing dose (10 percent of the ED_{95} of the nondepolarizing muscle relaxant followed in 3 minutes to 5 minutes by a large dose (2 times to 3 times the ED_{95}). Conceptually, the initial small dose binds "spare" receptors without any significant effect on awake patients such that the onset of neuromuscular blockade is facilitated after administration of the larger "intubating" dose. Efficacy of the priming principle has been difficult to document, but some recommend its use based on the argument that little is lost and something can be gained.

MONITORING THE EFFECTS OF MUSCLE RELAXANTS

The most satisfactory and reliable method for monitoring effects of muscle relaxants at the neuromuscular junction is use of a peripheral nerve stimulator and visual observation of the mechanically evoked response produced by electrical stimulation. Most often electrodes or subcutaneous needles are placed over the ulnar nerve at the wrist or elbow, and a supramaximal electrical stimulation is delivered from the peripheral nerve stimulator (Fig. 8-7).[10] The adductor pollicis muscle is innervated solely by the ulnar nerve, accounting for the popularity of placing stimulating electrodes from the peripheral nerve stimulator over the ulnar nerve. Alternatively, the stimulating electrodes may be placed over the distribution of the facial nerve.

The four commonly used patterns of stimulation for monitoring neuromuscular blockade are single twitch, train-of-four, tetanus, and post-tetanic stimulation (Figs. 8-8 and 8-9).[10] These mechanically evoked responses are evaluated visually, by touch, or by recording. Depth of neuromuscular blockade may be defined as percent inhibition of twitch response and duration of blockade as the time from muscle relaxant administration until the twitch response recovers to a percent of control height (Tables 8-1, 8-4, and 8-5). Train-of-four

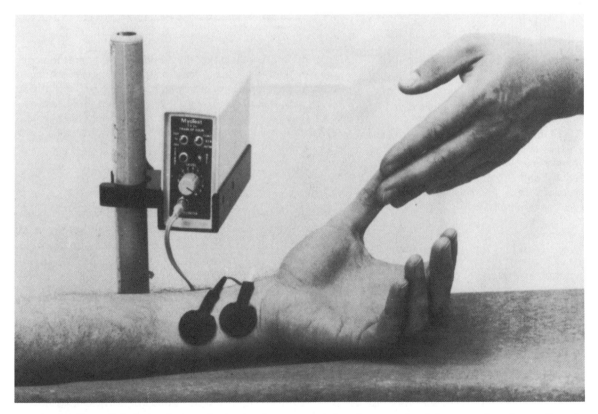

Fig. 8-7. Superficial stimulating electrodes from a peripheral nerve stimulator are placed over the ulnar nerve and the mechanical response evoked by electrical stimulation evaluated by touch or observation. (From Vigy-Mogensen,[10] with permission.)

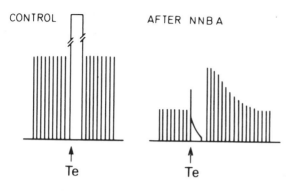

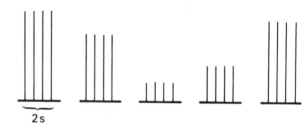

B/A = TOF-RATIO.

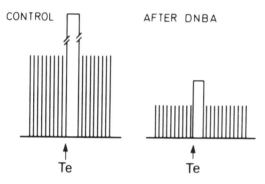

DEPOLARIZING NEUROMUSCULAR BLOCK

Fig. 8-8. A schematic illustration of the mechanically evoked response to tetanic and post-tetanic stimulation following injection of a nondepolarizing (upper panel, NNDA) and depolarizing (lower, panel, DNBA) muscle relaxant. Te = tetanic stimulation. (From Viby-Mogensen,[10] with permission.)

Fig. 8-9. A schematic illustration of the mechanically evoked response to train-of-four (TOF) nerve stimulation after injection of a nondepolarizing or depolarizing muscle relaxant. The train-of-four ratio (B/A) becomes less than 1 only in the presence of nondepolarizing neuromuscular blockade. (From Viby-Mogensen,[10] with permission.)

(four twitches at 2 Hz every 0.5 second) employs the concept that acetylcholine is depleted by successive stimulations. Only four twitches are necessary since additional stimulation fails to further alter release of additional acetylcholine. In the presence of nondepolarizing muscle relaxants, the height of the fourth twitch is less than the first twitch, allowing calculation of a train-of-four ratio (Fig. 8-9).[10] Recovery of the train-of-four ratio to greater than 0.7 correlates with complete return of a single twitch response. In the presence of depolarizing neuromuscular blockade, the train-of-four ratio remains near 1.0 as the height of all four responses are decreased a similar degree (Fig. 8-9).[10] A train-of-four ratio less than 0.3 in the presence of succinylcholine reflects phase II blockade (Table 8-1). Tetanus (continuous electrical stimulation for 5 seconds at about 50 Hz) is an intense stimulus for release of acetylcholine at the neuromuscular junction. In the presence of nondepolarizing muscle relaxants, the response to tetanus is not sustained (fades), whereas in the presence of succinylcholine the response is greatly reduced but does not fade (Fig. 8-8).[10] A sustained response to tetanic stimuli is present when the train-of-four ratio is greater than 0.7. At the end of tetanic stimuli, there is an increase in the immediately available store of acetylcholine such that subsequent twitch responses are transiently enhanced (post-tetanic facilitation).

Use of a peripheral nerve stimulator permits titration of muscle relaxant doses to produce optimal skeletal muscle relaxation. For example, greater than 90 percent depression of twitch response correlates with adequate skeletal muscle relaxation for intubation of the trachea or performance of intra-abdominal surgery in the presence of adequate concentrations or doses of anesthetic drugs. At the conclusion of surgery, responses evoked by the peripheral nerve stimulator are used to judge recovery from neuromuscular blockade that occurs spontaneously or after administration of anticholinesterases (see the section *Antagonism of Neuromuscular Blockade*). Attempts to judge recovery from the effects of muscle relaxants on clinical criteria (tidal volume, vital capacity, patient movement) without the aid of a peripheral nerve stimulator may result in failure to appreciate significant residual neuromuscular blockade (Table 8-6).[11] However, the most definitive indicator of no significant residual neuro-

muscular blockade is the head lift (i.e., the ability of a patient to lift the head for at least 5 seconds in the supine position).

ANTAGONISM OF NEUROMUSCULAR BLOCKADE

Pharmacologic antagonism of nondepolarizing muscle relaxants is achieved by the intravenous administration of anticholinesterases (edrophonium, neostigmine, or pyridostigmine) that inhibit the activity of acetylcholinesterase, leading to accumulation of acetylcholine at nicotinic (neuromuscular junction) and muscarinic sites (Table 8-7)[12] (see Chapter 3). The quaternary ammonium structure of these drugs greatly limits their entrance into the central nervous system such that selective antagonism of the effects of nondepolarizing muscle relaxants at the neuromuscular junction is possible. The peripheral cardiac muscarinic effects (bradycardia) of anticholinesterases are attenuated or prevented by the simultaneous intravenous administration of atropine or glycopyrrolate (Table 8-7).[12] If glycopyrrolate is given simultaneously with edrophonium, an initial bradycardia is likely due to the more rapid onset

Table 8-6. Comparison of Tests of Neuromuscular Function

Test	Estimated Receptors Occupied (%)	Disadvantages
Tidal volume	80	Insensitive
Twitch height	75–80	Insensitive, uncomfortable
Tetanic stimulation (30 Hz)	75–80	Insensitive, uncomfortable
Vital capacity	75–80	Insensitive, need patient cooperation
Train-of-four	75–80	Modestly sensitive
Tetanic stimulation (100 Hz)	50	Very painful
Inspiratory force	50	Difficult to perform especially in absence of tracheal tube
Head lift/hand grip	33	Need patient cooperation

Table 8-7. Comparative Effects of Anticholinesterases

	Edrophonium	Neostigmine	Pyridostigmine
Reversal dose (mg·kg^{-1})	0.5–1	.035–.070	0.15–0.35
Speed of onset	Rapid	Intermediate	Delayed
Duration (minutes)	60	60	90
Renal contribution to total clearance (percent)	66	54	76
Dose of atropine (μg·kg^{-1})^a	7	15	15
Dose of glycopyrrolate (μg·kg^{-1})^a	Not recommended	7	7

^{a} Administered simultaneously with anticholinesterase.

of action of edrophonium. Atropine with a more rapid onset of action is administered simultaneously with edrophonium. Furthermore, the dose of atropine is reduced when edrophonium is administered as it is less likely than neostigmine or pyridostigmine to cause bradycardia. Although edrophonium has a more rapid onset of action than does neostigmine or pyridostigmine, it may not be as effective as the other drugs when antagonism of an intense blockade (greater than 90 percent twitch depression) is required (Table 8-7).[10]

Antagonism of nondepolarizing muscle relaxants should not be initiated in the absence of a detectable twitch response. If an anticholinesterase is administered when only the first response in the train-of-four is present or twitch height is less than 5 percent of control, 15 minutes to 30 minutes will be required before twitch height reaches preblock height or the train-of-four ratio is greater than 0.7. If all four twitches from train-of-four stimulation can be felt, even though the ratio may be very low, reversal of neuromuscular blockade can usually be achieved in less than 10 minutes.

In the postoperative period, a peripheral nerve stimulator can be used in the differential diagnosis of a patient who is complaining of dyspnea. If the train-of-four ratio is greater than 0.7 and there is an absence of fade in response to tetanic stimulation or if head lift can be maintained for 5 seconds, it is unlikely that residual neuromuscular blockade is responsible for the patient's symptoms.

When the initial response to anticholinesterases seems inadequate, the following questions should be answered before additional antagonist drugs are administered:

1. Has enough time elapsed for the anticholinesterase to antagonize the muscle relaxant (15 minutes to 30 minutes)?
2. Is the degree of neuromuscular blockade too intense to be antagonized?
3. Is the acid-base and electrolyte status normal?
4. Is body temperature normal?
5. Is the patient receiving any drugs that may interfere with antagonism?
6. Has clearance of the muscle relaxant from the plasma been reduced by renal and/or hepatic dysfunction?

Answers to these questions will often provide the reason for failure of anticholinesterases to antagonize a nondepolarizing neuromuscular blockade.

REFERENCES

1. Drachman DA. Myasthenia gravis. N Engl J Med 1978;298:136–42.
2. Taylor P. Are neuromuscular blocking agents more efficacious in pairs? Anesthesiology 1985;63:1–3.
3. Lee C. Dose relationship of phase II, tachyphylaxis and train-of-four fade on suxamethonium-induced dual neuromuscular block in man. Br J Anaesth 1975;47:841–5.

4. Gronert GA, Theye RA. Pathophysiology of hyperkalemia induced by succinylcholine. Anesthesiology 1975;43:89–99.

5. Miller RD, Way WL, Hamilton WK. Succinylcholine-induced hyperkalemia in patients with renal failure? Anesthesiology 1972;36:138–41.

6. Libonati MM, Leahy JJ, Ellison N. The use of succinylcholine in open eye surgery. Anesthesiology 1985;62:637–40.

7. Stoelting RK. Pharmacology and Physiology in Anesthetic Practice. Philadelphia, JB Lippincott, 1987;169–216.

8. Savarese JJ, Ali HH, Basta SJ, et al. The clinical neuromuscular pharmacology of mivacurium chloride (BW 109OU). A short-acting nondepolarizing ester neuromuscular blocking drug. Anesthesiology 1988;68:723–32.

9. Ali HH, Savarese JJ. Monitoring of neuromuscular function. Anesthesiology 1976;45:216–49.

10. Viby-Mogensen J. Clinical assessment of neuromuscular transmission. Br J Anaesth 1982;54:209–23.

11. Viby-Mogensen J, Chraemmer-Jorgensen B, Ording H. Residual curarization in the recovery room. Anesthesiology 1979;50:539–41.

12. Cronnelly R, Morris RB. Antagonism of neuromuscular blockade. Br J Anaesth 1982;54:183–94.

Section III

Preoperative Preparation and Intraoperative Management

Chapter 9

Preoperative Evaluation and Choice of Technique of Anesthesia

Preoperative evaluation and preparation for anesthesia begins when the anesthesiologist reviews the patient's medical record and visits with the patient, ideally the day before elective surgery. Important aspects of the preoperative evaluation performed by the anesthesiologist include a history, review of current drug therapy, and a physical examination. Another important aspect of this preoperative visit is to inform the patient and other interested adults about events to expect on the day of surgery. The planned management of anesthesia and methods available for relief of postoperative pain are discussed with the patient, and informed consent is obtained. Indeed, the patient or guardian must sign a consent statement authorizing the administration of anesthesia. Informed consent does not require that the anesthesiologist describe to the patient remote risks associated with the administration of anesthesia, as this would serve only to alarm a patient who is most likely already apprehensive. The anesthesiologist should describe, however, specific potential complications if an unusual technique or drug is to be employed or if the physical condition of the patient makes adverse responses likely, such as dislodgement of loose or diseased teeth during direct laryngoscopy. The apprehension-allaying effect on the patient produced by the anesthesiologist's preoperative visit is an important aspect of preoperative medication (see Chapter 10).

After the preoperative visit, a summary of pertinent findings, including details of the history, current drug therapy, physical examination, and laboratory data, should be written in the patient's medical record. In addition, a physical status classification is assigned, and the technique of anesthesia that has been discussed with the patient is detailed. Specific potential complications associated with the administration of anesthesia that have been described to the patient should be noted. Finally, orders for the preoperative medication are written (see Chapter 10).

On occasion, based on the preoperative evaluation, it may be the anesthesiologist's opinion that the patient is not in optimal medical condition before elective surgery. This judgment should be discussed with the patient's primary physician and, if necessary, elective surgery deferred until the patient's medical condition improves. When surgery is urgent, however, the benefits of immediate treatment offset the hazards introduced by less than optimal medical preparation, and the surgery is not delayed.

HISTORY

The history obtained preoperatively should include details relating to previous anesthetics experienced by the patient or relatives as well as a careful review of organ system function as altered

---

Perioperative Events that Should be Discussed with the Patient Preoperatively

Preoperative insomnia and medication available for its treatment

Time, route of administration, and expected effects from the preoperative medication

Time of anticipated transport to operating room for surgery

Anticipated duration of surgery

Awakening after surgery in the recovery room

Likely presence of catheters on awakening (tracheal, gastric, bladder, venous, arterial)

Time of expected return to hospital room after surgery

Incidence of postoperative nausea and vomiting, pharyngitis, myalgia

Magnitude of postoperative discomfort and methods available for its treatment

---

Table 9-1. Specific Areas to Investigate in Preoperative History

Previous adverse responses related to anesthesia
  Allergic reactions
  Prolonged skeletal muscle paralysis
  Delayed awakening
  Nausea and vomiting
  Hoarseness
  Myalgia
  Hemorrhage
  Jaundice
  Postspinal headache
  Adverse responses in relatives
Central nervous system
  Cerebrovascular insufficiency
  Seizures
Cardiovascular system
  Exercise tolerance
  Angina pectoris
  Prior myocardial infarction
  Hypertension
  Rheumatic fever
  Claudication
  Tachydysrhythmias
Lungs
  Exercise tolerance
  Dyspnea and orthopnea
  Cough and sputum production
  Bronchial asthma
  Cigarette consumption
  Pneumonia
  Recent upper respiratory tract infection
Liver
  Ethanol consumption
  Hepatitis
Kidneys
  Nocturia
  Pyuria
Skeletal and muscular systems
  Arthritis
  Osteoporosis
  Weakness
Endocrine system
  Diabetes mellitus
  Thyroid gland dysfunction
  Adrenal gland dysfunction
Coagulation
  Bleeding tendency
  Easy bruising
  Hereditary coagulopathies
Reproductive system
  Menstrual history
  Sexually transmitted diseases
Dentition
  Dentures
  Caps

---

by co-existing diseases (Table 9-1). Co-existing diseases that influence the management of anesthesia may be related to the reason for surgery. Adverse events related to previous anesthetics should be specifically sought. Questions relating to major organ system function serve to elicit the presence and impact of co-existing diseases. The reader should consult specific sections of subsequent chapters for detailed discussions of the importance of co-existing diseases in the management of anesthesia.

A history of chronic atopy (asthma, food sensitivities, hay fever, drug allergies) may reflect a genetic predisposition to form immunoglobulin E antibodies against antigens as possibly represented by drugs administered intravenously during the perioperative period. Other than recognizing the possible increased likelihood of allergic reactions, however, there is no need to alter the drugs selected for administration during anesthesia to such patients. Certainly, a preoperative history of allergy to a specific drug mandates avoidance of that drug or the same class of drugs unless the anesthesiologist can be convinced the symptoms described by the patient do not represent an allergic reaction. Should an unexpected allergic reaction occur during the perioperative period, it is important to document the responsible drug (often several drugs have been administered in a narrow time frame) for the future safety of the patient.

CURRENT DRUG THERAPY

Current drug therapy must be carefully reviewed during the preoperative evaluation because adverse interactions of these medications with drugs administered in the perioperative period must be considered. For example, current drug therapy can alter anesthetic requirements (minimum alveolar concentration [MAC]) for volatile drugs, potentiate muscle relaxants, exaggerate responses to sympathomimetics, reduce peripheral sympathetic nervous system activity, or enhance or impair the metabolism of drugs (Table 9-2).[1–7] The reader should consult Chapters 3, 5, and 8 for detailed discussions of these drug interactions. Potential drug interactions, however, do not dictate the need to discontinue preoperatively drugs that are producing desirable therapeutic responses. Indeed, drug therapy (antihypertensives, antianginal drugs, digitalis, diuretics, anticonvulsants, hormone replacement) should be continued throughout the perioperative period. Nevertheless, the safety of maintaining current drug therapy is based on the anesthesiologist's awareness of potential adverse drug interactions and appropriate modifications in perioperative selection of drugs and doses, as well as techniques of monitoring.

PHYSICAL EXAMINATION

The physical examination performed by the anesthesiologist is primarily directed toward the cardiovascular system, lungs, and upper airway. Blood pressure obtained in the supine and standing position; heart rate and its regularity; and auscultation for cardiac murmurs, carotid artery bruits, and the presence of abnormal breath sounds, such as rales or expiratory wheezing, are part of the usual physical examination performed by the anesthesiologist. It is particularly important to listen

Table 9-2. Current Drug Therapy and Potential Interactions with Drugs Administered in the Perioperative Period

Increase anesthetic requirements (MAC) for volatile drugs
    Monoamine oxidase inhibitors
    Tricyclic antidepressants (?)
    Chronic ethanol abuse
    Acute dextroamphetamine
    Acute cocaine

Decrease anesthetic requirements (MAC) for volatile drugs
    Acute ethanol intoxication
    Alpha methyldopa
    Clonidine
    Chronic amphetamine
    Verapamil
    Cimetidine (?)

Potentiate neuromuscular blockers
    Magnesium
    Aminoglycoside antibiotics
    Lidocaine
    Quinidine
    Lithium

Exaggerate response to sympathomimetics
    Monoamine oxidase inhibitors
    Tricyclic antidepressants

Reduce peripheral sympathetic nervous system activity
    Alpha methyldopa
    Guanethidine
    Clonidine
    Propranolol or other beta-adrenergic antagonists

Enhance metabolism
    Barbiturates
    Phenytoin
    Chronic ethanol abuse
    Corticosteroids
    Isoniazid

Impair metabolism
    Monoamine oxidase inhibitors
    Disulfiram
    Echothiophate
    Organophosphates (insecticides)

for the murmur of aortic stenosis (systolic murmur at the right sternal border maximum in the second intercostal space) because patients with this valvular abnormality may be asymptomatic but vulnerable to unexpected cardiac dysrhythmias or adverse reductions in stroke volume should blood pressure, heart rate, or systemic vascular resistance change abruptly during anesthesia and surgery. The presence of orthostatic hypotension may reflect previously unrecognized hypovolemia or drug-induced impairment of peripheral sympathetic nervous system activity (see Chapters 3 and 18).

Physical characteristics of the patient that could make management of the airway difficult, such as obesity, short neck, limited temporomandibular and/or cervical spine mobility, and prominent central incisors, should be appreciated at this time (see Chapter 12). Availability of peripheral venous sites, including the external jugular veins, should be noted. The adequacy of collateral blood flow probably should be determined if the plan is to insert an arterial catheter in the perioperative period (see Chapter 16). It may be important to evaluate the effect of operative position on circulation. For example, extending or turning the head may not be tolerated in the presence of carotid or vertebral artery occlusive disease. Furthermore, patient immobility due to arthritis may limit positioning of the arms and/or legs during surgery. Finally, if regional anesthesia is planned, it is essential to inspect the likely site of local anesthetic injection for any anatomic abnormalities or signs of infection.

LABORATORY DATA

Many hospitals and departments of anesthesia have specific rules regarding which tests should or must be performed on all patients before anesthesia for elective surgery. Ideally, however, only those laboratory tests indicated on the basis of positive findings elicited during the history and physical examination of the patient should be ordered.[8] Likewise, the age of the patient and complexity of the planned operation should be considered in determining which laboratory tests must be undertaken preoperatively. Nevertheless, because patients frequently enter the hospital the evening before or morning of surgery, it has become common to order routine laboratory screening tests before the history and physical examination and regardless of the age of the patient or complexity of the planned surgery.

Hemoglobin Concentration

Routine determination of the hemoglobin concentration (or hematocrit) is indicated before anesthesia for elective surgery. It is difficult to justify

---

> **Examples of Laboratory Screening Tests Frequently Ordered Prior to Anesthesia for Elective Surgery**
>
> Hemoglobin concentration
> Blood chemistries
>   Blood glucose
>   Blood urea nitrogen
>   Serum glutamic oxalacetic transaminase
>   Serum potassium
> Coagulation studies
>   Prothrombin time
>   Plasma thromboplastin time
> Urinalysis
> Electrocardiogram
> Radiograph of the chest
> Pulmonary function studies
>   Arterial blood gases and pH
>   Forced exhaled volume in 1 second (FEV_1)
>   Vital capacity (VC)
> FEV_1/VC
>   Maximum breathing capacity

---

proceeding with an elective operation in the presence of anemia (hemoglobin less than 10 $g \cdot dl^{-1}$) due to an unknown cause discovered preoperatively by the measurement of the hemoglobin concentration. Nevertheless, no data confirm that treatment of moderate normovolemic anemia in the preoperative period leads to a decrease in perioperative morbidity or mortality.[8] Perhaps the duration of anemia is also important, for with time the cardiovascular system adjusts to the reduced concentration of hemoglobin by increasing the cardiac output so as to maintain tissue oxygen delivery despite reduced oxygen carrying capacity of the blood.

In contrast to anemia, there is evidence that the preoperative presence of polycythemia is associated with adverse perioperative events such as hemorrhage and/or thrombosis. Furthermore, the presence of unexpected polycythemia may be a clue preoperatively to the unexpected existence of chronic arterial hypoxemia or depletion of intravascular fluid volume related to diuretic therapy.

Blood Chemistries

Routine blood chemistry screening tests (SMA-12), in the absence of positive findings in the history or physical examination, reveal unexpected abnormal findings in about 2.5 percent of patients under 40 years of age. This incidence of unexpected abnormal findings increases to about 7.5 percent in patients over 60 years of age. About 70 percent of the unexpected abnormal findings are related to measurement of the blood glucose concentration and blood urea nitrogen concentration. Based on these data, the recommendation is to measure the blood glucose concentration and blood urea concentration before anesthesia for elective surgery even in the absence of positive findings in the history and physical examination.[8]

Determination of the serum glutamic oxalacetic transaminase concentration as a routine screening test for the detection of unexpected hepatocellular disease can be considered for adult patients. Indeed, about 1 in 750 otherwise healthy adults manifest unexpected abnormal liver function tests preoperatively, and one in three of these patients will subsequently become jaundiced.[9]

Serum potassium concentration should be measured routinely before anesthesia for elective surgery if the patient has been receiving chronic diuretic therapy.

Coagulation Studies

In the absence of positive findings in the history or physical examination suggesting the possibility of abnormal coagulation, the routine performance of prothrombin time and partial thromboplastin time before anesthesia for elective surgery is not necessary.

Urinalysis

Routine urinalysis as a screen before anesthesia for elective surgery offers little or no new information and in many respects only duplicates the blood chemistry measurements.

Electrocardiogram (ECG)

In the absence of positive findings in the history and physical examination, a routine resting ECG before anesthesia for elective surgery is not nec-

---

Unexpected Abnormalities Detected on a Preoperative Electrocardiogram

Atrial fibrillation
Atrioventricular heart block
ST–T changes suggestive of myocardial ischemia
Atrial premature contractions
Ventricular premature beats
Left or right ventricular hypertrophy
Prolonged Q–T interval
Tall peaked T waves
Evidence of preexcitation syndrome
Evidence of a prior myocardial infarction

---

essary in patients less than 40 years of age.[8] This recommendation assumes that careful observation of the ECG will take place in the operating room before the induction of anesthesia. Indeed, most if not all the important abnormalities that might alter the management of anesthesia should be recognizable on a single lead ECG as routinely observed before the induction of anesthesia. After 40 years of age, a routine ECG before anesthesia for elective surgery is recommended.

Radiography of the Chest

A routine radiograph of the chest before anesthesia for elective surgery reveals unexpected abnormal findings in about 1.5 percent of patients under 40 years of age, in approximately 5 percent of patients 40 years to 60 years of age, and in 6 percent to 30 percent of patients over 60 years of age.[8] There is no reason, therefore, to obtain a routine preoperative chest radiograph in patients less than 40 years of age with no evidence of chest disease in the history and physical examination.

Pulmonary Function Tests

Pulmonary function tests are not necessary in the absence of positive findings in the history and physical examination of patients undergoing elective surgery that does not involve the chest. Conversely, pulmonary function tests are useful in the preoperative preparation and subsequent intra-

---

Unexpected Abnormalities Detected on a Preoperative Radiograph of the Chest

Tracheal deviation
Mediastinal masses
Pulmonary masses
Pulmonary blebs
Aortic aneurysm
Pulmonary edema
Pneumonia
Atelectasis
Fractures of the ribs or vertebrae
Cardiomegaly
Dextrocardia

---

operative and postoperative management of patients with evidence of pulmonary disease and undergoing upper abdominal or intrathoracic operations (see Chapter 20).

PHYSICAL STATUS CLASSIFICATION

Assignment of a physical status classification (Class 1 through 5) is based on the physical condition of the patient independent of the planned operation (Table 9-3).[10] It is important to recognize that the physical status classification is not intended to represent an estimate of anesthetic risk. Instead, the physical status classification serves as a "common language" among different institutions for subsequent examination of anesthetic morbidity and mortality. Not surprisingly, intraoperative cardiac arrest is more frequent in the poor physical status classification, particularly if emergency surgery is necessary.

TECHNIQUES OF ANESTHESIA

After the preoperative evaluation, the anesthesiologist selects as the technique of anesthesia either a general anesthetic, regional anesthetic (see Chapter 13), or peripheral nerve block (see Chapter 14). The technique of anesthesia is determined by several considerations. In many instances, more than one technique of anesthesia may be accepta-

Table 9-3. Physical Status Classification of the American Society of Anesthesiologists (ASA)

Status	Disease State
ASA Class 1	No organic, physiologic, biochemical, or psychiatric disturbance
ASA Class 2	Mild to moderate systemic disturbance that may or may not be related to the reason for surgery
	Examples: Heart disease that only slightly limits physical activity, essential hypertension, diabetes mellitus, anemia, extremes of age, morbid obesity, chronic bronchitis
ASA Class 3	Severe systemic disturbance that may or may not be related to the reason for surgery
	Examples: Heart disease that limits activity, poorly controlled essential hypertension, diabetes mellitus with vascular complications, chronic pulmonary disease that limits activity, angina pectoris, history of prior myocardial infarction
ASA Class 4	Severe systemic disturbance that is life-threatening with or without surgery
	Examples: Congestive heart failure, persistent angina pectoris, advanced pulmonary, renal, or hepatic dysfunction
ASA Class 5	Moribund patient who has little chance of survival but is submitted to surgery as a last resort (resuscitative effort)
	Examples: Uncontrolled hemorrhage as from a ruptured abdominal aneurysm, cerebral trauma, pulmonary embolus
Emergency Operation (E)	Any patient in whom an emergency operation is required
	Example: An otherwise healthy 30-year-old woman who requires a dilation and curettage for moderate but persistent hemorrhage (ASA Class 1 E)

(From information in American Society of Anesthesiologists.[10])

ble. It is the responsibility of the anesthesiologist to evaluate the medical condition and unique needs of each patient and to select an appropriate technique of anesthesia.

General Anesthetic

Induction of general anesthesia is most often accomplished by the intravenous administration of a drug such as thiopental that produces the rapid onset of unconsciousness (see Chapter 6). Commonly, succinylcholine is also administered intravenously shortly after the induction drug to produce skeletal muscle relaxation so as to facilitate direct laryngoscopy for intubation of the trachea. The injection of drugs to produce unconsciousness followed immediately by succinylcholine is referred to as a "rapid sequence induction." Frequently, the patient is breathing oxygen via a mask (preoxygenation) before a rapid sequence induction. A typical rapid sequence induction includes preoxygenation, the intravenous administration of a defasiculating dose of a nondepolarizing muscle relaxant (d-tubocurarine 3 mg to 5 mg) followed 1 minute to 3 minutes later by thiopental (3 $mg \cdot kg^{-1}$ to 5 $mg \cdot kg^{-1}$) and succinylcholine (1 $mg \cdot kg^{-1}$ to 2 $mg \cdot kg^{-1}$). Direct laryngoscopy for intubation of the trachea may be initiated about 60 seconds after intravenous administration of succinylcholine. Preoxygenation minimizes the likelihood of arterial hypoxemia developing during the period of apnea necessary for insertion of

the tracheal tube. Alternatively, a nondepolarizing muscle relaxant can be substituted for succinylcholine, realizing that the onset of skeletal muscle paralysis that is considered ideal for intubation of the trachea may be delayed compared with the rapid onset of relaxation produced by succinylcholine. After intubation of the trachea, it may be prudent to insert a gastric tube through the mouth to decompress the stomach and remove any easily accessible fluid. This orogastric tube should be removed at the conclusion of anesthesia. When gastric suction is needed postoperatively, the tube should be inserted through the nares rather than the mouth.

An alternative to the rapid sequence induction of anesthesia is the inhalation of nitrous oxide plus a volatile anesthetic with or without the prior intravenous administration of a "sleep dose" of an induction drug (see Chapter 6). This is referred to as an "inhalation or mask induction." An inhalation induction is often employed in pediatric patients, particularly when prior insertion of a venous catheter is not practical. When an inhalation induction of anesthesia is selected, a depolarizing or nondepolarizing muscle relaxant is administered intravenously when it is deemed appropriate to intubate the trachea. Alternatively, skeletal muscle relaxation produced by the volatile anesthetic can be used to facilitate intubation of the trachea. Finally, it may be the decision of the anesthesiologist not to place a tube in the trachea, and anesthesia is then maintained by inhalation via a mask.

The objectives of maintenance of general anesthesia are analgesia, unconsciousness, skeletal muscle relaxation, and control of sympathetic nervous system responses evoked by noxious stimulation. These objectives are achieved most often by the use of a combination of drugs that may include inhaled and/or injected anesthetics with or without muscle relaxants. Each drug selected should be administered on the basis of a specific goal that is relevant to that drug's known pharmacologic effects at therapeutic doses. For example, it is not logical to administer high concentrations of volatile anesthetics to produce skeletal muscle relaxation when muscle relaxants are specific for achieving this goal. Likewise, it is not acceptable to obscure skeletal muscle movement due to insufficient doses of anesthetics by administering excessive amounts of muscle relaxants. The selective use of drugs for their specific effect permits the anesthesiologist to tailor the anesthetic to the patient's medical condition and any unique needs introduced by the surgery.

Despite its lack of potency, nitrous oxide is the most frequently administered inhaled anesthetic. Typically, nitrous oxide (50 percent to 70 percent inhaled concentration) is administered in combination with volatile anesthetics or opioids. It is important to remember that it is the partial pressure of an inhaled anesthetic (nitrous oxide, halothane, enflurane, isoflurane) that produces its pharmacologic effect. For example, 60 percent inhaled nitrous oxide administered at sea level exerts a partial pressure of 456 mmHg (60 percent of the total barometric pressure of 760 mmHg). The same inhaled concentration of nitrous oxide (or a volatile anesthetic) administered at an altitude where the barometric pressure is less than 760 mmHg exerts a reduced pharmacologic effect because the partial pressure of the anesthetic that can be achieved in the brain is less.

Volatile anesthetics have the advantage of high potency and they can be readily controlled in terms of the concentration delivered from the anesthetic machine, allowing titration of the dose to produce a desired response. Excessive sympathetic nervous system responses evoked by noxious stimulation are predictably attenuated by volatile anesthetics. Dose-dependent cardiac depression is a major disadvantage of volatile anesthetics (see Chapter 4). Indeed, a volatile drug is seldom administered as the sole anesthetic, but instead these drugs are more often administered in combination with nitrous oxide. Substitution of nitrous oxide for a portion of the dose of the volatile anesthetic allows a reduction in the delivered concentration of the volatile drug, which results in less cardiac depression despite the same total dose of anesthetic drugs (see Chapter 4).

In certain instances, it is acceptable to administer muscle relaxants to assure lack of patient movement and to permit a decrease in the delivered concentration of volatile anesthetics. This use of muscle relaxants, however, must not be interpreted as an endorsement for the administration of an inadequate dose of anesthetic that is obscured by skeletal muscle paralysis. Indeed, intraoperative awareness is a constant fear and risk of light anesthesia, especially when patient movement is obscured by muscle relaxant induced paralysis.

Opioids that generally do not depress the cardiovascular system are combined most often with nitrous oxide (see Chapter 6). In patients with normal left ventricular function, however, the lack of opioid-induced cardiovascular depression and absence of attenuation of sympathetic nervous system reflexes may lead to elevated blood pressure. When this occurs, the addition of low concentrations of volatile anesthetics to the delivered gases is often effective in returning the elevated blood pressure to acceptable levels. Muscle relaxants are often necessary even in the absence of the need for skeletal muscle relaxation because adequate doses of opioids with nitrous oxide are unlikely to prevent patient movement in response to painful stimulation. Another disadvantage of injected drugs compared with inhaled anesthetics is the inability to accurately titrate and maintain a therapeutic concentration of the injected drug. This disadvantage can be offset to some extent by continuous intravenous infusion of the injected anesthetic at a rate previously determined in other patients to be associated with therapeutic concentrations in the blood.

The methods and equipment necessary for accurate administration of inhaled gases and the vapors of volatile anesthetics are described in Chapter 11.

Regional Anesthetic

A regional anesthetic (spinal, epidural, caudal) is selected when maintenance of consciousness during surgery is desirable (see Chapter 13). Skeletal muscle relaxation and contraction of the gastrointestinal tract are also produced by a regional anesthetic. Patients may have preconceived and inaccurate conceptions about regional anesthesia that will require the anesthesiologist to reassure them about the safety of this technique. A regional anesthetic should not be performed against the wishes of the patient. Disadvantages of this technique of anesthesia include the occasional failure to produce adequate anesthesia for the surgical stimulus and the reduction in blood pressure that accompanies the peripheral sympathetic nervous system blockade produced by the regional anesthetic, particularly in the presence of hypovolemia.

A regional anesthetic technique is most often selected for surgery that involves the lower abdomen or lower extremities in which the level of sensory anesthesia required is associated with minimal sympathetic nervous system blockade. This should not imply that a general anesthetic is an unacceptable technique for similar types of surgery.

Peripheral Nerve Blocks

Peripheral nerve blocks are most appropriate as a technique of anesthesia for superficial operations on the extremities (see Chapter 14). Advantages of peripheral nerve blocks include maintenance of consciousness and continued presence of protective upper airway reflexes. The isolated anesthetic effect produced by peripheral nerve blocks is particularly attractive in patients with chronic pulmonary disease, severe cardiac impairment, or inadequate renal function. For example, insertion of a vascular shunt in the upper extremity for hemodialysis in a patient who often has associated pulmonary and cardiac disease is often accomplished with anesthesia provided by peripheral nerve block of the brachial plexus. Likewise, the avoidance of the need for muscle relaxants in this type of patient circumvents the possible prolonged effect produced by these drugs in the absence of renal function.

A disadvantage of peripheral nerve blocks as a technique of anesthesia is the unpredictable attainment of adequate sensory and motor anesthesia for performance of the surgery. The success rate of peripheral nerve blocks is often inversely related to the frequency with which the anesthesiologist employs this technique of anesthesia. Finally, patients must be cooperative for a peripheral nerve block to be effective. For example, acutely intoxicated and agitated patients are not ideal candidates for peripheral nerve blocks.

Table 9-4. Routine Preparation Before Induction of Anesthesia Regardless of Technique of Anesthesia Selected

Anesthetic machine
 Attach an anesthetic breathing system with a proper-sized face mask
 Occlude the patient end of the anesthetic breathing system and fill with oxygen from the anesthetic machine ("flush valve"). Applying manual pressure to the distended reservoir bag checks for leaks in the anesthetic breathing system and confirms the ability to provide positive pressure ventilation of the patient's lungs with oxygen.
 Check anesthetic breathing system valves
 Calibrate oxygen analyzer with air and oxygen and set alarm
 Check soda lime for color changes
 Check liquid level and content of vaporizers
 Confirm function of mechanical ventilator
 Confirm availability and function of wall suction
 Check final position of all flowmeter, vaporizer, and monitor (alarm) settings
Drugs
 Local anesthetic (lidocaine)
 Barbiturate (thiopental, thiamylal, or methohexital)
 Anticholinergic (atropine)
 Sympathomimetic (ephedrine, phenylephrine)
 Depolarizing muscle relaxant (succinylcholine)
 Nondepolarizing muscle relaxants (d-tubocurarine, pancuronium, atracurium, or vecuronium)
 Anticholinesterase (pyridostigmine, neostigmine, or edrophonium)
 Opioid antagonist (naloxone)
 Catecholamine to treat an allergic reaction (epinephrine)
Equipment
 Intravenous solution and connecting tubing
 Intracath or extracath for vascular cannulation
 Suction catheter
 Oral and/or nasal airway
 Laryngoscope
 Tracheal tube
 Nasogastric tube

PREPARATION FOR ANESTHESIA

Preparation for anesthesia after the preoperative medication has been administered and the patient is transported to the operating room is similar regardless of the technique of anesthesia that has been selected (Table 9-4). Upon arrival in the operating room, the patient is identified and the scheduled surgery reconfirmed. The nurse's notes are consulted by the anesthesiologist to learn of any unexpected changes in the patient's medical condition, vital signs, or body temperature and to determine that the preoperative medication has been administered. Likewise, any laboratory data that have become available since the anesthesiologist's prior visit should be reviewed.

Initial preparation for anesthesia, regardless of the technique of anesthesia selected, begins with insertion of a catheter in a peripheral vein and application of a blood pressure cuff. This initial preparation may be accomplished in a holding area or in the operating room. Use of separate rooms (induction rooms) distinct from the operating room for induction of anesthesia is not recommended by some because of the questionable safety of routinely moving anesthetized patients with the necessary attached equipment from one area to another. An exception to this recommendation may be the performance of peripheral nerve blocks in a holding area, thus allowing the block to be in place when the operating room becomes available. Monitors such as the pulse oximeter, ECG, peripheral nerve stimulator, and chest stethoscope are also applied while the patient is still awake. Immediately before the induction of anesthesia baseline vital signs (blood pressure, heart rate, cardiac rhythm, arterial oxygen saturation, breathing rate) are recorded.

Regardless of the technique of anesthesia selected, the anesthetic machine is present and functional and specific drugs and equipment are always immediately available (Table 9-4). It is mandatory to be able to suction the patient's pharynx followed by ventilation of the lungs with oxygen via cuffed tube placed in the trachea.

PROFESSIONAL LIABILITY

The anesthesiologist is responsible for the management of and recovery from anesthesia. Physicians administering anesthetics are not expected to guarantee a favorable outcome to the patient but are required to exercise ordinary or reasonable care or skill compared with other anesthesiologists.

That the anticipated result does not follow or that complications occur does not imply negligence. Furthermore, an anesthesiologist is not responsible for an error in judgment unless it is so gross as to be inconsistent with the skill expected of every physician. As a specialist, however, an anesthesiologist is responsible for making medical judgments that are consistent with national, not local, standards. Anesthesiologists carry professional liability (malpractice) insurance that provides financial protection should a court judgment against them occur.

A certified registered nurse anesthetist can be held legally responsible for the technical aspects of the administration of anesthesia. It is likely, however, that legal responsibilities for the actions of the nurse will be shared by the physician responsible for supervising the administration of anesthesia. If an anesthesiologist employs the nurse or advises the hospital as to the qualifications or conditions of employment, the anesthesiologist may be held responsible for the nurse's actions even though not directly concerned in supervision at the time of an alleged act of negligence.

Medical students and resident physicians are not immune to court action and should be protected by professional liability insurance in the same manner as the anesthesiologist or certified nurse anesthetist. Insurance coverage for the medical student or resident physician is most often provided by the institution that provides the course for credit for the medical student or who employs the resident physician.

An estimated 20 million anesthetics are administered annually in the United States. The risk of mortality due solely to the administration of anesthesia is extremely rare (about 1 in 10,000 administrations or 0.01 percent).[11] For the relatively healthy patient having a simple elective operation, the risk is even less, perhaps in the range of 1 in 50,000 to 100,000 anesthetic administrations. Regardless of the risk of anesthesia, it is estimated that 50 percent to 75 percent of anesthetic-related deaths are preventable. When adverse events do occur, it is often difficult to establish the exact mechanism. In many instances, it is impossible to separate an adverse event due to an inappropriate action of the anesthesiologist ("lapse of vigilance") from an unavoidable mishap (coincidental event) despite optimal care.[12-14] Although anesthetic medical liability claims make up only about 3 percent to 4 percent of the total in medicine, the indemnity paid exceeds 10 percent, emphasizing the severity of the associated injuries. Common mechanisms of avoidable adverse events include unrecognized (1) inadequate ventilation of the lungs, (2) esophageal intubation, (3) extubation of the trachea, (4) ventilator disconnects, and (5) relative or absolute drug overdoses. It is hoped that improved monitoring of anesthetized patients will serve to further enhance the vigilance of the anesthesiologist and reduce the role of human error in anesthetic morbidity and mortality. At the same time, it is importance to recognize that not all adverse events during anesthesia are a result of human error and therefore preventable.

The Anesthesia Patient Safety Foundation, formed in 1985, is dedicated to providing a better understanding of preventable anesthetic injuries and encouraging programs and practices that will reduce the number of anesthetic injuries. In this regard, a newsletter is distributed in an attempt to promote information about patient safety during anesthesia and grants are available to fund relevant research projects. The board of directors of this foundation includes representatives from anesthesia, insurance companies, hospitals, biomedical engineering, pharmaceutical industry, and the federal government.

Most patients and/or families are understanding and are satisfied by frank discussion of problems related to administration of anesthesia. In the event of an accident or complication related to the administration of anesthesia, the anesthesiologist should immediately document the facts on the patient's medical record. Patient treatment should be noted and consultation with other physicians sought when appropriate. The anesthesiologist should provide the hospital and the company that holds the physician's professional liability insurance with a complete account of the incident. Should a lawsuit be threatened or legal inquiry be made concerning a patient, the anesthesiologist should immediately notify the insurance company and, when appropriate, seek legal assistance.

Malpractice is a theory arising from tort law. A tort is a civil (not criminal) wrong for which a patient can seek compensation through legal action for an alleged act of negligence of the anesthesiologist. The patient who claims injury obtains legal counsel and files a malpractice suit. Depositions are taken by attorneys for both sides to elicit plantiffs', defendants', and witnesses' opinions as to the facts of the event; a court hearing is arranged, usually with a jury present; and witnesses, including experts, for the defendant (physician) and plantiff (patient) give testimony. The judge explains the points of law to the jury, and the jury then makes a decision and recommendation of compensation for damages. This chain of events may be interrupted at any point. For example, the plaintiff may drop the suit, or the defendant may be advised by counsel to make a settlement. A settlement can be arranged with the aid of the judge at any time during the trial before the jury verdict. Indeed, about 80 percent of malpractice suits are settled out of court, and, of those that go to court trial, physicians win more than they lose.

The best protection for the anesthesiologist against medicolegal action lies in the thorough and up-to-date practice of anesthesia coupled with interest in the patient by virtue of preoperative and postoperative visits plus detailed records of the course of anesthesia.

REFERENCES

1. Tinker JH, Tarhan S. Discontinuing anticoagulant therapy in surgical patients with cardiac valve prosthesis. JAMA 1978;239:138–9.
2. Miller RD, Way WL, Eger EI II. The effects of alpha-methyldopa, reserpine, guanethidine, and iproniazid on minimum alveolar anesthetic requirement (MAC). Anesthesiology 1968;29:1153–8.
3. Ghoneim MM, Long JP. The interaction between magnesium and other neuromuscular blocking agents. Anesthesiology 1970;32:23–7.
4. Sokoll MD, Gergis SD. Antibiotics and neuromuscular function. Anesthesiology 1981;55:148–59.
5. Edwards RP, Miller RD, Roizen MF, et al. Cardiac responses to imipramine and pancuronium during anesthesia with halothane or enflurane. Anesthesiology 1979;50:421–5.
6. El-Ganzouri AR, Ivankovich AD, Braverman B, McCarthy R. Monoamine oxidase inhibitors: Should

they be discontinued preoperatively? Anesth Analg 1985;64:592–6.

7. Rao TLK, El-Etr AA. Anticoagulation following placement of epidural and subarachnoid catheters. Anesthesiology 1981;55:618–20.

8. Roizen MF. Routine preoperative evaluation. In: Miller RD, ed. Anesthesia. 2nd Ed. New York, Churchill Livingstone, 1986;225–54.

9. Schemel WH. Unexpected hepatic dysfuncion found by multiple laboratory screening. Anesth Analg 1976;55:810–2

10. American Society of Anesthesiologists. New classification of physical status. Anesthesiology 1963;24:111.

11. Deaths during general anesthesia J Health Care Technol 1985;1:155–75.

12. Hamilton WK. Unexpected deaths during anesthesia: Wherein lies the cause? Anesthesiology 1979;7:25–32.

13. Keats AS. What do we know about anesthetic mortality? Anesthesiology 1979;50:387–92.

14. Keats AS. Anesthesia mortality—a new mechanism. Anesthesiology 1988;68:2–4.

Chapter 10

Preoperative Medication

Management of anesthesia begins with the preoperative psychological preparation of the patient and administration of a drug or drugs selected to elicit specific pharmacologic responses. This initial psychological and pharmacologic component of anesthetic management is referred to as preoperative medication.[1] Ideally, all patients should enter the preoperative period free from apprehension, sedated but easily arousable, and fully cooperative.

PSYCHOLOGICAL PREMEDICATION

Psychological premedication is provided by the anesthesiologist's preoperative visit and interview with the patient and family members (see Chapter 9). A thorough description of the planned anesthetic and events to anticipate in the perioperative period serves as a nonpharmacologic antidote to anxiety.[2,3] Indeed, the incidence of anxiety is reduced in patients visited by the anesthesiologist preoperatively compared with patients receiving only pharmacologic premedication and no visit (Table 10-1).[2] Likewise, a booklet designed to reassure patients about anesthesia is not as effective in reducing anxiety as is a preoperative visit and interview by the anesthesiologist.[3] Nevertheless, a shortage of time and the fact that some patients' problems do not lend themselves to reassurance may limit the value of the preoperative interview.

PHARMACOLOGIC PREMEDICATION

Pharmacologic premedication is typically administered orally or intramuscularly in the patient's hospital room 1 hour to 2 hours before the anticipated induction of anesthesia. For outpatient surgery, premedication is usually administered intravenously in the immediate preoperative period. The goals for pharmacologic premedication are multiple and must be individualized to meet each patient's unique requirements. Some previously acceptable goals of pharmacologic premedication are either no longer valid or are better achieved by intravenous administration of drugs at a time more likely to correspond to the period when pharmacologic effects are necessary. The best drug or drug combination to achieve the desired goals of pharmacologic premedication is not known and often is influenced by the individual physician's previous experience.

The appropriate drug(s) and doses to be used for pharmacologic premedication can be selected only after the psychological and physiologic condition of the patient have been evaluated. Drug choice and dose must take into account multiple factors. Certain types of patients should not receive depressant pharmacologic drugs in attempts to decrease preoperative anxiety and produce sedation (Table 10-2). The patient who requests to be

Table 10-1. Value of Preoperative Interview Compared with Pentobarbital

| | Percentage of Patients | | | |
	Interview Only	Pentobarbital[a] Only	Interview and Pentobarbital	No Interview or Pentobarbital
Feel nervous	40	61	38	58
Feel drowsy	26	30	38	18
Judged adequately sedated by anesthesiologist	65	48	71	35

[a] 2 mg·kg^{-1} intramuscularly 1 hour before surgery.
(Data from Egbert et al.[2])

"asleep" before being transported to the operating room must be assured that this is neither a desired nor safe goal of pharmacologic premedication.

DRUGS ADMINISTERED FOR PHARMACOLOGIC PREMEDICATION

Several classes of drugs are available to facilitate achievement of the desired goals for pharmacologic premedication in each individual patient (Table 10-3). These drugs are often administered intramuscularly, but when possible, the oral route of administration should be considered to improve patient comfort. The small amount of water used (up to 150 ml) to facilitate oral administration of drugs introduces no hazards related to gastric fluid volume (see the section *Fasting Before Elective Surgery*). Ultimately, the specific drugs selected are

---

Primary Goals for Pharmacologic Premedication

Anxiety relief

Sedation

Analgesia

Amnesia

Antisialogogue effect

Elevation of gastric fluid pH

Reduction of gastric fluid volume

Attenuation of sympathetic nervous system reflex responses

Reduction of anesthetic requirements

Prophylaxis against allergic reactions

Secondary Goals for Pharmacologic Premedication

Reduction of cardiac vagal activity—better achieved with the intravenous injection of an anticholinergic (atropine) just before the time of anticipated need.

Facilitate induction of anesthesia—not necessary in view of availability of potent intravenous induction drugs.

Postoperative analgesia—better achieved with the intravenous injection of an opioid (morphine) just before the time of anticipated need.

Prevention of postoperative nausea and vomiting—better achieved with the intravenous injection of an antiemetic (droperidol) just before the time of anticipated need.

Determinants of Drug Choice and Dose
Patient age and weight
Physical status
Level of anxiety
Tolerance for depressant drugs
Previous adverse experience with drugs used for preoperative medication
Allergies
Elective or emergency surgery
Inpatient or outpatient surgery

based on a consideration of desirable goals to be achieved balanced against the potential undesirable effects these drugs may produce.

Barbiturates

Advantages of using barbiturates for pharmacologic premedication include sedation, minimal ventilatory depressant effects, minimal circulatory depression, rarity of nausea and vomiting, and effectiveness when administered orally. Disadvantages include lack of analgesia; disorientation, especially if administered to patients in pain; and absence of a specific pharmacologic antagonist. Stimulation of hepatic microsomal enzyme activity is not a consideration with a one-time administra-

Table 10-2. Is Depressant Pharmacologic Premedication Indicated?

No	Yes
Less than 1 year of age	Cardiac surgery
Elderly	Cancer surgery
Decreased level of consciousness	Co-existing pain
	Regional anesthesia
Intracranial pathology	
Severe pulmonary disease	
Hypovolemia	

tion of barbiturates for preoperative medication. A patient with porphyria, however, should not receive barbiturates as these drugs may precipitate an acute exacerbation of this disease (see Chapter 23). Use of barbiturates for pharmacologic premedication has been largely replaced by benzodiazepines.

Opioids

Advantages of opioids as used for pharmacologic premedication include the absence of direct myocardial depression and the production of analgesia in patients who are experiencing pain preoperatively or who will require insertion of invasive monitors before the induction of anesthesia. Discomfort associated with institution of a regional anesthetic is another possible indication for use of an opioid as pharmacologic premedication. Inclusion of morphine in the preoperative medication reduces the likelihood that undesirable increases in heart rate will accompany surgical stimulation during administration of volatile anesthetics (Fig. 10-1).[4] Pharmacologic premedication with intramuscular administration of opioids may seem reasonable when a nitrous oxide-opioid anesthetic is planned. The opioid, however, may be just as logically given intravenously immediately before the induction of anesthesia.

Adverse effects of opioids as used for pharmacologic premedication include (1) depression of the medullary ventilatory center as evidenced by decreased responsiveness to carbon dioxide, and (2) orthostatic hypotension due to relaxation of peripheral vascular smooth muscle. Orthostatic hypotension will be further exaggerated if opioids are administered to patients with decreased intravascular fluid volumes. The euphoric effect of opioids in patients with pain may be dysphoria in the absence of pain. Nausea and vomiting most likely reflect opioid stimulation of the chemoreceptor trigger zone in the medulla. Recumbency seems to minimize nausea and vomiting after administration of opioids, suggesting that stimulation of the vestibular apparatus may also be important in production of this undesirable effect. Opioid-induced smooth muscle constriction may manifest as choledochoduodenal sphincter spasm,

Table 10-3. Drugs and Doses Used for Pharmacologic Premedication Before Induction of Anesthesia

Classification	Drug	Typical Adult (Dose, mg)[a]	Route of Administration
Barbiturates	Secobarbital	50–150	Orally, IM
	Pentobarbital	50–150	Orally, IM
Opioids	Morphine	5–15	IM
	Meperidine	50–100	IM
Benzodiazepines	Diazepam	5–10	Orally, IM
	Lorazepam	2–4	Orally, IM
	Midazolam	2.5–5	IM
	Flurazepam	15–30	Orally
	Temazepam	15–30	Orally
	Triazolam	0.125–0.25	Orally
Antihistamines	Diphenhydramine	25–75	Orally, IM
	Promethazine	25–50	IM
	Hydroxyzine	50–100	IM
Anticholinergics	Atropine	0.3–0.6	IM
	Scopolamine	0.3–0.6	IM
	Glycopyrrolate	0.2–0.3	IM
H$_2$ antagonists	Cimetidine	300	Orally, IM, IV
	Ranitidine	150	Orally, IM
Antacids	Particulate	15–30 ml	Orally
	Nonparticulate	10–20 ml	Orally
Stimulants of gastric motility	Metoclopramide	10–20	Orally, IM, IV

[a] Except for antacids.

IM, intramuscularly; IV, intravenously.

causing some anesthesiologists to question the use of opioids in patients with biliary tract disease (see Chapter 21). Pain associated with opioid-induced biliary tract spasm may be difficult to differentiate from angina pectoris. In this regard, nitroglycerin will relieve pain due to both etiologies, whereas administration of an opioid antagonist, naloxone, relieves only pain due to opioid-induced biliary tract spasm. An annoying side effect of opioids used as pharmacologic premedication is pruritus, which may be particularly prominent around the nose.

Benzodiazepines

Benzodiazepines act on specific brain receptors to produce selective antianxiety effects at doses that do not produce excessive sedation or cardiopulmonary depression (see Chapter 2). In addition,

these drugs, particularly lorazepam, produce suppression of recall of events that occur after (anterograde amnesia) their administration (Fig. 10-2).[5] Midazolam is also a potent amnestic drug. Suppression of recall for preceding events (retrograde amnesia) is less predictable. In animals, diazepam increases the seizure threshold for lidocaine, but there is no evidence in humans that doses of benzodiazepines as used for pharmacologic premedication reduce the likelihood of local anesthetic toxicity. Flurazepam, temazepam, and triazolam are examples of benzodiazepines used principally to treat insomnia that is often present the night before scheduled surgery.

Disadvantages of benzodiazepines as used for pharmacologic premedication include excessive and prolonged sedation in occasional patients. This is particularly likely in patients who receive lora-

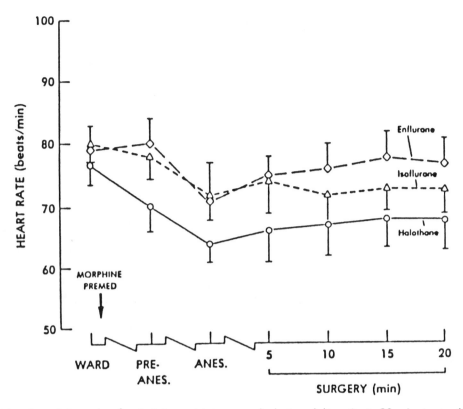

Fig. 10-1. Morphine 0.1 mg·kg⁻¹ administered intramuscularly to adult patients 30 minutes to 60 minutes before induction of anesthesia for elective surgery may contribute to a decrease in heart rate, even during surgery. Mean ± SE. (From Cahalan et al.,[4] with permission.)

zepam in doses that exceed 50 μg·kg⁻¹ (total dose should not exceed 4 mg). Physostigmine, and, in the future, specific antagonists, may be effective in reversing sedation produced by benzodiazepines. Pain on injection and occasional erratic absorption after intramuscular injection of diazepam reflects the presence of propylene glycol in the commercial preparation of this drug. In contrast, midazolam lacks these adverse effects as it is water soluble, obviating the need for propylene glycol.

Cimetidine has been shown to delay the clearance of diazepam from the plasma, introducing the theoretical possibility of an enhanced and prolonged benzodiazepine effect when these drugs are administered together for preoperative medication (Fig. 10-3).[6] The same concern is not relevant for lorazepam or midazolam as these drugs depend on glucuronidation in the liver, which is not influenced by cimetidine. Furthermore, their metabolites are inactive, in contrast to the significant pharmacologic activity of desmethyldiazepam, the major metabolite of diazepam.

Butyrophenones

The use of droperidol for pharmacologic premedication is limited because of the occasional production of dysphoria after its administration. These patients express a fear of death and may refuse a previously agreed to elective operative procedure. Another disadvantage of droperidol is production of dopaminergic receptor blockade, which may produce extrapyramidal symptoms in normal patients as well as those with co-existing paralysis agitans. Proponents of droperidol for use as preoperative medication cite its potential pro-

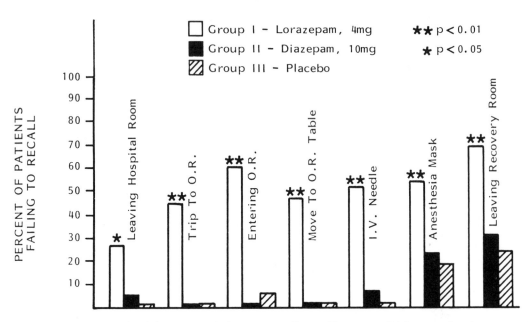

Fig. 10-2. The percentage of adult patients failing to recall specific events 24 hours after intramuscular injections of lorazepam, diazepam, or placebo was significantly greater in those receiving lorazepam. (From Fragen and Caldwell,[5] with permission.)

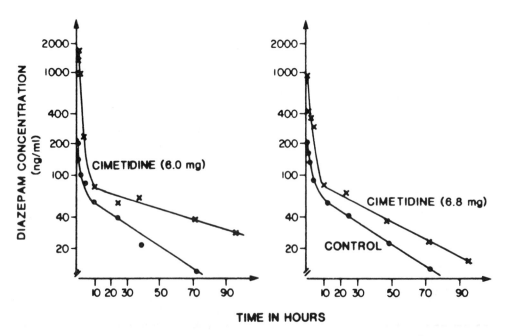

Fig. 10-3. The rate of decline in the plasma concentration of diazepam (0.1 mg·kg^{-1} administered intravenously) is slowed by prior administration of cimetidine (6 mg·kg^{-1} to 6.8 mg·kg^{-1}). (From Klotz and Reimann,[6] with permission.)

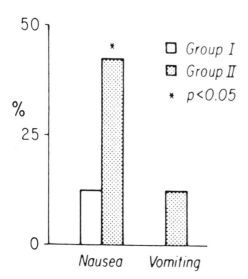

Fig. 10-4. The incidence of nausea and vomiting was significantly reduced postoperatively in patients receiving droperidol 2.5 mg administered intravenously near the end of surgery (group I) compared with those treated with a placebo (group II). (From Santos and Datta,[7] with permission.)

tection against epinephrine-induced cardiac dysrhythmias and production of a postoperative antiemetic effect. Indeed, intravenous administration of droperidol, 1.25 mg to 2.5 mg, just before conclusion of anesthesia is an effective antiemetic and is often recommended for patients considered to be at high risk for postoperative nausea and vomiting (ophthalmologic operations, gynecologic procedures) (Fig. 10-4).[7] This use of droperidol, however, has been associated with delayed recovery from anesthesia and an increased incidence of postoperative vertigo.[1]

Antihistamines

Antihistamines are used for pharmacologic premedication because of their sedative and antiemetic properties. Promethazine, combined with meperidine, does not increase depression of ventilation produced by meperidine or alter the incidence of nausea and vomiting but does produce an additive sedative effect.

Prophylaxis Against Allergic Reactions

Diphenhydramine (0.5 $mg \cdot kg^{-1}$ to 1 $mg \cdot kg^{-1}$ orally) has been recommended as a pharmacologic premedication to provide prophylaxis against intraoperative allergic reactions in patients with a history of chronic atopy or undergoing procedures (radiographic dye studies, chemonucleolysis) known to be associated with allergic reactions. Cimetidine (4 $mg \cdot kg^{-1}$ to 6 $mg \cdot kg^{-1}$ orally) should also be administered with diphenhydramine (see the section H_2-Antagonist). This combination of an H_1-antagonist (diphenhydramine) and H_2-antagonist (cimetidine) acts to occupy peripheral receptor sites normally responsive to histamine, thus reducing manifestations of any subsequent drug-induced release of histamine. Prednisone (50 mg every 6 hours for the 24 hours before surgery) may also be added to this prophylactic regimen.

Alpha-2 Agonist

Clonidine is a centrally-acting alpha-2 agonist that acts as a antihypertensive drug. Administered orally as preoperative medication, this drug attenuates autonomic nervous system reflex responses (e.g., increases in blood pressure and heart rate) associated with intraoperative stimulation.[8] Anesthetic requirements are also reduced in patients treated with clonidine.

Anticholinergics

Routine inclusion of anticholinergics as part of the pharmacologic premedication is not necessary.[9] The most frequent reasons for administering anticholinergics are (1) production of an antisialagogue effect, (2) production of sedative and amnesic effects, and (3) prevention of reflex bradycardia (Table 10-4). Anticholinergics are not predictably effective in elevating gastric fluid pH or lowering gastric fluid volume (Table 10-5).[1,10]

Antisialagogue Effect

The need for including an anticholinergic in the preoperative medication to produce an antisialagogue effect has been questioned, since currently used inhaled anesthetics do not stimulate excessive

Table 10-4. Comparative Effects of Anticholinergics Administered Intramuscularly as Pharmacologic Premedication

	Atropine	Scopolamine	Glycopyrrolate
Antisialagogue effect	+	+ + +	+ +
Sedative and amnesic effects	+	+ + +	0
Increased gastric fluid pH	0	0	±
Central nervous system toxicity	+	+ +	0
Relaxation of lower esophageal sphincter	+ +	+ +	+ +
Mydriasis and cycloplegia	+	+ + +	0

0, none; +, mild; + +, moderate; + + +, marked.

upper airway secretions. Nevertheless, reduced secretions during general anesthesia, particularly when a tracheal tube is in place, are a desirable effect of an anticholinergic administered preoperatively.[9] An antisialagogue effect is particularly important for intra-oral operations, bronchoscopies, or when topical anesthesia is necessary, as excessive secretions may interfere with the surgery or impair production of topical anesthesia by diluting the local anesthetic. Administration of an anticholinergic for an antisialagogue effect is not necessary when regional anesthesia is planned.

Scopolamine is about three times more potent as an antisialagogue than is atropine. For this reason, scopolamine is often selected when both an antisialagogue effect and sedation are desired results of preoperative medication. Glycopyrrolate is selected when an antisialagogue effect, in the absence of sedation, is desired. As an antisialagogue, glycopyrrolate is about twice as potent as

atropine and its duration of action is longer. To avoid the discomfort of a dry mouth and throat, an anticholinergic can be given just before the patient leaves the ward for transportation to the operating room. Nevertheless, anxiety, fluid deprivation before elective surgery, and other drugs used for pharmacologic premedication may produce a dry mouth and throat even in the absence of an anticholinergic.

Sedative and Amnesic Effects

Atropine and scopolamine are tertiary amines that can cross lipid barriers, including the blood-brain barrier. Resulting sedative and amnesic effects reflect penetrance of these drugs into the central nervous system. Scopolamine, more than atropine, produces useful sedative effects, particularly in combination with barbiturates, opioids, or benzo-

Table 10-5. Percentages of Patients with Gastric Fluid pH Below 2.5 and/or Volume Above 20 ml

	pH Below 2.5	Volume Above 20 ml	pH Below 2.5 and Volume Above 20 ml
Morphine	63	27	16
Morphine-atropine (0.4 mg)	58	27	17
Morphine-glycopyrrolate (0.2 mg)	52	23	16
Morphine-atropine-Riopan	0[a]	60[a]	0[a]

[a] $P < 0.05$
(From Stoelting,[10] with permission.)

Undesirable Effects of Anticholinergics

Central nervous system toxicity

Tachycardia

Lower esophageal sphincter relaxation

Mydriasis and cycloplegia

Body temperature elevation

Drying of airway secretions

Increased physiologic dead space

---

diazepines as used for pharmacologic premedication. It is estimated that scopolamine is eight times to ten times more potent than atropine in terms of its effects on the central nervous system. Glycopyrrolate, as a quaternary ammonium compound, cannot easily cross the blood-brain barrier and thus does not produce significant sedative or amnesic effects.

Prevention of Reflex Bradycardia

Use of anticholinergics in the pharmacologic premedication for prevention of reflex bradycardia is a secondary objective since the dose and timing of intramuscular administration is not appropriate. The most logical approach, particularly in children with increased vagal activity, is to administer atropine or glycopyrrolate intravenously shortly before the anticipated need.

Undesirable Side Effects

Undesirable side effects of anticholinergics are multiple and must be considered in the decision to use these drugs for pharmacologic premedication.

Central Nervous System Toxicity. Central nervous system toxicity (central anticholinergic syndrome) produced by anticholinergics manifests as delerium or prolonged somnolence after anesthesia. This undesirable response is more likely to follow administration of scopolamine than atropine, but the incidence should be low with the doses used for pharmacologic premedication. Nevertheless,

elderly patients may be uniquely susceptible to central nervous system toxicity secondary to atropine or scopolamine (see Chapter 30). Central nervous system toxicity is unlikely after the administration of glycopyrrolate since this drug cannot easily cross the blood-brain barrier. Finally, it must be remembered that toxicity attributed to the anticholinergic may also represent an uninhibited response to pain as the depressant effects of the anesthetic dissipate.

Central anticholinergic syndrome presumably reflects blockade of muscarinic cholinergic receptors in the central nervous system. Physostigmine, a tertiary amine anticholinesterase, administered in intravenous doses of 15 μg$\cdot$kg^{-1} to 60 μg$\cdot$kg^{-1} is a specific treatment for central nervous system toxicity due to scopolamine or atropine. Neostigmine and pyridostigmine are not effective anticholinesterase antidotes because their quaternary ammonium structure prevents these drugs from easily entering the central nervous system.

Tachycardia. Scopolamine and glycopyrrolate, which have minimal cardioaccelerator effects, are better selections than atropine for pharmacologic premedication when an increased heart rate would be undesirable as in patients with mitral stenosis and atrial fibrillation being treated with digitalis. Nevertheless, the most likely cardiac response after intramuscular administration of atropine, glycopyrrolate, or scopolamine for pharmacologic premedication is heart rate slowing, presumably reflecting a weak cholinergic agonist effect of these drugs. Previous speculation that heart rate slowing after administration of atropine reflected a central vagal action is not supported by similar heart rate changes after administration of glycopyrrolate, which cannot easily cross the blood-brain barrier.

Relaxation of the Lower Esophageal Sphincter. Intravenous administration of anticholinergics results in relaxation of the lower esophageal sphincter. Intramuscular administration of these drugs should also lower esophageal sphincter pressure. When barrier pressure (lower esophageal sphincter pressure minus gastric pressure) is less than 13 cm H_2O, the patient becomes vulnerable to gastroesophageal reflux and the hazards of aspiration pneumonitis. This remains a theoretical hazard of anticholinergics, however, as there is no evidence that the incidence of aspiration pneumonitis is increased in patients receiving these drugs as pharmacologic premedication.

Mydriasis and Cycloplegia. Atropine and scopolamine may produce mydriasis and cycloplegia, causing patients to experience visual impairment postoperatively. In this regard, scopolamine has a greater mydriatic effect than atropine. Conceivably, mydriasis could interfere with drainage of aqueous humor from the anterior chamber of the eye. There is no evidence, however, that inclusion of anticholinergics in the pharmacologic premedication is contraindicated for patients with glaucoma. Nevertheless, miotic eye drops should be continued throughout the perioperative period in these patients.

Elevation of Body Temperature. Anticholinergics may result in elevations of body temperature by suppressing sweat glands that are innervated by cholinergic nerves via the sympathetic nervous system. Prevention of sweating by this mechanism may be undesirable in the presence of co-existing increases in body temperature, particularly in children.

H₂-Antagonists

H₂-antagonists counter the ability of histamine to induce secretion of gastric fluid with high hydrogen ion concentrations. Therefore, these drugs offer a pharmacologic approach for increasing gastric fluid pH before the induction of anesthesia. Studies indicate that 40 percent to 80 percent of adult patients undergoing elective surgery with or without an anticholinergic included in the preoperative medication have a gastric fluid pH below 2.5 (Table 10-5).[1,10] Elevation of gastric fluid pH above 2.5 is desirable since the severity of aspiration pneumonitis is likely to be accentuated by inhalation of fluid with a pH below 2.5.

Routine inclusion of H₂-antagonists in the preoperative medication is appealing. Certainly, the use of H₂-antagonists would be particularly attractive for inclusion in the pharmacologic premedication of (1) parturients, (2) patients with symptoms of gastroesophageal reflux, (3) obese patients who tend to have low gastric fluid pH values, and

Table 10-6. Influence of Cimetidine on Gastric Fluid pH

	pH (percentage of patients)		
	Below 2.5	2.5–5.0	Above 5.0
Cimetidine (evening before operation)	22% (11)[a]	38% (19)	40% (20)
Cimetidine (preanesthetic medication)	16% (8)	24% (12)	60%[b][c] (30)
Control (no cimetidine)	60% (30)	34% (17)	6% (3)

[a] (n), number of patients.
[b] P < 0.05 vs. control.
[c] t, P < 0.05 preanesthetic medication vs. evening before operation.
(From Stoelting,[11] with permission.)

(4) outpatients who may have unexpectedly low gastric fluid pH values presumably reflecting the lack of a preoperative interview and medication to decrease anxiety. Intravenous administration of H₂-antagonists is a consideration for patients requiring emergency surgery, or those who cannot receive oral medications. An objection to routine inclusion of H₂-antagonists in the preoperative medication is the concept that all therapies should be individualized and tailored to fit individual patients, their diseases, and specific preoperative circumstances.

Despite convincing evidence that H₂-antagonists increase gastric fluid pH, increased patient safety has not been demonstrated when inhalation of gastric fluid occurs in those pretreated with cimetidine. Furthermore, these drugs are not 100 percent effective (e.g., an inherent failure rate) (Table 10-6).[11] H₂-antagonists will not alter the pH of gastric fluid that is present before administration of the drug, nor will they facilitate gastric emptying. In addition, cimetidine may be associated with adverse side effects including (1) central nervous system sedation; (2) decreased hepatic blood flow and enzyme activity with resulting delayed clearance of drugs such as diazepam, lidocaine, propranolol, and succinylcholine; (3)

increased airway resistance due to unopposed H_1-receptor mediated bronchoconstriction; and (4) cardiac dysrhythmias (Fig. 10-3).[1,6] These side effects may be less likely to occur after administration of ranitidine.

Under no circumstances can preoperative medication with H_2-antagonists be substituted for an anesthetic technique with a cuffed tracheal tube or maintenance of consciousness to protect the lungs from inhalation of gastric fluid (see Chapter 9). Aspiration is also a hazard at the conclusion of surgery when the trachea is extubated. In this regard, ranitidine with a longer duration of action than cimetidine, may be more likely to offer protection at the conclusion of operations lasting more than 3 hours.

Antacids

Antacids administered 15 minutes to 30 minutes before the induction of anesthesia are nearly 100 percent effective in elevating the gastric fluid pH above 2.5. The efficacy of antacids may be dependent to some extent on patient movement so as to facilitate complete mixing with gastric fluid. Inhalation of gastric fluid containing particulate antacids, however, may be associated with severe and persistent pulmonary dysfunction despite a high pH of the aspirated material.[1] In contrast, nonparticulate antacids, such as sodium citrate, effectively raise gastric fluid pH above 2.5 and do not produce significant pulmonary dysfunction should inhalation of fluid containing antacids occur.

Compared with H_2-antagonists, administration of antacids is effective in raising the pH of gastric fluid that is present in the stomach at the time of administration (i.e., no lag time). This desirable effect, however, is predictably associated with an increased gastric fluid volume that does not occur with H_2-antagonists. Furthermore, antacids may delay gastric emptying. Since the severity of aspiration pneumonitis is likely to depend on both the volume (greater than $0.4 \text{ ml} \cdot \text{kg}^{-1}$) and pH (below 2.5) of the inhaled fluid, the increased gastric fluid volume produced by the administration of antacids must be considered. Nevertheless, withholding antacids because of concern of increasing gastric fluid volume is not warranted, considering animal evidence that documents increased mortality after aspiration of low volumes of acidic gastric fluid compared with aspiration of large volumes of buffered gastric fluid (Table 10-7).[12]

Metoclopramide

Metoclopramide speeds gastric emptying by selectively increasing motility of the upper gastrointestinal tract and relaxing the pyloric sphincter. The onset of metoclopramide effect is 30 minutes to 60 minutes after oral administration and 1 minute to 3 minutes after intravenous injection. This drug may be useful in preoperative medication for use in reducing gastric fluid volume, particularly in patients with diabetes mellitus and associated gastroparesis, parturients, and patients who have recently ingested food and subsequently require

Table 10-7. Mortality Rates (Percentage) for Rats After Aspiration of Solutions of Various pHs and Volumes

Volume ($\text{ml} \cdot \text{kg}^{-1}$)	Fluid pH					
	1.0	1.4	1.8	2.5	3.5	5.8
0.2	20	0				
0.3	90	0	9			
0.4	90	40	9	0		
1.0	100	90	20	0	0	0
2.0	100	100	27	30	20	10
4.0	100	100	38	20	40	30

(From James et al.[12] with permission.)

Table 10-8. Volume of Gastric Contents and pH in Study Groups

	Metoclopramide (n-30)	Placebo (n-28)
Gastric volume (range)	24 + 2 ml[a] (3–60)	30 ± 5 ml (4–155)
Volume >25 ml	16[b] (53%)	15 (54%)
Gastric pH (range)	2.86 ± 0.27[a] (1–6)	2.55 ± 0.24 (1–5.5)
pH <2.5	12[b] (40%)	16 (57%)

[a] Mean ± SE.
[b] number of patients.
(From Cohen,[18] with permission.)

emergency surgery for disease unrelated to the gastrointestinal tract. Nevertheless, metoclopramide does not guarantee gastric emptying, and its beneficial effects may be offset by concomitant or prior administration of anticholinergics, opioids, or antacids (Table 10-8).[1,13] The ability of metoclopramide to increase lower esophageal sphincter tone may be negated by inclusion of atropine in the preoperative medication. Metoclopramide does not predictably alter gastric fluid pH. Side effects of metoclopramide include abdominal cramping if administered rapidly intravenously and occasional neurologic dysfunction reflecting passage into the central nervous system and production of dopaminergic receptor blockade.[1] Any antiemetic effect produced by this drug is likely to be due to antagonism of dopamine receptors in the central nervous system.

OUTPATIENTS

Administration of preoperative medication to outpatients must avoid introducing persistent drug effects that delay emergence from anesthesia or prevent early discharge after elective and usually minor surgery (see Chapter 24).

PEDIATRIC PATIENTS

Pediatric patients, like adults, benefit from attempts to tailor the preoperative medication to unique requirements of each child. Age is a par-

ticularly important aspect in considering psychological preparation of pediatric patients. In this regard, preschool children are often the most upset when separated from their family and benefit from having parents accompany them to the operating room. After about 5 years of age, it becomes easier to communicate with the child, allowing the anesthesiologist to explain expected events in the preoperative period and to offer reassurance. The attitude and behavior of the parents are also important in the psychological preparation of the child.

After about 1 year of age, children may benefit from pharmacologic attempts to reduce anxiety.[14] The oral route for administration of drugs is appealing, as most children abhor intramuscular injections. In preschool age children, the rectal administration of barbiturates, particularly methohexital, may be considered. Atropine, administered intravenously just before the induction of anesthesia, is often recommended to reduce elevated vagotonic activity characteristically present in pediatric patients.

EVALUATION OF DEPRESSANT DRUGS USED FOR PHARMACOLOGIC PREMEDICATION

Precise methods to evaluate the value of depressant drugs as used for pharmacologic premedication are not available. For example, anxiety is a subjective response that may be influenced by differences in the emotional states of patients, as well as what patients expect from the preoperative medication. Sedation is a more objective measurement, but drowsiness does not always parallel relief of anxiety. Comparison of studies on pharmacologic premedication is hampered by different drug doses, sites, and routes of administration and varying time for measuring responses. Despite these complexities, a well-controlled study suggested desirable (decreased anxiety, sedation) and undesirable effects (dry mouth, nausea, vomiting) of pharmacologic premedication were difficult to distinguish from placebo effects.[15] This casts doubt on the ability to measure and confirm the value of drugs used for pharmacologic premedication, but should not be accepted as evidence that pharmacologic premedication fails to produce more comfortable

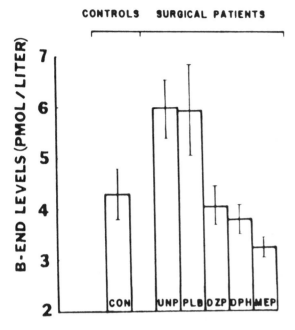

Fig. 10-5. Compared with control values (CON), plasma concentrations of beta endorphins (B-END) were decreased in presurgical patients receiving pharmacologic premedication with oral diazepam, 10 mg (DZP), intramuscular diphenhydramine 1 mg·kg⁻¹ (DPH), or intramuscular meperidine 1 mg·kg⁻¹ (MEP). Plasma concentrations of B-END were elevated in presurgical patients receiving no pharmacologic premedication (UNP) or intramuscular saline (PLB). Mean ± SE. Measurements were made 1 hour after treatment. (From Walsh et al.,[16] with permission.)

patients in the preoperative period. Indeed, plasma concentrations of beta-endorphins, as a reflection of the anterior pituitary response to stress before induction of anesthesia are lower in patients receiving pharmacologic premedication than in patients receiving placebo injections (Fig. 10-5).[16]

FASTING BEFORE ELECTIVE SURGERY

Fasting before elective surgery (non per os [NPO] after midnight) is recommended in the hope of minimizing gastric fluid volume at the time of induction of anesthesia. Nevertheless, complete emptying of the stomach can never be guaranteed.

Furthermore, foods pass through the stomach at variable and unpredictable rates, sometimes taking up to 12 hours. In contrast, water and crystalloid-containing solutions have a 50 percent emptying time of only 12 minutes to 20 minutes. Therefore, it may be illogical to have a single guideline for solid and liquid ingestion before induction of anesthesia for elective operations. Indeed, gastric fluid volumes are less in patients receiving 150 ml of water 2 hours to 3 hours before induction of anesthesia compared with patients who are fasted.[17] It is possible that a liquid bolus stimulates gastric peristalsis and thus gastric emptying. For this reason, it does not seem logical to forbid ingestion of small volumes of liquids before elective surgery. Clearly, this recommendation does not apply to solid foods or to patients at known risk for slow gastric emptying (obese, parturients, opioids included in preoperative medication, diabetes mellitus, gastrointestinal disease).

RECOMMENDED PREOPERATIVE MEDICATION FOR ADULT PATIENTS BEFORE ELECTIVE SURGERY

Preoperative medication begins with the anesthesiologist's interview and subsequent decision as to the need for and type of pharmacologic premedication. Timing of drug administration is as important as the drugs selected for pharmacologic premedication. Drugs administered to decrease anxiety and to produce sedation are more appropriately administered 1 hour to 2 hours before induction of anesthesia. A benzodiazepine and/or an H₂-antagonist is also conveniently administered orally at this time. Metoclopramide is a logical consideration for inclusion in the pharmacologic premedication when a predictable reduction in gastric fluid volume is important. Nevertheless, administration of an H₂-antagonist with up to 150 ml of water may be the most effective method to increase gastric fluid pH and decrease gastric fluid volume.[17] Emergency surgery requiring general anesthesia in patients who have recently eaten may be an appropriate situation for intravenous administration of cimetidine and metoclopramide. Intramuscular administration of morphine is an alternative to benzodiazepines if analgesia is an important objective of preoperative medication.

Suggestions for Preoperative Medication for Adults Before Elective Surgery (see Table 10-3 for doses)

1. Patient visit and interview by anesthesiologist the day before surgery.

2. Benzodiazepine (orally) to treat insomnia the night before surgery.

3. Benzodiazepine (preferably orally) 1 hour to 2 hours before surgery. Water up to 150 ml may stimulate gastric emptying.

4. Substitute opioid (intramuscularly) for number 3 if analgesia is desired. Opioids may delay gastric emptying.

5. Scopolamine (intramuscularly) 1 hour to 2 hours before surgery if reliable sedation and amnesia are desired; otherwise, follow recommendation number 7 or do not administer an anticholinergic.

6. Consider H_2 antagonist (orally) 1 hour to 2 hours before surgery. Administration with up to 150 ml of water may be the most predictable method to reduce gastric fluid volume and elevate gastric fluid pH.

7. Glycopyrrolate (intramuscularly) when patient is ready to be transported to the operating room if an antisialagogue effect is desired.

Intramuscular scopolamine administered at the same time as the drug selected to decrease anxiety is indicated when it is desirable to exploit the amnesic and sedative effects of this anticholinergic. For example, the combination of intramuscular morphine with or without oral benzodiazepines plus intramuscular scopolamine is useful for producing sedation in patients most deserving of aggressive pharmacologic premedication (Table 10-2).

An anticholinergic selected solely to produce an antisialagogue effect is most appropriately administered intramuscularly, immediately before patients are transported to the operating room. This timing minimizes the duration of the uncomfortable sensation of a dry mouth and throat experienced by patients before the induction of anesthesia. Glycopyrrolate is the most logical drug to select if an antisialagogue response without central nervous system effects is desired.

Drugs that decrease vagal activity (atropine, glycopyrrolate), protect against postoperative nausea and vomiting (droperidol) or provide postoperative analgesia are most logically administered intravenously at a time just preceding that of the desired effect.

REFERENCES

1. White PF. Pharmacologic and clinical aspects of preoperative medication. Anesth Analg 1986;65:963–74.
2. Egbert LD, Battit GE, Turndorf H, Beecher HK. The value of the preoperative visit by an anesthetist. JAMA 1963;185:553–5.
3. Leigh JM, Walker J, Janaganthan P. Effect of preoperative anesthetic visit on anxiety. Br Med J 1977;2:987–9.
4. Cahalan MK, Lurz FW, Eger EI II, Schwartz LA, Beaupre PN, Smith JS. Narcotics decrease heart rate during inhalational anesthesia. Anesth Analg 1987;66:166–70.
5. Fragen RJ, Caldwell N. Lorazepam premedication: Lack of recall and relief of anxiety. Anesth Anagl 1976;55:792–6.
6. Klotz U, Reimann I. Delayed clearance of diazepam due to cimetidine. N Engl J Med 1980;302:1012–4.
7. Santos A, Datta S. Prophylactic use of droperidol for control of nausea and vomiting during spinal anesthesia for cesarean section. Anesth Analg 1984;63:85–7.
8. Ghignone M, Calvillo O, Quintin L. Anesthesia and hypertension. The effect of clonidine on perioperative hemodynamics and isoflurane requirements. Anesthesiology 1987;67:3–10.
9. Falick YS, Smiler BG. Is anticholinergic premedication necessary? Anesthesiology 1975;43:472–3.
10. Stoelting RK. Response to atropine, glycopyrrolate, and Riopan of gastric fluid pH and volume in adult patients. Anesthesiology 1978;48:367–9.
11. Stoelting RK. Gastric fluid pH in patients receiving cimetidine. Anesth Analg 1978;57:675–7.
12. James CF, Modell JH, Gibbs CP, Kuck EJ, Ruiz BC. Pulmonary aspiration-effects of volume and pH in the rat. Anesth Analg 1984;63:665–8.
13. Cohen SE, Jasson J, Talafre M-L, Chauvelot-Moachon L, Barrier G. Does metoclopramide de-

crease the volume of gastric contents in patients undergoing cesarean section? Anesthesiology 1984;61:604–7.

14. Brzustowicz RM, Nelson DA, Betts EK, Rosenberry KR, Swedlow DB. Efficacy of oral premedication for pediatric outpatient surgery. Anesthesiology 1984; 60:475–7.

15. Forrest WH, Brown CR, Brown BW. Subjective responses to six common preoperative medications. Anesthesiology 1977;47:241–7.

16. Walsh J, Puig MM, Lovitz MA, Turndorf H. Premedication abolishes the increase in plasma beta-endorphin observed in the immediate preoperative period. Anesthesiology 1987;66:402–5.

17. Sutherland AD, Maltby JR, Sale JP, Reid CRG. The effect of preoperative oral fluid and ranitidine on gastric fluid volume and pH. Can J Anaesth 1987; 34:117–21.

18. Cohen SE: Antiemetic efficacy of droperidol and metoclopramide. Anesthesiology 1984;60:67–9.

Chapter 11

Anesthetic Equipment and Breathing Systems

Delivery of known concentrations of inhaled anesthetics and oxygen to the patient requires appropriate equipment including an anesthetic machine, vaporizer, and anesthetic breathing system. An understanding of the principles governing the performance of this anesthetic equipment is mandatory to assure maximal patient safety. Furthermore, the implications of bacterial contamination of anesthetic equipment and the role of anesthetic equipment in pollution of the atmosphere with anesthetic gases should be considered.

ANESTHETIC MACHINE

Anesthetic machines, regardless of their manufacturer, consist of the same basic components (700 or more individual parts integrated to perform as a single unit) (Figs. 11-1 and 11-2).[1] These include (1) a source of compressed gases, (2) flowmeters to assure delivery of known flows and concentrations of these gases into an anesthetic breathing system, and (3) means to vaporize and deliver known concentrations of the vapor of liquid anesthetics. The anesthetic machine may be equipped with a mechanical ventilator and devices to monitor the electrocardiogram, blood pressure, body temperature, arterial hemoglobin saturation with oxygen, and inhaled and exhaled concentrations of oxygen and carbon dioxide. Alarm systems to signal apnea or disconnection of the anesthetic

breathing system from the patient as reflected by an oxygen supply pressure below 30 psi are included (see Chapter 16). Anesthetic machines are equipped with a fail-safe valve designed to prevent delivery of hypoxic gas mixtures from the machine due to failure of the oxygen supply. This valve shuts off or proportionally decreases flow of all gases when the pressure in the oxygen delivery line decreases below about 30 psi. This will protect against an unrecognized exhaustion of oxygen delivery from a cylinder attached to the anesthetic machine or from a central source. This valve, however, does not prevent the delivery of pure nitrous oxide when the oxygen flowmeter is turned off but pressure in the circuit of the anesthetic machine is maintained by an open oxygen cylinder or central supply source. In this situation, an oxygen analyzer is necessary to detect the delivery of an hypoxic gas mixture. Far superior to the fail-safe valve or oxygen analyzer is the continuous presence of a vigilant anesthesiologist.

Compressed Gases

Gases used in the administration of anesthesia are available in cylinders attached to the anesthetic machine (Table 11-1). Compression of gas to a liquid offers the most economic and practical volume for storage. Oxygen is stored in cylinders in the operating room as a gas because the tem-

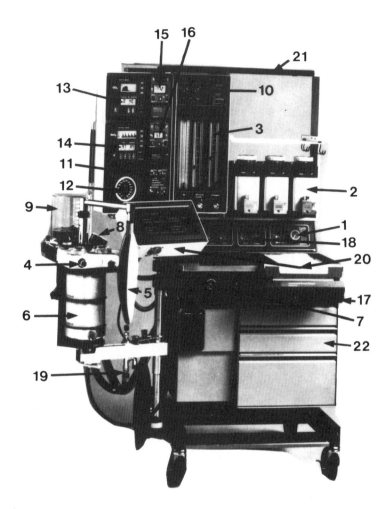

Fig. 11-1. An anesthetic machine (1) on-off electrical/pneumatic switch, (2) agent specific vaporizers, (3) flowmeters, (4) connections for a circle anesthetic breathing system, (5) reservoir bag, (6) canister for granules to absorb carbon dioxide, (7) oxygen flush valve, (8) airway pressure gauge, (9) ventilator, (10) ventilator controls, (11) airway pressure monitor and alarm, (12) blood pressure gauge, (13) capnograph, (14) pulse oximeter, (15) tidal volume monitor, (16) oxygen analyzer, (17) yokes for compressed gas cylinders, (18) pressure gauges, (19) gas evacuation (scavenging system), (20) automated anesthesia record, (21) shelf for portable equipment; and (22) drawers for storage. Noninvasive blood pressure monitors, pulse oximeters, and capnographs are examples of equipment that may be built into the design of the anesthetic machine or, alternatively, remain portable units that are added to the machine (see Chapter 16).

perature (critical temperature) at which oxygen exists as a liquid is far below room temperature. Nevertheless, liquid oxygen stored in large insulated containers (5 atm to 10 atm, minus 150° Celsius) can be vaporized for supply throughout the hospital. Unlike oxygen, nitrous oxide is compressible to a liquid at a temperature far above room temperature.

Oxygen and nitrous oxide may be piped to the operating room from a central source for delivery to the anesthetic machine via pressure tubing. Oxygen or air from a central source may also be used to drive the ventilator on the anesthetic machine. Gas used for this purpose does not enter the circuitry of the anesthetic machine. Even with a central source, cylinders of oxygen and nitrous

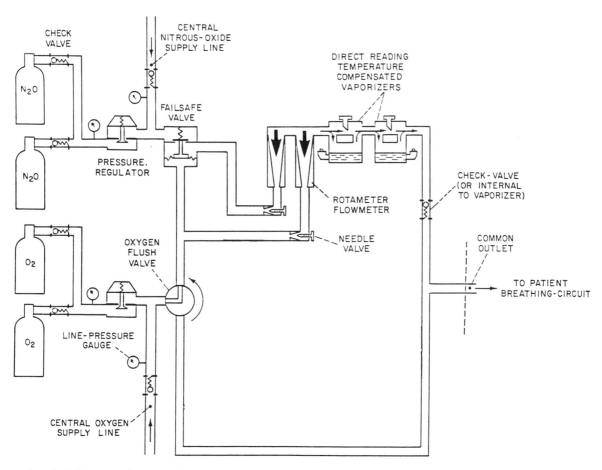

Fig. 11-2. Schematic diagram of internal circuitry of an anesthetic machine. Oxygen and nitrous oxide enter the anesthetic machine from gas cylinders attached to yokes on the machine or from a central supply line. Check valves prevent transfilling of gas cylinders or flow of gas from the cylinders into the central supply line. Pressure regulators reduce pressure in the tubing from gas cylinders to about 50 psi. The fail-safe valve prevents flow of nitrous oxide if the pressure in the oxygen supply circuit decreases below about 30 psi. Needle valves control gas flows to rotameters (flowmeters). Vaporizers (agent-specific, temperature-compensated) provide a reliable means to deliver preselected concentrations of volatile anesthetics. An interlock allows only one vaporizer to be on at a time. After mixing in the manifold of the anesthetic machine, the total fresh gas flow enters the anesthetic breathing system (circuit), for delivery to the patient. (Adapted from Check-Out,[1] with permission.)

oxide should be attached to the anesthetic machine should the central supply fail. Gas cylinders are attached to yokes on the anesthetic machine. The position of two metal pins on the yoke corresponds to holes in the valve casing of the gas cylinder (pin-index), which makes it impossible to attach the gas cylinder to the wrong yoke. Otherwise, a cylinder containing nitrous oxide could be attached to the oxygen yoke, resulting in the delivery of

nitrous oxide when the oxygen flowmeter was activated. Anesthetic machines usually have double yokes so that two cylinders of oxygen and nitrous oxide can be attached. Check valves prevent one gas cylinder from transfilling the other. This valve allows exchange of empty gas cylinders for full ones while the other tank is in use. Imprinted letters and numbers near the top of the gas cylinder refer to cylinder size (E,H), maximal permissible

Table 11-1. Characteristics of Compressed Gases Stored in E Size Cylinders that May Be Attached to the Anesthetic Machine

Charateristics	Oxygen	Nitrous Oxide	Carbon Dioxide	Air
Cylinder color	Green[a]	Blue	Gray	Yellow[a]
Physical state in cylinder	Gas	Liquid	Liquid	Gas
Cylinder contents (L)	625	1590	1590	625
Cylinder weight empty (kg)	5.90	5.90	5.90	5.90
Cylinder weight full (kg)	6.76	8.80	8.90	
Cylinder pressure full (psi)	2000	750	838	1800

[a] The World Health Organization specifies that cylinders containing oxygen for medical use be painted white but United States manufacturers use green. Likewise, the international color code for air is white and black, whereas cylinders in the United States are color-coded as yellow.

pressure in psi, manufacturer's serial number, and date of original and retest dates for pressure tolerance. The contents of the gas cylinder are not designated by any permanent notation on the tank. Instead, the contents of the gas cylinder are indicated only by a detachable label and the color of the cylinder (green for oxygen, blue for nitrous oxide).

Color-coded pressure gauges (green for oxygen, blue for nitrous oxide) on the anesthetic machine indicate the pressure of the gas in the corresponding gas cylinder. The pressure in an oxygen cylinder is directly proportional to the volume of oxygen in the cylinder. For example, a full oxygen cylinder (E size) contains about 625 L oxygen at a pressure of 2000 psi, and one-half this volume when the pressure is 1000 psi. Therefore, it is possible to calculate accurately how long a given flow rate of oxygen can be maintained before the cylinder is empty. In contrast to oxygen the pressure gauge for nitrous oxide does not indicate the amount of gas remaining in the cylinder. This occurs because the pressure in the gas cylinder remains at 750 psi as long as any liquid nitrous oxide is present. When nitrous oxide as a vapor leaves the cylinder, additional liquid is vaporized to maintain an unchanging pressure in the cylinder. When all the liquid nitrous oxide is vaporized, the pressure begins to decrease, and it can be assumed that about 75 percent of the contents of the gas cylinder have been exhausted. Because a

full nitrous oxide cylinder (E size) contains about 1590 L, approximately 400 L remain when the pressure gauge begins to decrease from its previously constant value of 750 psi. Vaporization of a liquified gas (nitrous oxide), as well as the expansion of a compressed gas (oxygen), absorbs heat, which is extracted from the metal cylinder and the surrounding atmosphere. For this reason, atmospheric water vapor often accumulates as frost on gas cylinders and in valves, particularly during high flows. Internal icing does not occur because compressed gases are free of water vapor.

When gas leaves the cylinder, it enters metal tubing in the anesthetic machine and is directed through a pressure-reducing valve or regulator. This device lowers and maintains pressure constant at 50 psi before delivery of the gas to the flowmeters. If the gases are delivered from a central source, the reducing valve is usually located at this site and the line pressure maintained at about 50 psi.

Flowmeters

Flowmeters measure the flow of gases based on the principle that flow past a resistance is proportional to pressure. Typically, gas flow enters the bottom of a vertically positioned and tapered (cross-sectional area increases upward from site of gas entry) glass tube. Gas flow into the flowmeter raises a bobbin- or ball-shaped float. The float comes to rest when gravity is balanced by the fall in pressure caused by the float. The upper end of the bobbin or equator of the ball indicates the gas flow in ml·min^{-1} or L·min^{-1}. Proportionality between pressure and flow is determined by the shape of the tube (resistance) and physical properties (density and viscosity) of the gas. The flowmeters are initially calibrated for the indicated gas at the factory. Since few gases have the same density and viscosity, flowmeters are not interchangeable with other gases. The scale accompanying an oxygen flowmeter is green, and the scale for the nitrous oxide flowmeter is blue.

Gas flow exits the flowmeters and passes into a manifold (mixing chamber) located at the top of the flowmeters (Fig. 11-2). To ensure against accidental decreases in the delivered oxygen concentration, the oxygen flowmeter should be the last in the sequence of flowmeters and thus the last gas added to the manifold. This arrangement assures that leaks in the apparatus proximal to oxygen inflow cannot diminish the delivered oxygen concentration, whereas leaks distal to that point result in loss of volume without a qualitative change in the mixture. Gases mix in the manifold and flow to an outlet port on the anesthetic machine where they are directed into either a vaporizer or an anesthetic breathing system. For emergency purposes, provision is made for delivery to the outlet port of a large volume of oxygen through an oxygen flush valve that bypasses the flowmeters and manifold to deliver pure oxygen at 35 L·min^{-1} to 75 L·min.$^{-1}$

VAPORIZERS

Potent inhaled anesthetics (halothane, enflurane, isoflurane) are liquids at room temperature and atmospheric pressure. Vaporization, which is the conversion of a liquid to a vapor, is accomplished in a closed container, which is referred to as a vaporizer. The vapor concentration resulting from vaporization of a volatile liquid anesthetic must be delivered to the patient with the same accuracy and predictability as other gases (nitrous oxide, oxygen). The safe use of vaporizers for this purpose requires an understanding of the physics of vaporization.

Physics of Vaporization

Molecules comprising a liquid are in constant random motion. In a vaporizer containing a volatile liquid anesthetic, there is an asymmetric arrangement of intermolecular forces applied to the molecules at the liquid-oxygen interface. The result of this asymmetric arrangement is a net attractive force pulling the surface molecules into the liquid phase. This force must be overcome if surface molecules are to enter the gas phase where their relatively sparse density constitutes a vapor. Energy necessary for molecules to escape from the liquid is supplied as heat. Heat of vaporization of a liquid is the number of calories required at a specific temperature to convert 1 gram of a liquid into a vapor. Heat of vaporization necessary for molecules to leave the liquid phase is greater when the temperature of the liquid decreases.

Vaporization in the closed confines of a vaporizer ceases when equilibrium is reached between the liquid and vapor phases such that the number of molecules leaving the liquid phase is the same as the number re-entering. The molecules in the vapor phase collide with each other and the walls of the container, creating a pressure. This pressure is termed vapor pressure. Vapor pressure is unique for each volatile anesthetic (see Chapter 2). Furthermore, vapor pressure is temperature dependent such that a reduction in temperature of the liquid is associated with a lower vapor pressure and fewer molecules in the vapor phase. Cooling of the liquid anesthetic reflects a loss of heat (heat of vaporization) necessary to provide energy for vaporization. This cooling is undesirable, as it lowers the vapor pressure and limits the attainable vapor concentration.

Vaporizer Classification and Design

Vaporizers (Ohmeda Tec 4, Drager Vapor 19.1) are classified as agent-specific, variable bypass, flow-over, temperature-compensated, out-of-circuit vaporizers (Fig. 11-3).[2,3] Variable bypass describes splitting of the total fresh gas flow through the vaporizer into two portions (Fig. 11-4).[2] The first portion of the fresh gas flow (20 percent or less) passes into the vaporizing chamber of the vaporizer where it becomes saturated (flow-over)

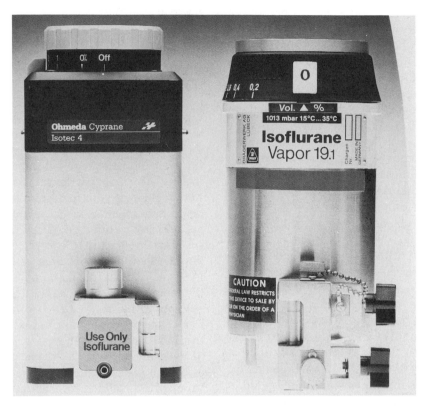

Fig. 11-3. Ohmeda Tec 4 and Drager Vapor 19.1 are examples of agent-specific vaporizers. Note the low position of the filler port to minimize the likelihood of overfilling the vaporizer chamber and the window near the filler port to permit visual verification of the level of liquid anesthetic in the vaporizing chamber.

with the vapor of the liquid anesthetic. The second portion of the fresh gas flow passes through the bypass chamber of the vaporizer. Both portions of the fresh gas flow mix at the patient outlet side of the anesthetic machine. The proportion of fresh gas flow diverted through the vaporizing chamber, and thus the concentration of volatile anesthetic delivered to the patient is determined by the concentration control dial. The scale on the concentration control dial is in volumes percent for the specific anesthetic drug. Vaporizer output is not influenced by fresh gas flows until very low flow rates (less than 250 ml·min^{-1}) are used. At these low fresh gas flows, vaporizer output is less than the concentration dial setting. This reflects the relatively high specific gravity of volatile anesthetics such that insufficient pressure is gener-

ated at low flow rates in the vaporizing chamber to upwardly advance the molecules. At high fresh gas flows (15 L·min^{-1} and greater) incomplete mixing in the vaporizing chamber also results in vaporizer output that is less than the concentration control dial setting.

A temperature sensitive bimetallic strip or an expansion element influences proportioning of total gas flow between the vaporizing and bypass chambers as vaporizer temperature changes (temperature compensated) (Fig. 11-4).[2] For example, as temperature of the liquid anesthetic in the vaporizer chamber decreases, the temperature sensing elements allow increased gas inflow into this chamber to offset the effect of reduced anesthetic liquid vapor pressure. Vaporizers are often constructed of metals with high thermal conduc-

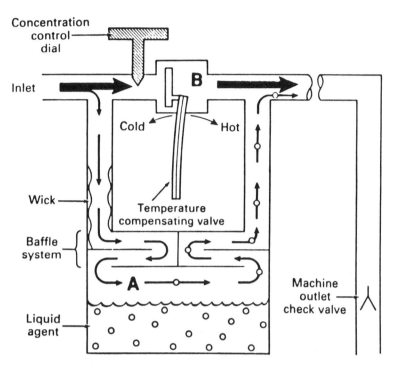

Fig. 11-4. Schematic diagram of the agent-specific Ohmeda Tec 4 vaporizer. Counterclockwise rotation of the concentration control dial diverts a portion of the total fresh gas flow through the vaporizing chamber (A) where wicks saturated with liquid anesthetic (agent) assure a large gas-liquid interface for efficient vaporization. A temperature compensating valve diverts more or less fresh gas flow through the vaporizing chamber to offset the effect of change in temperature of the liquid anesthetic on its vapor pressure (i.e., temperature compensated). Gases saturated with the vapor of the liquid anesthetic join gases that have passed through the chamber not containing liquid anesthetic (B) (bypass chamber) and are delivered to the machine outlet check valve. When the concentration control dial is in the off position, no fresh gas inflow passes into the vaporizing chamber.

tivity (copper, bronze) to further minimize heat loss. As a result, vaporizer output is nearly linear between 20° Celsuis and 35° Celsuis.[3] Designation of vaporizers as agent-specific and out-of-circuit emphasizes that these devices are designed to accommodate a single volatile anesthetic and are located outside the circuit. Copper kettle vaporizers (bubble through, nontemperature compensated, multiple drug, out-of-circuit vaporizers) are no longer manufactured.

Intermittent back pressure (pumping effect) transmitted to the vaporizing chamber as associated with positive pressure ventilation of the lungs or oxygen flush could increase vaporizer output. Design of the Ohmeda Tec 4 and Drager Vapor 19.1 vaporizers minimize the influence of this pumping effect.[2,3] Composition of the total gas flow (i.e., presence or absence of nitrous oxide) does not influence output of these vaporizers. Tipping of vaporizers can cause liquid anesthetic to spill from the vaporizing chamber into the bypass chamber with resulting increased vapor concentrations exiting from the vaporizer. Leaks associated with vaporizers are most often due to a loose filler cap.

Commonly two to three agent-specific vaporizers (enflurane, isoflurane, halothane) are present on the anesthetic machine. A safety interlock mechanism insures that only one vaporizer can be turned on simultaneously. Turning on a vaporizer requires depression of a release button on the concentration dial followed by counterclockwise rotation of the dial. This prevents accidental movement of the dial from the off to the on position. The low location of the filler port on the vaporizer minimizes the likelihood of overfilling of the vaporizing chamber (greater than 125 ml) with anesthetic liquid (Fig. 11-3). A window near the filler port permits visual verification of the level of liquid anesthetic in the vaporizing chamber. Use of an agent-specific keyed filler device prevents placement of a liquid anesthetic into the vaporizing chamber that is different from the drug for which the vaporizer was calibrated. Nevertheless, similar vapor pressures of halothane and isoflurane mean the concentration dial settings on agent-specific vaporizers for either of these liquids will also be accurate with the other liquid. Interchanging these liquids, however, is not recommended, since this practice would condone deliberate filling of the vaporizing chamber with the "wrong anesthetic." Furthermore, an overdose of halothane (MAC 0.75 percent) is possible should the concentration dial settings be used as if the administered anesthetic is isoflurane (MAC 1.15 percent). As with anesthetic machines, periodic maintenance (every 6 months to 12 months) is recommended by the manufacturers of vaporizers.

ANESTHETIC BREATHING SYSTEMS

Anesthetic breathing systems consist of the components necessary to deliver anesthetic gases and oxygen from the anesthetic machine to the patient.[4] Conceptually, the anesthetic breathing system is a tubular extension of the patient's upper airway. Because peak inspiratory flows as high as 60 L·min^{-1} are reached during spontaneous inspiration, anesthetic breathing systems can add considerable resistance to inhalation. The resistance imparted by an anesthetic breathing system is influenced by unidirectional valves and connectors. Minimizing resistance to breathing requires that components of the anesthetic breathing system, particularly the trachael tube connector, have the largest possible lumen. Increased airway resistance due to sharp bends produced by right-angle connectors is minimized by replacing these devices

with curved connectors. Finally, increased resistance to breathing due to the anesthetic breathing system can be offset by substituting controlled ventilation of the lungs for spontaneous breathing.

Anesthetic breathing systems are classified as open, semiopen, semiclosed, and closed, according to the presence or absence of (1) a gas reservoir bag in the system, (2) rebreathing of exhaled gases, (3) means to chemically neutralize exhaled carbon dioxide, and (4) unidirectional valves (Table 11-2).[5] In addition, the composition and flow rate of the inflow gases should be stated when describing an anesthetic breathing system.

Open Anesthetic Breathing System

An open anesthetic breathing system is characterized by the absence of a gas reservoir bag and the absence of rebreathing of exhaled gases (Table 11-2). The absence of a physical connection of this anesthetic breathing system to the patient results in spillage of anesthetic gases into the atmosphere (see the section *Pollution of the Atmosphere with Anesthetic Gases*) and an inability to assist or control ventilation of the lungs. The depth of anesthesia provided by an open anesthetic breathing system is unstable. For example, light anesthesia and the associated increase in ventilation results in increased dilution of the inhaled gases with room air such that even lighter levels of anesthesia result. Conversely, as the level of anesthesia deepens, the patient's tidal volume decreases and less dilution with room air occurs, resulting in deeper anesthesia.

Examples of open anesthetic breathing systems are insufflation and open drop administration of anesthetic gases.

Insufflation

Insufflation is the delivery of gases from the anesthetic machine via a delivery tube or mask held above the patient's face. During inspiration, the inhaled mixture is composed of gases delivered from the anesthetic machine plus room air. This is a useful technique for the induction of anesthesia in pediatric patients. During maintenance of anesthesia, as during bronchoscopy or laryngoscopy, insufflation of anesthetic gases and oxygen into the pharynx is facilitated by the use of a delivery

Table 11-2. Classification of Anesthetic Breathing Systems

System	Gas Reservoir Bag	Rebreathing of Exhaled Gases	Chemical Neutralization of Carbon Dioxide	Unidirectional Valves	Fresh Gas Inflow Rate[b]
Open					
Insufflation	No	No	No	None	Unknown
Open drop	No	No	No	None	Unknown
Semiopen					
Mapleson A, B, C, D	Yes	No[a]	No	One	High
Bain	Yes	No[a]	No	One	High
Mapleson E	No	No[a]	No	None	High
Jackson-Rees	Yes	No[a]	No	One	High
Semiclosed					
Circle	Yes	Partial	Yes	Three	Moderate
Closed	Yes	Total	Yes	Three	Low

[a] No rebreathing of exhaled gases only when fresh gas inflow is adequate.
[b] High, greater than 6 L·min^{-1}; moderate, 3 L·min^{-1} to 6 L·min^{-1}; low, 0.3 L·min^{-1} to 0.5 L·min^{-1}.

device that fits on the corner of the mouth (insufflation hook) so as to direct gases into the pharynx.

Open Drop Administration

Open drop administration of an anesthetic (most often ether but possible with all volatile anesthetics) is achieved by dripping the anesthetic liquid onto layers of gauze stretched over a wire frame in the shape of a face mask. Placement of this mask firmly on the patient's face may introduce some degree of rebreathing of exhaled gases. The carbon dioxide trapped under the mask also dilutes the inhaled concentration of oxygen. The decrease in oxygen concentration is offset by flowing oxygen under the mask (250 ml·min^{-1} to 500 ml·min^{-1}), but it must be appreciated that this flow reduces the inhaled concentration of anesthetic. The inhaled gases are cold, reflecting cooling of the gauze consequent to heat of vaporization. Open drop administration of anesthetic gases is rarely used, but its portability and simplicity favors its use in disaster situations.

Semiopen Anesthetic Breathing System

A semiopen anesthetic breathing system includes a gas reservoir bag and use of a unidirectional valve and/or high fresh gas inflow rates to prevent rebreathing of exhaled gases (Table 11-2).[5] These systems are lightweight, portable, easy to clean, and offer low resistance to breathing. Their principal advantage, however, is that the absence of rebreathing of exhaled gases results in a composition of the inspired gases that approximates that delivered by the anesthetic machine. As a result, an accurate estimate of the concentration of anesthetic gases and oxygen being delivered to the patient is possible. The presence of a gas reservoir bag enables assisted or controlled ventilation of the lungs. Like the open anesthetic breathing system, there is no conservation of respiratory moisture and body heat and the operating room atmosphere is contaminated with anesthetic gases (see the section *Pollution of the Atmosphere with Anesthetic Gases*).

Unidirectional Valve

The presence of a unidirectional valve in the semiopen anesthetic breathing system functions to direct fresh gases into the patient and exhaled gases out of the system. As a result, the total fresh gas inflow can be reduced often to a flow that equals the patient's minute ventilation. Disadvantages of a unidirectional valve include increased resistance to breathing and valve malfunction due to condensation of moisture. In addition, respiratory obstruction with a subsequent pneumothorax can occur in the presence of a unidirectional valve when the patient's minute ventilation exceeds fresh gas inflow into the anesthetic breathing system. Construction of the unidirectional valve to allow room air to enter when the patient's minute ventilation exceeds fresh gas inflow (Steen valve) prevents this adverse effect but results in dilution of the concentration of anesthetic gases and oxygen. Semiopen anesthetic breathing systems employing a unidirectional valve are frequently used in equipment designed for cardiopulmonary resuscitation (see Chapter 34).

High Fresh Gas Inflow

Semiopen anesthetic breathing systems that lack a unidirectional valve to prevent rebreathing of exhaled gases require high fresh gas inflow rates. These systems are classified as Mapleson A through E, depending on the location of the fresh gas inflow relative to the patient or overflow valve (Fig. 11-5).[6] The arrangement of these components influences the efficiency of the elimination of carbon dioxide. Mapleson systems are most often used in pediatric patients up to about 10 kg body weight. The limiting factor in the use of

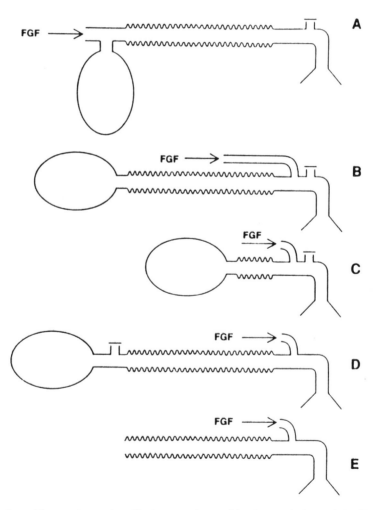

Fig. 11-5. Anesthetic breathing systems classified as semiopen Mapleson A through E. (From Willis et al.,[6] with permission.)

these systems is the fresh gas inflow rate (often based on ml·kg^{-1} or a multiple of the patient's minute ventilation) required to prevent rebreathing of exhaled gases. The high fresh gas inflow rates reduce the usefulness of these systems as body weight increases.

Mapleson A System

The Mapleson A system (Magill attachment) is characterized by placement of the overflow valve near the patient and separation of the gas reservoir bag from this valve by a corrugated tube (Fig. 11-5).[6] Fresh gas inflow is into the gas reservoir bag. This placement of the overflow valve and fresh gas inflow is the most efficient for elimination of carbon dioxide during spontaneous ventilation. Elimination of carbon dioxide reflects the preferential spillage of alveolar gas that contains carbon dioxide through the overflow valve during exhalation (Fig. 11-6).[7] For example, during exhalation, physiologic dead space gas followed by alveolar gas flows back into the corrugated tube. Pressure increases in the corrugated tube as exhaled gases

meet fresh gas inflow. When the pressure is sufficiently elevated, the overflow valve opens and the last gas to be exhaled (alveolar gas containing carbon dioxide) is preferentially vented to the atmosphere. Indeed, rebreathing of exhaled gases containing carbon dioxide does not occur using this system until fresh gas inflow decreases to a value equal to the patient's alveolar ventilation. Conservation of physiologic dead space gas is desirable, because this gas resembles fresh gas inflow in that carbon dioxide has not been added and anesthetic gases and oxygen have not been removed.

Compared with spontaneous ventilation, the Mapleson A system is less efficient during assisted or controlled ventilation of the lungs. This reflects the need to tighten the overflow valve to permit production of positive airway pressure when the gas reservoir bag is manually compressed. As a result, gases exit from the system during manually produced inspiration rather than during exhalation, leading to rebreathing of exhaled alveolar gas. The fresh gas inflow required to prevent

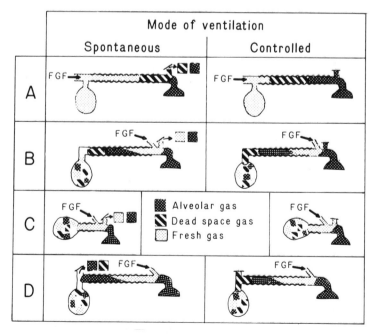

Fig. 11-6. Gas disposition at end-exhalation during spontaneous or controlled ventilation of the lungs using semiopen Mapleson A through D anesthetic breathing systems (Modified from Sykes,[7] with permission.)

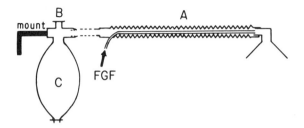

Fig. 11-7. Schematic diagram of the Bain system showing fresh gas flow (FGF) into a narrow tube within the corrugated expiratory limb (A). The only valve in the system (B) is an adjustable pressure-limiting valve (overflow valve) located near the FGF inlet and reservoir bag (C). (Modified from Bain and Spoerel,[8] with permission.)

rebreathing during assisted or controlled ventilation of the lungs using this system is difficult to estimate. Therefore, the Mapleson A system is best used in the presence of spontaneous ventilation.

Mapleson B System

The Mapleson B system is characterized by placement of the fresh gas inflow just distal to the overflow valve, which is located near the patient (Fig. 11-5).[6] This location of the fresh gas inflow results in a system that is less efficient than the Mapleson A system during spontaneous ventilation. In contrast to the Mapleson A system, however, the Mapleson B system behaves in a similar manner during spontaneous, assisted, or controlled ventilation of the lungs (Fig. 11-6).[7] A fresh gas inflow equal to at least twice the patient's minute ventilation is recommended to prevent rebreathing of exhaled gases.

Mapleson C System

The Mapleson C system is a Mapleson B system in which the expiratory limb has been shortened (Fig. 11-5).[6] As a result, the inhaled gases contain more alveolar gas (Fig. 11-7).[6] Therefore, the fresh gas inflow rate should be at least twice the patient's minute ventilation to prevent rebreathing of exhaled gases. The Mapleson C system may be used with any mode of ventilation.

Mapleson D System

The Mapleson D system resembles the Mapleson A system except that the locations of the fresh gas inflow and the overflow valve are reversed (Fig. 11-5).[6] Placement of the fresh gas inflow near the patient produces efficient elimination of carbon dioxide, regardless of the mode of ventilation (Fig. 11-6).[7] When the fresh gas inflow rate is equal to twice the patient's minute ventilation, the amount of rebreathing of exhaled gases is negligible.

Bain System

The Bain system is a coaxial version of a Mapleson D system in which the fresh gas inflow enters through a narrow tube within the corrugated expiratory limb (Fig. 11-7).[8] Advantages claimed for the Bain system include (1) warming of the fresh gas inflow by the surrounding exhaled gases in the expiratory limb, (2) improved humidification as a result of partial rebreathing, and (3) ease of scavenging waste anesthetic gases from an overflow valve. Availability of this system as a disposable item facilitates sterility, and its light weight is particularly important when anesthetic equipment must be far removed from the airway, as during head and neck surgery.

During controlled ventilation of the lungs using a Bain system, a fresh gas inflow rate equal to about 70 ml·kg^{-1} will maintain normocarbia.[6] Similiar fresh gas inflow rates during spontaneous ventilation of the lungs may result in hypercarbia because the patient may not be able to sufficiently increase alveolar ventilation in the presence of anesthetic induced depression of ventilation. Therefore, fresh gas inflow rates of 100 ml·kg^{-1} to 300 ml·kg^{-1} have been recommended when the Bain system is used during spontaneous ventilation.[9] In addition to hypercarbia, other complications associated with the use of the Bain system include increased resistance to breathing, rebreathing of exhaled gases due to unrecognized disconnection of the inner tube, and absence of fresh gas inflow due to unrecognized kinking of the inner tube.

Mapleson E System

The Mapleson E system consists of an expiratory limb connected to an Ayre's T piece (Fig. 11-5).[6] The Ayre's T piece is a metal tube with an internal diameter of 1 cm that receives fresh gas inflow via a side arm. During exhalation both exhaled and fresh gases flow down the open expiratory limb. During inspiration, varying ratios of fresh and exhaled gases can be inhaled, depending on the fresh gas inflow rate and the volume of the expiratory limb. For example, a fresh gas inflow rate equal to three times the patient's minute ventilation avoids rebreathing of exhaled gases during spontaneous ventilation when the volume of the expiratory limb is one-third the patient's tidal volume. Although there is no gas reservoir bag, ventilation of the lungs can be controlled by intermittent manual occlusion of the expiratory limb that forces gas into the patient's trachea.

Jackson-Rees Modification of the Ayre's T Piece

The addition of a gas reservoir bag with an adjustable overflow valve to the expiratory limb of a Mapleson E system is designated the Jackson-Rees modification of the Ayre's T piece (Fig. 11-8).[10] The advantage of this arrangement is ease of instituting assisted or controlled ventilation of the lungs, as well as monitoring ventilation by movement of the gas reservoir bag during spontaneous breathing. This system is particularly popular for pediatric patients because of its minimal dead space and low resistance to breathing. Furthermore, this system can be used with a face mask or a tracheal tube. Scavenging systems can be adapted to this system to reduce pollution of the atmosphere with anesthetic gases. The major disadvantage of this system is the need to deliver a fresh gas inflow rate equal to at least twice the patient's minute ventilation so as to assure the absence of rebreathing of exhaled gases.

Semiclosed Anesthetic Breathing System

A semiclosed anesthetic breathing system is the most commonly used system for delivery of anesthetic gases and oxygen to children and adults. This system has a gas reservoir bag and provides for partial rebreathing of exhaled gases (Table 11-2).[5] Rebreathing of exhaled gases is acceptable because of the use of chemical neutralization of carbon dioxide. As a result of partial rebreathing of exhaled gases, there is some conservation of airway moisture and body heat. Furthermore, the fresh gas inflow rate can be less than the patient's minute ventilation, which diminishes pollution of the surrounding atmosphere with anesthetic gases. The price paid for these desirable characteristics includes increased resistance to breathing (due to unidirectional valves and carbon dioxide canister), bulkiness with loss of portability, and enhanced opportunity for malfunction of a more complex apparatus.

Circle System

The most commonly used semiclosed anesthetic breathing system, the circle system is a true breathing circuit; anesthetic gases and oxygen circulate in one direction entirely within the confines of the components of the system. Essential components of this system are (1) unidirectional inspiratory and expiratory valves, (2) inspiratory and expiratory corrugated ("elephant") tubes, (3) carbon dioxide canister, (4) gas reservoir bag, and (5) adjustable pressure limiting (overflow) valve on

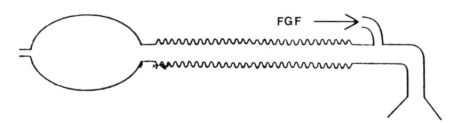

Fig. 11-8. Schematic diagram of the Jackson-Rees modification of the Ayre's T-piece showing fresh gas flow (FGF) entering near the patient and an adjustable pressure limiting (overflow) valve on the distal end of the gas reservoir bag.

the expiratory side (Fig. 11-9).[1] An airway pressure gauge, oxygen analyzer, and scavenging system are also included in the circuitry of a circle anesthetic breathing system (Fig. 11-9).[1]

The two unidirectional valves are situated so that one tube is for inhalation and the other for exhalation. This arrangement eliminates the inhalation of exhaled gases until they have passed through the carbon dioxide canister (see the section *Elimination of Carbon Dioxide*) and have had their oxygen content replenished. Incompetence or absence of a unidirectional valve permits breathing back and forth in one tube, resulting in rebreathing of exhaled gases and development

of hypercarbia. The two corrugated tubes serve as the conduits to deliver anesthetic gases and oxygen to the patient. These large lumen tubes (22 mm) provide minimal resistance to breathing and are corrugated to prevent kinking. The gas reservoir bag maintains an available reserve volume to satisfy inspiratory flow rates of the patient (up to 60 L· min^{-1}), which greatly exceed conventional fresh gas flows (3 L·min^{-1}) from the anesthetic machine. The adjustable pressure-limiting valve allows the anesthesiologist to increase pressure in the anesthetic breathing system (depicted on the airway pressure oxygen gauge) so as to provide assisted or controlled ventilation of the lungs by

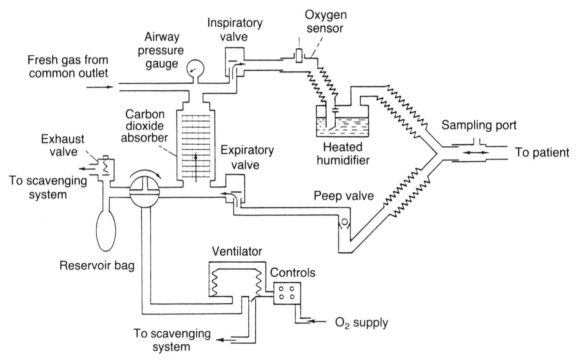

Fig. 11-9. Schematic diagram showing essential components (unidirectional inspiratory and expiratory valves, inspiratory and expiratory corrugated tubes, carbon dioxide canister [absorber], gas reservoir bag and adjustable pressure limiting [exhaust or overflow] valve) of a circle anesthetic breathing system. An oxygen analyzer (sensor) is placed in the inspiratory or expiratory side of the system. An airway pressure gauge reflects pressure in the system that is potentially being transmitted to the patient's airway. Excess gases are prevented from entering the atmosphere by continuous suction to a scavenging system. Optional components and their location in the circle anesthetic breathing system include a heated humidifer and PEEP (positive end-expiratory pressure) valve. Note the separate circuit for an oxygen driven ventilator that may be substituted for the gas reservoir bag by clockwise rotation of a valve. (From Check-Out,[1] with permission.)

manual compression of the gas reservoir bag. Alternatively, the anesthesiologist may provide controlled ventilation of the lungs by turning a valve that eliminates the gas reservoir bag from the circle anesthetic breathing system and substitutes intermittent positive airway pressure delivered from a mechanical ventilator (Fig. 11-9).[1]

Prevention of rebreathing of exhaled gases using a circle system mandates that a unidirectional valve be placed between the patient and gas reservoir bag on both the inspiratory and expiratory limbs of the circuit.[4] The most efficient arrangement of components for both spontaneous and controlled ventilation of the lungs is placement of the (1) unidirectional valves near the patient, (2) adjustable pressure-limiting valve near the patient just distal to the exhalation valve, and (3) fresh gas inflow entering between the carbon dioxide absorber and inhalation valve. In this arrangement, fresh gas inflow preferentially expels ("flushes") alveolar gas (as in the Mapleson A system) while conserving physiologic dead space gas. Nevertheless, this optimal arrangement is impractical, as the bulky unidirectional valves and overflow valve are located near the patient. A more practical but less efficient arrangement is placement of the unidirectional valves and adjustable pressure-limiting valve more distal to the patient (Fig. 11-9).[1]

Rebreathing of exhaled gases using a semiclosed anesthetic breathing system influences the inhaled anesthetic concentrations of these gases. For example, when uptake of an anesthetic gas is high, as during induction of anesthesia, rebreathing of exhaled gases depleted of anesthetic greatly dilutes the concentration of anesthetic in the fresh gas inflow. This dilutional effect of uptake is offset clinically by increasing the delivered concentration of anesthetic. As uptake of anesthetic diminishes, the impact of dilution on the inspired concentration produced by rebreathing of exhaled gases is lessened. A circle system can be semiopen, semiclosed, or closed, depending on the fresh gas inflow.

Closed Anesthetic Breathing System

A closed anesthetic breathing system is present when the fresh gas inflow into a circle system is decreased sufficiently to permit closure of the overflow valve, and all the exhaled carbon dioxide is neutralized in the carbon dioxide absorber. The fresh gas inflow for a closed system (150 ml·min^{-1} to 500 ml·min^{-1}) satisfies the patient's metabolic oxygen requirements (150 ml·min^{-1} to 250 ml·min^{-1} during anesthesia) and replaces anesthetic gases lost by virtue of tissue uptake.

Advantages of the closed anesthetic breathing system compared with the semiclosed anesthetic breathing system include (1) maximal humidification and warming of inhaled gases, (2) less pollution of the surrounding atmosphere with anesthetic gases, and (3) economy in the use of anesthetics. A disadvantage of the closed anesthetic breathing system is the inability to rapidly change the delivered concentration of anesthetic gases and oxygen due to the low fresh gas inflow. The principal dangers of a closed anesthetic breathing system are delivery of (1) unpredictable and possibly insufficient amounts of oxygen, and (2) unknown and possibly excessive concentrations of potent anesthetic gases.

Unpredictable Amounts of Oxygen

Unpredictable and possibly insufficient concentrations of oxygen using a closed anesthetic breathing system are particularly likely when nitrous oxide is included in the fresh gas inflow. For example, decreased tissue uptake of nitrous oxide with time in the presence of continued and unchanged uptake of oxygen can result in a decreased concentration of oxygen in the alveoli (Table 11-3). Therefore, the use of an oxygen analyzer placed on the inspiratory or expiratory limb of the circle system is mandatory when nitrous oxide is delivered using a closed anesthetic breathing system.

Unknown Concentrations of Potent Anesthetic

Exhaled gases, freed of carbon dioxide, form a major part of the inhaled gases when a closed anesthetic breathing system is used. This means the composition of the inhaled gases is influenced by the concentration present in the exhaled gases. The concentration of anesthetic in exhaled gases reflects tissue uptake of the anesthetic. Initially, tissue uptake is maximal and the concentration of anesthetic in the exhaled gases is reduced. Subsequent rebreathing of these exhaled gases dilutes

Table 11-3. Alveolar Gas Concentration Using a Closed Circle Anesthetic Breathing System

Example 1

Gas inflow is nitrous oxide 300 ml·min^{-1} and oxygen 300 ml·min^{-1} for 15 minutes. Nitrous oxide uptake by tissues at this time is 200 ml·min^{-1}, and oxygen consumption is 250 ml·min^{-1}. Alveolar gas after tissue uptake consists of 100 ml nitrous oxide and 50 ml oxygen. The alveolar concentration of oxygen ($F_{A}O_2$) is

$$F_{A}O_2 = \frac{50 \text{ ml oxygen}}{100 \text{ ml nitrous oxide} + 50 \text{ ml oxygen}} \times 100 = 33\%$$

Example 2

Gas inflow as in Example 1 but duration of administration is 1 hour. At this time, tissue uptake of nitrous oxide has decreased to 100 ml·min^{-1}, but oxygen consumption remains unchanged at 250 ml·min^{-1}. Alveolar gas after tissue uptake consists of 200 ml nitrous oxide and 50 ml oxygen. The alveolar concentration of oxygen ($F_{A}O_2$) is

$$F_{A}O_2 = \frac{50 \text{ ml oxygen}}{200 \text{ ml nitrous oxide} + 50 \text{ ml oxygen}} \times 100 = 20\%$$

the inhaled concentration of anesthetic delivered to the patient. Therefore, high inflow concentrations of anesthetic are necessary to offset maximal tissue uptake. Conversely, little or no anesthetic needs to be added to the inflow gases when tissue uptake is reduced. The unknown impact of tissue uptake on the concentration of anesthetic in the exhaled gases makes it difficult to estimate the inhaled concentration delivered to the patient using a closed anesthetic breathing system. This disadvantage can be partially offset by administering higher fresh gas inflows (3 L·min^{-1}) for about 15 minutes before instituting use of a closed anesthetic breathing system. This approach permits elimination of nitrogen from the lungs and corresponds to the time of greatest tissue uptake of anesthetic.

ELIMINATION OF CARBON DIOXIDE

Elimination of carbon dioxide from an anesthetic breathing system can be achieved by venting all exhaled gases to the atmosphere, as occurs during

Table 11-4. Composition of Carbon Dioxide Absorbents

Soda Lime (Percentage of Wet Weight)	Baralyme (Percentage of Wet Weight)
Sodium hydroxide, 4%	Barium hydroxide, 20%
Potassium hydroxide, 1%	Calcium hydroxide, 80%
Water, 14%–19%	Water, bound water of crystallization in the octahydrate salt of barium hydroxide
Silica, 0.2%	Silica, none
Calcium hydroxide, balance	

the use of an open or semiopen anesthetic breathing system. More often, however, partial (semiclosed anesthetic breathing system) or total (closed anesthetic breathing system) rebreathing of exhaled gases is permitted and carbon dioxide is eliminated by chemical neutralization. Chemical neutralization of carbon dioxide is achieved by directing exhaled gases through a container (canister) containing a carbon dioxide absorbent such as soda lime or baralyme.

Soda Lime

Soda lime granules consist of calcium hydroxide plus smaller amounts of sodium hydroxide and potassium hydroxide that are present as activators (Table 11-4). A specific water content of soda lime granules is necessary to assure optimal activity. Silica is added to the granules to give hardness and thus minimize the formation of alkaline dust. Formation of this alkaline dust must be prevented because its inhalation can produce irritation of the airways, manifesting as bronchospasm.

Neutralization of carbon dioxide begins with the reaction of this gas with the water present in soda lime granules and exhaled gases to form carbonic acid. Carbonic acid then reacts with the hydroxides present in soda lime granules to form carbonates, water, and heat. The water formed by the neutralization of carbon dioxide is useful for humidifying the inhaled gases and for dissipating some of the heat generated in the exothermic neutrali-

---

Chemical Neutralization of Carbon Dioxide

Soda lime

$$CO_2 + H_2O \rightarrow H_2CO_3$$
$$H_2CO_3 + NaOH \rightarrow Na_2CO_3 \text{ (rapid)} +$$
$$2H_2O + Heat$$
$$H_2CO_3 + Ca(OH)_2 \rightarrow CaCO_3 \text{ (slow)} +$$
$$2H_2O + Heat$$

Baralyme

$$CO_2 + H_2O \rightarrow H_2CO_3$$
$$H_2CO_3 + Ba(OH)_2 \rightarrow BaCO_3 \text{ (rapid)} +$$
$$2H_2O + Heat$$
$$H_2CO_3 + Ca(OH)_2 \rightarrow CaCO_3 \text{ (slow)} +$$
$$2H_2O + Heat$$

---

zation reaction. Accumulation of this highly alkaline water in the bottom of the canister can produce burns on contact with the skin. The heat generated during neutralization of carbon dioxide can be detected by warmness of the canister. Failure of the canister to become warm to touch should alert the anesthesiologist to the possibility that chemical neutralization of carbon dioxide is not taking place.

Baralyme

Baralyme granules consist of barium hydroxide and calcium hydroxide (Table 11-4). Unlike soda lime, the addition of silica to baralyme granules is not necessary to assure hardness. This inherent hardness of baralyme granules reflects the presence of bound water of crystallization in the octahydrate salt of barium hydroxide. This bound water also accounts for the more reliable performance of baralyme than soda lime in dry environments. As with soda lime, the neutralization of carbon dioxide by baralyme results in the formation of carbonates, water, and heat.

Efficiency of Carbon Dioxide Neutralization

Efficiency of carbon dioxide neutralization is influenced by the size of the carbon dioxide absorbent granules and presence or absence of channeling in the canister containing the carbon dioxide ab-

sorbent. In addition, optimal absorptive conditions provide that the equivalent of the patient's tidal volume be accommodated entirely within the void space of the canister. Therefore, about one-half the volume of a properly packed canister should consist of intergranular spaces.

A pH-sensitive dye is added to soda lime or baralyme by the manufacturer. A change in color of the absorbent granules is produced when this dye is activated by carbonic acid that accumulates due to exhaustion of the activity of absorbent granules. If the exhausted absorbent granules are not replaced with fresh granules, the color change often disappears during disuse. Minimal regeneration of absorbent granule activity, however, will have occurred and, upon reuse, the dye quickly produces the color change again.

The maximum volume of carbon dioxide that can be absorbed is approximately 26 L of carbon dioxide per 100 g of absorbent granules. Usually, considerably less carbon dioxide is absorbed due to factors such as canister design and the specific end-point used to detect exhaustion of absorbent granule activity. For example, only 10 L to 15 L of carbon dioxide per 100 g of absorbent are neutralized in a single-chambered canister, whereas 18 L to 20 L are absorbed in a dual-chambered (jumbo) canister. In the jumbo canister, the chamber through which the exhaled gases flow first is replaced with new absorbent granules when the indicator dye changes color and at the same time the canister is inverted so that the second chamber is moved to the position occupied by the first canister. This sequence is intended to maximally use the activity of the absorbent granules in both canisters.

Absorbent Granule Size

Absorbent granule size is designated as mesh size. For example, an absorbent granule size of 8 mesh (2.5 mm) will pass through a screen having 8 or fewer wires per 2.5 cm. Empirically, the optimal absorbent granule size of soda line or baralyme has been found to be 4 mesh to 8 mesh. This absorbent granule size represents a compromise between absorptive activity and resistance to air flow through the canister. Absorptive activity increases as absorbent granule size decreases because total surface area increases. The smaller the absorbent granules, however, the smaller the interstices through which gases must flow, resulting in increased resistance to flow.

Channeling

Channeling is the preferential passage of exhaled gases through the canister via pathways of low resistance such that the bulk of the carbon dioxide absorbent granules are bypassed. Loose packing of the absorbent granules in the canister is the most frequent cause of channeling. Shaking the canister gently before use to assure firm packing of the absorbent granules reduces the likelihood of channeling without substantially increasing resistance to flow of gases. In addition, the absorbent granules are held in place with screens and baffles to facilitate uniform dispersion of gas flow.

HUMIDIFICATION

Humidification is a form of vaporization in which water vapor (moisture) is added to the gases delivered by the anesthetic breathing system. Normally,

air passing through the nose is warmed to body temperature and saturated with water vapor before reaching the carina. Administration of dry anesthetic gases and oxygen at room temperature via an anesthetic breathing system that bypasses the nose leads to cytologic damage to the respiratory epithelium within 1 hour.[11] Breathing dry gases for several hours can result in drying of secretions and, when a trachael tube is used, airway obstruction from inspissated secretions in the tube. In addition, breathing dry and unwarmed gases is associated with water and heat loss from the patient (see Chapter 31). More important than water loss, however, is the heat loss, which may lead to adverse reductions in body temperature, particularly in infants and children who are rendered poikilothermic by general anesthesia. Indeed, the most important reason to provide heated humidification during general anesthesia is to reduce heat loss and associated decreases in body temperature (Fig. 11-10).[12]

The simplest method for raising the water content of inhaled gases is passing these gases through

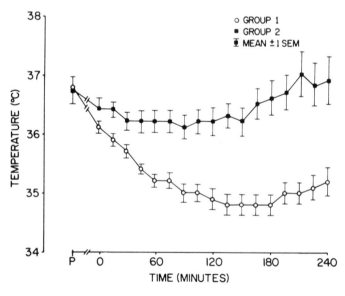

Fig. 11-10. Nasopharyngeal temperature was measured in 10 patients breathing gases that were heated to 37° Celsius and 100 percent humidified (group 1) and 10 patients breathing gases delivered at room temperature (group 2). Preoperative oral temperatures (P) and nasopharyngeal temperatures immediately after induction of anesthesia (0 time) were similar in both groups of patients. Subsequently, nasopharyngeal temperature decreased only in patients not receiving warmed and humidified gases. (From Stone et al.,[12] with permission.)

the canister used for carbon dioxide absorption. Heating due to the exothermic reaction produced by the neutralization of carbon dioxide enables the inhaled gases to hold more water. The most reliable way to warm and humidify anesthetic gases and oxygen is to use specially designed humidifiers placed in the anesthetic breathing circuit (Fig. 11-9)[1] (see Chapter 31).

BACTERIAL CONTAMINATION OF ANESTHETIC EQUIPMENT

The role of bacterial contamination of the anesthetic machine and equipment and the subsequent development of pulmonary infection and cross-infection between patients is controversial.[13] Nevertheless, it is assumed that equipment used to deliver anesthesia is a potential source of bacterial contamination to patients. Based on this assumption, the use of disposable anesthetic breathing systems has become popular. The incidence, however, of postoperative pulmonary infection is not altered by the use of a sterile disposable anesthetic breathing system as compared with the use of a reusable system that is cleaned with basic hygienic techniques but not sterilized between uses. Likewise, the incidence of postoperative pulmonary infection is not altered by inclusion of a bacterial filter in the anesthetic breathing system.

The reason anesthetic equipment has not been implicated as a cause of infection, in contrast to the undeniable role of respiratory therapy equipment (particularly nebulizers), involves the low likelihood of airborne transmission of bacteria from the host. Furthermore, the environment presented to organisms that may be present in the anesthetic machine and breathing system is not conducive to bacterial survival.

Airborne Transmission

During anesthesia and quiet breathing only a small number of bacteria are likely to be liberated from the host. Indeed, the administration of anesthesia to patients with known colonization of gram-negative bacteria does not result in contamination of the anesthetic breathing system. Bacteria that are released from the airway during violent forms of exhalation originate almost exclusively from the

anterior portion of the oropharynx and rarely the nose or pharynx, which harbors respiratory pathogens. Furthermore, even low concentrations of oxygen are lethal to airborne bacteria.

Environment Presented to Bacteria

Airborne bacteria released into a circle anesthetic breathing system are exposed to shifts in humidity and temperature. Bacteria, particularly gram-negative organisms, are sensitive to both these changes. In fact, shifts in humidity and temperature are probably the most important factors responsible for bacterial killing that occurs within the anesthetic breathing system.

Most studies have shown that clinical concentrations of general anesthetics have little influence on the survival of bacteria in the anesthetic breathing system. However, bacteria placed in vaporizers containing liquid anesthetics do not survive. The role of anesthetic equipment in transmitting viral illnesses is not known. If patients with known viral infections, such as acquired immunodeficiency syndrome, require anesthesia, it would seem prudent to use a disposable anesthetic breathing system including the soda lime canister and ventilator bellows. Disinfection of nondisposable equipment including laryngoscope blades is with sodium hypochlorite (bleach), which destroys the human immunodeficiency virus.

Metallic ions of metals (copper, zinc, chromium, brass) present in the anesthetic machine and other equipment have a highly lethal effect on bacteria. A practical use for this effect has been the insertion of copper mesh or sponges into the expiratory limb of ventilators to prevent infection from contaminated respiratory therapy equipment.

Transmission of Tuberculosis

There has been no documented transmission of tuberculosis from a contaminated anesthetic machine or anesthetic breathing system to a patient.[13] Nevertheless, of all bacterial forms, acid-fast bacilli are the most adaptable and resistant to destruction. Therefore, a greater degree of vigilance should be observed in dealing with patients with pulmonary disease conceivably due to tuberculosis. This vigilance should include use of a disposable anesthetic breathing system and disinfection of nondisposable equipment with an appropriate chemical such as glutaraldehyde (Cidex).

POLLUTION OF THE ATMOSPHERE WITH ANESTHETIC GASES

Chronic exposure to low concentrations of anesthetics that result from spillage of these gases into the atmosphere from the anesthetic machine and anesthetic breathing system constitutes a health hazard to operating room personnel[14] (see Chapter 5). For this reason removal (scavenging) of trace concentrations of anesthetic gases present in the atmosphere of the operating rooms is recommended. In addition, dental and veterinary settings should be provided with gas scavenging capabilities. The National Institute of Occupational Safety and Health (NIOSH) has proposed that nitrous oxide concentrations in the atmosphere should be less than 22 ppm (parts per million) and less than 5 ppm for volatile anesthetics. It must be recognized, however, that there is no evidence these proposed levels are either desirable or less hazardous than higher concentrations. Nevertheless, nitrous oxide concentrations in excess of 200 ppm as determined by gas chromatography or infrared analysis should alert personnel to search for leaks and/or consider alterations in anesthetic techniques.

Source of Anesthetic Gases in the Environment

High pressure system leakage of anesthetic gases into the atmosphere occurs when a gas, such as nitrous oxide, escapes from tanks attached to the anesthetic machine (faulty yokes) or from tubing or connectors necessary for the delivery of nitrous oxide to the anesthetic machine from a central gas supply (faulty quick-coupler connector). Low pressure leakage is characterized by escape of anesthetic gases from sites located between the flowmeters of the anesthetic machine and the patient, including spillage from the anesthetic breathing system.

Control of Gas Leakage

Control of gas spillage into the environment requires (1) periodic maintenance of anesthetic equipment, (2) removal of excess gases vented from the anesthetic breathing system by the process known as scavenging, (3) attention to technique of anesthesia, and (4) adequate ventilation of the operating rooms.[15]

Periodic Maintenance

Periodic maintenance of the anesthetic machine by a qualified service representative is the best protection against persistence of leaks in the high or low pressure system of the anesthetic machine and anesthetic breathing system. Spillage from high or low pressure system components can be detected by applying a soap solution to suspected areas of spillage. The presence and amount of leakage using a circle anesthetic breathing system can be determined by closing the overflow valve, occluding the patient end of the system, and noting the oxygen inflow required to maintain a pressure of 30 cm H_2O. Leakage varies linearly with pressure such that a 150 ml·min^{-1} leakage rate at 30 cm H_2O will manifest as 50 ml·min^{-1} spillage at 10 cm H_2O, which is the typical average pressure in a circle anesthetic breathing system during controlled ventilation of the lungs. Leakage of 50 ml·min^{-1} contributes less than 5 ppm to the average operating room concentration of anesthetic gases. Correction of leakage often involves simple steps such as replacing a worn canister gasket or removing a deformed washer on a yoke.

Scavenging

Scavenging is the term applied to collection and removal of excess gases that normally exit via the overflow valve of the anesthetic breathing system. Removal of these excess gases is accomplished by attaching a gas capturing device that includes suction to the anesthetic breathing system. Captured gases are most often delivered to the central vacuum system of the hospital for disposal. Attachment of this device to the anesthetic breathing system introduces the risk of removal of excessive volumes of gas from the system unless the fresh gas inflow is greater than the suction rate. The presence of an excessive rate of suction most often manifests as collapse of the gas reservoir bag. Conversely, occlusion of the gas disposal route may allow excessive pressure increases to occur in the anesthetic breathing system and lead to barotrauma. For these reasons, a pressure-balancing capability is included in the gas capturing device so as to prevent the development of negative or positive pressure in the anesthetic breathing system.

Technique of Anesthesia

Poor fit of the face mask and allowing anesthetic gases to flow before placement of the mask on the patient's face or during intubation of the trachea, result in spillage of anesthetic gases into the atmosphere. Administration of oxygen at the conclusion of anesthesia serves to eliminate anesthetic gases from the patient and anesthetic breathing system and thus reduce spillage into the atmosphere. The use of low flow or closed system techniques diminishes but does not eliminate operating room pollution with waste anesthetic gases. Care should be exercised in filling vaporizers, as spillage of liquid anesthetic results in substantial pollution. For example, if halothane spillage is detectable by smell, the level of contamination is likely to exceed 30 ppm.

Room Ventilation

The efficiency of operating room ventilation in terms of room air turnovers per hour should be determined and ventilation filters checked at periodic intervals by the hospital engineer.

REFERENCES

1. Check-Out. A guide for preoperative inspection of an anesthetic machine. Chicago, American Society of Anesthesiologists, 1987:1–14.
2. Tec 4 continuous flow vaporizer. Operators manual. Steeton, England. Ohmeda, The BOC Group, Inc. 1986.
3. Vapor 19.1 operating manual. Lubeck, Federal Republic of Germany. Dragerwerk, 1985.
4. Eger EI II. Anesthetic systems: Construction and function. In: Anesthetic Uptake and Action. Baltimore, Williams & Wilkins, 1974:206–7.
5. Hamilton WK. Nomenclature of inhalation anesthetic systems. Anesthesiology 1964;25:3–5.
6. Willis BA, Pender JW, Mapleson WW. Rebreathing in a T-piece: Volunteer and theoretical studies of the Jackson-Rees modification of Ayre's T piece during spontaneous respiration. Br J Anaesth 1975; 47:1239–46.
7. Sykes MK. Rebreathing circuits: A review. Br J Anaesth 1968;40:666–74.
8. Bain JA, Spoerel WE. A streamlined anesthetic system. Can Anaesth Soc J 1972;19:426–35.
9. Rose DK, Byrick RJ, Froese AB. Carbon dioxide elimination during spontaneous ventilation with a modified Mapleson D system: Studies in a lung model. Can Anaesth Soc J 1978;25:353–65.
10. Jackson-Rees G. Anaesthesia in the newborn. Br Med J 1950;2:1419–22.
11. Chalon J, Loew DAY, Malebranche J. Effect of dry anesthetic gases on tracheobronchial ciliated epithelium. Anesthesiology 1972;37:338–43.
12. Stone DR, Downs JB, Paul WL, Perkins HM. Adult body temperature and heated humidification of anesthetic gases during general anesthesia. Anesth Analg 1981;60:736–41.
13. duMoulin GC, Hedley-Whyte J. Bacterial interactions between anesthesiologists, their patients, and equipment. Anesthesiology 1982;57:37–41.
14. Vessey MP. Epidemiological studies of the occupational hazards of anaesthesia—a review. Anaesthesia 1978;33:430–8.
15. Lecky JH. Anesthetic pollution in the operating room. A notice to operating room personnel. Anesthesiology 1980;52:157–9.

Chapter 12

Airway Management

Intubation of the trachea (translaryngeal intubation) is a safe and common practice in patients undergoing general anesthesia. Atraumatic intubation of the trachea requires a knowledge of the anatomy of the upper airway and appropriate use of equipment and drugs, particularly muscle relaxants.

PREOPERATIVE EVALUATION

Preoperative evaluation of the patient determines the route (oral or nasal) and method (awake or anesthetized) for intubation of the trachea. This evaluation includes an assessment of anatomic characteristics that may make intubation of the trachea difficult, a thorough dental examination, and an evaluation of temporomandibular joint and cervical spine mobility.

Anatomic Characteristics

Anatomic characteristics that impair alignment of oral, pharyngeal, and laryngeal axes (Fig. 12-1) and make visualization of the glottic opening difficult by direct laryngoscopy include (1) a short muscular neck and a full set of teeth, (2) a receding mandible, (3) protruding maxillary incisors, and (4) poor mandibular mobility.[1] Visualization of the glottic opening by direct laryngoscopy is predictably difficult if the distance from the lower border of the mandible to the thyroid notch with the neck fully extended is less than 6.5 cm. If nasotracheal intubation is planned, the patency of the nares can be evaluated by asking the patient to breathe through each naris while the examiner occludes the other.

Dental Examination

Teeth and dental prostheses are vulnerable to damage or dislodgement by the laryngoscope blade during direct laryngoscopy. Therefore, the preoperative dental examination should ascertain the presence of (1) loose teeth, (2) dental prostheses, and (3) co-existing dental abnormalities.[2]

Loose Teeth

Newly erupted deciduous or permanent teeth initially have little support because the roots are only partially formed. Deciduous teeth begin to erupt at about 6 months of age, and permanent teeth start to appear at about 6 years of age. As a permanent tooth erupts, the root portion of the overlying deciduous tooth undergoes resolution such that just before exfoliation, it may be held in place only by fibrous tissue. Children 6 years to 12 years of age are considered to be in the mixed dentition stage. In adults, loosening of teeth most often reflects peridontal disease and loss of bony support.

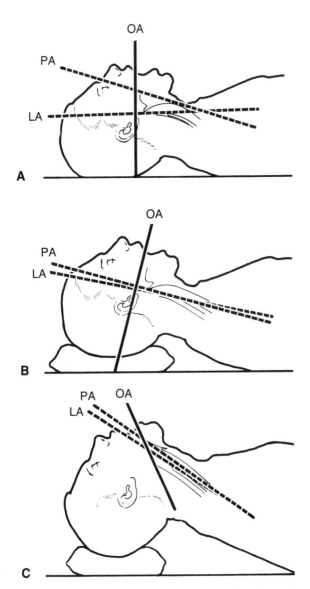

Fig. 12-1. Schematic diagram demonstrating head position for intubation of the trachea. (A) Successful exposure of the glottic opening using direct laryngoscopy requires alignment of the oral, pharyngeal, and laryngeal axes. (B) Elevation of the head with pads under the occiput with the shoulders remaining on the table aligns the pharyngeal and laryngeal axes. (C) Subsequent head extension at the altanto-occipital joint serves to create the shortest distance and most nearly straight line from the incisor teeth to glottic opening.

Dental Prostheses

The position of fixed or removable dental prostheses should be determined preoperatively. An individual crown (cap) is affixed to an underlying natural tooth and is difficult to detect, particularly if it is porcelain. A permanent (nonremovable) bridge fills a gap between one or more missing permanent teeth and prosthetic appliances are attached to the bridge. Nonpermanent bridges or dentures may be removed preoperatively or left in place until after induction of anesthesia so as to facilitate a mask fit to the face.

Co-Existing Dental Abnormalities

The position of missing teeth and chips or fractures (especially on maxillary incisors) is important to detect preoperatively. Otherwise, subsequent discovery of these abnormalities may be incorrectly attributed to damage produced by the laryngoscope blade. It must be appreciated that protruding maxillary incisors are particularly vulnerable to damage from levering effects exerted by the laryngoscope blade.

Temporomandibular Joint Mobility

Temporomandibular joint mobility can be evaluated by having the patient open his or her mouth as widely as possible. Normal mandibular opening in an adult is in the range of 40 mm or at least two finger breadths.[3] Limitation of mandibular mobility is most often due to involvement of the temporomandibular joint by arthritis. As a result, difficulty may be experienced in opening the mouth wide enough to permit direct laryngoscopy for intubation of the trachea.

Cervical Spine Mobility

Cervical spine mobility as demonstrated by flexion and extension of the head is essential for proper positioning in preparation for direct laryngoscopy (Fig. 12-1). The normal range of flexion-extension of the head decreases approximately 20 percent by 75 years of age.[4]

INDICATIONS FOR OROTRACHEAL INTUBATION

Orotracheal intubation may be considered for every patient receiving general anesthesia. There are also specific indications for intubation of the

---

Indications for Orotracheal Intubation

Provide patent airway
Prevent inhalation (aspiration) of gastric
 contents
Need for frequent suctioning
Facilitate positive pressure ventilation of the
 lungs
Operative position other than supine
Operative site near or involving the upper
 airway
Airway maintenance by mask difficult
Disease involving upper airway

---

trachea in surgical patients. Specific indications for placement of a cuffed tracheal tube include provision of a patent airway and prevention of the inhalation (aspiration) of gastric contents, blood, or secretions into the lungs. Intubation of the trachea is mandatory in patients who have recently ingested food or in whom intestinal obstruction is present. Any patient requiring frequent tracheal suctioning is best managed with a tracheal tube in place. Operations in which positive pressure ventilation of the lungs is required (thoracotomy, presence of neuromuscular blockade) or in which prolonged controlled ventilation of the lungs is necessary are most reliably managed in the presence of a tracheal tube. Maintenance of a patent upper airway or controlled ventilation of the lungs is not reliable in the absence of a tracheal tube when operations are performed in other than the supine position (e.g., sitting, prone, lateral, lithotomy, or head-down position). Operations about the head, neck, or upper airway require a tracheal tube for both airway maintenance and/or removal of anesthetic equipment from the operative site. Difficult maintenance of a patent airway by mask may be an indication for tracheal intubation. For example, the upper airway of an edentulous patient is difficult to maintain using a face mask, but intubation of the trachea is technically easy. Finally, disease involving the upper airway mandates placement of a tracheal tube when unconsciousness is to be produced with anesthetic drugs.

TECHNIQUE FOR OROTRACHEAL INTUBATION

Orotracheal intubation using direct laryngoscopy in anesthetized patients is routinely chosen unless specific circumstances dictate a different approach. Equipment and drugs used in accomplishing intubation of the trachea include a proper sized tracheal tube, laryngoscope, functioning suction catheter, appropriate anesthetic drugs, and facilities to provide positive pressure ventilation of the lungs with oxygen. If a cuffed tracheal tube is chosen, the cuff should be checked for air-tightness. Techniques for induction of anesthesia before intubation of the trachea are described in Chapter 9.

Head Position for Orotracheal Intubation

Elevating the head about 10 cm with pads under the occiput (shoulders remaining on the table) and extension of the head at the atlanto-occipital joint serves to align the oral, pharyngeal, and laryngeal axes such that the passage from the lips to glottic opening is most nearly a straight line (Fig. 12-1). This posture is described as the "sniffing position." Extension of the head, without elevation of the occiput, increases the distance from the lips to glottic opening, rotates the larynx anteriorly, and may necessitate leverage on the maxillary teeth or gums with the laryngoscope blade in order to expose the glottic opening. The height of the operating table should be adjusted such that the patient's face is at the level of the standing anesthesiologist's xiphoid cartilage. If not opened by extension of the head, the patient's mouth may be manually opened by depressing the mandible with the right thumb. Simultaneously, the patient's lower lip can be rolled away with the right index finger to prevent its bruising by the laryngoscope blade.

Use of the Laryngoscope

The laryngoscope consists of a battery-containing handle to which blades with a light source may be attached and removed interchangeably (Fig. 12-2). The laryngoscope is held in the anesthesiologist's left hand near the junction between the handle and blade of the laryngoscope. The blade

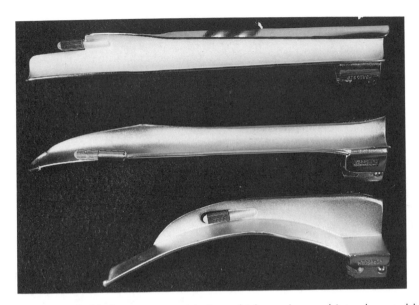

Fig. 12-2. Examples of detachable laryngoscope blades, which can be used interchangeably on the same handle include the straight blade (uppermost), straight blade with a curved distal tip (middle), and curved blade (lowermost).

is then inserted on the right side of the patient's mouth so as to avoid the incisor teeth and deflect the tongue to the left, away from the lumen of the blade. Pressure on the teeth or gums must be avoided as the blade is advanced forward and centrally toward the epiglottis. A protective plastic shield placed over the upper teeth may limit damage to teeth. The wrist is held rigid to prevent using the upper teeth or gums as a fulcrum with the blade of the laryngoscope as a lever. The laryngoscope handle must never be levered toward the anesthesiologist. Once the epiglottis is visualized, the next step depends on the type of laryngoscope blade being used.

Curved (MacIntosh) Blade

The tip of the curved blade is advanced into the space between the base of the tongue and the pharyngeal surface of the epiglottis (Fig. 12-3A). Forward and upward movement of the blade exerted along the axis of the laryngoscope handle, while avoiding any temptation to lever the blade on the teeth or gums by pulling back on the handle, serves to stretch the hypoepiglottic ligament, and,

in turn, to elevate the epiglottis and expose the glottic opening.

Straight (Jackson-Wisconsin) or Straight with Curved Tip (Miller) Blade

The tip of the straight blade is passed beneath the laryngeal surface of the epiglottis (Fig. 12-3B). Forward and upward movement of the blade exerted along the axis of the laryngoscope handle while avoiding any temptation to lever the blade on the teeth or gums by pulling back on the handle serves to directly elevate the epiglottis and expose the glottic opening. Depression or lateral movement of the patient's thyroid cartilage externally on the neck with the anesthesiologist's right hand may facilitate exposure of the glottic opening.

Choice of Laryngoscope Blade

The choice of laryngoscope blade is often based on personal preference. Advantages cited for the curved blade include less trauma to teeth with more room for passage of the tube and less bruising of the epiglottis because the tip of the blade should not touch this structure. Advantages cited

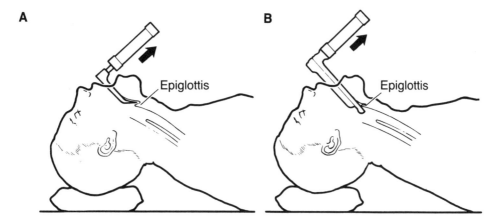

Fig. 12-3. Schematic diagram depicting proper position of the laryngoscope blade for exposure of the glottic opening. (A) The distal end of the curved blade is advanced into the space between the base of the tongue and the pharyngeal surface of the epiglottis. (B) The distal end of the straight blade is advanced beneath the laryngeal surface of the epiglottis. Regardless of blade design, forward and upward movement exerted along the axis of the laryngoscope handle, as denoted by the arrows, serves to elevate the epiglottis and expose the glottic opening.

for the straight blade include better exposure of the glottic opening and less need for a stylet to direct a tube into an anterior glottic opening.

Tracheal Tube Size and Length

Tracheal tube sizes are specified according to internal diameter (ID), which is marked on each tube (Table 12-1) (Fig. 12-4). Tracheal tubes are available in 0.5 mm internal diameter increments. Most adult tracheas (after 14 years of age) readily accept a cuffed 8.0 mm to 9.0 mm internal diameter tracheal tube. The tracheal tube also has lengthwise centimeter markings starting at the distal tracheal end to permit accurate determination of the tube length inserted past the lips. The letters I.T. (implantation tested) or Z-79 indicate that the tracheal tube material has been determined to be free of any tissue irritant or toxic properties. Tracheal tube material should also be radiopaque to facilitate demonstration of tube position relative to the carina and transparent to permit visualization of secretions or of air flow as evidenced by condensation of water vapor in the tube lumen (breath-fogging) during exhalation.

Tracheal Tube Cuff

Inflatable cuffs are built into the distal end of tracheal tubes (Fig. 12-4). The cuff is inflated with air to create a seal against the underlying tracheal mucosa. This seal facilitates positive pressure ventilation of the lungs and reduces the likelihood of aspiration of pharyngeal or gastric secretions. Cuffs are classified as high pressure or low pressure.[5]

High Pressure Cuffs

High pressure cuffs must be inflated to high intraluminal cuff pressures (180 mmHg to 250 mmHg) before they expand sufficiently to create a seal between the tube and tracheal mucosa. This high cuff pressure is partially transmitted to the underlying tracheal mucosa. Ischemia of the tracheal mucosa may occur whenever the pressure on the tracheal wall exceeds capillary arteriolar pressure (about 32 mmHg). Persistent ischemia of the tracheal mucosa may cause damage, which in extreme cases manifests as destruction of cartilaginous tracheal rings. High pressure cuffs also tend to inflate asymmetrically, deforming the trachea and ultimately producing tracheal dilation.

Table 12-1. Size and Length of Tracheal Tubes Relative to Airway Anatomy

Age	Internal Diameter (mm)	Distance Inserted from Lips to Place Distal End in Midtrachea (cm)[a]	Diameter of Trachea (mm)	Length of Trachea (cm)	Distance from Lips to Carina (cm)
Premature	2.5	10			
Full term	3.0	11			
1–6 months	3.5	11	5	6	13
6–12 months	4.0	12			
2 years	4.5	13			
4 years	5.0	14			
6 years	5.5	15			
8 years	6.5	16	8	8	18
10 years	7.0	17–18			
12 years	7.5	18–20			
14 years and over	8.0–9.0	20–22	20[b] 15[c]	14[b] 12[c]	28[b] 24[c]

[a] Add 2–3 cm for nasal tubes.
[b] Males.
[c] Females.

Low Pressure Cuffs

Low pressure cuffs inflate symmetrically, adapting to the contour of the tracheal wall and producing a seal with the tracheal mucosa at low intraluminal cuff pressures. The resulting tracheal wall pressures have been found to equal peak airway pressures (15 mmHg to 30 mmHg) during positive pressure ventilation of the lungs. These characteristics make tracheal mucosa ischemia and tracheal dilation less likely than with high pressure cuffs. Indeed, low pressure cuffs decrease the severity of tracheal injury observed at the cuff site.[6] Tracheal tubes with low pressure cuffs are often recommended when intubation of the trachea is anticipated to be required for longer than 48 hours. Nevertheless, there is probably no period of tracheal intubation that does not produce some laryngotracheal damage. For example, ciliary denudation has been found to occur predominantly over the tracheal rings and underlying cuff site with only 2 hours of intubation and tracheal wall pressures less than 25 mmHg.[6]

Placement of a Tracheal Tube

The glottic opening is recognized by its triangular shape and pale white vocal cords (Fig. 12-5). The tracheal tube is held in the anesthesiologist's right hand like a pencil and introduced on the right side of the patient's mouth with the built in curve directed anteriorly. Attempts to insert the tube in the midline of the mouth and then down the lumen of the laryngoscope blade usually obscure vision of the glottic opening. The tube is advanced past the vocal cords until the cuff just disappears, which should correspond to the distance predicted to place the distal end of the tube midway between the vocal cords and carina. At this point, the laryngoscope blade is removed from the mouth. The tracheal tube cuff is next inflated with air to just a no leak volume during positive pressure ventilation of the lungs. Distension of the small pilot balloon attached to the inflation tube leading to the cuff confirms cuff inflation.

Confirmation of placement of the tube in the trachea, rather than the esophagus, is verified by several different observations.[7] Symmetric bilat-

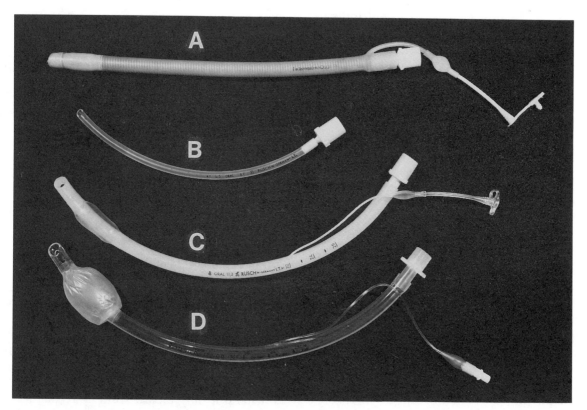

Fig. 12-4. Various types of tracheal tubes and cuffs. Tube (A) is an armored or anode tube with built-in spiral wire to minimize the opportunity of collapse or kinking. Tubes (B, C, and D) are tubes made of smooth plastic and are recommended for single use. Tube B is uncuffed and is a size appropriate for children. Tubes C and D are appropriate for adults. Tubes A and C are equipped with built-in high pressure cuffs. Tube D is constructed to include a low pressure cuff. These cuffs are inflated by attaching an air-filled syringe to the small diameter tube that leads to the cuff. Distension of the small balloon near the attachment for the syringe confirms inflation of the cuff. Numbers and letters visible on tubes B, C, and D denote the internal diameter, length from the distal tracheal end, and confirmation that the tubes have been tested for tissue compatibility.

eral movements of the chest with manual compression of the reservoir bag combined with the presence of bilateral breath sounds upon apical and/or midaxillary auscultation of the lungs are commonly established after tracheal intubation. A characteristic feel of the reservoir bag associated with normal lung compliance during manual inflation of the lungs and the presence of expiratory refilling of the bag is evaluated. The presence of carbon dioxide in the exhaled gases from the tracheal tube as detected by capnography or mass spectrometry may be the most reliable confirmatory sign of tracheal placement of the tube.[7] Carbon dioxide will not be persistently present in exhaled gases from a tube accidently placed in the esophagus. Declines in arterial oxygen saturation as evident on a pulse oximeter may alert the anesthesiologist to a previously unrecognized esophageal intubation. Noting the depth of insertion as determined by the centimeter markings on the tracheal tube at the lips helps predict a midtrachea position of the distal end of the tube. For

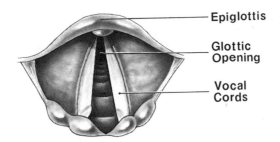

Fig. 12-5. Schematic view of glottic opening as seen during direct laryngoscopy when the epiglottis is elevated with a curved or straight laryngoscope blade. The glottic opening is recognized by its triangular shape bordered by the pale white vocal cords.

example, insertion of a tracheal tube 20 cm to 22 cm beyond the lips of an adult should reliably place the distal end of the tube in the midtrachea. Furthermore, if a cuffed tube is properly placed in the midtrachea, the anesthesiologist can easily detect, by external palpation, cuff distension in the suprasternal notch during rapid inflation of the cuff. Finally, the tube is secured in position with tape placed around the tube and applied

---

Observations Used to Verify Tracheal Placement of Tube

Direct visualization of tube in glottic opening
Symmetric bilateral chest movement with manual ventilation
Presence of bilateral breath sounds with auscultation
Absence of air movement during epigastric auscultation
Compliance of reservoir bag during manual inflation
Refilling of reservoir bag during exhalation
Reservoir bag movement during spontaneous ventilation
Condensation of water vapor in the tube lumen during exhalation
Presence of carbon dioxide in exhaled gases
Maintenance of arterial oxygen saturation

---

above and below the lips, extending over the cheeks.

ALTERNATIVES TO OROTRACHEAL INTUBATION DURING GENERAL ANESTHESIA

Alternatives to orotracheal intubation during general anesthesia include awake orotracheal intubation, nasotracheal intubation, and intubation using a fiberoptic laryngoscope. These alternatives are considered when orotracheal intubation during general anesthesia might be unsafe (recent food ingestion, bowel obstruction, upper airway disease) or impossible because of altered anatomy (see the section *Anatomic Characteristics*.)

Awake Orotracheal Intubation

Local anesthesia for awake orotracheal intubation using direct laryngoscopy may include (1) topical spray of the lips, tongue, palate and pharynx; (2) superior laryngeal nerve block; and (3) transtracheal injection of a local anesthetic, most often lidocaine. It is helpful to reduce oropharyngeal secretions with an anticholinergic. When vomiting is a hazard, only topical spray is recommended, thus avoiding anesthesia of areas necessary to protect against pulmonary aspiration.

Nasotracheal Intubation

Nasotracheal intubation may be performed electively for intraoral operations, when anatomic abnormalities or disease of the upper airway make direct laryngoscopy difficult or impossible and when long-term intubation of the trachea is anticipated. Advantages cited for nasotracheal intubation include (1) more stable tube fixation, (2) less chance for tube kinking, (3) greater comfort in awake patients, and (4) fewer oropharyngeal secretions.

Awake Blind Nasotracheal Intubation

Awake blind nasotracheal intubation is usually reserved for situations in which direct laryngoscopy or ventilation of the lungs would be impossible or induction of anesthesia before intubation of the trachea would be hazardous. To insure maximum patient comfort and nasal patency and to minimize the chance of epistaxis, the nasal mucosa should be anesthetized and constricted with topical cocaine. If cocaine is not available, constriction, but not anesthesia of the nasal mucosa, can be produced with topical phenylephrine. Either naris may be chosen, depending on the history and physical examination, but the right naris is preferable because the bevel of most tracheal tubes when introduced through the right naris will face the flat nasal septum, reducing damage to the turbinates. Tracheal tubes can be used interchangeably for nasal or oral intubation of the trachea (Table 12-1). In adults, 7.0 mm to 7.5 mm internal diameter tubes are usually adequate. After passage through the naris into the oropharynx, the tracheal tube is advanced toward the glottic opening as long as breath sounds are maximal as determined by listening to exhaled air passing from the proximal end of the tube. Ideally, the tracheal tube is swiftly passed through the glottic opening just before inspiration because the vocal cords are most open during this time and the risk of vocal cord trauma is thus minimized. Successful placement of the tube in the trachea is confirmed by continued breathing through the tube.

Nasotracheal Intubation During General Anesthesia

Nasotracheal intubation during general anesthesia is acceptable when vomiting is not a hazard and ventilation of the lungs can be maintained by a mask. General anesthesia is produced following vasoconstriction of the nasal mucosa with topical cocaine or phenylephrine. If blind nasotracheal intubation is to be performed, it is mandatory to maintain spontaneous ventilation in the patient so as to permit identification of the glottic opening as evidenced by exhaled air passing from the proximal end of the tube. Alternatively, nasotracheal intubation may be accomplished using direct laryngoscopy to expose the glottic opening. When this approach is selected, succinylcholine or a short-acting nondepolarizing muscle relaxant is administered to produce skeletal muscle relaxation, and the tracheal tube is placed through the right naris into the oropharynx. The glottic opening is then visualized using direct laryngoscopy and the tracheal tube guided through the glottic opening

under vision by manually advancing it at the proximal end. Alternatively, the tracheal tube may be grasped in the oropharynx with intubating forceps (Magill forceps) and directed so that pressure on the proximal end causes the tube to pass between the vocal cords. The right naris is preferred because a left nasotracheal tube is clumsy to advance under direct vision with the anesthesiologist's left hand holding the laryngoscope.

Complications Unique to Nasotracheal Intubation

Complications unique to nasotracheal intubation include (1) epistaxis, (2) dislodgement of pharyngeal tonsils (adenoids), (3) eustachian tube obstruction, (4) maxillary sinusitis, and (5) bacteremia.[8] Epistaxis most likely reflects avulsion of nasal mucosa covering the turbinates. Shrinkage of nasal mucosa with cocaine or phenylephrine and use of small and generously lubricated tracheal tubes should minimize this complication. When pharyngeal tonsils are prominent, as in children, it is preferable to perform all nasotracheal intubations using direct laryngoscopy to expose the glottic opening so as to prevent unrecognized delivery into the trachea of a dislodged piece of tonsil. Bacteremia is not predictably associated with trauma to the nasal mucosa nor is it reliably prevented by prior use of topical vasoconstrictors.[9] Prophylactic antibiotics are indicated when nasotracheal intubation is planned in patients with heart disease.

Intubation Using a Fiberoptic Laryngoscope

The fiberoptic laryngoscope consists of glass fibers that are bound together to provide a flexible unit for transmission of images and light (Fig. 12-6). Intubation of the trachea using a flexible fiberoptic laryngoscope is useful for patients in whom the glottic opening cannot be visualized because of anatomic abnormalities. After topical anesthesia as described for awake blind nasotracheal intubation, the tracheal tube is passed through the naris into the oropharynx. The lubricated fiberoptic laryngoscope is then passed through the tracheal tube (tube must be about 8 mm internal diameter to allow easy passage of the fiberoptic laryngoscope; pediatric fiberoptic bronchoscope will pass through a 5 mm internal diameter tracheal tube)

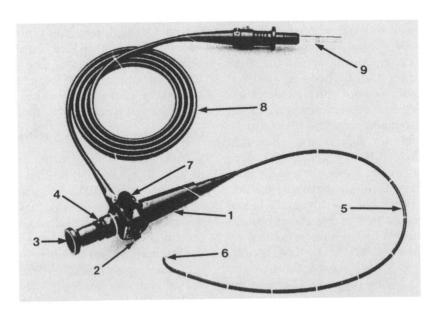

Fig. 12-6. Flexible fiberoptic laryngoscope consists of (1) control unit, (2) tip deflection control lever, (3) eyepiece, (4) diopter adjustment ring, (5) flexible insertion cord, (6) bending tip responsive to the control level, (7) working channel sleeve and plug, (8) light guide cable, and (9) light guide plug. The working channel can be used to administer inhaled or topical anesthetics, deliver supplemental oxygen, and suction secretions. The length of the flexible insertion cord is 500 mm to 600 mm, the diameter for adult fiberoptic laryngoscopes is 4 mm to 6 mm, and the diameter for the pediatric bronchoscope is 3.5 mm. The diameter of the working channel is 1.2 mm to 2 mm. Upward and downward deflection of the bending tip in response to the control lever is about 120 degrees.

until the epiglottis and glottic opening are visualized. Compared with the view seen using direct laryngoscopy, the depth of the vocal cords may seem exaggerated and the true vocal cords not seen until the false vocal cords have been passed with the fiberoptic laryngoscope. The visual field often becomes limited as the fiberoptic laryngoscope nears the glottic opening while secretions, blood, or fogging of the lens may further obscure the view. Immersion of the tip of the fiberoptic laryngoscope in warm water or application of silicone spray to the lens may reduce the likelihood of fogging or adherence of secretions. Inclusion of anticholinergics in the preoperative medication is useful as upper airway secretions obscure visibility using the fiberoptic laryngoscope. It is important to keep the fiberoptic laryngoscope in the midline to avoid entering the pyriform sinus. A

helpful sign that the trachea has been entered is the glow seen over the anterior neck from transillumination of the larynx and trachea as the tip of the fiberoptic laryngoscope passes through the glottic opening. The tracheal tube is then advanced into the trachea using the fiberoptic laryngoscope as a guide. Oral intubation of the trachea is accomplished in a similar manner by placing the fiberoptic laryngoscope behind the base of the tongue often with limited traction using a laryngoscope blade. Alternatively, a plastic oropharyngeal airway with a cylindric passage (Airway Intubator) that permits passage of the tracheal tube containing the fiberoptic laryngoscope may be used.[10] This airway can be placed in awake patients following appropriate topical anesthesia. Use of the fiberoptic laryngoscope is facilitated in awake patients, as tissue tone is maintained and the tongue

---

Possible Indications for Use of a Fiberoptic Laryngoscope

Upper airway obstruction
   Tumor
   Abscess
   Prior surgery

Mediastinal mass

Subglottic stenosis

Congenital upper airway abnormalities
   Mandibular hypoplasia
   Craniofacial synostosis
   Kippel-Feil syndrome

Immobile cervical vertebrae
   Arthritis
   Traction
   Verify position of a double lumen tracheal
      tube

---

and epiglottis do not relax to obscure the vocal cords.

OROTRACHEAL INTUBATION IN CHILDREN

Orotracheal intubation in children differs from adults because of anatomic differences in pediatric patients, as well as the need to more carefully select the size and length of tracheal tube inserted in these young individuals (see Chapter 27).

Anatomic Differences from Adults

The newborn head and tongue are large and the neck is short. The larynx is more cephalad than in the adult. For example, the lower border of the cricoid cartilage is opposite the 4th cervical vertebra at birth and opposite the 5th cervical vertebra at age 6. The epiglottis is U-shaped and stiff. These anatomic differences result in difficulty aligning the oral, pharyngeal, and tracheal axes and elevating the epiglottis to expose the glottic opening (Fig. 12-1). As such, the glottic opening of the newborn tends to be anterior compared with the adult. It must be remembered that the cricoid cartilage is the narrowest point in the larynx of children such that a tube that passes through the glottic opening may subsequently resist advancement at this site.

Tracheal Tube Size and Length

Selection of the appropriate tracheal tube size and length is critical in children, as the margin for error is small. Excessive tube size is responsible for unnecessary laryngotracheal trauma, which may manifest as laryngeal edema when the tube is removed from the trachea. Likewise, the short glottis to carina distance in children necessitates careful calculation of correct tube length to assure a midtrachea position of the distal end of the tube. One must be aware that head flexion or change from the supine to head-down position may shift the carina upward, converting a midtrachea tube placement to an endobronchial intubation while head extension may place the distal end of the tube in the pharynx.

A tracheal tube one size above and below the calculated size should be available with the final choice made when the glottic opening is visualized and the tube is inserted into the trachea. Cuffed tubes are probably not necessary before 5 years of age because the narrow subglottic tracheal diameter insures an adequate seal between the tube and tracheal mucosa. Resistance to breathing is a consideration for the small lumen tracheal tubes and connectors necessary in children. When increased airway resistance is a concern, the best approach is placement of a proper (not the largest possible) sized tube in the trachea and controlled ventilation of the lungs to prevent excessive work of breathing.

Technique for Tracheal Intubation

Orotracheal intubation is routinely chosen for short-term intubation of the trachea in children. Awake orotracheal intubation of the newborn is preferable. After about 2 weeks of age, infants are sufficiently strong to resist awake intubation of the trachea, and anesthesia may be produced before direct laryngoscopy. A straight laryngoscope blade often provides better exposure of the glottic opening than the curved blade, especially in children less than 3 years of age.

EXTUBATION OF THE TRACHEA

Extubation of the trachea following general anesthesia is ideally accomplished while the patient is still adequately anesthetized so as to diminish the likelihood of coughing or laryngospasm (reflex closure of the vocal cords). This assumes that adequate ventilation of the lungs is present or can be maintained without the tracheal tube in place and that the presence of gastric contents is not a likely hazard. Suctioning of the pharynx should be performed before extubation of the trachea so that secretions proximal to the tube cuff do not drain into the trachea when the cuff is deflated. After the cuff is deflated, the tube is removed often with simultaneous pressure on the reservoir bag so the lungs are inflated and the initial gas flow is outward. This maneuver may facilitate a cough and expulsion of any aspirated material. When the presence of gastric contents is predictable at the conclusion of anesthesia, the trachea should not be extubated until protective laryngeal reflexes have returned. Vigorous reaction to the tracheal tube ("bucking") signals the return of the protective cough reflex, and at this point the trachea must be extubated or further sedation instituted to permit tolerance of the tube.

Laryngospasm and vomiting are the most serious immediate hazards after extubation of the trachea. Therefore, oxygen, succinylcholine, equipment for reintubation of the trachea, and suction must be immediately available.

COMPLICATIONS OF TRACHEAL INTUBATION

Complications of tracheal intubation are rare and should not influence the decision to place a tracheal tube. Certainly, the benefits of a properly placed and patent tracheal tube far exceed the risks of intubation of the trachea. Complications of tracheal intubation may be categorized as those occurring (1) during direct laryngoscopy and intubation of the trachea, (2) while the tracheal tube is in place, and (3) after extubation of the trachea either immediately or after a delay.[8]

Complications of Tracheal Intubation

During direct larygoscopy and intubation of the trachea
   Dental and oral soft tissue trauma
   Hypertension and tachycardia
   Cardiac dysrythmias
   Inhalation (aspiration) of gastric contents

While tracheal tube is in place
   Tracheal tube obstruction
   Endobronchial intubation
   Esophageal intubation
   Accidental extubation
   Increased resistance to breathing
   Tracheal mucosa ischemia

Immediate and delayed complications after extubation of the trachea
   Laryngospasm
   Inhalation (aspiration) of gastric contents
   Pharyngitis (sore throat)
   Laryngitis
   Laryngeal or subglottic edema
   Laryngeal ulceration with or without granuloma formation
   Tracheitis
   Tracheal stenosis
   Vocal cord paralysis
   Arytenoid cartilage dislocation

Complications During Direct Laryngoscopy and Intubation of the Trachea

Dental trauma is the most serious and frequent type of damage related to direct laryngoscopy. Use of a plastic shield placed over the upper teeth and avoidance of using the laryngoscope blade as a lever on the teeth will minimize the hazard of dental trauma. Should injury occur, immediate consultation with a dentist is indicated. A dislodged tooth must be recovered, but, if the search is unsuccessful, appropriate radiographs of the chest and abdomen should be taken to assure that the tooth has not passed through the glottic opening.

Hypertension and tachycardia frequently accompany direct laryngoscopy (regardless of type of laryngoscope blade used) and intubation of the trachea.[11] These responses are usually transient and innocuous. In patients with co-existing hypertension or those with coronary artery disease, however, these changes may be exaggerated or may jeopardize the balance between myocardial oxygen requirements and delivery. In these types of patients, it is particularly important to minimize the duration of direct laryngoscopy to less than 15 seconds. Serious or persistent cardiac dysrhythmias during intubation of the trachea are unlikely, particularly if adequate oxygenation during the period of apnea associated with direct laryngoscopy is assured by prior inflation of the lungs with oxygen.

Complications While the Tracheal Tube is in Place

Obstruction of the tracheal tube may occur due to the accumulation of secretions in the tube and kinking of the tube. Inadvertent endobronchial intubation is minimized by calculating the proper tracheal tube length for every patient and then noting the centimeter marking on the tube at the point of fixation at the lips. Flexion of the head may advance the tube up to 1.9 cm, converting a tracheal placement into an endobronchial intubation.[12] Conversely, extension of the head can withdraw the tube up to 1.9 cm and result in a pharyngeal intubation. Lateral rotation of the head moves the distal end of the tracheal tube about 0.7 cm from the carina.

Immediate and Delayed Complications After Extubation of the Trachea

Laryngospasm and/or inhalation of gastric contents are the two most serious potential immediate complications after extubation of the trachea. Laryngospasm is unlikely if the depth of anesthesia is sufficient during extubation of the trachea or the patient is allowed to awaken before extubation. The patient who is lightly anesthetized at the time of extubation of the trachea is most at risk. If laryngospasm occurs, oxygen under positive pressure via a face mask and forward displacement of the mandible using the index fingers to apply pressure at the temporomandibular joints may be sufficient treatment. Administration of intravenous (alternatively, intramuscular) succinylcholine

is indicated if laryngospasm persists. Inhalation of gastric contents is most likely to occur in the debilitated patient or in the presence of recent food ingestion or gastrointestinal obstruction. Pharyngitis (sore throat) is a frequent complaint after extubation of the trachea, particularly in females, presumably because of the thinner mucosal covering over the posterior vocal cords compared with males.[8] Skeletal muscle myalgia associated with administration of succinylcholine may manifest in the peripharyngeal muscles as postoperative sore throat, which is incorrectly attributed to prior intubation of the trachea.[13] Use of large (8.5 mm to 9.0 mm) versus small (6.5 mm to 7 mm) tracheal tubes may increase the likelihood of sore throat. Regardless of the mechanism, sore throat usually disappears spontaneously in 48 hours to 72 hours without any treatment. Symptomatic laryngeal or subglottic edema is most likely in children because a small amount of swelling greatly reduces the lumen of the larynx. The likely causes of laryngeal edema in children include traumatic intubation of the trachea, use of an oversized tracheal tube, or the presence of an upper respiratory tract infection. Even with ideal conditions, however, laryngeal edema may still occur. Laryngeal incompetence may be present in some patients in the first 4 hours to 8 hours after extubation of the trachea, leading to an increased risk of pulmonary aspiration.[14]

The major complication of prolonged intubation of the trachea (greater than 48 hours) is damage to the tracheal mucosa, which may progress to destruction of cartilaginous rings and subsequent circumferential cicatrical scar formation and tracheal stenosis. Stenosis becomes symptomatic when the adult tracheal lumen is reduced to less than 5 mm.

REFERENCES

1. McIntyre JWR. The difficult tracheal intubation. Can J Anaesth 1987;34:204–13.
2. Wright RB, Manfield FFV. Damage to teeth during the administration of general anesthesia. Anesth Analg 1974;53:405–8.
3. Block C, Brechner VL. Unusual problems in airway management II: The influence of the temporomandibular joint, the mandible, and associated structures

on endotracheal intubation. Anesth Analg 1971; 50:114–23.

4. Brechner VL. Unusual problems in the management of airways: I. Flexion-extension mobility of the cervical vertebrae. Anesth Analg 1968;47:363–73.

5. Carroll R, Hedden M, Safar P. Intratracheal cuffs: Performance characteristics. Anesthesiology 1969; 31:275–81.

6. Klainer AS, Turndorf H, Wen-Hsien WU, Maewal H, Allender P. Surface alterations due to endotracheal intubation. Am J Med 1975;58:674–83.

7. Buckingham PK, Cheney FW, Ward RJ. Esophageal intubation: A review of detection techniques. Anesth Analg 1986;65:886–91.

8. Blanc VF, Tremblay NAG. The complications of tracheal intubation. A new classification with a review of the literature. Anesth Analg 1974;53:202–13.

9. Dinner M, Tjeuw M, Artusio JF. Bacteremia as a complication of nasotracheal intubation. Anesth Analg 1987;66:460–2.

10. Rogers SN, Benumof JL. New and easy techniques for fiberoptic endoscopy-aided tracheal intubation. Anesthesiology 1983;59:569–71.

11. Stoelting RK. Blood pressure and heart rate changes during short duration laryngoscopy for tracheal intubation. Influence of viscous or intravenous lidocaine. Anesth Analg 1978;57:197–9.

12. Conrardy PA, Goodman LR, Lainage F, et al. Alteration of endotracheal tube position. Flexion and extension of the neck. Crit Care Med 1976;4:8–12.

13. Capan LM, Bruce DL, Patel KP, et al. Succinylcholine-induced postoperative sore throat. Anesthesiology 1983;59:202–5.

14. Bishop MJ, Weymuller EA, Fink RB. Laryngeal effects of prolonged intubation. Anesth Analg 1984; 63:335–42.

Chapter 13

Spinal, Epidural, and Caudal Blocks

Spinal, epidural, and caudal blocks are commonly referred to as regional or conduction block anesthesia.[1,2] Spinal block is produced by injection of local anesthetic solutions into the lumbar subarachnoid space. Epidural block is produced by injection of local anesthetic solutions into the epidural space, most often at the lumbar level. A caudal block results when local anesthetic solutions are placed in the epidural space via a needle introduced through the sacral hiatus.

Regional anesthesia produces anesthesia selective for the surgical site in contrast to general anesthesia, which produces total body anesthesia. Patients may remain awake or sedated by intravenous administration of drugs such as benzodiazepines (e.g., midazolam) and/or opioids (e.g., fentanyl). Skeletal muscle relaxation is profound without the need for administration of muscle relaxants. Despite these advantages, patients may be fearful of "needle sticks" or being "awake" during surgery. Alleged stories of paralysis following regional anesthesia can be effectively discounted but nevertheless remain a concern to some patients.[3] Even some surgeons are biased against regional blocks on the grounds they may fail and delay start of surgery while general anesthesia is instituted.

The efficacy of opioids placed into the epidural or subarachnoid space for providing postoperative analgesia and chronic pain relief has been one of the most important recent advances in medicine.[4] This approach has created many new options in the area of pain relief, including the development of postoperative pain management services (see Chapter 30).

ANATOMY

The spinal canal extends from the foramen magnum to the sacral hiatus (Fig. 13-1).[1] The vertebral column consists of seven cervical, twelve thoracic, and five lumbar vertebrae. The sacrum and coccyx are distal extensions of the vertebral column. Each vertebrae consists of a vertebral body and a bony arch. The body consists of two pedicles anteriorly and two laminae posteriorly. The transverse processes are formed by the junction of the pedicles and laminae, whereas the spinous process is formed by joining of each lamina. In the lumbar regions the spinous processes are nearly horizontal such that needles introduced at this site may be directed at right angles to the sagittal plane.

The laminae of the vertebrae are connected by the ligamentum flavum, and the posterior spinous processes are connected by the interspinous ligaments (Fig. 13-2).[1] The supraspinous ligaments connect the tips of the spinous processes. Intervertebral foramina are openings between the vertebral pedicles through which the spinal nerves pass. Each spinal nerve supplies a specific region

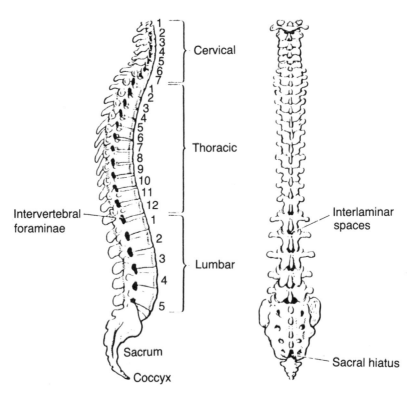

Fig. 13-1. Vertebral column from a lateral (left) and posterior view (right) illustrating curvatures (maximum thoracic kyphosis at T6) and interlaminar spaces. The spinal cord ends at L1–2 and the dura mater extends to S2. (From Bridenbaugh and Green,[1] with permission.)

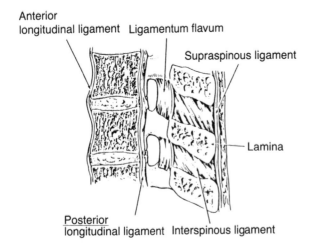

Fig. 13-2. Sagittal section of vertebral column. (From Bridenbaugh and Greene,[1] with permission.)

of skin (dermatome) and skeletal muscles (Fig. 13-3). Preganglionic nerves of the sympathetic nervous system originate from the spinal cord (T1–L2) and travel with the spinal nerves before leaving to form the sympathetic chain (Fig. 13-4). The sympathetic chain extends the entire length of the spinal column along the anterolateral aspects of the vertebral bodies, giving rise to the stellate ganglion, splanchnic nerves, and celiac plexus.

The spinal canal contains the spinal cord and its coverings, the pia mater, arachnoid mater, and dura mater. The spinal cord extends from the foramen magnum to L1–2. Because the spinal cord ends at L1–2, the lower lumbar and sacral nerves extend for some distance in the spinal canal as the cauda equina. The pia mater is adherent to the spinal cord and nerves. The space between the arachnoid mater and dura mater contains cerebrospinal fluid and is known as the subarachnoid

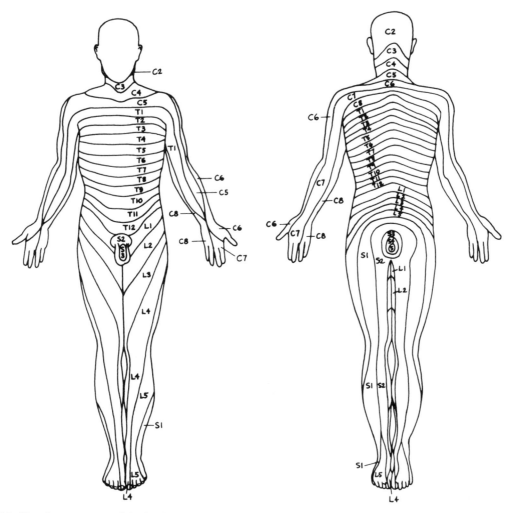

Fig. 13-3. The dermatomes of the body shown in an orderly progression from the cranial to caudal aspects of the body.

space. Local anesthetic solutions are injected into the subarachnoid space to produce a spinal blockade.

The epidural space is located between the dura mater and connective tissues covering the vertebrae and ligamentum flavum. This is a potential space, being normally filled with connective and adipose tissue. Venous plexuses are prominent but no free fluid exists in the epidural space. Local anesthetic solutions injected into the epidural space to produce an epidural block spread freely in all directions.

PREOPERATIVE PREPARATION

Preoperative preparation for regional anesthesia does not differ from general anesthesia (see Chapter 9). Under no circumstances, however, should patients be encouraged against their wishes to accept the anesthesiologist's recommendation for a regional anesthetic. Examination of the back to rule out deformities or infection is uniquely important when regional anesthesia is planned. Coagulation status (determined by history and/or specific tests) should be determined, as perfor-

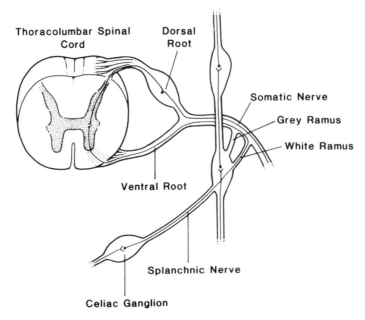

Fig. 13-4. Cell bodies in the thoracolumbar portion of the spinal cord (T1–L2) give rise to the peripheral sympathetic nervous system. Efferent fibers travel in the ventral root and then via the white ramus communicans to paravertebral sympathetic ganglia or more distant sites such as the celiac ganglion. Afferent fibers from paravertebral sympathetic ganglia travel via the gray ramus communicans to join somatic nerves, which pass to the dorsal root and the spinal cord.

mance of regional blocks in the presence of abnormal clotting is controversial. Because of profound sympathetic nervous system blockade regional anesthesia may not be a logical selection in patients who are hypovolemic due to acute hemorrhage.

Preoperative medication is dependent on each individual patient's level of anxiety (see Chapter 10). Inclusion of an opioid may be useful for reducing pain associated with the needle insertions required to perform a regional block. Anticholinergics are probably not needed when regional blocks are planned, as the resulting dry mouth will be uncomfortable for awake patients. Patients must be reassured that medications will be administered intravenously as needed to assure their comfort during the surgery. An intravenous infusion is started before performance of the block; and all the equipment, drugs, and monitors normally present for a general anesthetic are also required for regional anesthesia.

SPINAL BLOCK

The principal landmarks for performance of a spinal block are the vertebral spinous processes and the iliac crests (Fig. 13-5). The spinous processes identify the midline, and a line drawn between the iliac crests crosses the fourth lumbar vertebrae. The interspace above this line represents the L3–4 interspace and the interspace below the L4–5 interspace. These interspaces are commonly selected for insertion of the spinal needle, remembering that the spinal cord ends at the L1–2 level.

Technique

Spinal block is typically instituted with the patient in the lateral decubitus or the sitting position (Fig. 13-5). The needle is inserted in the midline (i.e., midline approach) at an easily palpable interspace below L2 (usually L3–4 or L4–5). The lateral decubitus position (knees and head flexed on the

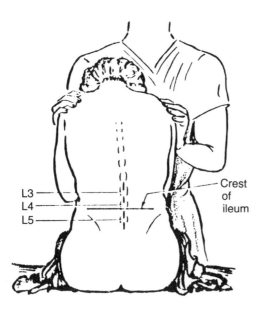

Fig. 13-5. A line drawn between the iliac crests crosses the fourth lumbar (L4) vertebra.

chest) is useful for ill or heavily sedated patients, and the sitting position is used when there is difficulty in separating the lumbar spinous processes or a low level of spinal anesthesia is desired. The area of skin over the selected area is prepared with an antiseptic solution (e.g., 1 percent iodine) and the anesthesiologist wears sterile gloves. A skin wheal of local anesthetic is raised and a 22-gauge or 25-gauge needle is inserted at this site parallel to the spinous processes. The needle is advanced with a slightly cephalad angle until it is firmly lodged in the supraspinous ligament after which it is no longer possible to change the direction of the needle tip by bending the distal shaft of the needle. Continued needle advancement transverses the ligamentum flavum and the dura mater. A distinct "pop" is felt by the fingers of the anesthesiologist as the needle passes through the dura mater. Subarachnoid placement of the needle is confirmed by the appearance of cerebrospinal fluid at the hub. At this point, the needle is stabilized by grasping the hub of the needle between the thumb and forefinger with the dorsum of the hand resting against the patient's back. A syringe containing local anesthetic solution is attached and after aspiration of a small amount of cerebrospinal fluid into the syringe to confirm continued subarachnoid placement, the entire contents are injected over 3 seconds to 5 seconds. Occasionally, blood-tinged cerebrospinal fluid will appear at the hub of the spinal needle. If blood-tinged cerebrospinal fluid continues to flow, the needle should be removed and reinserted at a different interspace. Should blood-tinged cerebrospinal fluid still persist, the attempt to produce spinal anesthesia should be terminated and the patient further evaluated. Conversely, if clear cerebrospinal fluid is obtained, the spinal anesthetic can be completed. After completion of the injection, the syringe and needle are removed as a single unit.

The incidence of postspinal headache is less after puncture of the dura mater with a 25-gauge compared with a 22-gauge needle. For this reason, a 25-gauge needle is likely to be selected when spinal block is selected for younger patients who are more likely than elderly patients to experience postspinal headache. Use of the flexible 25-gauge needle may be facilitated by its placement through a larger introducer needle that has been previously placed into the interspinous ligament. The larger and more rigid 22-gauge needle does not require use of an introducer needle and cerebrospinal fluid spontaneously appears at the hub of the needle when the subarachnoid space is entered. The small lumen of the 25-gauge needle may require syringe aspiration to confirm presence of cerebrospinal fluid. Equipment and drugs necessary for performance of a spinal block are most often provided by prepackaged and sterile kits (Fig. 13-6).

Lateral (Paramedian) Approach

The spinal needle is introduced through the skin wheal at a site 1 cm to 2 cm lateral to the midline opposite the center of the chosen interspace. The needle is directed medial and cephalad at an angle of 15 degrees to 20 degrees until it passes through the ligamentum flavum into the subarachnoid space. Compared with the midline approach, the lateral approach is less dependent on patients being able to flex their backs (parturients, prone position) and circumvents calcified ligaments often encountered in the midline of elderly patients.

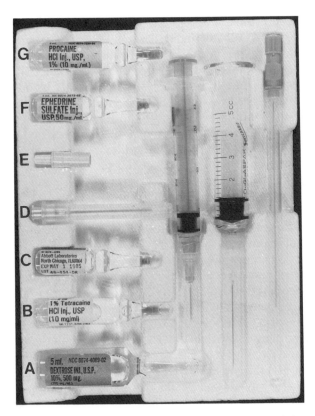

Fig. 13-6. A typical prepackaged and sterile disposable kit for institution of a spinal block. The contents of the glass vials are (A) 5 ml of 10 percent dextrose, (B) 2 ml of 1 percent tetracaine, (C) one ampule of epinephrine 1:1000 (1 mg·ml⁻¹), (D) a thin-walled introducer needle, (E) a 5 micron filter, (F) 1 ml of ephedrine 50 mg·ml⁻¹, and (G) 2 ml of 1 percent procaine.

Lumbosacral (Taylor) Approach

The largest interspace in the vertebral column is the L5–S1 interspace. To enter this space, the spinal needle is introduced through the skin wheal approximately 1 cm medial and 1 cm cephalad to the posterior superior iliac spine. The spinal needle is directed medial and cephalad to enter the subarachnoid space in the midline at the L5–S1 interspace. Advantages of this approach are similar to the lateral approach.

Level and Duration

Distribution of local anesthetic solutions in cerebrospinal fluid is principally influenced by the (1) baricity of the solution, (2) contour of the spinal

canal, and (3) position of the patient during and in the first few minutes after placement of drug into the subarachnoid space. Assuming an appropriate dose is selected, the duration of spinal block depends on the drug selected (tetracaine and bupivacaine last longer than lidocaine, which lasts longer than procaine) and the presence or absence of a vasoconstrictor (epinephrine or phenylephrine) in the local anesthetic solution (Table 13-1).

Local anesthetics produce different intensities of sensory and motor blockade. For example, sensory anesthesia below L1 seems to be more intense in the presence of bupivacaine (e.g., reduced frequency of tourniquet pain), whereas motor blockade is greatest after injection of tetracaine. Lidocaine is useful for short duration (30 minutes to 60 minutes) surgical and obstetrical procedures. Tetracaine is commonly used for abdominal surgery lasting up to 5 hours. Bupivacaine is useful for lower extremity vascular and orthopaedic operations lasting up to 5 hours. During recovery, anesthesia regresses from the highest dermatome in a caudad direction.

Baricity and Position of the Patient

Baricity is the density of the local anesthetic solution divided by the density of cerebrospinal fluid (1.001 to 1.005) at 37° Celsius. Local anesthetic solutions are characterized as hyperbaric, hypobaric, or isobaric relative to cerebrospinal fluid. Understanding baricity allows the anesthesiologist to "direct" the local anesthetic solution in the subarachnoid space toward the spinal nerves innervating the surgical site (Table 13-1).[5]

Hyperbaric Solutions. Hyperbaric solutions are prepared by adding glucose in sufficient amounts to increase the density of the local anesthetic solution above that of cerebrospinal fluid. A common hyperbaric solution is tetracaine 0.5 percent plus 5 percent dextrose obtained by the anesthesiologist mixing equal volumes of 1 percent tetracaine and 10 percent dextrose. Lidocaine 5 percent and bupivacaine 0.75 percent are premixed with dextrose to provide a commercial hyperbaric solution (Table 13-1). Being heavier than cerebrospinal fluid, hyperbaric local anesthetic solutions settle to the most dependent aspect of the subarachnoid

Table 13-1. Local Anesthetic Solutions Used for Spinal Block

	Concentration (%)	Carrier	Baricity	Dose (mg)		Volume (ml)	Onset (min)	Duration (min)[a]	
				T10	T4			No Epi	Epi (0.2 mg)
Procaine	2.5	DW	Hypo						
	5		Hyper	100–150	150–200	3	5–10	30–45	60–75
Lidocaine	2	S	Iso						
	5	G	Hyper	30–50	75–100	1–2	2–4	45–60	60–90
Tetracaine	0.5	G	Hyper	6–10	12–16	1–3	4–6	60–90	120–180
Bupivacaine	0.5	S	Iso			3			
	0.5–0.75	G	Hyper	6–10	12–16	1–2		90	140

Dose, volume, onset, and duration are estimates.
DW, distilled water; S, saline; G, glucose; Hypo, hypobaric; Hyper, hyperbaric; Iso, isobaric; Epi, epinephrine.
[a] Satisfactory analgesia.

space, which is determined by the position of the patient. In supine patients, hyperbaric solutions gravitate to the thoracic kyphosis (low point is T6 in an average adult patient), assuring an adequate level of spinal anesthesia for intra-abdominal surgery (Fig. 13-1). Conversely, injection of hyperbaric local anesthetic solutions in the sitting position allows production of low levels (saddle block) of anesthesia as commonly employed for vaginal delivery (see Chapter 26). Hyperbaric solutions are the most commonly used preparations for spinal block. This popularity reflects the belief among anesthesiologists that it is easier to control the spread of these solutions.

Hypobaric Solutions. Hypobaric solutions are prepared by adding 6 ml to 8 ml of sterile water to the local anesthetic solution. After injection into the subarachnoid space, the hypobaric solution "floats" up to the nerves innervating the surgical site. For example, patients undergoing hemorrhoidectomy in the jack-knife prone position or hip arthroplasty in the lateral position may be positioned before production of a spinal block knowing that subsequently injected local anesthetic solutions will rise to nondependent areas in the subarachnoid space.

Isobaric Solutions. Isobaric solutions are produced by diluting local anesthetic solutions with cerebrospinal fluid. Commercially available local anesthetic solutions are commonly formulated with sodium chloride and are isobaric. Spinal block can be induced in the most convenient position for the patient and the anesthesiologist, and the patient can then be placed in the position required by the surgery. Surgery performed on areas innervated by nerves below L1 (e.g., hip surgery) are often performed using isobaric local anesthetic solutions.

Vasoconstrictors

Epinephrine (0.1 mg to 0.2 mg; 0.1 ml to 0.2 ml of a 1:1000 solution) or phenylephrine (2 mg to 5 mg; 0.2 ml to 0.5 ml of a 1 percent solution) are frequently added to local anesthetic solutions before their injection into the subarachnoid space (Table 13-1). Vasoconstrictors are presumed to prolong spinal block up to 50 percent by localized vasoconstriction, which decreases spinal cord blood flow and subsequent vascular absorption of the local anesthetic.[6] As a result, more of the local anesthetic remains in contact with neural tissue for a longer time creating a more intense block. A direct antinociceptive action may also be contributing to prolonged spinal block.[6]

Vasoconstrictors seem to be most useful in prolonging the duration of spinal block below L1 with all local anesthetics. This most likely reflects the high concentration of drugs in this site because of the lumbar site of injection. For abdominal surgery, vasoconstrictors added to solutions containing lidocaine or bupivacaine may not be as efficacious as when added to solutions containing tetracaine for prolonging the duration of anesthesia.[6]

Documentation of Block

Within 30 seconds to 60 seconds after subarachnoid injection of local anesthetic solutions, an attempt should be made to determine the developing level of spinal anesthesia. The desired level of spinal block is dependent on the type of surgery (Table 13-2). Because the sympathetic nerves are usually the first ones to be blocked, an early indication of the level of a spinal block can be obtained by evaluating the patient's ability to discriminate temperature changes as produced by an alcohol sponge.[7] In the area blocked by the spinal anesthetic, the alcohol sponge produces a warm or neutral sensation rather than the cold sensation perceived in the unblocked areas. It is important to remember that the level of sympathetic nervous system blockade usually exceeds the level of sensory blockade, which in turn exceeds the level of motor blockade (see the section *Physiology*). The level of sensory blockade is often evaluated by the patient's ability to discriminate sharpness as produced by a needle touched to the abdomen or chest. Skeletal muscle power is tested by asking the patient to dorsiflex the foot (S1–2), raise the knees (L2–3), or tense the abdominal rectus muscles (T6–12).

Physiology

Spinal blockade interrupts sensory, motor and sympathetic nervous system innervation. According to the classic concept, local anesthetics injected

Table 13-2. Sensory Level of Spinal Block Necessary for Certain Surgical Procedures

Level	Type of Surgery	Local Anesthtic and Dose (Estimate)
S2–5 (perineal)	Rectal surgery Hemorrhoidectomy	Lidocaine 50 mg
L2–3 (knee)	Foot surgery	Tetracaine
L1 (inguinal ligament)	Lower extremity	6 mg
T10 (umbilicus)	Hip surgery	Lidocaine 50–75 mg
	Transurethral resection or prostate	Tetracaine 6–8 mg
	Vaginal delivery	
T6 (xiphoid process)	Lower abdominal surgery	Lidocaine 75–100 mg
T4 (nipple)	Upper abdominal surgery	Tetracaine 12–16 mg

into the subarachnoid space block small-diameter, unmyelinated (sympathetic) fibers before interrupting conduction via larger myelinated (sensory and motor) fibers. This reflects the anatomy of the spinal nerves in which unmyelinated small-diameter nerve fibers are close to the surface and thus the first fibers exposed to local anesthetic solutions. In fact, large-diameter myelinated somatic sensory fibers are more susceptible to local anesthetic blockade, but their location deep in the nerve increases the diffusion distance and delays the onset of sensory and motor blockade relative to sympathetic nervous system blockade. Sympathetic nervous system blockade typically exceeds somatic sensory blockade by two dermatomes. This may be a conservative estimate, with sympathetic nervous system blockade sometimes exceeding somatic sensory blockade by as many as six dermatomes.[6] This explains why hypotension may accompany even low levels of a spinal block (see the section *Complications*).

Sympathetic nervous system blockade produced by injection of local anesthetic solutions into the subarachnoid space is responsible for decreased venous return and bradycardia with resultant hypotension (see the section *Complications*). Spinal blockade has little if any effect on resting ventilation (arterial blood gases unchanged), but high levels of motor blockade that produce paralysis of abdominal and intercostal muscles can lead to decreased ability to cough and clear secretions. Patients may complain of difficulty in breathing during spinal block, reflecting the lack of proprioception in abdominal and thoracic muscles. Spinal blockade above T5 inhibits sympathetic nervous system innervation to the gastrointestinal tract, and the resulting unopposed parasympathetic nervous system activity results in contracted intestines and relaxed sphincters. The ureters are contracted and the ureterovesical orifice is relaxed. Block of afferent impulses from the surgical site by the spinal block is consistent with the absence of an adrenocortical response to painful stimulation. Decreased bleeding during regional blocks and certain types of surgery (hip surgery, transurethral resection of the prostate) may reflect reductions in arterial blood pressure, and increased blood flow to lower extremities after sympathetic nervous system blockade has been proposed as an explanation for the decreased incidence of thromboembolic complications after hip surgery.[8] There is no difference in perioperative mortality between regional block or general anesthesia administered to relatively healthy patients scheduled for elective surgery.

Complications

Complications associated with spinal blockade are usually predictable and acceptable, considering the merits of this anesthetic technique for individual patients. Neurologic complications, although a common concern among patients, are nearly nonexistent with this technique (zero incidence of paralysis in over 582,000 spinal blocks).[3]

Hypotension

Sympathetic nervous system blockade produced by a spinal block results in venous pooling with subsequent decreases in venous return (preload).

> ## Complications Associated with a Spinal Block
>
> Hypotension
> Bradycardia
> Postspinal headache
> High spinal
> Nausea
> Urinary retention
> Backache
> Neurologic sequelae (extremely unlikely)

As a result, the cardiac output may decline, leading to hypotension. Bradycardia due to block of cardioaccelerator fibers may contribute to further reductions in cardiac output. The degree of hypotension thus parallels the level of the spinal block and the intravascular fluid volume of the patient. Indeed, the magnitude of hypotension produced by a spinal block is greatly exaggerated by co-existing hypovolemia. During a spinal block, systemic vascular resistance is only slightly decreased.

Treatment. Spinal-block-induced hypotension is treated physiologically by restoration of venous return so as to increase cardiac output. In this regard, the internal autotransfusion produced by a modest head-down position (5 degrees to 10 degrees) will facilitate venous return without greatly exaggerating the cephalad spread of the spinal block. Adequate hydration before institution of the spinal block is important for minimizing the effects of venodilation due to sympathetic nervous system blockade. Excessive hydration in attempts to prevent or treat spinal-block-induced hypotension, however, may be undesirable in patients with coronary artery disease if hemodilution reduces the hematocrit sufficiently to decrease myocardial oxygen delivery. Occasionally, sympathomimetics with positive inotropic and venoconstrictor effects, such as ephedrine (5 mg to 10 mg administered intravenously), are required to maintain perfusion pressures at acceptable levels in the first few minutes after institution of the spinal block. In this regard, some anesthesiologists recommend prophylactic administration of ephedrine (25 mg to

50 mg administered intramuscularly) before institution of a spinal block. Sympathomimetics, such as phenylephrine, which increase systemic vascular resistance and may decrease the cardiac output, do not specifically correct the decreased venous return responsible for spinal-block-induced hypotension. Nevertheless, anesthesiologists have long used phenylephrine successfully to treat decreases in blood pressure associated with spinal block administered to nonparturients.

Postspinal Headache

Postspinal headache is characterized as frontal or occipital, made worse by the sitting position, improved by the supine position, and sometimes accompanied by diplopia. Tinnitus and decreased hearing acuity may accompany postspinal headache. A headache without a postural component is not a postspinal headache. Postspinal headache is believed to be due to decreased cerebrospinal fluid pressures and resulting tension on meningeal vessels and nerves due to leakage of cerebrospinal fluid through the needle hole in the dura mater created by the lumbar puncture. Diplopia is presumed to be due to traction on the abducens nerve. In support of the cerebrospinal fluid leakage theory is the observation that the incidence of postspinal headache is less when 25-gauge needles rather than 22-gauge needles are used for spinal block. Young females, especially parturients, seem most likely to develop postspinal headache.

Treatment of postspinal headache is initially with bedrest, analgesics, and oral/intravenous hydration (3L or more daily). Hydration is intended to increase cerebrospinal fluid production to levels that exceed loss through the needle hole in the dura mater. If postspinal headache persists after 24 hours to 48 hours of conservative therapy, it is a common recommendation to perform a lumbar epidural "blood patch" with 10 ml to 20 ml of the patient's blood (obtained with strict asepsis).[9] Prompt relief of the postspinal headache after the epidural blood patch is presumed to reflect sealing of the hole in the dura mater and re-establishment of normal pressures in the subarachnoid space. Epidural saline does not appear to be as efficacious as blood for treatment of a persistent postspinal headache. Alternatively, intravenous administration of caffeine sodium benzoate, 500 mg, has been effective in alleviating postpsinal headache in about 70 percent of patients.

High Spinal

High spinal is the term used to describe a block that is T3 or higher. There is often an undesired excessive level of sensory and motor anesthesia associated with difficulty breathing or apnea leading to arterial hypoxemia and hypercarbia. Hypotension is frequent and patients become nauseated and agitated. These symptoms must immediately alert the anesthesiologist to the possible presence of a high spinal. Treatment is support of breathing and circulation. Positive pressure ventilation of the lungs with oxygen via an anesthetic face mask and support of circulation by administration of fluid intravenously and sympathomimetics are indicated. Intubation of the trachea after induction of general anesthesia is indicated for patients at increased risk for aspiration (i.e., parturients). High spinal block usually manifests soon after injection of the local anesthetic solution into the subarachnoid space.

Nausea

Nausea occurring shortly after initiation of the spinal block must alert the anesthesiologist to the possible presence of hypotension sufficient to produce cerebral ischemia. Treatment of hypotension with sympathomimetics should eliminate nausea. Another cause of nausea during spinal block is a predominance of parasympathetic nervous system activity due to selective blockade of sympathetic nervous system innervation to the gastrointestinal tract. In this instance, administration of atropine 0.4 mg intravenously may be effective therapy.

Urinary Retention

Because a spinal block interferes with innervation of the bladder, administration of large amounts of fluids intravenously can cause bladder distension, which may require catheter drainage. For this reason, it seems prudent to minimize fluid replacement to patients undergoing minor surgery with a spinal block.

Backache

Backache is infrequent after a spinal block and may be more related to the position required for the surgery. Ligament strain may be more likely when anesthesia and skeletal muscle relaxation produced by the spinal block permits positioning of patients for surgery in positions that might otherwise be uncomfortable.

Neurologic Sequelae

Neurologic sequelae are extremely rare, due in part to use of prepackaged and sterile kits and the small doses of local anesthetics employed.[3] When a neurologic complication follows a spinal block, it is important to consult a neurologist and seek to establish the cause (errantly placed spinal needle, injection of the wrong substance, exacerbation of co-existing neurologic disease, surgical retractors, pressure on peripheral nerves due to positioning during surgery, birth trauma). In the absence of a hematoma or abscess, treatment is usually symptomatic.

Hypoventilation

Exaggerated hypoventilation may accompany intravenous administration of drugs to produce a sleeplike state during spinal block.[10] It is conceivable that depressant effects of drugs on ventilation are enhanced in patients in whom spinal block has produced sympathetic nervous system blockade and reductions in external stimulation. Constant vigilance by the anesthesiologist that is enhanced by monitors, such as the pulse oximeter, is important to promptly recognize dangerous hypoventilation during spinal block.

EPIDURAL BLOCK

Epidural block follows placement of local anesthetic solutions into the epidural space most often at the lumbar level.

Technique

Epidural block is typically instituted with the patient in the lateral decubitus position using needles and drugs from prepackaged and sterile kits. The skin of the back is prepared with an antiseptic solution, and the needle is inserted through a local anesthetic skin wheal into a previously selected lumbar interspace using landmarks as described for midline spinal block (see the section *Spinal Block, Technique*). A 17-gauge or 18-gauge Tuohy needle with a curved distal end is designed to decrease the likelihood of accidental puncture of the dura mater and to facilitate passage of a plastic catheter into the epidural space.

A common method for identifying the epidural space is the loss of resistance technique reflecting the presence of negative pressure in this space. After the epidural needle is positioned in the interspinous ligament, a glass syringe with a freely moveable plunger is attached (Fig. 13-7).[2] If the needle is properly positioned, it will be difficult to inject air or saline and the plunger of the syringe will "spring back" to its original position. The needle is advanced in a slightly cephalad direction while continuous pressure is exerted on the plunger of the syringe. The dorsum of the anesthesiologist's noninjecting hand rests on the patient's back and the thumb and index finger grasp the hub of the needle (Fig. 13-7). As the needle passes through the ligamentum flavum into the epidural space, there is a sudden loss of resistance to pressure being exerted on the plunger of the

syringe. A sterile plastic catheter is placed through the needle and 2 cm to 3 cm into the epidural space to allow repeated injections of local anesthetic solutions. This allows anesthesia for operations of unpredictable duration as well as provision of postoperative analgesia. The needle is withdrawn over the catheter taking care not to move the catheter. No attempt should be made to withdraw a catheter back through the needle, as this may result in shearing of a portion of the catheter in the epidural space. The catheter is taped to the patient's back and a test dose of local anesthetic solution (3 ml of 1.5 percent lidocaine with 1:200,000 epinephrine) is injected. Failure of the test dose to produce sensory (saddle area) or motor blockade after 3 minutes to 5 minutes confirms the absence of an accidental subarachnoid placement of the catheter. Absence of a heart rate effect due to epinephrine in the local anesthetic solution suggests that the drugs were not injected intravascularly. The calculated dose and volume of local anesthetic solution appropriate for the planned surgical procedure is then injected over 1 minute to 3 minutes (Table 13-3). Documentation of the level of sympathetic nervous system blockade and sensory anesthesia is determined as described for spinal block (see the section *Documentation of Block*).

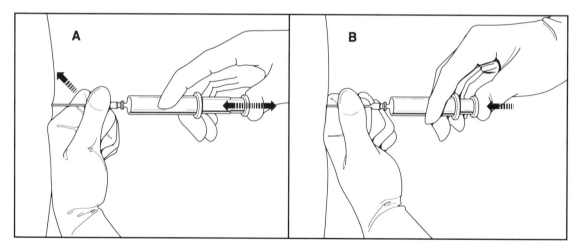

Fig. 13-7. (A) During location of the epidural space when the needle is in the interspinous ligament, it is difficult to inject air or saline, and the plunger of the syringe will "spring back" to its original position. (B) Entrance into the epidural space is confirmed by ease of depression of the plunger in the syringe (i.e., loss of resistance). (From Cousins and Bromage,[2] with permission.)

Table 13-3. Local Anesthetic Solutions for Epidural Block

	Concentration (%)	Dose (mg·segment-1)[a]	Onset (min)	Duration[b] (min)
Chloroprocaine	2–3	45	5–15	30–90
Lidocaine	1–2	25	5–15	60–120
Bupivacaine	0.25–0.75	7	10–20	120–240

[a] Generally 1 ml to 1.5 ml·segment-1 of local anesthetic solution are required.
[b] Sensory analgesia.
Dose, onset, and duration are estimates.

It is acceptable to inject local anesthetic solutions into the epidural space through the epidural needle (single-shot technique) when only a brief duration of anesthesia is required.

Level and Duration

Level and duration of epidural block depends on the (1) dose, volume, and concentration of local anesthetic; and (2) presence or absence of epinephrine (1:200,000 dilution, 5 μg·ml^{-1}) in the local anesthetic solutions (Table 13-3). The dose of local anesthetic seems to be more important than variations in the volume or concentration of the local anesthetic solution in determining onset, intensity, and duration of the block. Weight, height, age, and rate of injection do not seem to influence distribution of local anesthetic solutions in the epidural space.[11] In contrast to spinal block, the baricity of local anesthetic solutions does not influence the level of epidural block. Likewise, position is less important for the level of sensory anesthesia produced by an epidural block. Nevertheless, it is likely that the dependent portion of the body will manifest more intense block than the nondependent side.

Local anesthetics used for epidural block include (1) chloroprocaine (rapid onset and short duration), (2) lidocaine (intermediate onset and duration), and (3) bupivacaine slow onset and prolonged duration of action (Table 13-3). Procaine and tetracaine are rarely used for epidural block because of their slow onset of action. Lumbar epidural administration usually requires volumes of 15 ml to 25 ml to achieve sensory levels for surgery. Cephalad spread occurs more easily than caudad spread after lumbar epidural injections, due in part to transmission of negative intrathoracic pressure and the resistance to spread produced by narrowing of the epidural space at the lumbosacral junction.

Addition of epinephrine to local anesthetic solutions reduces vascular absorption of drug from the epidural space, thus maintaining effective anesthetic concentrations at the nerve roots for more prolonged periods of time. Epinephrine seems to potentiate epidural block produced by lidocaine more than that produced by bupivacaine.

Physiology

The major site of action of local anesthetic solutions placed in the epidural space appears to be the spinal nerve roots where the dura mater is relatively thin. A spinal nerve root site of action is consistent with the often observed delay in onset or absence of anesthesia in the S1–2 region, presumably reflecting the covering of these nerve roots with connective tissue. To a lesser extent, diffusion of local anesthetic solutions from the epidural space into the subarachnoid space produces spinal cord blockade.

Sympathetic nervous system, sensory, and motor blockade follow injection of local anesthetic solutions into the epidural space. In contrast to spinal block, the onset of sympathetic nervous system blockade produced by epidural block is often slower, and the likelihood of abrupt hypotension is less. Relatively large volumes of local anesthetics are required for an epidural block. Vascular absorption of local anesthetic solutions may be sufficient to produce systemic toxicity (see the section *Complications*). Beta agonist effects from low plasma concentrations that result from systemic absorption of this catecholamine produce sufficient vasodilation to accentuate blood pressure declines compared with those produced by local anesthetics alone.[12] When epinephrine is not included in local anesthetic solutions, changes in blood pressure and calculated systemic vascular resistance are minimal. Effects of epidural block on breathing and the gastrointestinal tract resemble those produced by spinal block.

Complications

Complications of epidural block resemble those described for spinal block with the added risks of accidental dural puncture and local anesthetic toxicity. Epidural hematoma formation is a theoretical complication of epidural block, although the incidence is almost nonexistent even in the presence of bleeding abnormalities as may result from platelet dysfunction due to aspirin therapy. Patients on anticoagulants, however, may be at increased risk for this complication.

Hypotension

Hypotension, as with a spinal block, parallels the degree of sympathetic nervous system blockade produced by the epidural block. Due to the slower onset of sympathetic nervous system blockade, however, an excessive fall in blood pressure does not usually accompany epidural block administered to normovolemic patients. Treatment of hypotension is as described for that produced by spinal block.

High Spinal

Accidental subarachnoid injection of the large volumes of local anesthetic solutions used for epidural block produces rapid evidence of a high spinal block (i.e., greater than a T3 level). Unrecognized injection of drug in the subdural space may produce a slower onset of high spinal block than that following accidental subarachnoid injection.

Accidental Dural Puncture

Accidental dural puncture is always a potential risk when performing an epidural block. Appearance of cerebrospinal fluid (warm when allowed to drop on the anesthesiologist's forearm in con-

trast to saline that may be injected during determination of loss of resistance) at the hub of the epidural needle should be ample evidence of an accidental dural puncture. At this point, the anesthetic may be converted to a spinal block, or the epidural block can be attempted at a different lumbar interspace. Development of a postspinal headache is likely, considering the relatively large hole in the dura mater made by the needle used for the epidural block.

Local Anesthetic Toxicity

The high doses of local anesthetics required for epidural block plus the presence of numerous venous plexuses in the epidural space increase the likelihood of substantial blood levels of local anesthetics after an epidural block. Nevertheless, these blood levels are rarely sufficient to produce systemic toxicity, especially if epinephrine is added to the local anesthetic solution in an attempt to minimize vascular absorption. The accidental intravascular injection of local anesthetic solutions results in local anesthetic toxicity, manifesting principally as cardiovascular collapse, apnea, seizures, and unconsciousness (see Chapter 7).

CAUDAL BLOCK

Caudal block is instituted with the patient in the prone position. The sacral hiatus (in the midline about 5 cm from the tip of coccyx between the sacral cornu) is identified and a needle is introduced perpendicular to the skin through the sacrococcygeal ligament until the sacrum is contacted (Fig. 13-8). The needle is then slightly withdrawn and the angle reduced before advancing it about 2 cm into the caudal canal (Fig. 13-8). Confirmation that the needle is actually in the caudal canal can be made by injecting 4 ml to 5 ml of air through the needle and palpating the skin for a crepitation. Although infection is rare, the nearness of this approach to the rectum suggests caution. A subarachnoid injection is a risk if the caudal needle extends beyond S2, which is the termination of the dural sac. Because of abnormalities in the anatomy of the caudal canal, the failure rate with a caudal block can be as high as 10 percent. As a result the lumbar rather than sacral (caudal) ap-

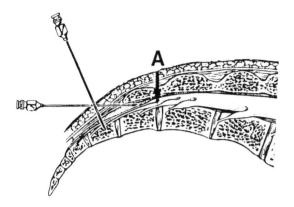

Fig. 13-8. A caudal block is initiated by insertion of a needle through the sacral hiatus until the sacrum is contacted. The needle is then slightly withdrawn and the angle reduced before advancing it through the sacrococcygeal membrane and into the caudal canal (A).

proach to the epidural space is often preferred, as the former is more predictable and easier to perform.

REFERENCES

1. Bridenbaugh PO, Greene NM. Spinal (subarachnoid) neural blockade. In: Cousins MJ, Bridenbaugh PO, eds. Neural Blockade in Clinical Anesthesia and Management of Pain. Philadelphia, JB Lippincott, 1988;213–52.
2. Cousins MJ, Bromage PR. Epidural neural blockade. In: Cousins MJ, Bridenbaugh PO, eds. Neural blockade in Clinical Anesthesia and Management of Pain. Philadelphia, JB Lippincott, 1988;253–360.
3. Lund PC. Principles and practices of spinal anesthesia. Springfield, IL, Charles C Thomas, 1971.
4. Cousins MJ, Mather LE. Intrathecal and epidural administration of opiates. Anesthesiology 1984; 61:276–310.
5. Lambert DH, Covino BG. Hyperbaric, hypobaric and isobaric spinal anesthesia. Res Staff Phys 1987;33:79–86.
6. Armstrong IR, Littlewood DG, Chambers WA. Spinal anesthesia with tetracaine-effect of added vasoconstrictor. Anesth Analg 1983;62:793–5.
7. Chamberlain DP, Chamberlain BDL. Changes in skin temperature of the trunk and their relationship to sympathetic blockade during spinal anesthesia. Anesthesiology 1986;65:139–43.
8. Modig J, Hjelmstedt A, Sahlstedt B, Maripuu E. Comparitive influences of epidural and general anaesthesia on deep vein thrombosis and pulmonary embolism after total hip replacement. Acta Chir Scand 1981;147:125–8.
9. Szeinfeld M, Ihmeidan IH, Moser MM, Machado R, Klose KJ, Serafini AN. Epidural blood patch: Evaluation of the volume and spread of blood injected into the epidural space. Anesthesiology 1986;64:820–2.
10. Caplan RA, Ward RJ, Posner K, Cheney FW. Unexpected cardiac arrest during spinal anesthesia: A closed claims analysis of predisposing factors. Anesthesiology 1988;68:5–11.
11. Park WY, Massengale M, Kim S-I, Poon KC, Macnamara TE. Age and spread of local anesthetic solutions in the epidural space. Anesth Analg 1980;59:768–71.
12. Ward RJ, Bonica JJ, Freund FG. Epidural and subarachnoid anesthesia. JAMA 1965;191:275–8.

Chapter 14

Peripheral Nerve Blocks

Peripheral nerve blocks are used for (1) anesthesia, (2) postoperative analgesia, and (3) diagnosis and treatment of chronic pain syndromes. Advantages and disadvantages of peripheral nerve blocks for anesthesia must be considered when advising patients as to the choice of anesthesia (see Chapter 9). Patients are often more receptive to peripheral nerve blocks when they are reassured that supplemental sedation can be administered if they become uncomfortable during surgery. During the preoperative evaluation the patient should be examined for bony landmarks, which are required to perform peripheral nerve blocks. The presence of skin infections in the area to be used for insertion of needles must be recognized preoperatively. Confirmation of normal coagulation (either by history and/or specific tests) is considered by many to be essential before performance of peripheral nerve blocks.

PREPARATION FOR NERVE BLOCKS

Patients scheduled for peripheral nerve blocks are evaluated medically in the same way as are patients scheduled for general or regional anesthesia (see Chapter 9). Preoperative medication is useful for decreasing apprehension and providing analgesia during needle insertions necessary to perform the block. When the needle comes in contact with the desired nerve, the patient will experience paresthesias ("electric shocks") in the peripheral distri-

bution of that nerve. Although this serves to identify the nerve to be blocked, it is an uncomfortable sensation that may be better accepted by patients who have received preoperative medication. Paresthesias during injection of local anesthetic solutions suggest that the needle is intraneural and are an indication to reposition the needle before continuing the injection.

A holding area for performing nerve blocks may be useful for minimizing any delay once the operating room becomes available. This area must have available appropriate monitors, equipment, and drugs should toxic reactions to local anesthetics occur. Also for this reason, an intravenous catheter should usually be in place before performance of the nerve block. Prepackaged and sterile trays are often used for performance of peripheral nerve blocks. In the operating room, the anesthesiologist must be prepared to provide appropriate supplemental sedation and analgesia or to induce general anesthesia should the peripheral nerve block be inadequate. Sedation can also be provided by allowing patients to inhale nitrous oxide. This approach permits termination of sedation within minutes after surgery.

CERVICAL PLEXUS BLOCK

The cervical plexus is formed by the first four cervical nerves, which pass behind the vertebral artery and lie in the nerve sulci of the transverse

Peripheral Nerve Blocks

Cervical plexus
Brachial plexus

   Interscalene
   Supraclavicular
   Axillary

Median nerve
Ulnar nerve
Radial nerve
Intercostal nerves
Sciatic nerve
Femoral nerve
Lateral femoral cutaneous nerve
Obturator nerve
Stellate ganglion
Celiac plexus
Lumbar sympathetic nerves
Intravenous regional block

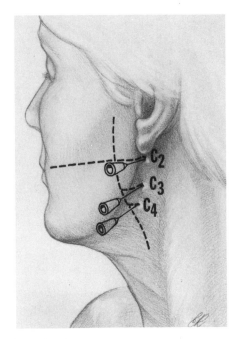

Fig. 14-1. Superficial landmarks necessary for block of the cervical plexus.

processes of the cervical vertebrae. With the patient's head turned to the opposite side, a line connecting the tip of the mastoid process of the temporal bone and the anterior tubercle of the 6th cervical vertebra (Chassaignac's tubercle, which is the most prominent of the cervical transverse processes) identifies the approximate plane in which the cervical transverse processes lie (Fig. 14-1). The transverse processes of C2–4 are identified and 3 ml to 5 ml of local anesthetic solution are injected. Blockade of the phrenic nerve is common but rarely requires treatment, as the intercostal muscles are able to compensate fully. Care must be taken to avoid intravascular injections because this region is highly vascular and the vertebral artery is located nearby. A Horner's syndrome (ptosis, miosis, enophthalmos, and anhydrosis) is possible, and hoarseness occurs when the recurrent laryngeal nerve is blocked by diffusion of local anesthetic solutions. Subcutaneous injection of local anesthetic solutions along the posterior lateral border of the sternocleidomastoid muscle blocks branches of the superficial cervical plexus.

Anesthesia includes the area from the inferior surface of the mandible to the level of the second rib. Skeletal muscles of the neck are profoundly relaxed. Cervical plexus block is used most often to provide anesthesia in an otherwise conscious patient undergoing carotid endarterectomy surgery.

BRACHIAL PLEXUS

The brachial plexus arises from the anterior rami of C5–8 and T1. These rami unite to form three trunks in the space between the anterior and middle scalene muscles and then pass over the first rib and under the midpoint of the clavicle to enter the apex of the axilla (Fig. 14-2).[1] All of the motor and nearly all of the sensory function (skin over the shoulders supplied by the cervical plexus and posterior medial aspect of the arm supplied by the intercostobrachial branch of the second intercostal nerve) of the upper extremity is via the brachial plexus. Approaches to the brachial plexus for performance of nerve blocks are designated as interscalene, supraclavicular, and axillary (Table 14-1).[2]

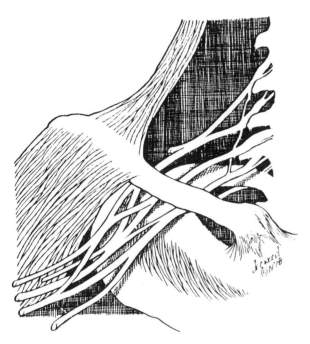

Fig. 14-2. Schematic depiction of the brachial plexus in its course from the intervertebral foramina over the first rib and under the clavicle into the axilla. (From Bridenbaugh,[1] with permission.)

Interscalene Block

Interscalene block of the brachial plexus is achieved by injecting 10 ml to 40 ml of local anesthetic solution into the interscalene groove opposite the transverse process of C6 (external jugular vein often overlies this area) (Fig. 14-3).[1] A line extended laterally from the cricoid cartilage intersects the interscalene groove at C6. Paresthesias must be elicited before injection of local anesthetic solutions, keeping in mind that the transverse process is superficial (1.5 cm to 2 cm). Injection of 40 ml of local anesthetic solution will anesthetize the cervical plexus and brachial plexus, permitting surgery on the acromioclavicular joint. This block can be performed with the arm at the patient's side, and the risk of pneumothorax is remote. Epidural block and spinal block are possible using this approach, and the vertebral artery is located nearby. If local anesthetics are accidentally injected into the vertebral artery, convulsions are likely to follow.

Supraclavicular Block

Supraclavicular block of the brachial plexus is achieved by injecting 15 ml to 25 ml of local anesthetic solution at a point just behind the midpoint of the clavicle where the nerves cross the first rib (Fig. 14-4).[1] The midpoint of the clavicle is confirmed by palpating the subclavian artery pulse or by extending an imaginary straight line from the end of the external jugular vein. Paresthesias should be elicited before injection of local anesthetic solution. Pneumothorax is the most common complication of supraclavicular block (about a 1 percent incidence), manifesting initially as cough, dyspnea, and pleuritic chest pain. Block of the phrenic nerve occurs frequently but usually causes no symptoms. Bilateral supraclavicular blocks are not recommended for fear of bilateral pneumothoraces or phrenic nerve paralysis. Likewise, patients with chronic obstructive airways disease may not be ideal candidates for supraclavicular block. Advantages of the supraclavicular block are the need for small volumes of local anesthetic solutions, as the brachial plexus is most compact at this site; rapid onset; and ability to perform the block with the arm in any position.

Axillary Block

Axillary block (perivascular axillary infiltration) of the brachial plexus is achieved by injecting 20 ml to 40 ml of local anesthetic solution into the axillary sheath in the axilla (Fig. 14-5).[1] The arm is abducted to 90 degrees and externally rotated (Fig. 14-5).[1] The axillary artery is palpated and traced as far as possible toward the axilla. As the finger of one hand palpates the artery, the needle is inserted just anterior to the vessel into the axillary sheath (Fig. 14-5).[1] Entrance of the needle into the axillary sheath transmits a "popping" sensation to the anesthesiologist's fingers and the needle pulsates with arterial pulsations. Paresthesias are useful but not mandatory for confirming correct placement of the needle. Digital pressure applied distal to the needle during and after injection promotes proximal flow of local anesthetic solutions within the sheath toward the site where the musculocutaneous nerve exits. An alternative approach to locating the axillary sheath is identifi-

Table 14-1. Advantages to Various Approaches to the Brachial Plexus

Location	Nerve Roots					
	C5	C6	C7	C8	T1	T2
Shoulder						
Interscalene	+++	+++	+++	+++	+	0
Supraclavicular	++	++	++	++	+	0
Axillary	0	0	0	0	0	0
Elbow						
Interscalene	+++	+++	+++	+++	++	0
Supraclavicular	++	++	++	++	++	0
Axillary	+	+	++	++	++	0
Wrist and Hand						
Interscalene	+++	+++	++	+	+	0
Supraclavicular	++	+++	+++	+++	++	0
Axillary	+	+	++	++	++	

+++, marked blockade; ++, moderate blockade; +, slight blockade; 0, no blockade.

cation of the axillary artery with the exploring needle. The needle is then withdrawn or inserted further until blood is no longer aspirated. Since the nerves of the brachial plexus are adjacent to the axillary artery, it is presumed that injection of the local anesthetic using this "transarterial approach" will result in a successful block. Regardless of the approach, frequent aspirations during injection of the local anesthetic are essential to ensure that the needle remains outside the axillary artery. A small amount of local anesthetic solution is deposited in the subcutaneous tissue (a cuff over the proximal medial aspect of the axilla) during withdrawal of the needle to block the intercostobrachial nerve.

Axillary block provides excellent conditions for surgery on the forearm and hand. Surgery on the shoulder, upper arm, or elbow, however, is usually impossible with this block. The musculocutaneous nerve is sometimes missed because it leaves the sheath proximal to the point of injection. This nerve is important because of its extensive area of innervation on the radial side of the forearm extending onto the thenar eminence. Block of the musculocutaneous nerve, as it emerges between the biceps and brachialis muscles 5 cm proximal to the elbow crease, is usually performed as a supplement to an axillary plexus block.

DISTAL NERVE BLOCKS OF THE UPPER EXTREMITY

Reliable brachial plexus anesthesia has reduced the need for block of individual nerves distal to the axilla.[1] Little can be gained by blocking nerves at the elbow as opposed to the wrist. For example, only anesthesia of the hand results from blocking the median, ulnar, or radial nerves at the elbow because the forearm cutaneous nerves arise in the upper arm.

Median Nerve Block

Injection of 3 ml to 5 ml of local anesthetic solution just medial to the brachial artery in the flexion crease of the elbow will block the median nerve. At the wrist, the median nerve is blocked by 3 ml to 5 ml of local anesthetic solution injected just lateral to the palmaris longus tendon (Fig. 14-6).

Ulnar Nerve Block

Injection of 5 ml to 8 ml of local anesthetic solution proximal to the medial epicondyle of the elbow will block the ulnar nerve. At the wrist, the ulnar nerve is blocked by 3 ml to 5 ml of local anesthetic solution injected at the flexor carpi ulnaris tendon (Fig. 14-6).

Radial Nerve Block

Injection of 4 ml to 10 ml of local anesthetic solution along the lateral border of the humerus at the junction of its middle and lower third will block the radial nerve. Paresthesias are highly desirable since the landmarks for this block are not precise. At the wrist, the radial nerve is blocked by 2 ml to 3 ml of local anesthetic solution injected lateral to the radial artery (Fig. 14-6). In addition, a subcutaneous cuff of anesthesia is produced on the lateral and dorsal aspects of the radial side of the wrist to anesthetize those branches of the radial nerve that have left the parent trunk in the lower third of the forearm.

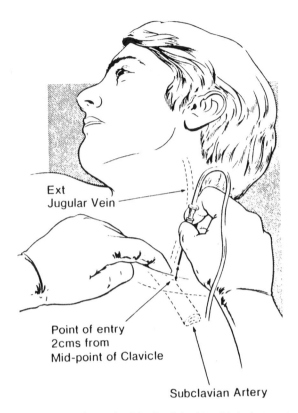

Fig. 14-4. Supraclavicular block of the brachial plexus. An imaginary line from the end of the external jugular vein crosses the midpoint of the clavicle beneath which passes the compact nerves of the brachial plexus. For convenience of injection and minimal displacement of the needle from its correct position, the needle can be connected by tubing to a syringe containing the local anesthetic solution. (From Bridenbaugh,[1] with permission.)

INTERCOSTAL BLOCKS

Intercostal nerves (12 pairs) pursue a circumferential course in the inferior groove of each rib supplying skin and abdominal wall skeletal muscles. Each nerve is accompanied by an intercostal vein and artery, which lie superior to the nerve in the inferior groove (Fig. 14-7).[3] The location of these vessels explains the frequent occurrence of high plasma concentrations of local anesthetics after performance of intercostal nerve blocks.

Intercostal nerve blocks are optimally performed

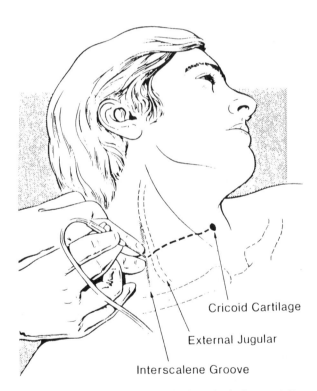

Fig. 14-3. Interscalene block of the brachial plexus. A line drawn from the cricoid cartilage crosses the approximate location of the transverse process of C6. For convenience of injection and minimal displacement of the needle from its correct position, the needle can be connected by tubing to a syringe containing the local anesthetic solution. (From Bridenbaugh,[1] with permission.)

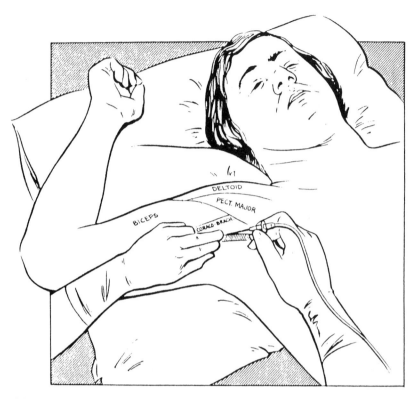

Fig. 14-5. Axillary block of the brachial plexus. The needle is inserted just anterior to the axillary artery while the fingers of the other hand provide compression, so as to facilitate central spread of the local anesthetic solution. A distally placed tourniquet may also be used to facilitate central spread of the local anesthetic solution. For convenience of injection and minimal displacement of the needle from its correct position, the needle can be connected by tubing to a syringe containing the local anesthetic solution. (From Bridenbaugh,[1] with permission.)

with the patient in the prone position and the needle inserted about 8 cm from the midline posteriorly where the rib can be palpated. Lateral cutaneous branches of intercostal nerves arise at the midaxillary line and may not be blocked if the needle is inserted too far laterally. The needle is advanced until the rib is contacted at which point the needle is redirected caudad and "walked off" the inferior border of the rib (Fig. 14-7).[3] The needle is then advanced an additional 2 mm to 3 mm, and 5 ml of local anesthetic solution is injected with frequent aspiration to minimize the likelihood of accidental intravascular injections. Multiple intercostal blocks may be performed to provide postoperative analgesia after thoracic or abdominal surgery or to relieve pain related to rib frac-

tures. Supplementation of intercostal nerve blocks with other blocks (celiac plexus block, brachial plexus block) is usually necessary when surgical procedures are planned. The principal risks of intercostal nerve blocks are pneumothorax and accidental intravascular injection of local anesthetic solutions.

BLOCKS OF THE LOWER EXTREMITY

Unlike the compactness of the brachial plexus, the lower extremity is supplied by nerves that are widely separated from each other as they enter the thigh. Major nerves to the lower extremity include the sciatic, femoral, lateral femoral cutaneous, and obturator nerves.[4] The sciatic nerve

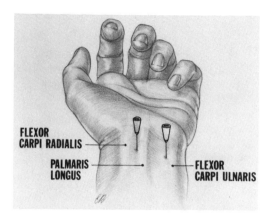

Fig. 14-6. An illustration of the approach to blocking the radial, median, and ulnar nerves at the wrist.

divides in the popliteal fossa into the tibial portion passing medially and the common peroneal nerve passing laterally. In many respects, it is easier to perform an epidural or spinal block than to attempt to achieve the same degree of anesthesia with multiple peripheral nerve blocks.

Sciatic Nerve Block

The sacral plexus (L4–5, S1–3) gives rise to the sciatic nerve, which is nearly 2 cm in width as it leaves the pelvis. The classic approach to sciatic nerve block is with the patient lying on the side opposite the one to be blocked (Fig. 14-8). A line is drawn from the posterior iliac spine and the greater trochanter. The needle is inserted about 5 cm caudad from the midsection of this line and 10 ml to 30 ml of local anesthetic solution injected after elicitation of a paresthesia. Sciatic nerve block is usually combined with other nerve blocks to provide complete anesthesia.

Femoral Nerve Block

Femoral nerve block is produced by injection of 10 ml to 20 ml of local anesthetic solution immediately lateral to the femoral artery just below the midpoint of the inguinal ligament. A line drawn from the anterior superior iliac spine to the symphysis pubis will approximate the inguinal ligament.

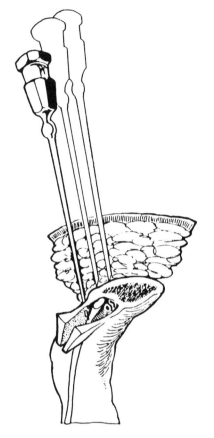

Fig. 14-7. Schematic depiction of the intercostal nerve as it travels in the inferior groove of the rib accompanied by an intercostal vein and artery. The needle is inserted over the rib and then "walked off" the inferior border of the rib. (From Thompson and Moore,[3] with permission.)

Lateral Femoral Cutaneous Nerve Block

The lateral femoral cutaneous nerve is blocked by injection of 5 ml to 10 ml of local anesthetic solution at a point 2 cm medial and 2 cm below the anterior superior iliac spine. This block may provide suitable anesthesia for removal of small skin grafts but is most often used to supplement sciatic nerve block, femoral nerve, and obturator nerve blocks for surgery on or above the knee.

Obturator Nerve Block

Obturator nerve block is performed by introducing a needle 1 cm to 2 cm below and lateral to the pubic tubercle. When the pubic bone is reached,

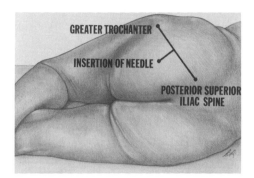

Fig. 14-8. The sciatic nerve is blocked by identifying the midpoint of a line joining the posterior iliac spine and the greater trochanter. Needle insertion is about 5 cm caudad from the midsection of this line.

the needle is withdrawn and redirected cephalad to identify the obturator canal where 10 ml to 15 ml of local anesthetic solution are placed. Successful obturator nerve block is evidenced by paresis of the abductor muscles because the cutaneous distribution is small and inconsistent. This block is useful for diagnosing painful conditions of the hip and is sometimes necessary to supplement sciatic, femoral, and lateral femoral cutaneous nerve blocks for surgery on or above the knee.

Inguinal Paravascular Technique of Lumbar Plexus Block

Blockade of the femoral, obturator, and lateral femoral cutaneous nerves is achieved with a single injection (thus the description as a "3-in-1 block").[5] The lumbar plexus can be blocked because a fascial envelope surrounds the femoral nerve, which serves as a conduit for carrying local anesthetic solution injected below the inguinal ligament cephalad to the level where the lumbar plexus forms.

Combined Lumbosacral Plexus Block

If the approaches described earlier are not possible, the lumbar and sacral plexuses can be blocked by a lumbar paravertebral approach.[5] This technique is similar to a paravertebral block at L4, except that a paresthesia must be obtained and a total of 40 ml of local anesthetic solution injected. Obviously, it may be easier to perform a spinal anesthetic in a patient who needs a lower extremity anesthetized. However, if a patient refuses a spinal

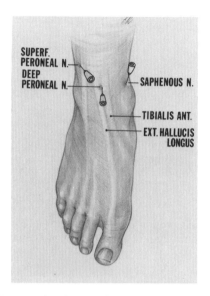

Fig. 14-9. Nerve distribution for innervation of the foot. Block of the saphenous nerve, superficial peroneal nerve, and deep peroneal nerve is illustrated. (From Bridenbaugh,[4] with permission.)

block or is anticoagulated, this approach can be considered.

DISTAL NERVE BLOCKS OF THE LOWER EXTREMITY

Major nerves that can be blocked at the level of the knee are the saphenous, common peroneal, and tibial nerves. The saphenous nerve is the cutaneous extension of the femoral nerve. Despite the known anatomic courses of these nerves, there remains an unexplained lack of interest among anesthesiologists in pursuing techniques for interrupting nerve conduction at these sites.[4] For surgical procedures on the foot that do not require a leg tourniquet, anesthesia can be provided by blocking appropriate nerves as they cross the ankle joint (Figs. 14-9 and 14-10).[4]

STELLATE GANGLION BLOCK

The cervical sympathetic chain consists of superior, middle, and inferior cervical ganglia. The inferior cervical ganglion and first thoracic ganglion often fuses to form the stellate ganglion. Sympathetic

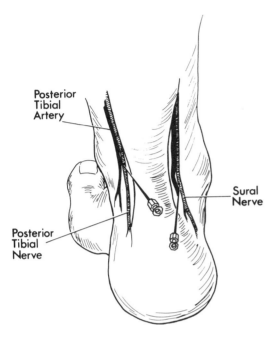

Posterior
Tibial
Artery

Sural
Nerve

Posterior
Tibial
Nerve

Fig. 14-10. Needle placement for block of the posterior tibial nerve and sural nerve.

nervous system fibers that traverse the stellate ganglion supply the head and arm. Techniques to block the stellate ganglion require large volumes of local anesthetic solutions (e.g., 10 ml) to assure adequate sensory anesthesia and thus may be more appropriately described as cervicothoracic sympathetic block rather than stellate ganglion block.[6]

A common approach to stellate ganglion block is the anterior or paratracheal technique. With the patient supine and the head extended on a pillow, the anesthesiologist retracts the sternomastoid muscle laterally and locates the transverse process of the 6th cervical vertebra (Chassignac tubercle), which is typically at the level of the cricoid cartilage. The needle is inserted through the skin over this transverse process and advanced 2.5 cm to 4 cm until it makes contact with bone, at which point the needle is withdrawn 2 mm to 3 mm, and 15 ml to 20 ml of local anesthetic solution is injected. Successful interruption of sympathetic nervous system impulses to the head is evidenced by the occurrence of a Horner's syndrome. Increased

skin temperature is the only sure evidence of interruption of sympathetic nervous system innervation to the upper extremity. A Horner's syndrome alone does not assure complete sympathetic denervation of the upper extremity, which may receive sympathetic fibers from as low as T9. Risks of causing stellate ganglion block are accidental intravascular injections (vertebral artery) or injection of local anesthetic solutions into the dural sheath enclosing cervical nerve roots, leading to diffusion of drug into the cervical subarachnoid space. Common indications for stellate ganglion block are diagnosis and treatment of reflex sympathetic dystrophies (see Chapter 33) and management of circulatory insufficiency in the upper extremity.

CELIAC PLEXUS BLOCK

The celiac plexus is the largest plexus of the sympathetic nervous system, providing innervation to abdominal organs (pancreas, liver, stomach). A needle is inserted about 8 cm from the midline at the inferior edge of the 12th rib and advanced until it contacts the lateral body of the L1 vertebra at an average depth of 10 cm to 12 cm (Fig. 14-11).[3] The needle is then withdrawn and redirected so that it will slide off the anterolateral side of the vertebral body. Many anesthesiologists recommend radiographic or computed tomography to confirm proper needle placement before injection of a 2 ml test dose of local anesthetic solution.[3] Assuming the absence of unexpected sensory blockade following the test dose, the remaining 25 ml to 35 ml of local anesthetic solution is injected.

Complications of celiac plexus block include hypotension due to extensive sympathetic nervous system blockade (exaggerated in chronically ill hypovolemic patients); accidental intravascular, epidural, or subarachnoid injection; and retroperitoneal hematoma secondary to bleeding from the aorta, inferior vena cava, or puncture of viscera. Pneumothorax is a potential but rare complication following a celiac plexus block. The complexity and risks of this block suggest that it should be performed only by anesthesiologists experienced in its use. Celiac plexus block with alcohol or

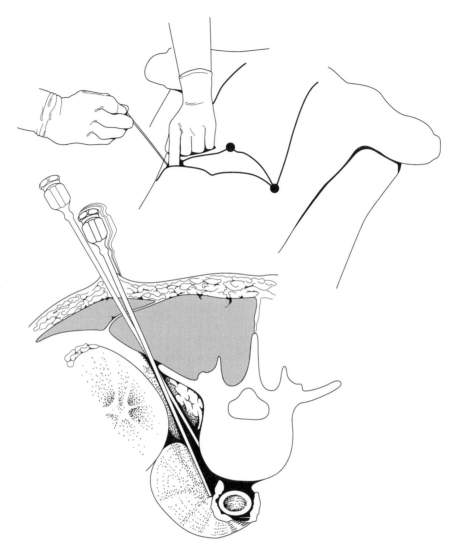

Fig. 14-11. Landmarks for performance of a celiac plexus block. A needle is inserted at the inferior edge of the 12th rib about 8 cm from the midline and advanced 10 cm to 12 cm until it contacts the body of the L1 vertebra. The needle is then withdrawn and redirected so that it passes to the anterolateral side of the vertebral body. (From Thompson and Moore,[3] with permission.)

phenol is the most effective block for treatment of pancreatic cancer pain (see Chapter 33).

LUMBAR SYMPATHETIC BLOCK

The lumbar sympathetic chain is located on the anterolateral aspects of the vertebral bodies. With the patient in the lateral position, needles are inserted opposite the spinous processes of L2–4, about 8 cm lateral to the midline. Each needle is advanced until the transverse process of the vertebra lying above it is contacted. The needle is then withdrawn and redirected to reach the sympathetic chain on the anterolateral aspects of the vertebral bodies. Lumbar sympathetic block is useful for increasing blood flow to the lower extremity.

INTRAVENOUS REGIONAL BLOCK

Intravenous regional block (Bier block) is a simple method of producing anesthesia of the arm or leg by injection of large volumes of local anesthetic solutions intravenously while the circulation to that extremity is occluded by a tourniquet.[7] A venous catheter is placed in a distal portion of the involved extremity and the arm or leg is exsanguinated by wrapping with an Esmarch bandage (Fig. 14-12).[7] The tourniquet is then inflated to about 50 mm Hg above the patient's systolic blood pressure and local anesthetic solution (25 ml to 50 ml for the upper extremity and 100 ml to 200 ml for the lower extremity) is injected. A double tourniquet technique can be used to eliminate tourniquet pain. The proximal tourniquet is initially inflated and when the patient subsequently experiences pain, the more distal tourniquet over anesthetized skin is inflated and the proximal cuff is then deflated.

Commonly used local anesthetic solutions for intravenous regional blocks are 0.5 percent lidocaine or prilocaine. Chloroprocaine is not used for intravenous regional blocks because of its association with thrombophlebitis, and bupivacaine is avoided because of concern of systemic toxic ef-

fects, especially on the heart, when the drug enters the circulation. Onset of anesthesia is rapid and skeletal muscle relaxation is profound. The duration of anesthesia depends on the time the tourniquet is inflated and not the local anesthetic selected. Technically, this block is easier to perform than a brachial plexus block or lower extremity blocks and is readily applicable to all age groups, including pediatric patients.

The principal risk of intravenous regional block anesthesia is the potential systemic toxicity that may occur when the tourniquet is deflated and local anesthetic solutions from the previously isolated extremity enter the circulation. For this reason, slow or intermittent deflations and inflations of the tourniquet at the conclusion of surgery are recommended in attempt to prevent excessive plasma concentrations of local anesthetics from developing. Likewise, limitation of extremity movement after release of the tourniquet is useful for minimizing anesthetic blood levels. Rapid metabolism of prilocaine is advantageous for reducing the likelihood of systemic toxicity. Significant methemoglobinemia is unlikely to accompany metabolism of prilocaine when the total dose of this local anesthetic administered to adults is less than 600 mg (see Chapter 7).

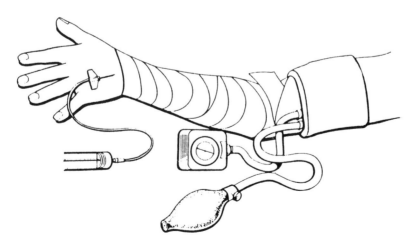

Fig. 14-12. Exsanguination of the arm with an Esmarch bandage before inflation of the tourniquet and injection of the local anesthetic solution through the distally placed intravenous needle. (From Holmes,[7] with permission.)

REFERENCES

1. Bridenbaugh LD. The upper extremity: Somatic blockade. In: Cousins MJ, Bridenbaugh PO, eds. Neural Blockade in Clinical Anesthesia and Management of Pain. Philadelphia, JB Lippincott, 1988:387–416.
2. Winnie AP. Plexus Anesthesia I: The perivascular technique of brachial plexus block. Philadelphia, WB Saunders, 1983.
3. Thompson GE, Moore DR. Celiac plexus, intercostal and minor peripheral blockade. In: Cousins MJ, Bridenbaugh PO, eds. Neural Blockade in Clinical Anesthesia and Management of Pain. Philadelphia, JB Lippincott, 1988:503–532.
4. Bridenbaugh PO. The lower extremity: Somatic blockade. In: Cousins MJ, Bridenbaugh PO, eds. Neural Blockade in Clinical Anesthesia and Management of Pain. Philadelphia, JB Lippincott, 1988:417–42.
5. Winnie AP, Ramamurthy S, Durrani Z. The inguinal paravascular technique of lumbar plexus anesthesia. Anesth Analg 1973;52:989–96.
6. Lofstrom JB, Cousins MJ. Sympathetic neural blockade of upper and lower extremity. In: Cousins MJ, Bridenbaugh PO, eds. Neural Blockade in Clinical Anesthesia and Management of Pain. Philadelphia, JB Lippincott, 1988:461–502.
7. Holmes C McK. Intravenous regional neural blockade. In: Cousins MJ, Bridenbaugh PO, eds. Neural Blockade in Clinical Anesthesia and Management of Pain. Philadelphia, JB Lippincott, 1988:443–60.

Chapter 15

Positioning

During surgery and anesthesia, patients are positioned so as to offer optimal surgical exposure. From the standpoint of surgical exposure, however, these desirable positions may evoke undesirable changes, which manifest most often as impaired venous return to the heart and interference with ventilation to perfusion relationships in the lungs. Peripheral nerve injury is an ever present danger in anesthetized patients. Despite the multiple complications that may occur, most of them are preventable with careful positioning of patients and proper use of equipment.

PERIPHERAL NERVE INJURY

The principal cause of peripheral nerve injuries in anesthetized patients is ischemia of the intraneural vasa nervorum.[1] This results primarily from stretching of the nerve and secondarily from compression of a nerve rendered vulnerable to the effects of ischemia by stretching. Stretching and compression of nerves are more likely to occur in anesthetized patients than in awake patients for two reasons. First, skeletal muscle tone is reduced during anesthesia, especially when muscle relaxants are administered, thus enhancing susceptibility to unphysiologic positions. Second, anesthetized patients cannot complain about postural positions that would not be tolerated when awake. For

example, in awake patients, abduction of the arm to more than 90 degrees in a steep head-down position becomes painful and intolerable in a few minutes. The same patient in the anesthetized state could not warn the anesthesiologist as to the unacceptability of this position. Other factors contributing to nerve injuries include congenital anomalies (cervical rib), co-existing diseases (diabetic neuropathy), anticoagulant therapy and hematomas that compress nerves, hypothermia, hypotension, and prolonged (usually greater than 3 hours) application of a tourniquet.[1]

Brachial Plexus

The brachial plexus, because of its long superficial course in the axilla between two points of fixation and proximity to freely moveable bony structures, is susceptible to damage from stretching and compression. Indeed, brachial plexus damage is the most common nerve injury in anesthetized patients. Stretching of the brachial plexus in the abducted arm is increased by dorsal extension and lateral flexion of the head to the opposite side (Fig. 15-1).[2] The brachial plexus may be compressed between the clavicle and first rib when shoulder braces are not placed properly over the acromioclavicular joint, but rather placed too far medially, where they depress the clavicle into the retroclavicular space (Fig. 15-2).[2] Lateral place-

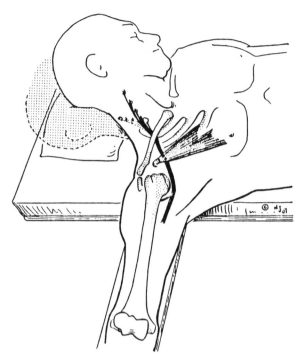

Fig. 15-1. Dorsal extension and lateral flexion of the head to the opposite side produces undesirable stretch on the brachial plexus. (From Britt and Gordon,[2] with permission.)

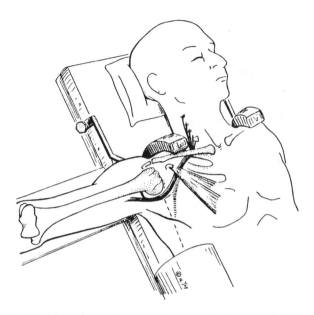

Fig. 15-2. Shoulder rests placed too medially and abduction of the arm in the head-down position cause compression of the brachial plexus between the depressed clavicle and first rib. (From Britt and Gordon,[2] with permission.)

ment of the shoulder rests may depress the head of the humerus, causing it to stretch the brachial plexus (Fig. 15-3).[2]

Radial Nerve

The radial nerve may be injured if the arm slips off the side of the surgical table or if pressure is applied to the nerve as it traverses the spiral groove of the humerus (Fig. 15-4).[2] Clinically, radial nerve injury is manifested by wrist drop, inability to extend the metacarpophalangeal joints, and weakness of abduction of the thumb (Fig. 15-5).[3] There is diminished sensation over the dorsal surface of the lateral 3½ fingers and adjacent hand.

Median Nerve

The median nerve, which runs adjacent to the medial cubital and basilic veins in the antecubital fossa, may be injured during intravenous injection of drugs such as thiopental, either by the needle

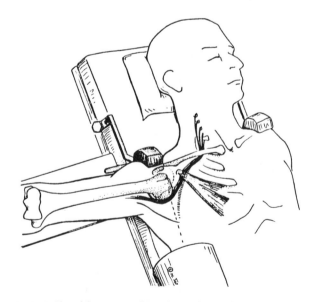

Fig. 15-3. Shoulder rests placed too far laterally and abduction of the arm in the head down position cause compression of the brachial plexus below the head of the humerus, which has been forced down into the axilla. (From Britt and Gordon,[2] with permission.)

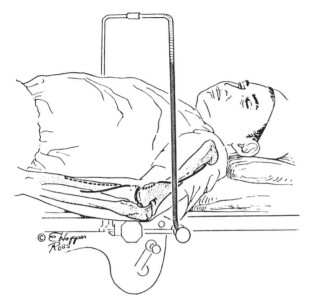

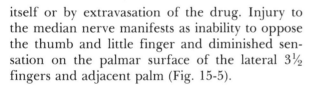

Fig. 15-4. The radial nerve may be compressed against the humerus and the metal brace at the patient's head. (From Britt and Gordon,[2] with permission.)

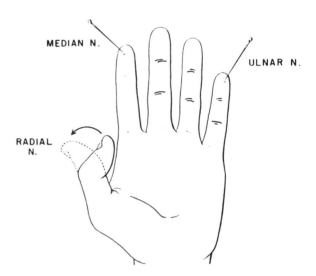

Fig. 15-5. Schematic diagram for the rapid identification of peripheral nerve injuries to the upper extremity. (From Nicholson and McAlpine,[3] with permission.)

itself or by extravasation of the drug. Injury to the median nerve manifests as inability to oppose the thumb and little finger and diminished sensation on the palmar surface of the lateral 3½ fingers and adjacent palm (Fig. 15-5).

Ulnar Nerve

The ulnar nerve is most likely to be injured when the nerve is compressed against the posterior aspect of the medial epicondyle of the humerus, often by the sharp edge of an operating room table (Fig. 15-6). Injury to the ulnar nerve manifests as inability to abduct or oppose the little finger, diminished sensation over both surfaces of the medial 1½ fingers and adjacent hand, and eventually atrophy of the thenar eminence and intrinsic muscles of the hand (claw hand) (Fig. 15-5).[3]

Sciatic Nerve

The sciatic nerve may be injured by compression as the nerve passes under the piriformis muscle or by stretching, as the distance between points of fixation of the nerve (sciatic notch and fibula) is

increased by external rotation of the legs or extension of the knees. Stretch of the sciatic nerve is most likely to occur when patients are placed improperly into lithotomy position (see the section *Lithotomy Position*). To minimize stretch of the sciatic nerve, the patient should be positioned such that external rotation of the legs is minimal and the knees should be flexed. Intramuscular injections into the buttock may damage the sciatic nerve, especially when needle placement is not in the recommended upper outer quadrant of the buttock. For this reason, intramuscular injections into the lateral aspect of the thigh may be the preferred approach. Injury to the sciatic nerve manifests as weakness of all the skeletal muscles below the knee and diminished sensation over the lateral half of the leg and almost all of the foot, with the exception of the inner border of the arch.

Common Peroneal Nerve

The common peroneal nerve, which is a branch of the sciatic nerve, is the most frequently damaged nerve in the lower extremity. Most often this

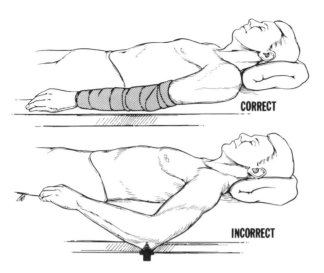

Fig. 15-6. If the arm is allowed to hang over the edge of the operating table in the supine position, an ulnar nerve neuropathy may result.

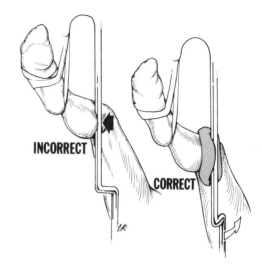

Fig. 15-7. In the lithotomy position, the saphenous nerve can be compressed by the stirrups used to elevate the legs when padding is inadequate. (Adapted from Britt and Gordon,[2] with permission.)

damage reflects compression of the nerve between the head of the fibula and the metal brace used in the lithotomy position. Proper padding greatly reduces the likelihood of this complication. Injury to the common peroneal nerve manifests as foot drop, loss of dorsal extension of the toes, and inability to evert the foot.

Anterior Tibial Nerve

Foot drop may manifest postoperatively if the feet are plantar-flexed for extended periods during anesthesia. Patients in the sitting position should have a foot support under their feet, and patients in the prone position should have a roll placed under the anterior aspect of the ankle to maintain the extended position.

Femoral Nerve

The femoral nerve may be compressed at the pelvic brim by the blade of a self-retaining retractor as used during a laparotomy or by excessive angulation of the thigh when the patient is placed in the lithotomy position. On examination, there is loss of flexion of the hip and extension of the knee due to quadriceps femoris injury. Sensation is absent to diminished over the superior aspect of the thigh and medial and anteromedial side of the leg. The possibility of femoral nerve injury due to these mechanisms must be considered when

neurologic deficits in the postoperative period are attributed to a prior regional anesthetic.

Saphenous Nerve

The saphenous nerve is a branch of the femoral nerve and can be damaged by compression against the medial tibial condyle if the foot is suspended lateral to a vertical brace (Fig. 15-7).[2] This complication is minimized by appropriate padding between the legs and metal leg brace.

Obturator Nerve

Damage to the obturator nerve manifests as inability to abduct the leg and diminished sensation over the medial side of the thigh. This nerve may be damaged during difficult forceps delivery or by excessive flexion of the thigh to the groin.

NON-NEURAL INJURY

Injury to the skin, eyes, and appendages are examples of non-neural damage related to positioning during anesthesia.

Skin

Excessive pressure over an area of skin may result in ischemia and localized ulceration. In severe cases, a skin graft may be required. In essence, any area of skin upon which excessive pressure has been exerted, as over bony prominences (medial malleoli, heels, supraorbital ridge), is vulnerable to ischemic damage. Taping an endotracheal tube may cause ulceration of skin at the corner of the mouth. Care must be taken to ensure that orthopaedic frames used to support patients during hip procedures are well padded to prevent pressure necrosis, especially in the groin.

Eyes

Pressure on the eye, as may occur in the prone position, may cause thrombosis of the central retinal artery with permanent blindness. The likelihood of this complication is increased when deliberate or accidental hypotension accompany the anesthetic. Care must be exercised by the anesthesiologist to assure that the orbit of the eye can be felt in its entirety so as to assure absence of pressure on the eye.

Appendages

Whenever parts of a surgical table are being moved, the possibility of a finger or toe being damaged in a progressively narrowing gap between the main portion and the part of the table being moved must be appreciated. The most likely problem is trauma to the fingers when the foot of the adjustable surgical table is returned to the horizontal position from the lithotomy position. Finally, the ear may be damaged if it is forcibly folded between the patient's head and the mattress of the surgical table.

DAMAGE RELATED TO THE ANESTHETIC FACE MASK

Improper application of the anesthetic face mask may result in several complications. For example, loss of hair of the outer third of the eyebrow (does not grow back) may reflect pressure from the face mask strap (Fig. 15-8). The likelihood of this complication is reduced by placing a gauze pad beneath the face mask strap to avoid discrete pressure on the outer third of the eyebrow. Another complication from the face mask strap is pressure on the buccal branch of the facial nerve, resulting in paresis of the obicularis oris muscle. Pressure from the anesthetic face mask may cause necrosis of the bridge of the nose. The likelihood of this complication is minimized by removing the

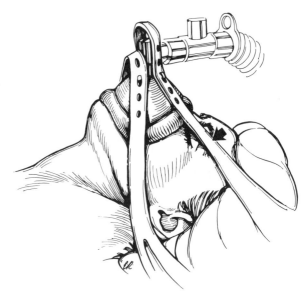

Fig. 15-8. Several complications can occur from excessive pressure with application of an anesthetic face mask and mask strap. The outer third of the eyebrow can disappear with excessive compression from the strap. The buccal branch of the facial nerve can be injured from the mask strap; also, necrosis of the bridge of the nose can occur from excessive pressure by the anesthetic mask.

mask from the face periodically and massaging the bridge of the nose to restore circulation to the compressed area.

Compression of the supraorbital nerve by the tracheal tube connector manifests as decreased sensation over the forehead and pain in the eye (Fig. 15-9). The facial nerve may be damaged by compression between the anesthesiologist's fingers and the ascending ramus of the patient's mandible if extreme and prolonged manual forward pressure is required to maintain a patent upper airway.

SURGICAL POSITIONS

Commonly used surgical positions are the supine, prone, head-down, lateral decubitus, sitting, and lithotomy positions. Decubitus is used to indicate the part of the patient that is in contact with the operating table.

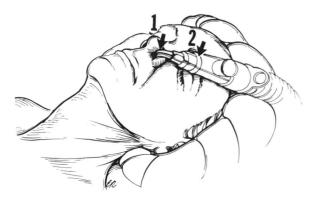

Fig. 15-9. The supraorbital nerve can be compressed by a tracheal tube connector, especially when padding is insufficient. Pressure on the nasal opening by the connector can result in tissue ischemia and damage.

Supine

Nerve injuries in the supine position most often involve the brachial plexus and ulnar nerve. Proper positioning of the arm during anesthesia is mandatory to reduce the likelihood of these complications (see the sections *Brachial Plexus* and *Ulnar Nerve*). The supine position produces minimal effects on circulation and perfusion of the lung tends to be homogenous. Functional residual capacity declines about 800 ml when changing from the standing to supine position. Subsequent administration of muscle relaxants further decreases functional residual capacity, reflecting accentuation of the cephalad displacement of the diaphragm and compression of the adjacent lung.[4] Loss of skeletal muscle tone in the chest wall reduces opposition to the inherent elastic recoil of pulmonary tissues further contributing to reductions in lung volumes. These adverse effects on lung volumes are offset by intermittent positive pressure ventilation of the lungs. Otherwise minimal circulatory effects may be exaggerated in the presence of an abdominal mass (ascites, gravid uterus) that compresses the inferior vena cava sufficiently to impede venous return, resulting in decreased cardiac output and hypotension.

In the supine position, the hips and knees should be flexed slightly (lawn-chair position). This position facilitates venous drainage from the lower extremities and shortens the xiphoid-to-pubis distance, which reduces anterior abdominal wall tension during surgical closure. The legs must remain uncrossed and the heels are padded. Pressure on the occiput of the head with the risk of focal alopecia is prevented by appropriate use of pillows.

Head-Down

The head-down (Trendelenburg) position does not predictably improve cardiac output in hypotensive and hypovolemic patients. Presumably, displacement of abdominal viscera pushes the diaphragm against the heart resulting in decreases in stroke volume, and in some patients, accentuation of co-existing hypotension.[5] Furthermore, this position accentuates compression of the lung bases by abdominal viscera. In vulnerable patients, the head-down position will increase intracranial pressure by elevating venous pressures leading to decreased venous outflow from the brain. Placement of patients in the head-down position requires use of shoulder braces to prevent cephalad movement of the entire body. Proper placement of these shoulder braces is mandatory to avoid peripheral nerve injuries (see the section *Peripheral Nerve Injury*).

Prone

Pressure from the mattress of the surgical table on the abdominal walls of prone patients results in cephalad displacement of the diaphragm, impediment of downward descent of the diaphragm, and compression of the inferior vena cava and aorta. Positive pressure ventilation of the lungs may offset undesirable effects of the prone position on breathing, but associated increases in venous pressure may further jeopardize venous return and cardiac output. Turning of the head necessitated by the prone position may obstruct jugular venous drainage and vertebral artery blood flow and be responsible for postoperative neck pain or, in rare cases, thrombosis. Protection of the prominent aspects of the face and eyes must be assured when patients are placed in the prone position. The patient's arms are placed at the side or extended alongside the head on arm boards, taking care to avoid compression of the ulnar nerves (Figs. 15-10 and 15-11). Firm rolls (bolsters) are placed under the patient's sides from the clavicle to iliac crest (Fig. 15-10). These rolls serve to

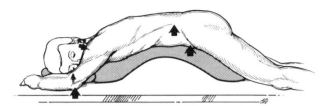

Fig. 15-10. This position indicates the multiple problems that can occur with an improperly positioned patient in the flexed prone position. If excessively stretched, the brachial plexus can be damaged. The ulnar nerve can be damaged by inadequate padding of the elbow. Inadequate padding under the head can cause eye damage or undue pressure to the face or lower eyelid. Excessive compression to the inferior vena cava can be minimized by padding under the inferior iliac spine.

relieve abdominal compression by the mattress of the surgical table, thus facilitating venous return to the heart and ease of ventilation of the lungs. The legs are often fitted with elastic stockings to minimize pooling of blood, which is particularly likely to occur when flexion as needed for laminectomy is added to the prone position. Movement of patients into and from the prone position requires sufficient assistance and is accomplished slowly to allow time for compensatory cardiovascular responses to minimize undesirable reduc-

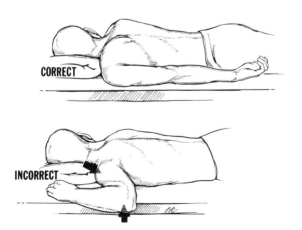

Fig. 15-11. Proper padding in the prone position can minimize damage to the brachial plexus, especially the ulnar nerve.

tions in blood pressure. During this time, the anesthesiologist is responsible for stabilizing the patient's head and assuring continued proper position of the tracheal tube.

There are several variations of the prone position, such as the knee-chest position, and many devices are used to achieve these positions. The principles, including padding of pressure points (i.e., knees and face), free abdominal and chest expansion, and no greater than 90 degrees of abduction of the arms, apply to all of these variations of the prone position.

Lateral Decubitus

The lateral decubitus position may be associated with significant circulatory and ventilatory effects during positive pressure ventilation of the lungs. Compression of the inferior vena cava may occur, especially if the kidney rest (properly placed under the dependent iliac crest) is elevated. The dependent lung tends to be underventilated because it is compressed by the pressure of the abdominal contents and the weight of the mediastinum. The nondependent lung is relatively overventilated because the compliance of this lung is increased, particularly when the corresponding hemothorax is opened. At the same time, gravity favors distribution of pulmonary blood flow to the underventilated dependent lung. The accentuated mismatching of ventilation to perfusion introduced by the lateral decubitus position may manifest as unexpected arterial hypoxemia.

To avoid compression of the dependent neurovascular bundle in the axilla, a roll should be placed under the thorax just caudal to the axilla (Fig. 15-12). It is useful to periodically check the radial pulse to assure absence of neurovascular compression. A pulse oximeter can be used to ensure adequate perfusion of the dependent hand. A pillow beneath the head minimizes stretch on the dependent brachial plexus, and a pillow between the knees, with the dependent leg flexed at the knee, minimizes pressure on bony prominences and stretch on nerves of the lower extremity (Figs. 15-12 and 15-13). The nondependent arm can be positioned on an elevated board bent in front of the patient's face or suspended from a well-padded

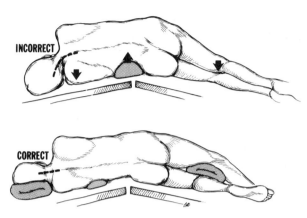

Fig. 15-12. In the lateral decubitus position, pillows between the legs and elbows help distribute the weight of the upper extremity to that of the lower extremity.

support bar with care taken to avoid stretch on the brachial plexus (Fig. 15-14).[2]

Sitting

The sitting position is most often used for posterior fossa craniotomy, as this position facilitates venous drainage and improves surgical exposure. The cardiovascular effects of the sitting position are complex and may include decreases in cardiac output, cerebral perfusion pressure, and intrathoracic blood volume.[6] Venous return from dependent extremities is enhanced by placing the legs in elastic stockings. Venous air embolism is the principal hazard of the sitting position (see Chapter 24).

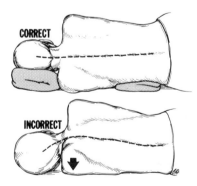

Fig. 15-13. Injury to the nondependent brachial plexus can be minimized by proper padding underneath the head.

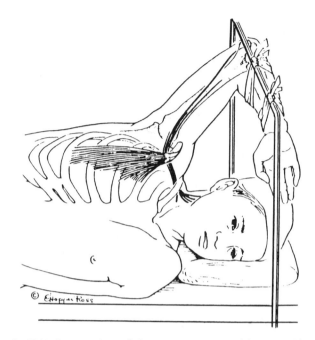

Fig. 15-14. Suspension of the arm on a metal brace with extreme abduction of the arm and pronation of the forearm depresses the brachial plexus posteriorly behind the tendon of the pectoralis major muscle. (From Britt and Gordon,[2] with permission.)

Lithotomy

Circulatory effects of the lithotomy position are not detrimental unless an abdominal mass (ascites, gravid uterus) contributes to obstruction of the inferior vena cava. The effect of this position on breathing is manifest as cephalad displacement of the diaphragm by abdominal viscera.

Injury to peripheral nerves (sciatic, common peroneal, femoral, saphenous, obturator) are the principal hazards of the lithotomy position (see the section *Peripheral Nerve Injury*). Injury to these peripheral nerves is unlikely when proper padding between the metal leg braces and the patient's legs is assured. When positioning the patient, both legs should be elevated and flexed simultaneously to avoid stretching of peripheral nerves. The thigh should be flexed at no more than 90 degrees before rotating the stirrups laterally.

REFERENCES

1. Britt BA, Joy N, Mackay MB. Positioning trauma. In: Orkin FK, Cooperman LH, eds. Complications of Anesthesia. Philadelphia, JB Lippincott, 1983;646–70.
2. Britt BA, Gordon RA. Peripheral nerve injuries associated with anaesthesia. Can Anaesth Soc J 1964;11:514–36.
3. Nicholson MJ, McAlpine FS. Neural injuries associated with surgical positions and operations. In: Martin JT, ed. Positioning in anesthesia and surgery. Philadelphia, WB Saunders, 1978;193–224.
4. Froese AB, Bryan AC. Effects of anesthesia and paralysis on diaphragmatic mechanisms in man. Anesthesiology 1974;41:242–7.
5. Baskerville J. The Trendelenburg position: Hemodynamic effects in hypotensive and normotensive patients. Crit Care Med 1979;7:218–24.
6. Dalrymple DG, MacGowan SW. Cardiorespiratory effects of the sitting position in neurosurgery. Br J Anaesth 1979;51:1079–82.

Chapter 16

Monitoring

Monitoring of anesthetized patients is designed to collect data that reflect (1) physiologic homeostasis, allowing prompt recognition of adverse changes; (2) responses to therapeutic interventions; and (3) proper functioning of anesthetic equipment.[1] Monitoring as such provides an early warning of adverse changes or trends before irreversible damage occurs. The most important monitor in the operating room is the anesthesiologist, who continuously obtains subjective and objective information from the anesthetized patient. Subjective monitoring depends on the anesthesiologist's senses (visual, touching, auditory, "sixth sense") and past experience. For example, an experienced anesthesiologist often assesses the patient's status using principally clinical signs. This continual vigilance (awareness) on the part of the anesthesiologist is enhanced by the use of monitoring equipment designed to provide objective data relevant to the anesthetized patient's well-being. Indeed, human vigilance is not infallible, which emphasizes the importance of using monitors beyond the anesthesiologist's subjective observation.[2]

Standards for basic intraoperative monitoring have been endorsed by the American Society of Anesthesiologists (see Appendix). Depending on the patient's medical condition and complexity of the surgery, this basic intraoperative monitoring is expanded to include more technologically sophisticated and often "invasive" monitors. The inherent risk in the use of all monitors, especially invasive monitors, must be weighed against the potential benefits in selecting their use for individual patients.

COMMONLY EMPLOYED MONITORS IN ANESTHETIZED PATIENTS

Commonly employed monitors in anesthetized patients include those considered appropriate for every patient (routine monitors) and others that are indicated only in selected patients. Routine monitors for every anesthetized patient include (1) devices for measurement of arterial blood pressure, (2) use of either a precordial or esophageal stethoscope, and (3) continuous visual display of the electrocardiogram (ECG). Pulse oximetry, which provides continual assessment of the patient's oxygenation, has become a routine monitor. Capnography, which reflects the adequacy of ventilation and provides early warning of an accidental esophageal intubation, is a commonly employed but not routine monitor (see Chapter 12). In some institutions, mass spectrometry serves to monitor delivered and exhaled concentrations of inhaled anesthetics while also providing information otherwise available only from oxygen analyzers and capnography.[3] Neuromuscular blockade is evaluated by use of a peripheral nerve stimulator (see

Chapter 8). Renal function is monitored by measurement of urine output in selected patients. Body temperature is commonly measured, especially in children. Arterial blood gases and pH may be measured in certain patients (see Chapter 17).

Intactness of the anesthetic breathing system is sensed by disconnect alarms, and proper function of anesthetic machines is assessed by fail-safe mechanisms and oxygen analyzers placed in the anesthetic breathing system.

Noninvasive Arterial Blood Pressure Monitoring

Arterial blood pressure may be measured noninvasively by palpation, auscultation, or by using the oscillometric method. Regardless of the method used, the size of the blood pressure cuff must be appropriate for the patient. The width of the blood pressure cuff should be about 40 percent of the circumference of the arm. Too small a cuff or a

---

Monitors Used in Anesthetized Patients

Routine
  Blood pressure
  Precordial or esophageal stethoscope
  Electrocardiogram
  Pulse oximeter
  Disconnect alarm
  Oxygen analyzer

Common but not routine
  Capnography
  Peripheral nerve stimulator
  Tidal volume
  Urine output
  Body temperature
  Arterial blood gases and pH
  Mass spectrometry

Invasive
  Intra-arterial blood pressure
  Central venous pressure
  Pulmonary artery catheter

Nervous system
  Electroencephalogram
  Evoked potentials

Monitoring That Requires No Instrumentation

Inspection
  Skin—color, capillary refill, rash, edema
  Nail beds—color, capillary refill
  Mucous membranes—color, moisture, edema
  Surgical field—color of tissues and blood, rate of blood loss, skeletal muscle relaxation
  Movement—purposeful or reflex
  Eyes—conjunctiva (color and edema), pupils (size, reactivity)

Palpation
  Skin—temperature and texture
  Pulse—fullness, rate, and regularity
  Skeletal muscle—tone.

Percussion
  Gastric—distension
  Chest—pneumothorax

Auscultation
  Chest—ventilation and cardiac sounds
  Blood pressure—sphygmomanometry

---

cuff that is too loosely wrapped around the arm will result in a falsely elevated blood pressure reading.

Automated Arterial Blood Pressure Devices

Arterial blood pressure in anesthetized patients is most commonly monitored by oscillometric devices, such as the Dinamapp. Such a device automatically measures and displays mean arterial pressure, systolic pressure, diastolic pressure, and heart rate (Fig. 16-1). Advantages of oscillometric devices are use of a cuff that is both an actuator and a transducer. A separate transducer is not needed, cuff application is simple, and the system is not sensitive to electrosurgical interference. Automatic determination of arterial blood pressure allows the anesthesiologist to continue other tasks without interruption. Determination of arterial blood pres-

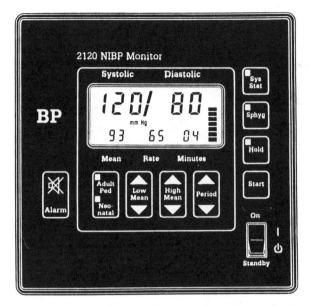

Fig. 16-1. Example of a noninvasive automatic monitoring device providing digital display of blood pressure and heart rate.

sure with oscillometric devices requires 20 seconds to 45 seconds. Frequent blood pressure measurements can result in edema of the extremity distal to the cuff, emphasizing the importance of not cycling the device more frequently than every 1 minute to 3 minutes. Oscillometric methods are accurate even in neonates.[4] When monitoring patients with very low blood pressures, oscillometric devices may display mean arterial pressure but not systolic and diastolic blood pressures. This is due to low level pressure deflections in the cuff caused by low amplitudes in the systolic/diastolic wave form. Mean arterial pressure, however, is probably accurate.

Precordial or Esophageal Stethoscope

A weighted precordial stethoscope is commonly applied over the suprasternal notch or heart before the induction of anesthesia and is connected by tubing to a monaural earpiece worn by the anesthesiologist (Fig. 16-2). This arrangement allows continuous monitoring of heart sounds and breath sounds by the anesthesiologist and leaves the other ear available for operating room communication.

After intubation of the trachea, an esophageal stethoscope is commonly inserted. This stethoscope has the advantage of being close to the heart where both breath sounds and heart sounds are clearly audible. Routine use of an esophageal stethoscope during maintenance of anesthesia facilitates early detection of (1) changes in heart rate, (2) onset of cardiac dysrhythmias, (3) development of increased airway resistance, and (4) failure to ventilate the lungs of a paralyzed patient.

Electrocardiogram

Continuous visual display of the anesthetized patient's ECG on an oscilloscope is useful for detection of (1) cardiac dysrhythmias, (2) myocardial ischemia as reflected by ST segment depression, and (3) electrolyte changes, particularly potassium. Heart rate is often calculated from the ECG tracing. The ability to retain a portion of the ECG on the oscilloscope screen or obtain a hard copy recording is helpful for more detailed analysis of the tracing. An audible indicator for each QRS complex allows the anesthesiologist to carry on other activities while listening for changes in heart rate or cardiac rhythm.

Lead II is commonly used for detection of cardiac dysrhythmias because it parallels the P-wave vector, resulting in maximum amplitude of the P wave on the ECG. Inferior wall myocardial ischemia may be reflected by ST segment depression in lead II. More common sites of myocardial ischemia, however, are the anterior and lateral walls, which are best monitored by a precordial lead in the V5 position (5th intercostal space along the anterior axillary line). For this reason, a V5 lead is often used when the goal is to monitor the ECG for the detection of myocardial ischemia. The equivalent of a V5 lead can be obtained using three electrodes by placing the left arm electrode in the V5 position and selecting lead aVL on the monitor.

It must be recognized that the ECG reflects only the electrical activities occurring in the heart and in no way is a measure of heart function. For example, normal ECG complexes may persist on the oscilloscope in the absence of an effective cardiac output (electromechanical dissociation).

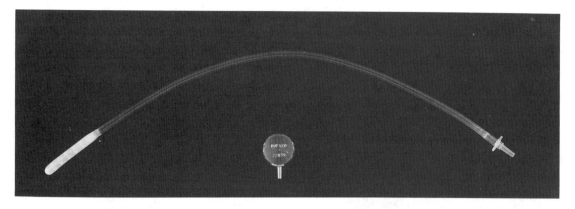

Fig. 16-2. A typical weighted precordial stethoscope and esophageal stethoscope.

Pulse Oximetry

Pulse oximetry provides continuous noninvasive monitoring of arterial oxygen saturation, thus providing an early warning of hypoxemia in anesthetized patients.[5] A light-emitting diode that detects light absorbance differences between reduced hemoglobin and oxyhemoglobin is most commonly placed on a finger or ear. A computer calculates arterial oxygen saturation and displays the value on a screen (Fig. 16-3). Because the technique uses light absorbance changes produced by arterial pulsations, any event that significantly reduces vascular pulsations (hypotension, hypothermia, vasoconstriction) will reduce the ability

of the instrument to obtain and process the signal and thus calculate arterial oxygen saturation. Even an anesthetized patient with a normal core temperature (as measured by an esophageal stethoscope) may have cold fingers and, therefore, inaccurate readings by pulse oximetry. Keeping the patient's hand warm will prevent these problems. Maintenance of arterial oxygen saturations above 90 percent assures a PaO_2 of 90 mmHg or greater.

Transcutaneous PO_2 (PtcO$_2$)

Transcutaneous oxygen sensors use polarographic oxygen electrodes to measure oxygen that diffuses to the skin surface (heated to at least 43° Celsius) from the dermal capillaries beneath the electrode.

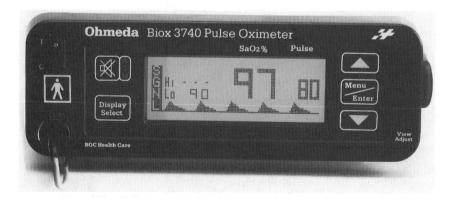

Fig. 16-3. Example of a pulse oximeter providing a visual display of the arterial pulse wave form and a digital display of arterial oxygen saturation (SaO2) and heart (pulse) rate.

A decreasing $PtcO_2$ implies either a decrease in PaO_2 or a decline in skin blood flow due to a low cardiac output (hypovolemia). Considering the need for calibration and occasional drift from calibration, as well as the risk introduced by the requirement to heat the skin, it seems unlikely that transcutaneous oxygen measurements will challenge the popularity of pulse oximetry.[5]

Capnography

Capnography allows continuous measurement of carbon dioxide concentrations in the inhaled and exhaled gases of the patient (Fig. 16-4). This measurement permits evaluation of alveolar ventilation and to a lesser extent the status of circulation.[6] Absence of carbon dioxide in the patient's exhaled gases alerts the anesthesiologist to events such as esophageal intubation or disconnection of a paralyzed patient from the anesthesia delivery circuit (also detected by disconnect alarm) (see Chapter 11). A gradual decline in exhaled carbon dioxide concentrations over several breaths may reflect a partial leak in the anesthesia delivery system or decreased pulmonary blood flow as may accompany hypotension, pulmonary embolism, or cardiac arrest. Hypoventilation or unexpected increases in carbon dioxide production as associated with malignant hyperthermia will be promptly reflected by increases in the exhaled concentrations of carbon dioxide. Rebreathing of carbon dioxide due to an exhausted carbon dioxide absorber or malfunctioning inspiratory or expiratory values will manifest as elevated inspired and exhaled concentrations of carbon dioxide. It must be appreciated that an alveolar-to-arterial difference for carbon dioxide due to dead space venti-

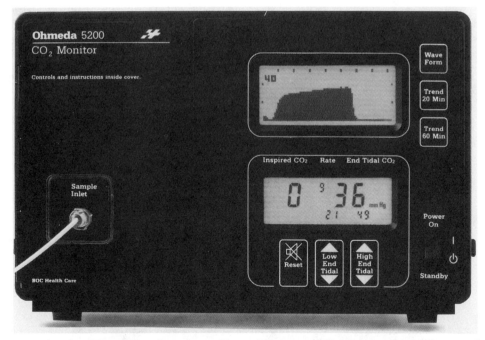

Fig. 16-4. Example of a CO_2 monitor (capnograph) providing a graphic display of the CO_2 wave form and a digital display of the inspired and end-tidal CO_2 concentrations, as well as rate of breathing. The normal capnogram depicts the various phases of the breathing cycle. For example, there is a rapid return to baseline (zero CO_2) during inspiration. As exhalation begins, the dead space gas contains little or no CO_2, but this gas is rapidly displaced by CO_2-containing alveolar gas, resulting in a sustained plateau until the beginning of the next breath.

lation often results in underestimation of the $PaCO_2$ based on exhaled gas analyses.

Mass Spectrometry

Mass spectrometry permits intermittent or continuous measurement of airway gas composition including inhaled anesthetics during inhalation and exhalation (Fig. 16-5). Use of mass spectrometry, particularly if continuous measurement is possible, reduces or eliminates the need for oxygen analyzers and capnography.

Tidal Volume

A ventimeter or respirometer placed in the anesthetic breathing system (commonly on the exhalation limb) measures tidal volume and permits calculation of minute ventilation (rate of breathing times tidal volume). All leaks in the anesthetic breathing system must be eliminated for accurate measurement of tidal volume.

Airway Pressure

Airway pressure created by mechanical ventilation of the lungs is measured by a gauge on the anesthesia machine (see Fig. 11-1). When the maximum inspiratory pressure does not reach prede-

termined levels, an alarm sounds that warns the anesthesiologist that a large leak or disconnect is present. Excessive airway pressures measured on this gauge reflect low pulmonary compliance or obstruction in the anesthetic breathing system (e.g., closed adjustable pressure limiting valve). The gas reservoir bag is designed to expand into a sphere when pressures exceed about 50 cm H_2O preventing transmission of higher pressures to the patient's airways. When a mechanical ventilator is used, the gas reservoir bag is excluded from the anesthetic delivery system making it possible to deliver pressures in excess of 50 cm H_2O to the airways.

Clinical Monitoring of Breathing

When patients breath spontaneously during general anesthesia, the pattern of breathing (rate, depth, regularity) should be continuously monitored by the anesthesiologist. This is accomplished by visual and tactile (hand on the bag) monitoring of the movements of the reservoir bag on the anesthetic breathing system, by observing chest movement, and by auscultation of the chest via either a precordial or esophageal stethoscope. The

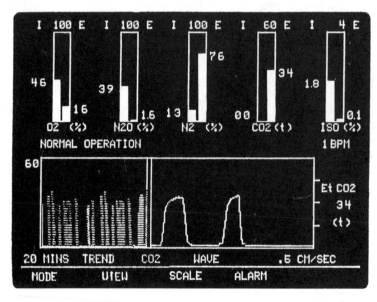

Fig. 16-5. Example of a mass spectrometer screen and graphic display of inhaled (I) and exhaled (E) concentrations of O_2, N_2O, N_2, CO_2 (trend and wave form also displayed) and a volatile anesthetic (ISO, isoflurane).

character of respiratory movements is helpful in assessing depth of anesthesia. Also, by correlating chest movements to movements of the reservoir bag, a judgment can be made regarding the presence or absence of upper airway obstruction. Breathing is often rapid and shallow in the presence of inhaled anesthetics, whereas opioids usually decrease breathing frequency while tidal volume may be increased.

Renal Function

In selected patients, measurement of urine output can be a useful guide to intravascular fluid volume (see Chapter 22). Monitoring urine output also permits early detection of hemoglobinuria, which is an initial sign of hemolytic transfusion reactions.

Body Temperature

Appropriate equipment to measure body temperature should be available for every patient (see Appendix to Chapter 16). Body temperature often decreases 1° Celsius to 4° Celsius during anesthesia and surgery performed in cold operating rooms.[7] Although this decrease in body temperature is usually not serious, postoperative awakening may be delayed, and shivering, when it occurs, may increase oxygen demand by as much as 400 percent.

Sites for monitoring body temperature are the esophagus, nasopharynx, rectum, bladder, and tympanic membrane. A temperature probe in the lower third of the esophagus (often placed via an esophageal stethoscope) accurately reflects blood temperature. Nasopharyngeal temperature is accurate when a cuffed tube in the trachea prevents artificial cooling of the nasopharynx by respiratory gases. Epistaxis is a risk when a temperature probe is inserted into the nasopharynx. Tympanic membrane temperature reflects the temperature of blood perfusing the brain. Risks of tympanic membrane temperature probes are external auditory canal bleeding and perforation of the tympanic membrane.

Oxygen Analyzers

Oxygen analyzers are routinely used to ensure that the anesthesia machine is delivering adequate concentrations of oxygen. An oxygen analyzer is mandatory for low flow or closed circuit administration of anesthetic mixtures containing nitrous oxide

(see Chapter 11). The sensor for the oxygen analyzer may be placed on the inspiratory or expiratory side of the anesthetic breathing system. A common placement is in the inspiratory limb distal to the one-way valve. The oxygen analyzer is calibrated with room air and pure oxygen with an alarm set to sound should the oxygen concentration decline below a certain level, typically 25 percent to 30 percent.

INVASIVE MONITORING OF THE CARDIOVASCULAR SYSTEM

Invasive monitoring of the cardiovascular system is reserved for complex and sometimes prolonged operations often in patients with significant co-existing medical diseases. Intra-arterial, central venous pressure, and pulmonary artery catheters (Swan Ganz) are examples of invasive monitors placed and used by anesthesiologists. The risk-to-benefit ratio and cost are important considerations in the selection of these monitors for individual patients. It is recommended that the anesthesiologist responsible for inserting invasive monitors wear gloves and protective eyeglasses to minimize the risk of transmission of blood-borne diseases from the patient.

Intra-arterial Blood Pressure

Continuous recording of blood pressure from a catheter placed in a peripheral artery allows beat-to-beat monitoring and provides a reliable access site to obtain samples for analyses of arterial blood gases, pH, and electrolytes. Although several peripheral arteries are available for cannulation (radial, brachial, femoral, dorsalis pedis, superficial temporal), the radial artery is most commonly selected. Before cannulation, an Allen's test may be performed to determine the adequacy of collateral flow from the ulnar artery. The Allen's test is performed by simultaneously occluding the radial and ulnar arteries and asking the patient to make a tight fist, which forces blood from the hand such that the palmar surface becomes blanched and appears pale. Pressure over only the ulnar artery is then released, and the patient is instructed to open his or her hand, avoiding hyperextension of the fingers. Return of color to the palmar surface of the hand within 5 seconds to 15 seconds is considered to represent adequate collateral blood flow in the hand. Traditionally, inadequate collateral ulnar arterial blood flow, as suggested by the Allen's test, has been considered a relative contraindication to insertion of a catheter into a radial artery. Nevertheless, there is evidence that adverse events do not follow cannulation of the radial artery in the presence of an abnormal Allen's test.[8] Furthermore, decreased or absent radial arterial blood flow after removal of the catheter (presumably due to emboli) are of little or no clinical significance.[9] The inescapable conclusion is that radial artery cannulation is a low-risk, high-benefit monitoring technique that deserves frequent use.

Cannulation of the radial artery is performed with the wrist dorsiflexed 40 degrees to 60 degrees over a towel or gauze sponges (Fig. 16-6). Tape is used to immobilize the hand and the course of the radial artery palpated. The selected entry site is prepared with an antiseptic solution such as 70 percent alcohol, and if the patient is awake, the anticipated entry site is infiltrated with a small amount of local anesthetic. Sometimes it is helpful to make a superficial incision to avoid damaging the tip of the catheter as it is introduced through the skin. Typically, small gauge (20 gauge in adults, 22 gauge to 24 gauge in children) Teflon catheters are selected. The catheter is inserted at a 15 degree to 30 degree angle and advanced slowly until the lumen of the artery is entered as evidenced by appearance of blood at the distal end (hub) of the

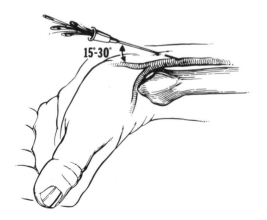

Fig. 16-6. A diagramatic illustration of an approach to cannulating the radial artery.

catheter (Fig. 16-6). After successful placement, the catheter should be flushed continuously with a solution containing 1 unit to 2 units of heparin in saline at a rate of 1 ml·hr^{-1} to 3 ml·hr^{-1}. This continuous flush is important in minimizing thrombus formation and for maintaining adequate arterial blood pressure wave forms.

Central Venous Pressure

Catheterization of the central veins has become an important maneuver both for measuring central venous pressure and for providing long-term intravenous feedings, especially hyperalimentation. Furthermore, in an emergency, such as after acute hemorrhage with peripheral vasoconstriction, it may be impossible to catheterize a peripheral vein percutaneously and only a central vein may be available to infuse fluids for rapid restoration of blood volume. The four veins commonly used for catheterization are the basilic (arm veins), subclavian, external jugular, and internal jugular. The relative advantages and disadvantages of using each vein are summarized on Table 16-1.

Cannulation of the basilic vein is associated with a low complication rate, but advancement of a catheter centrally via this route can be time-consuming and often unsuccessful. For example, it is often difficult to entice the catheter to turn the corner around the shoulder and enter the superior vena cava. The subclavian vein is a continuation of the axillary vein beginning at the outer border of the first rib. It may be cannulated by using either a supraclavicular or infraclavicular approach. The subclavian vein has a wide caliber, is held open by surrounding tissue even in severe circulatory collapse, and is easily accessible to the anesthesiologist during a surgical procedure. The use of the subclavian vein allows the catheter to be securely fixed on the chest wall. Most clinicians report a high success rate for central placement, but serious complications occur much more frequently with cannulation of the subclavian vein than with other routes. Pneumothorax is the most common complication, so the technique should be used with caution, if at all, in patients with severe lung disease. After an unsuccessful cannulation attempt, it is prudent to avoid attempts at cannulation of the opposite subclavian vein because of the risk of producing bilateral pneumothoraxes.

Table 16-1. Advantages of Different Approaches to Central Vein Catheterization[a]

	Vein			
	Basilic	Subclavian	External Jugular	Internal Jugular
Ease of insertion and safety for inexperienced	1	4	1	3
Complications	1	3	1	2
Ability to insert a central venous or pulmonary artery catheter	4	1	3	1

[a] In each category 1 = best; 4 = poorest

The external jugular vein is usually visible and easy to cannulate. It is therefore a useful alternative to arm veins. Passage of the catheter inserted through the external jugular vein into the superior vena cava is facilitated by prior placement of flexible J-shaped wire.[10] This J-wire is manipulated into the superior vena cava and the venous catheter is then threaded over the J-wire.

The internal jugular vein is probably preferred to the subclavian vein because there is a lower incidence of major complications. The nursing management of neck catheters, however, may be difficult. The right internal jugular vein is ideal as it forms a shorter, straighter line than the left internal jugular vein to the superior vena cava. Furthermore, potential damage to the thoracic duct is eliminated by selecting the right internal jugular vein. Techniques in which the needle is inserted well above the clavicle are less likely to cause major complications and, therefore, are most often selected. Although various approaches can be used to locate the internal jugular vein, several points of management are common to all techniques (Fig. 16-7). The vein can first be located with a small (23-gauge) "seeker" needle to avoid unnecessary trauma. A larger needle is then introduced using the small needle as a guide. Saline should be injected through the larger needle, after puncturing the skin, to clear the needle of any tissue. The primary complication of this approach is puncture of the carotid artery and hematoma formation. Although other complications are rare, thrombophlebitis, infection, pneumothorax, nerve damage, thoracic duct injury (left internal jugular

vein cannulation), hematoma, neck tenderness, tracheal tube cuff puncture, venous air embolism, vocal cord paralysis, mediastinal infiltration, cardiac dysrhythmias, and cardiac tamponade have been reported.

From a clinical point of view, the central venous pressure or right atrial pressure is influenced by the right ventricular volume. If the right ventricle fails to empty because of pulmonary hypertension or, more often, left heart failure, the central venous pressure will be elevated and may incorrectly infer that the patient's blood volume is

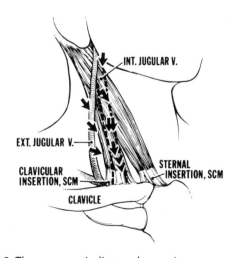

Fig. 16-7. The arrows indicate the various approaches used to cannulate the internal jugular vein. The position of the internal jugular vein is indicated by the dashed lines.

expanded. If left heart failure is suspected, additional monitoring, such as a pulmonary artery catheter, is needed.

Pulmonary Artery Catheter

A flow-directed, balloon-tipped pulmonary artery catheter enables catheterization of the right heart for measurement of pressures without requiring the manipulative and radiologic control demanded by other methods of cardiac catheterization. The pulmonary artery occlusion (wedge) pressure reflects left atrial pressure because at no flow, the pressures can equilibrate between the distal end of the pulmonary artery catheter and the left atrium. The flow-directed pulmonary artery catheter measures cardiac output by the thermodilution technique. Specifically, a thermistor in the distal end of the pulmonary artery catheter senses the change in blood temperature produced by the rapid injection of iced (or room temperature) solution administered through the proximal (central venous pressure) port of the catheter. Cardiac output is inversely proportional to the area under the time–temperature curve (calculated by the cardiac output computer and expressed as $L \cdot min^{-1}$) because blood flow is the source of the thermal dilution. The output of only the right ventricle is measured by this technique. Specially designed pulmonary artery catheters are capable of providing cardiac pacing or fiberoptic oximetry with the ability to constantly monitor mixed venous oxygen saturations. When metabolic oxygen requirements are unchanging, the mixed venous oxygen saturation is directly proportional to the cardiac output.

Pulmonary artery catheters are often inserted percutaneously via the right internal jugular vein. Insertion of the catheter requires continuous displays of pressures and recognition of characteristic wave forms (Fig. 16-8). The balloon on the distal end of the catheter is inflated with 1 ml to 1.5 ml of air only after a right atrial tracing has been confirmed. The inflated balloon facilitates passage (flotation) of the distal end of the catheter with blood flow into the pulmonary artery. A right ventricular tracing should appear after the catheter is inserted 28 cm to 32 cm and a pulmonary artery occlusion pressure tracing is evident after insertion of the catheter 45 cm to 50 cm. The balloon is deflated at this point and a pulmonary artery pressure tracing should again appear. Reinflation of the balloon with about 1.0 ml of air should result in reappearance of the pulmonary artery occlusion tracing. Rigid adherence to these insertion distances will minimize the likelihood of catheter loops or intracardiac knot formation. The balloon should not be left in the inflated position except during actual measurement of pulmonary artery occlusion pressure so as to minimize the likelihood of pulmonary ischemia or infarction. Other risks of pulmonary artery catheter insertion are as described for insertion of central venous pressure catheters. A rare but catastrophic complication associated with use of pulmonary artery catheters is pulmonary artery perforation.

It is important to minimize the number of balloon inflations. Because the pulmonary artery diastolic pressure agrees well with the pulmonary

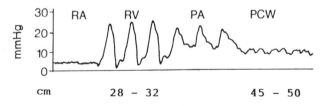

Fig. 16-8. Schematic depiction of pressure wave forms as a pulmonary artery catheter passes through the right atrium (RA), right ventricle (RV), and pulmonary artery (PA). Note the narrowing of pulse pressure ("diastolic step-up") as the catheter enters the PA. Loss of a pulsatile pressure trace as the catheter is advanced through the PA reflects the pulmonary capillary wedge (PCW) pressure or pulmonary artery occlusion pressure (PAo). Insertion of the catheter through the right internal jugular vein should result in an RV tracing at 28 cm to 32 cm and a PCW tracing at 45 cm to 50 cm.

Indications for Insertion of a Pulmonary Artery Catheter
Impaired left ventricular function
Evaluation of response to fluid administration or therapeutic interventions (inotropes, vasodilators)
Hemorrhagic shock
Sepsis
Massive trauma
Major vascular surgery, especially if cross-clamping of abdominal aorta required
Severe respiratory failure

Table 16-2 Normal Pressures of Various Cardiovascular Sites

Location	Abbreviation	Pressure (mmHg)
Central venous	CVP	6
Right atrial	RAP	4
Right ventricular		
Systolic	—	24
Diastolic	RVEDP	4
Pulmonary artery		
Systolic	PAsP	24
Diastolic	PAdP	10
Mean	PAP	16
Pulmonary artery occlusion	PAo	9
Left atrial	LAP	7
Left ventricular		
Systolic	—	120
Diastolic	LVEDP	7

artery occlusion pressure in the absence of pulmonary hypertension, it is logical to use the diastolic pressure as an indirect measurement of left atrial pressure.

Indications for use of pulmonary artery catheters are numerous and often controversial. For example, the need for intravascular fluid volume replacement, as well as the response to intravenous fluid infusion, is commonly monitored with a pulmonary artery catheter. Measurement of cardiac output and calculation of systemic and pulmonary vascular resistance are essential information for evaluating the response to inotropes and/or vasodilators in patients with valvular heart disease or coronary artery disease. Subendocardial myocardial ischemia may manifest as V waves on the tracing of the pulmonary artery occlusion pressure even before changes in the ECG suggest myocardial ischemia. Normal pressures in various sites of the cardiovascular system are summarized in Table 16-2, and the interpretation of various disease states are summarized in Table 16-3.

MONITORING THE NERVOUS SYSTEM

The electroencephalogram (EEG) is used to monitor the central nervous system, and evoked potentials provide a method to evaluate the intactness of neural pathways.

Electroencephalogram

The EEG is a monitor of cerebral function that provides early evidence of cerebral ischemia as during carotid endarterectomy or cardiopulmonary bypass. The EEG has also been advocated to monitor depth of anesthesia. The complexity of the EEG and its interpretation, plus variable and often unpredictable effects of events (e.g., changes in body temperature, alterations in $PaCO_2$), and anesthetic drugs on the EEG tracing detract from the frequent use of this monitor.

Evoked Potentials

Evoked potentials are the electrophysiologic responses of the nervous system to sensory stimulation (somatic, auditory, visual) that allow assessment of the functional integrity of neural pathways during anesthesia. For example, somatosensory evoked potentials are produced by application of small electrical currents that stimulate a peripheral nerve, such as the median nerve at the wrist or posterior tibial nerve at the ankle. The resulting recorded evoked potential reflects the intactness (or interruption) of neural pathways from the peripheral nerve through the spinal cord to the somatosensory cortex. This type of monitoring is

Table 16-3.   Use of a Pulmonary Artery Catheter in the Interpretation of Various Low
Cardiac Output States

Cause of Low Cardiac Output	CVP	PAo	PAdP vs. PAo Pressure
Hypovolemia	Decreased	Decreased	PAdP = PAo
Left ventricular failure	Increased	Increased	PAdP = PAo
Right ventricular failure	Increased	No change	PAdP = PAo
Pulmonary embolism	Increased	No change	PAdP > PAo
Cardiac tamponade	Increased	Increased	PAdP = PAo

CVP, central venous pressure; PAo, pulmonary artery occlusion pressure; PAdP, pulmonary artery
diastolic pressure.

particularly useful in confirming intactness of the spinal cord in anesthetized patients undergoing Harrington rod procedures for treatment of scoliosis. Volatile anesthetics, especially in high concentrations, and hypothermia may produce changes in the latency period and amplitude of evoked potentials that are similar to alterations produced by neural ischemia. Opioids produce the least change in evoked potentials and may be selected for this reason to provide a portion of the anesthetic maintenance in patients undergoing operations that benefit from use of this form of monitoring. As with the EEG, the complexity and cost of evoked potential monitoring limits its frequent use.

ELECTRICAL HAZARDS

Electrical monitoring equipment that is connected to a patient may result in delivery of leakage (extraneous) currents that produce thermal injury (burns) or cardiac dysrhythmias (ventricular fibrillation). Prevention of electrical injury to patients and operating room personnel requires elimination of extraneous voltage sources, especially in the presence of connections (electrolyte filled connecting tubing to a central venous pressure monitor) that result in complete circuits through tissues. For example, as little as 20 μA of 60 Hz applied directly to the endocardium can produce ventricular fibrillation. The high frequency current produced by the electrosurgical unit, however, does not produce cardiac dysrhythmias.

Monitors must be designed such that leakage currents are conducted to ground and not to the patient. Line isolation monitors detect leakage current and alert the anesthesiologist, by virtue of an audible alarm and appearance of a red warning light, to discontinue use of the malfunctioning monitor until appropriate repairs are performed. Indeed, periodic preventive maintenance of electrical equipment is a recommended practice. It is important to recognize, however, that isolation transformers limit the hazard of macroshock but not microshock to the patient. Battery powered monitors present little chance of electrocution to the patient or anesthesiologist because leakage currents do not occur.

The active electrode of the electrosurgical unit cuts or coagulates with intense heat produced by electrical current that flows through a small area. When this current exits from the body via a large ground plate attached to the patient, the current density is small and thermal injury does not occur. If the ground wire is broken or disconnected, the electrical current seeks alternative exits (electrodes for the ECG or peripheral nerve stimulator, contact sites with metal table) such that a high current density occurs at these small surface area sites with resultant burns.

RECORDING OF INTRAOPERATIVE DATA (ANESTHESIA RECORD)

The anesthesia record is a required and indispensable part of anesthetic care (Fig. 16-9). As in all aspects of medicine, the anesthetic and surgical events need to be documented for medical and

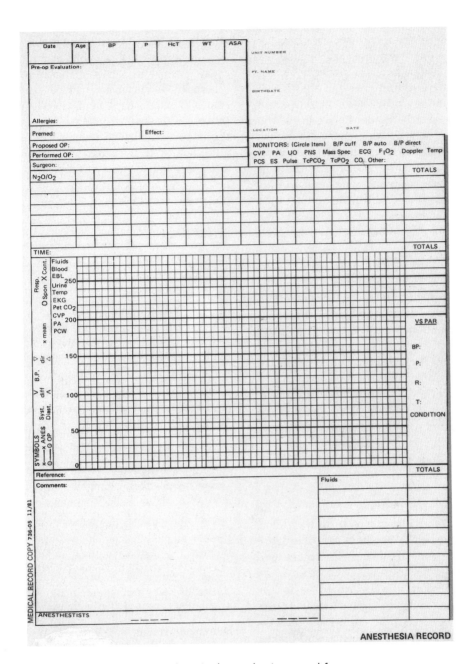

Fig. 16-9. A typical anesthesia record form.

legal purposes. The anesthesia record is the only continuous record that provides a detailed account of the intraoperative course of patients. This intraoperative record provides documentation of drugs and fluids that have been given. This information, for example, correlated with urinary output, can aid in predicting future drug and intravascular fluid needs. Also, recording of the vital signs and analgesic responses to opioids will aid the ward physicians in estimating opioid tolerance.

In essence, the anesthesia record provides a mechanism by which patient responses can be analyzed and appropriate action taken. Furthermore, this record can provide a reminder to the anesthesiologist that observations other than cardiopulmonary variables need to be made. For example, the anesthesia record may provide spaces to record fluid and blood replacement, estimated blood loss, urinary output, body temperature, ECG findings, end-tidal PCO_2, arterial blood gases and pH, arterial oxygen saturation, and central venous pressure. Also, if the anesthesiologist becomes distracted, a record exists as to when the last vital signs were determined.

Although patient care should take priority over making a neat and current anesthesia record, every effort should be made to keep the anesthesia record as current as possible. There can be no doubt that information recorded based on someone's memory will be suspect. To facilitate this process, automated anesthesia record-keeping systems are commercially available.

Retrospective review of anesthesia records can provide valuable information. For example, the effects, hazards, and disadvantages of a particular anesthetic technique can be assessed. Questions such as the magnitude of hypotension after spinal anesthetics and how many of these patients required vasopressor therapy can be quantitated. An overall assessment of anesthetic techniques and drugs used in a particular hospital can be determined. Also, a particular problem can be quantitated. Also, a particular problem can be assessed by analyzing multiple anesthesia records. As an example, the question may be raised as to the adequacy of monitoring for a particular procedure. By analysis of all past anesthesia records, the current practice can be established and quality assurance requirements met.

When litigation becomes a factor in assessing an anesthetic, it is essential that the anesthesia record be as complete as possible. An incomplete anesthesia record makes it difficult for attorneys to ascertain an accurate course of perioperative events. The anesthesiologist needs to develop work habits consistent with providing complete anesthesia records, which are properly dated, timed, and signed. It is further recommended that the anesthesiologist make postanesthesia rounds and record on the patient's chart findings relevant to the prior anesthetic.

REFERENCES

1. Watt R. OR patient monitoring. Med Instrum 1983;17:383–8.
2. Cooper JB, Newbower RS, Kitz RJ. An analysis of major errors and equipment failures in anesthesia management: Considerations for prevention and detection. Anesthesiology 1984;60:34–42.
3. Ozanne GM, Young WG, Mazzel WS, Serveringhaus JW. Multipatient anesthetic mass spectrometry. Anesthesiology 1981;56:62–70.
4. Kimble KJ, Darnall RA, Yelderman M, Ariagno RL, Ream AK. An automated oscillometric technique for estimating mean arterial pressure in critically ill newborns. Anesthesiology 1981;54:423–5.
5. Neil SG, Lam AM, Turnbull KW, Tremper KK. Monitoring of oxygen. Can J Anaesth 1987;34:56–63.
6. Swedlow DB. Capnometry and capnotraphy: The anesthesia disaster early warning system. Semin in Anesth 1986;5:194–205.
7. Morris RH. Operating room temperature and the anesthetized, paralyzed patient. Arch Surg 1971;102:95–7.
8. Slogoff S, Keats AS, Arlund C. On the safety of radial artery cannulation. Anesthesiology 1983;59:42–7.
9. Bedford RF. Radial arterial function following percutaneous cannulation with 18- and 20-gauge catheters. Anesthesiology 1977;47:37–9.
10. Blitt CD, Wright WA, Petty WC, Webster TA. Central venous catheterization via the external jugular vein. A technique employing the J-wire. JAMA 1974;229:817–8.

Appendix
Standards For Basic Intra-Operative Monitoring

(Approved by House of Delegates of the American Society of Anesthesiologists on October 21, 1986)

These standards apply to all anesthesia care although, in emergency circumstances, appropriate life support measures take precedence. These standards may be exceeded at any time based on the judgement of the responsible anesthesiologist. They are intended to encourage high quality patient care, but observing them cannot guarantee any specific patient outcome. They are subject to revision from time to time, as warranted by the evolution of technology and practice. This set of standards addresses only the issue of basic intra-operative monitoring, which is one component of anesthesia care. In certain rare or unusual circumstances, 1) some of these methods of monitoring may be clinically impractical, and 2) appropriate use of the described monitoring methods may fail to detect untoward clinical developments. Brief interruptions of continual† monitoring may be unavoidable. *Under extenuating circumstances, the responsible anesthesiologist may waive the requirements marked with an asterisk (*); it is recommended that when this is done, it should be so stated (including the reasons) in a note in the patient's medical record.* These standards are not intended for application to the care of the obstetrical patient in labor or in the conduct of pain management.

STANDARD I

Qualified anesthesia personnel shall be present in the room throughout the conduct of all general anesthetics, regional anesthetics and monitored anesthesia care.

Objective

Because of the rapid changes in patient status during anesthesia, qualified anesthesia personnel shall be continuously present to monitor the patient and provide anesthesia care. In the event there is a direct known hazard, e.g., radiation, to the anesthesia personnel which might require intermittent remote observation of the patient, some provision for monitoring the patient must be made. In the event that an emergency requires the temporary absence of the person primarily responsible for the anesthetic, the best judgement of the anesthesiologist will be exercised in comparing the emergency with the anesthetized patient's condition and in the selection of the person left responsible for the anesthetic during the temporary absence.

---

† Note that "continual" is defined as "repeated regularly and frequently in steady rapid succession" whereas "continuous" means "prolonged without any interruption at any time."

STANDARD II

During all anesthetics, the patient's oxygenation, ventilation, circulation, and temperature shall be continually evaluated.

Oxygenation

Objective

To ensure adequate oxygen concentration in the inspired gas and the blood during all anesthetics.

Methods

1. Inspired gas: During every administration of general anesthesia using an anesthesia machine, the concentration of oxygen in the patient breathing system shall be measured by an oxygen analyzer with a low oxygen concentration limit alarm in use.*
2. Blood oxygenation: During all anesthetics, adequate illumination and exposure of the patient is necessary to assess color. While this and other qualitative clinical signs may be adequate, there are quantitative methods, such as pulse oximetry, which are encouraged.

Ventilation

Objective

To ensure adequate ventilation of the patient during all anesthetics.

Methods

1. Every patient receiving general anesthesia shall have the adequacy of ventilation continually evaluated. While qualitative clinical signs such as chest excursion, observation of the reservoir breathing bag, and auscultation of breath sounds may be adequate, quantitative monitoring of the CO_2 content and/or volume of expired gas is encouraged.
2. When an endotracheal tube is inserted, its correct positioning in the trachea must be verified. Clinical assessment is essential and end-tidal CO_2 analysis, in use from the time of endotracheal tube placement, is encouraged.
3. When ventilation is controlled by a mechanical ventilator, there shall be in continuous use a device that is capable of detecting disconnection of components of the breathing system. The device must give an audible signal when its alarm threshold is exceeded.
4. During regional anesthesia and monitored anesthesia care, the adequacy of ventilation shall be evaluated, at least, by continual observation of qualitative clinical signs.

Circulation

Objective

To ensure the adequacy of the patient's circulatory function during all anesthetics.

Methods

1. Every patient receiving anesthesia shall have the electrocardiogram continuously displayed from the beginning of anesthesia until preparing to leave the anesthetizing location.*
2. Every patient receiving anesthesia shall have arterial blood pressure and heart rate determined and evaluated at least every five minutes.*
3. Every patient receiving general anesthesia shall have, in addition to the above, circulatory function continually evaluated by at least one of the following: palpation of a pulse, auscultation of heart sounds, monitoring of a tracing of intraarterial pressure, ultrasound peripheral pulse monitoring, or pulse plethysmography or oximetry.

Body Temperature

Objective

To aid in the maintenance of appropriate body temperature during all anesthetics.

Methods

There shall be readily available a means to continuously measure the patient's temperature. When changes in body temperature are intended, anticipated or suspected, the temperature shall be measured.

Chapter 17

Acid-Base Balance and Blood Gas Analysis

All living organisms depend on maintenance of acid-base equilibrium and oxygenation for survival. Regulation of acid-base balance is actually regulation of the hydrogen ion (H^+) and bicarbonate ion (HCO_3^-) concentrations in body fluids. Maintenance of the H^+ concentration over a narrow range is necessary to (1) ensure the optimal function of enzymes; (2) maintain the proper distribution of electrolytes; (3) optimize myocardial contractility; and (4) maintain an optimal saturation of hemoglobin. The normal H^+ concentration in the arterial blood and extracellular fluid is 36 $nmol \cdot L^{-1}$ to 44 $nmol \cdot L^{-1}$, which is equivalent to an arterial pH (pHa) of 7.44 to 7.36, respectively. The normal plasma concentration of HCO_3^- is 24 ± 2 $mEq \cdot L^{-1}$.

MAINTENANCE OF THE HYDROGEN ION CONCENTRATION

All body fluids are provided with buffer systems, which represent the first line of defense against changes in pHa produced by excess acid or alkali. The bicarbonate buffer system is the most important and readily available buffer system, representing over 50 percent of the total buffering capacity of the body. The most important nonbicarbonate buffer system is hemoglobin, which is responsible for about 35 percent of the buffering capacity in blood. The remainder of buffering capacity is provided by phosphates and plasma proteins.

The bicarbonate buffer system depends on the hydration of carbon dioxide to carbonic acid (H_2CO_3) in the plasma and erythrocytes (Fig. 17-1). Hydration of carbon dioxide in the plasma is a slow process, whereas in erythrocytes this reaction is greatly accelerated by the presence of the enzyme carbonic anhydrase. The H^+ formed by dissociation of H_2CO_3 in the erythrocytes and plasma is buffered by reduced hemoglobin. Hemoglobin can also transport carbon dioxide as carbaminohemoglobin. The HCO_3^- formed by dissociation of H_2CO_3 in erythrocytes enters the plasma where it functions as a buffer. At the same time, chloride ions enter the erythrocytes (chloride shift) to maintain electrical neutrality.

In addition to buffers, other compensatory

$$CO_2 + H_2O \xrightleftharpoons[\text{anhydrase}]{\text{carbonic}} H_2CO_3 \rightleftharpoons H^+ + HCO_3^-$$

Fig. 17-1. Carbon dioxide (CO_2) formed from aerobic metabolism undergoes hydration to form carbonic acid (H_2CO_3). Hydration of CO_2 in the plasma is a slow process, whereas in erythrocytes this reaction is greatly accelerated by the presence of the enzyme carbonic anhydrase. Dissociation of H_2CO_3 to hydrogen ions (H^+) and bicarbonate ions (HCO_3^-) is spontaneous.

229

mechanisms necessary for maintenance of an appropriate pHa include (1) alterations in the alveolar ventilation; (2) reabsorption of HCO_3^- by renal tubule cells; and (3) secretion of H^+ by renal tubule cells; (Figs. 17-2 and 17-3). Ultimately, the kidneys are the most powerful of the acid-base

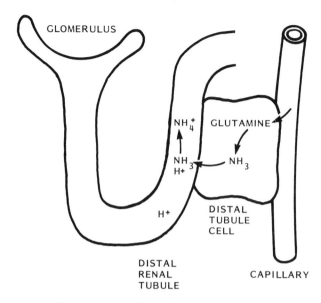

Fig. 17-3. The formation of ammonia (NH_3) from glutamine in distal renal tubule cells facilitates the elimination of hydrogen ions (H^+) in the urine as ammonium (NH_4^+). Neutralization of H^+ in the urine by formation of NH_4^+ is essential because secretion of H^+ by proximal renal tubule cells (Fig. 17-2) ceases when the urine pH is less than 4.5. Renal disease may impair the ability of distal renal tubule cells to form NH_3, resulting in decreased secretion of H^+ by renal tubule cells as the urine pH decreases below 4.5.

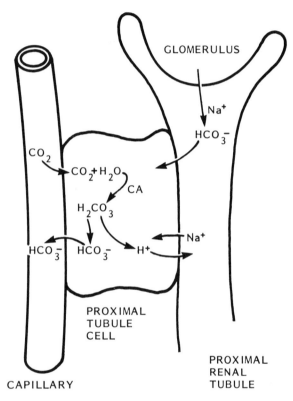

Fig. 17-2. Proximal renal tubule cells can regulate acid-base equilibrium by acidifying or alkalinizing the urine via reabsorption of bicarbonate ions (HCO_3^-) and/or secretion of hydrogen ions (H^+). In addition to reabsorption of HCO_3^-, proximal renal tubule cells are able to synthesize new HCO_3^- via hydration of CO_2 and subsequent dissociation of H_2CO_3. Hydration of CO_2 in these cells is accelerated by the presence of the enzyme carbonic anhydrase (CA). Reabsorbed and newly synthesized HCO_3^- can pass from renal tubule cells into capillaries to replenish that lost due to buffering. H^+ ion formed by dissociation of H_2CO_3 in proximal renal tubule cells are secreted into the urine in exchange for a cation, usually sodium (Na^+) so as to maintain electrical neutrality.

regulatory systems but in contrast to the instantaneous action of buffers and rapid adjustments in ventilation (1 minute to 3 minutes), the compensation via the kidneys requires 12 hours to 48 hours.

The Henderson-Hasselbalch equation emphasizes that a normal pHa depends on maintenance of an optimal 20 to 1 ratio of the concentration of HCO_3^- to carbon dioxide (Table 17-1). Acid-base disturbances characterized by changes in the plasma concentration of HCO_3^- are predictably accompanied by appropriate compensatory changes in the $PaCO_2$ secondary to alterations in alveolar ventilation. If changes in the plasma concentration of HCO_3^- and $PaCO_2$ are proportional such that a 20 to 1 ratio is maintained, the pHa will remain near or within the normal range despite disturbances of acid-base balance. For ex-

Table 17-1. Henderson-Hasselbalch Equation[a]

$$pHa = pK + \log \frac{HCO_3^-}{0.03 \times PaCO_2}$$

pHa = negative logarithm of the arterial concentration of hydrogen ions

pK = 6.1 at 37° Celsius

HCO_3^- = concentration of bicarbonate ions

0.03 = solubility coefficient for CO_2 in plasma

$PaCO_2$ = arterial partial pressure of CO_2

[a] Substitution of normal values for pHa (7.4) and $PaCO_2$ (40 mmHg) results in a calculated HCO_3^- concentration of 24 mEq·L^{-1}. Maintenance of this concentration of HCO_3^- relative to the concentration of CO_2 (0.03 × 40) results in an optimal 20 to 1 ratio. Likewise, alterations in HCO_3^- or the concentration of CO_2 will not significantly change the pHa if the 20 to 1 ratio is preserved.

ample, acid-base disturbances due to respiratory acidosis or alkalosis are compensated for by renal-induced changes in the plasma concentration of HCO_3^- such that the 20 to 1 ratio is maintained. As a result, the pHa in the presence of chronic respiratory acid-base disturbances is near normal despite persistent abnormalities of the $PaCO_2$. Likewise, acid-base disturbances due to metabolic abnormalities are compensated for by adjustments in alveolar ventilation in an effort to place the $PaCO_2$ in a range that preserves the 20 to 1 ratio.

DIFFERENTIAL DIAGNOSIS OF ACID-BASE DISTURBANCES

The differential diagnosis of acid-base disturbances (respiratory acidosis, respiratory alkalosis, metabolic acidosis, metabolic alkalosis) is based on the direct measurement of the pHa and $PaCO_2$ plus a derived estimate of the plasma concentration of HCO_3^- using a nomogram (Table 17-2, Fig. 17-4)[1,2]. Acidemia is present when the pHa is less than 7.36; alkalemia is present when the pHa is greater than 7.44. A $PaCO_2$ greater than 44 mmHg is defined as hypoventilation; hyperventilation is present when the $PaCO_2$ is less than 36 mmHg. Hypoventilation is synonymous with respiratory acidosis and hyperventilation is synonomous with respiratory alkalosis. Acidemia and alkalemia characterized by deviations of the HCO_3^- concentration above or below 24 mEq·L^{-1} are considered to be primary metabolic disturbances. Predictable adverse responses accompany acidemia and alkalemia.

Direct effects of alkalemia on myocardial contractility are less striking than those of acidemia. Although acidemia reduces myocardial contractility, little clinical effect occurs until pHa declines below 7.2. Because acidemia also induces release of catecholamines, much of the direct myocardial depressant effects are mitigated in mild acidemia. When pHa is below 7.1, however, myocardial

Table 17-2. Differential Diagnosis of Acid-Base Disturbances

Disturbance	pHa (7.36 to 7.44)	$PaCO_2$ (36 to 44 mmHg)	HCO_3^- (24 mEq·L^{-1})
Respiratory acidosis			
Acute	Moderate decrease	Marked increase	Slight increase
Chronic	Slight decrease to no change	Marked increase	Moderate increase
Respiratory alkalosis			
Acute	Moderate increase	Marked decrease	Slight decrease
Chronic	Slight increase to no change	Marked decrease	Moderate decrease
Metabolic acidosis			
Acute	Moderate to marked decrease	Slight decrease	Marked decrease
Chronic	Slight decrease	Moderate decrease	Marked decrease
Metabolic alkalosis			
Acute	Marked increase	Moderate increase	Marked increase
Chronic	Marked increase	Moderate increase	Marked increased

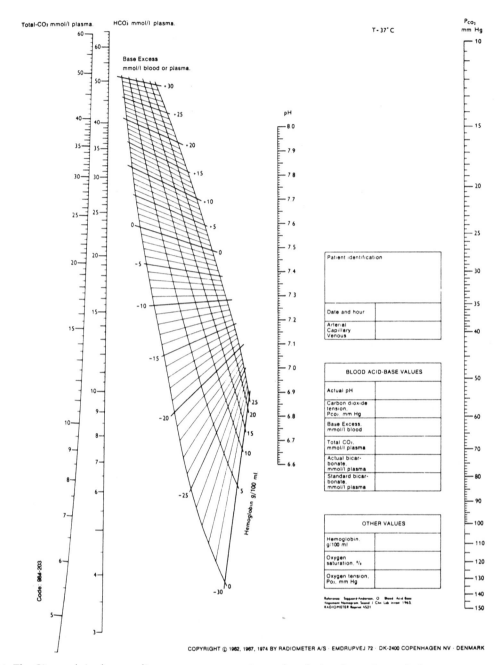

Fig. 17-4. The Siggard-Andersen alignment nomogram is used to derive the estimated plasma concentration of bicarbonate ions (HCO$_3^-$) or alternatively determination of base excess. A line connecting the measured partial pressure of carbon dioxide (PCO$_2$) and pH will transect the vertical column representing the plasma concentration of HCO$_3^-$ or base excess. (From Siggard-Andersen,[2] with permission.)

Adverse Effects of Respiratory or Metabolic Acidosis

Increased serum potassium concentration

Central nervous system depression

Cardiovascular depression due to direct depressant effects on the vasomotor center, arteriolar smooth muscle, and myocardial contractility (offset until severe acidosis by increased secretion of catecholamines and elevated plasma concentrations of ionized calcium)

Increased incidence of cardiac dysrhythmias

Decreased precapillary and increased post-capillary sphincter tone, leading to hypovolemia

---

Adverse Effects of Respiratory or Metabolic Alkalosis

Decreased serum potassium concentrations

Decreased ionized calcium concentrations (altered neuromuscular function manifesting as tetany, decreased myocardial contractility)

Central nervous system excitation

Decreased cerebral blood flow

Coronary artery vasoconstriction

Decreased availability of oxygen to tissues due to leftward shift of the oxyhemoglobin dissociation curve (Bohr effect)

Increased incidence of cardiac dysrhythmias

Increased airway resistance and right-to-left intrapulmonary shunting (respiratory alkalosis only)

Table 17-3. Normalization of Plasma Concentration of Bicarbonate for Alveolar Ventilation

Change in $PaCO_2$ from 40 mmHg	Change in HCO_3^- Concentration from 24 $mEq \cdot L^{-1}$
Acute 10 mmHg increase	Increase 1 $mEq \cdot L^{-1}$
Acute 10 mmHg decrease	Decrease 2 $mEq \cdot L^{-1}$
Chronic 10 mmHg increase	Increase 3 $mEq \cdot L^{-1}$
Chronic 10 mmHg decrease	Decrease 5 $mEq \cdot L^{-1}$

responsiveness to catecholamines decreases and compensatory increases in myocardial contractility are diminished. Interpretation of the plasma concentration of HCO_3^- as derived from the nomogram requires an adjustment for the impact of ventilation (Fig. 17-4). For example, an increased $PaCO_2$ will lead to the hydration of carbon dioxide with a subsequent increase in the plasma concentration of HCO_3^- (Fig. 17-1). Normalization of the HCO_3^- concentration above or below 24 mEq $\cdot L^{-1}$ in the presence of an increased or decreased $PaCO_2$ is achieved by applying a correction factor that is dependent on the rapidity and direction of change in the $PaCO_2$ (Table 17-3).

In discussing abnormalities of acid-base balance, primary alterations should be distinguished from changes that reflect compensatory responses. Compensation is the restoration of pHa toward 7.4 despite the continued presence of the primary acid-base abnormality. Indeed, compensatory responses frequently result in mixed acid-base disturbances. Ultimately, differentiation between primary respiratory or metabolic causes of acid-base disturbances is necessary to ensure proper treatment.

RESPIRATORY ACIDOSIS

Respiratory acidosis is present when the $PaCO_2$ exceeds 44 mmHg (Table 17-2). Measurement of the pHa or estimate of the plasma concentration of HCO_3^- provides evidence as to the chronicity of the acid-base disturbance and gives an indication as to the primary or compensatory nature of the respiratory change (Table 17-2). An increased $PaCO_2$ is due either to decreased elimination of

---

Causes of Respiratory Acidosis

Decreased elimination of carbon dioxide by
the lungs (hypoventilation)
  Central nervous system depression due to
  drugs (anesthetics)
  Decreased skeletal muscle strength (diseases, skeletal muscle relaxants)
  Intrinsic pulmonary disease
  Rebreathing of exhaled gases (exhausted
  soda lime, incompetent one-way valve in
  anesthetic breathing system)

Increased metabolic production of carbon
dioxide
  Hyperthermia

  Increased glucose load (hyperalimentation)

---

carbon dioxide by the lungs (hypoventilation) or
increased metabolic production of carbon dioxide.

The initial effect of an increase in the $PaCO_2$ is
a decreased pHa due to hydration of carbon
dioxide (Fig. 17-1). The reduction in pH occurs
to a similar extent in arterial blood and cerebrospinal fluid (CSF) because carbon dioxide rapidly
crosses lipid barriers such as the blood-brain barrier. The response to a reduction in pHa is stimulation of ventilation via the carotid bodies,
whereas the decreased pH of the CSF stimulates
medullary chemoreceptors located in the fourth
cerebral ventricle. With time, stimulation of ventilation via medullary chemoreceptors is eliminated
as the CSF pH is restored to normal by the active
transport of HCO_3^- into the CSF.[3] Therefore,
the volume of ventilation after restoration of the
CSF pH to normal is less than that present during
the initial phase of respiratory acidosis. It should
be appreciated that volatile anesthetics greatly
reduce the carotid body mediated responses to
acidemia.

Compensatory Responses

The absolute reduction in pHa produced by respiratory acidosis depends on the degree of compensation provided by the secondary increase in

the plasma concentration of HCO_3^-. It is estimated that the hydration of carbon dioxide increases the plasma concentration of HCO_3^- about
1 $mEq \cdot L^-$ for every 10 mmHg increase of the
$PaCO_2$ above normal (Table 17-3). This compensatory increase in the plasma concentration of
HCO_3^- occurs within seconds after the increase
in $PaCO_2$. In addition, hydration of carbon dioxide
in proximal renal tubule cells promotes secretion
of H^+ into the urine (Fig. 17-2). At the same time,
sodium is exchanged for H^+, which facilitates
reabsorption of HCO_3^- (Fig. 17-2). Likewise, distal
renal tubule cells secrete H^+ (Fig. 17-3). This renal
compensation requires 12 hours to 48 hours but
eventually increases the plasma HCO_3^- concentration by about 2 $mEq \cdot L^{-1}$ for every 10 mmHg
elevation in the $PaCO_2$ above normal (Table 17-
3). Thus, the total increase in the plasma concentration of HCO_3^- produced by hydration of carbon dioxide and renal reabsorption of HCO_3^- is
about 3 $mEq \cdot L^{-1}$ for every 10 mmHg increase of
the $PaCO_2$ above normal (Table 17-3). The net
effect of this compensatory response is a return
of the pHa to normal or near normal in patients
with chronic elevations in the $PaCO_2$. Acute respiratory acidosis is recognized by a reduced pHa
and less than the predicted increase in the plasma
concentration of HCO_3^- (Table 17-2).

Treatment

Treatment of chronic respiratory acidosis is by
correction of the disorder responsible for decreased elimination of carbon dioxide by the lungs
or increased metabolic production of carbon dioxide. Mechanical ventilation of the lungs will be
necessary when acute or chronic elevation of the
$PaCO_2$ is marked. Rapid lowering of a chronically
elevated $PaCO_2$, however, can result in metabolic
alkalosis and central nervous system irritability
because total body carbon dioxide washout occurs
more rapidly than the kidneys can produce a
corresponding reduction in the plasma concentration of HCO_3^-. Therefore, it is mandatory to
slowly reduce a chronically elevated $PaCO_2$ so as
to assure time for renal elimination of excess
HCO_3^-. Hypochloremia due to augmentation of
renal excretion of chloride in order to enhance

proximal renal tubule cell reabsorption of HCO_3^- may require treatment in some patients.

Mixed Acid-Base Disturbance

Respiratory acidosis complicated by metabolic acidosis is evidenced by an increase in the plasma concentration of HCO_3^-, which is less than 3 $mEq\cdot L^{-1}$ for every 10 mmHg increase of the $PaCO_2$. An increase in the plasma concentration of HCO_3^- that exceeds 3 $mEq\cdot L^{-1}$ for every 10 mmHg elevation of the $PaCO_2$ above normal suggests the presence of respiratory acidosis complicated by metabolic alkalosis. Metabolic alkalosis complicating respiratory acidosis is likely in the presence of hypochloremia and/or hypokalemia. Treatment of metabolic alkalosis associated with respiratory acidosis is with the intravenous administration of potassium chloride and avoidance of mechanical hyperventilation of the lungs.

RESPIRATORY ALKALOSIS

Respiratory alkalosis is present when the $PaCO_2$ is less than 36 mmHg (Table 17-2). Measurement of the pHa or estimate of the plasma concentration of HCO_3^- provides evidence as to the chronicity of the acid-base disturbance and gives an indication as to the primary or compensatory nature of the respiratory change (Table 17-2). A decreased $PaCO_2$ is due either to increased elimination of carbon dioxide by the lungs (hyperventilation) or decreased metabolic production of carbon dioxide. The initial effect of a decrease in the $PaCO_2$ is an increased pHa due to decreased hydration of carbon dioxide (Fig. 17-1). The decreased $PaCO_2$ and increased pHa reduces the stimulus to breath normally mediated by the carotid bodies and medullary chemoreceptors. Active transport of HCO_3^- out of the CSF subsequently restores the CSF pH to normal.[3] As a result, the activity of the medullary chemoreceptors becomes normal and the volume of ventilation is increased, despite persistence of a decreased $PaCO_2$. By the same mechanism, mechanical hyperventilation of the lungs during anesthesia can result in the initiation of spontaneous ventilation at a lower $PaCO_2$ than is present before hyperventilation (Fig. 17-5).[4] This initiation of ventilation reflects a normal CSF pH, which main-

tains ventilation via stimulation from the medullary chemoreceptors despite persistence of a decreased $PaCO_2$. Likewise, continued hyperventilation after returning to sea level from altitude reflects maintenance of ventilation by the medullary chemoreceptors exposed to a normal CSF pH.

Compensatory Responses

Three events occur simultaneously to reduce the plasma concentration of HCO_3^- and thus offset the increase in pHa that accompanies respiratory alkalosis. There is an immediate response via the bicarbonate buffer system, resulting in the production of carbon dioxide (Fig. 17-1). In addition, alkalosis stimulates the activity of phosphofructokinase enzyme, which results in glycolysis and generation of lactic acid. These two mechanisms operate rapidly to reduce the plasma concentration of HCO_3^- by about 2 $mEq\cdot L^{-1}$ for every 10 mmHg decrease in the $PaCO_2$ below normal (Table 17-3). The third compensatory mechanism is decreased reabsorption of HCO_3^-, which becomes maximal by 12 hours to 48 hours (Fig. 17-2). The reduction in the plasma concentration of HCO_3^- produced by these three compensatory mecha-

---

Causes of Respiratory Alkalosis

Increased elimination of carbon dioxide by the lungs (hyperventilation)
 Iatrogenic-mechanical or self-induced
 Pain
 Anxiety
 Decreased barometric pressure
 Central nervous system injury
 Arterial hypoxemia
 Pulmonary vascular disease
 Cirrhosis of the liver
 Sepsis
 Hyperthermia

Decreased metabolic production of carbon dioxide
 Hypothermia
 Skeletal muscle paralysis

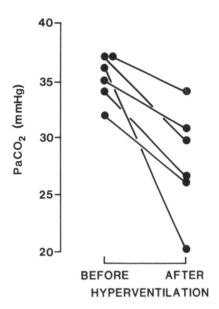

Fig. 17-5. The $PaCO_2$ present during spontaneous ventilation before and after mechanical hyperventilation to
a $PaCO_2$ of 20 mmHg for 2 hours was measured in six
adult patients. The return of spontaneous ventilation at
a lower $PaCO_2$ after mechanical hyperventilation of the
lungs reflects restoration of the cerebrospinal fluid pH
to normal despite persistent reductions in the $PaCO_2$.
This is equivalent to resetting the threshold of the medullary chemoreceptors for carbon dioxide. (Based on
data from Edelist and Osorio.[4])

nisms is about 5 mEq·L^{-1} for every 10 mmHg
decrease in the $PaCO_2$ below normal (Table 17-3).
This degree of metabolic compensation is sufficient to return the pHa to normal or near normal
in patients with chronic reductions in the $PaCO_2$
(Table 17-2). Chronic respiratory alkalosis complicated by metabolic acidosis is reflected by less
than a 5 mEq·L^{-1} decrease in the plasma concentration of $HCO_3{}^-$.

Treatment

Treatment of chronic respiratory alkalosis is directed at correcting the underlying disorder responsible for the increased elimination of carbon
dioxide by the lungs or decreased metabolic production of carbon dioxide. During anesthesia,
treatment of acute respiratory alkalosis is most
often accomplished by adjustment of the mechan-

ical ventilator to decrease the alveolar ventilation.
In addition, rebreathing of exhaled gases that
contain carbon dioxide can be provided by adding
dead space to the anesthetic breathing system.
Finally, carbon dioxide delivered from a metered
source can be added to the inhaled gases in attempts to re-establish a normal $PaCO_2$.

METABOLIC ACIDOSIS

Metabolic acidosis is present when the pHa is less
than 7.36 and the plasma concentration of $HCO_3{}^-$
is decreased below 24 mEq·L^{-1} (Table 17-2). Measurement of the $PaCO_2$ supplies evidence as to the
chronicity of the acid-base disturbance and gives
an indication as to the primary or compensatory
nature of the metabolic change (Table 17-2). A
decreased pHa, in association with a reduced
plasma concentration of $HCO_3{}^-$, is due either to
decreased elimination of H^+ by renal tubule cells
or to increased metabolic production of H^+ relative to $HCO_3{}^-$.

Compensatory Responses

Compensatory responses initiated by metabolic
acidosis include secretion of H^+ by renal tubule
cells with reabsorption of $HCO_3{}^-$ (Figs. 17-2 and
17-3) and increased alveolar ventilation due to
stimulation of the carotid bodies by H^+. The
reduction in $PaCO_2$ produced by increased alveolar
ventilation is rapidly reflected as a corresponding
decrease in the $PaCO_2$ in the CSF. As a result, the
CSF pH increases, leading to an inhibition of the
activity of the medullary chemoreceptors and a
blunting of the increase in ventilation produced
by the carotid bodies.[3] With time, however, the
CSF pH normalizes, reflecting the active transport
of $HCO_3{}^-$ into the CSF. Therefore, inhibition of
ventilation provided by the medullary chemoreceptors is removed and there is a further, although
delayed, increase in alveolar ventilation. As with
respiratory acidosis, volatile anesthetics blunt the
carotid body mediated response to metabolic acidosis. Another compensatory mechanism is the use
of buffers present in bone to neutralize nonvolatile
acids present in the circulation. Indeed, chronic
metabolic acidosis, as associated with chronic renal

Causes of Metabolic Acidosis

Decreased renal tubule elimination of hydrogen ions
　Renal failure
　Cirrhosis of the liver with decreased conversion of lactate to glucose

Increased metabolic production of hydrogen ions
　Anaerobic glycolysis due to decreased delivery of oxygenated blood to tissues
　Diabetic ketoacidosis
　Metabolism of amino acids in hyperalimentation solutions
　Idiopathic
　Excessive loss of gastrointestinal fluids formed distal to the pylorus (diarrhea, ileostomy) leading to a relative excess of hydrogen ions
　Renal tubular acidosis (inability of kidneys to reabsorb bicarbonate ions present in the glomerular filtrate results in a relative excess of hydrogen ions)

---

failure, is commonly associated with loss of bone mass.

Patients with lactic acidosis hyperventilate to a greater degree than do patients with other forms of metabolic acidosis such as ketoacidosis. This may reflect the brain's participation in lactic acid production, thereby directly exposing chemoreceptors to acid. In contrast to lactic acidosis, ketoacids produced by diabetics are only synthesized in the liver and must be transported across the blood-brain barrier before stimulation of ventilation occurs.

A useful guideline is that a 1 mmHg change in $PaCO_2$ above or below 40 mmHg results in a 0.008 unit pH change in the opposite direction. Therefore, a patient with a $PaCO_2$ of 30 mmHg and a pHa of 7.38 has a "corrected" pHa of 7.30. Routine use of this rule in the initial interpretation of the $PaCO_2$ and pHa permits rapid recognition of an acid-base abnormality due to a metabolic disturb-

Table 17-4. Calculation of the Dose of Sodium Bicarbonate to Treat Metabolic Acidosis

Dose of sodium bicarbonate = Body weight (kg)
　× Deviation of HCO_3^- from 24 $mEq \cdot L^{-1a}$
　× Extracellular fluid volume as a fraction
　　　　　　　　of body mass (0.2)

a The normal value for HCO_3^- (24 $mEq \cdot L^{-1}$) must be adjusted for deviations in the $PaCO_2$ from 40 mm Hg (see Table 17-3).

---

ance. Another useful guideline is that $PaCO_2$ will decrease about 1 mmHg for every $mEq \cdot L^{-1}$ reduction in the plasma concentration of HCO_3^- below 24 $mEq \cdot L^{-1}$. When metabolic acidosis is complicated by respiratory acidosis, the magnitude of reduction in the $PaCO_2$ is less than 1 mmHg for each $mEq \cdot L^{-1}$ reduction in the plasma concentration of HCO_3^-.

Treatment

Treatment of metabolic acidosis is removal of the cause for the accumulation of nonvolatile acids in the circulation. In addition, intravenous administration of sodium bicarbonate is indicated if metabolic acidosis is associated with myocardial depression or cardiac dysrhythmias. Calculation of the dose of sodium bicarbonate (Table 17-4) requires use of a nomogram to determine the plasma concentration of HCO_3^- or, alternatively, the base excess (Fig. 17-4).[2] A common approach is to administer about one-half of the calculated dose of sodium bicarbonate followed by a repeat measurement of the pHa to evaluate the impact of therapy.

METABOLIC ALKALOSIS

Metabolic alkalosis is present when the pHa is greater than 7.44 and the plasma concentration of HCO_3^- is increased above 24 $mEq \cdot L^{-1}$ (Table 17-2). Measurement of the $PaCO_2$ supplies evidence as to the chronicity of the acid-base disturbance and gives an indication as to the primary or compensatory nature of the metabolic change (Table 17-2). An increased pHa due to metabolic alkalosis reflects events that result in an excess of HCO_3^- relative to H^+. An example of an event that results in a relative excess of HCO_3^- is

---

Causes of Metabolic Alkalosis

Vomiting or nasogastric suction, resulting in excessive loss of hydrogen ions to bicarbonate ions

Chronic hypercarbia

Chloride and/or potassium depletion due to diuretics

Metabolism of lactate in lactated Ringer's solution, citrate in stored whole blood, or acetate in hyperalimentation solutions to bicarbonate ions

Depletion of intravascular fluid volume

Hyperaldosteronism leading to increased sodium reabsorption by distal renal tubule cells that results in increased hydrogen ion secretion

---

Effects of Hypokalemia that Contribute to Metabolic Alkalosis

Increased proximal renal tubule cell reabsorption of bicarbonate ions

Increased distal renal tubule cell secretion of hydrogen ions

Increased distal renal tubule cell synthesis of ammonia

---

conversion of citrate in the liver to HCO_3^-. Indeed, metabolic alkalosis is not an infrequent finding after administration of large amounts of stored whole blood containing citrate anticoagulant.[5]

Depletion of intravascular fluid volume is often the most important factor in maintenance of metabolic alkalosis. In this regard, hypovolemia should be considered in postoperative patients who develop metabolic alkalosis. Clinically, metabolic alkalosis correlates with reductions in the total body concentrations of chloride and potassium. For example, diuretics that facilitate chloride loss via renal tubule cells are associated with increased reabsorption of HCO_3^- to maintain electrical neutrality. Likewise, hypokalemia secondary to diuretic therapy is associated with similar renal changes that contribute to metabolic alkalosis.

Compensatory Responses

Compensatory responses initiated by metabolic alkalosis include increased reabsorption of H^+ by renal tubule cells (Fig. 17-2), decreased secretion of H^+ by renal tubule cells (Fig. 17-3), and alveolar hypoventilation. The efficiency of the renal compensatory mechanism is dependent on the presence of cations (sodium, potassium) and chloride (Figs. 17-2 and 17-3). Depletion of these ions, as occurs with vomiting, impairs the ability of the kidneys to excrete excess HCO_3^-, resulting in incomplete renal compensation for metabolic alkalosis. Hypoventilation in an attempt to compensate for metabolic alkalosis will initially stimulate the medullary chemoreceptors and thus offset the compensatory effect of decreased alveolar ventilation. With time, the CSF pH is normalized by active transport of HCO_3^- into the CSF and the volume of ventilation decreases, despite the persistence of a compensatory increase in the $PaCO_2$.[3] If the $PaCO_2$ increases again, however, the CSF pH will fall and the same sequence will be repeated. Indeed, respiratory compensation for pure metabolic alkalosis, in contrast to metabolic acidosis, is never more than 75 percent complete. As a result, the pHa remains elevated in patients with primary metabolic alkalosis (Table 17-2). Furthermore, a $PaCO_2$ above 55 mmHg is beyond the normal compensatory mechanism for metabolic alkalosis and reflects concomitant respiratory acidosis.

Treatment

Treatment of metabolic alkalosis is directed at resolution of the process responsible for the acid-base derangement plus intravenous infusion of potassium chloride, which allows the kidneys to excrete excess HCO_3^-. On occasion, intravenous infusion of H^+ in the form of ammonium chloride or 0.1 N hydrochloric acid (no greater than 0.2 $mEq \cdot kg^{-1} \cdot hr^{-1}$) is used to facilitate the return of pHa to near normal. Administration of acid requires insertion of a central venous catheter, as peripheral injections can cause sclerosis of veins and hemolysis.

MEASUREMENT OF ARTERIAL BLOOD GASES

Technological advances that permit the analysis of arterial and mixed venous blood gases (PO_2, PCO_2), as well as pH have contributed greatly to the management of patients during anesthesia and in the intensive care unit (see Chapter 32). Ability to obtain blood gas values within a few minutes permits moment-to-moment adjustments in the care of these patients. The small volume of blood required for the measurement (as little as 0.1 ml) extends this technique to the care of premature infants as well as to children and adults.

Sampling of Blood

Arterial blood is most often obtained percutaneously from the radial, brachial, or femoral artery. Arterialized venous blood may be an alternative when arterial sampling is not possible. Blood is drawn into a plastic or glass syringe that contains heparin sufficient to fill the dead space of the syringe. Heparin is acidic and excessive amounts of this anticoagulant in the sampling syringe could falsely lower the measured pH. Elimination of air bubbles from the syringe after obtaining the sample is important because equilibration of oxygen and carbon dioxide in the blood with the corresponding partial pressures in the air bubble could influence the measured results. Before analysis, the blood sample may be placed on ice to retard metabolism, which could consume oxygen and produce carbon dioxide.

Temperature Correction

In the past, it was recommended that blood gases and pH should be corrected for temperature if the temperature of the measuring electrode (usually 37° Celsius) differed from the patient's body temperature. This recommendation is based on the knowledge that the solubilities of oxygen and carbon dioxide in the blood are temperature-dependent. Therefore, placing blood from a patient with a body temperature less than 37° Celsius

into an electrode maintained at 37° Celsius means that more molecules enter the gas phase to be sensed as partial pressure than would be present in vivo at the lower body temperature of the patient. Nomograms are available to correct blood gases and pH measurements for temperature; however, the need to correct PCO_2 and pH measurements for body temperature has been challenged.[6] It is argued that a normal PCO_2 and pH measured at an electrode temperature of 37° Celsius reflects an unperturbed acid-base status of the patient, regardless of the body temperature that existed at the time the sample was drawn. This argument is based on the concept that maintenance of electrochemical neutrality (pH = pOH) requires the pH to rise with reductions in body temperature. Conversely, as body temperature increases, the neutral point falls and maintenance of electrochemical neutrality requires a decrease in pH. If this concept is accepted, it is not necessary to correct PCO_2 and pH for variations in body temperature from the temperature of the electrodes, which are usually maintained at 37° Celsius. Temperature correction of the PO_2 remains important, however, for assessing oxygenation. As a guideline, the measured PO_2 should be decreased 6 percent for every degree Celsius the patient's body temperature is below the temperature of the electrode (37° Celsius). The PO_2 is increased 6 percent for every degree Celsius the body temperature exceeds 37° Celsius. Furthermore, calculation of the alveolar-to-arterial difference for oxygen ($AaDO_2$) requires temperature correction of the PaO_2 and $PaCO_2$ (Table 17-5).

Blood Gas pH Electrodes

The oxygen electrode (Clark electrode) used to measure PO_2 is a polarographic cell consisting of a silver reference anode and a platinum cathode charged to minus 0.5 volts.[7] The platinum surface is covered with an oxygen permeable membrane (polyethylene) on the other side of which is placed the unknown sample. Electrical current passing through the polarographic cell is directly proportional to the PO_2 outside the membrane.

The carbon dioxide electrode (Severinghaus electrode) used to measure PCO_2 uses a carbon dioxide permeable membrane (Teflon), which per-

Table 17-5. Calculation of the Alveolar-to-Arterial Difference for Oxygen

$$A\text{-}aDO_2 = P_AO_2 - PaO_2$$

$$P_AO_2 = (P_B - P_{H_2O})F_IO_2 - \frac{PaCO_2}{0.8}$$

$A\text{-}aDO_2$ = alveolar-to-arterial difference for oxygen, mmHg

P_AO_2 = alveolar partial pressure of oxygen, mmHg

PaO_2 = arterial partial pressure of oxygen, mmHg

P_B = barometric pressure, mmHg

P_{H_2O} = partial pressure of water vapor, 47 mmHg at 37° Celsius

F_IO_2 = inspired concentration of oxygen

$PaCO_2$ = arterial partial pressure of carbon dioxide, mmHg

0.8 = respiratory exchange ratio to compensate for the fact that less carbon dioxide is transferred into the alveolus than oxygen is removed from the alveolus

Example. Arterial blood gases are PaO_2 310 mmHg and $PaCO_2$ 40 mmHg breathing pure oxygen (F_IO_2 = 1.0). The P_B is 747 mmHg and the P_{H_2O} is 47 mmHg. The $A\text{-}aDO_2$ is:

$$P_AO_2 = (747 - 47)1.0 - 40/0.8$$
$$P_AO_2 = 700 - 50$$
$$P_AO_2 = 650 \text{ mmHg}$$

$$A\text{-}aDO_2 = 650 - 310$$
$$A\text{-}aDO_2 = 340 \text{ mmHg}^a \text{ (normal less than 60 mmHg)}$$

[a] Assuming each 20 mmHg $A\text{-}aDO_2$ represents venous admixture equivalent to 1% of the cardiac output, it can be estimated that 17% of the cardiac output is shunted past the lungs without exposure to ventilated alveoli.
(Modified from Stoelting et al.,[11] with permission.)

mits carbon dioxide to diffuse from the unknown sample into a buffer solution containing bicarbonate bathing a conventional glass pH electrode.[8] The measured pH in the bathing solution is altered in direct proportion to the PCO_2.

Measurement of pH employs a glass electrode that senses the concentration of H^+ in the unknown sample. This H^+ concentration produces a proportional change in voltage between the glass and reference electrode.

Information Provided by Blood Gases and pH

Minimum information for assessment of oxygenation and ventilation requires the measurement of PaO_2 and $PaCO_2$. As an alternative to arterial samples, blood from veins on the back of the hand, which reflects primarily cutaneous blood, can be used to estimate arterial blood gases and pH. Indeed, the combination of cutaneous vasodilation and increased cutaneous blood flow associated with general anesthesia is often sufficient to arterialize

peripheral venous blood.[9] As a result, the peripheral venous PCO_2 and pH measured during general anesthesia approximate arterial values closely enough to permit estimation of the adequacy of ventilation and acid-base status. For example, venous PCO_2 is only 4 mmHg to 6 mmHg higher and pH only 0.03 units to 0.04 units lower than arterial values. The calculated bicarbonate concentration in venous blood is therefore only about 2 $mEq \cdot L^{-1}$ higher. The peripheral venous PO_2, however, does not reliably parallel the PaO_2. Nevertheless, when the peripheral venous PO_2 exceeds 60 mmHg, the absence of arterial hypoxemia is confirmed. Additional measurements and calculations that further define the efficiency of oxygenation and ventilation include the (1) $AaDO_2$, (2) arterial-to-alveolar PO_2 ratio (a/A), (3) mixed venous PO_2, (4) arterial and mixed venous content of oxygen, (5) position of the oxyhemoglobin dissociation curve, and (6) deadspace-to-tidal-volume ratio (V_D/V_T). The anesthesiologist must be familiar with these measurements and able to rapidly adjust patient care based on information derived from blood gases and pH measurements.

Oxygenation

Oxygenation is assessed by measurement of the PaO_2. Arterial hypoxemia, as reflected by decreases in PaO_2 below 60 mmHg, may be caused by (1) a low PO_2 in the inhaled gases (altitude, accidental during anesthesia); (2) hypoventilation; and (3) venous admixture.

Hypoventilation. Reductions in PaO_2 due to hypoventilation reflect encroachment of the $PaCO_2$ on the space available in the alveolus for oxygen. Decreases in PaO_2 are roughly equivalent to increases in alveolar PCO_2.

Venous Admixture. Venous admixture as a cause of decreased PaO_2 may reflect right-to-left intrapulmonary shunts (atelectasis, pneumonia), intracardiac shunts (congenital heart disease), or mismatching of ventilation to perfusion (chronic obstructive airways disease). A right-to-left shunt is defined as passage of blood from the pulmonary circulation to the systemic circulation without coming into contact with alveolar gases. Arterial hypoxemia due to right-to-left shunts represents dilution of oxygenated arterial blood with shunted and desaturated venous blood. In this instance, inhalation of pure oxygen produces minimal, if any, effect on the PaO_2. Mismatching of ventilation to perfusion as a cause of venous admixture and arterial hypoxemia reflects underventilation of alveoli relative to their blood flow. Inhalation of pure oxygen eventually eliminates residual nitrogen from poorly ventilated alveoli such that blood coming from these alveoli is well-oxygenated. This is the reason that even small increases in inhaled oxygen concentrations (24 percent to 30 percent) may correct arterial hypoxemia due to mismatching of ventilation to perfusion characteristic of patients with chronic obstructive airways disease. This therapeutic response to supplemental oxygen helps distinguish arterial hypoxemia that is due to right-to-left shunts from that due to mismatching of ventilation to perfusion. Diffusion limitation to the passage of oxygen from the alveoli to blood has not been documented to be a cause of arterial hypoxemia in humans.

AaDO2

The magnitude of venous admixture may be estimated in the clinical setting by calculation of the $AaDO_2$ (Table 17-5). For example, when the PaO_2 is above 150 mmHg, so that hemoglobin is completely saturated with oxygen, the magnitude of venous admixture can be estimated to be equivalent to 1 percent of the cardiac output for every 20 mmHg of $AaDO_2$. Below a PaO_2 of 150 mmHg or when cardiac output is increased relative to metabolism, this guideline will underestimate the actual amount of venous admixture. It must be appreciated that the normal $AaDO_2$ breathing air is 5 mmHg to 10 mmHg, reflecting right-to-left intracardiac shunting of 2 percent to 5 percent of the cardiac output via bronchial, pleural, and thebesian veins.

a/A Ratio

A disadvantage of $AaDO_2$ is the normal range changes with varying concentrations of inhaled oxygen. For this reason, the a/A ratio may be more useful because it remains relatively constant regardless of the concentration of oxygen (Table 17-6).[10] For example, a patient with an a/A ratio of 0.5 will have a PaO_2 equal to 50 percent of the alveolar PO_2, regardless of the inhaled concentration of oxygen.

Table 17-6. Calculation of the Ratio of Arterial to Alveolar Oxygen Partial Pressure

$$a/A = PaO_2/PAO_2$$

Example. Arterial blood gases are PaO_2 310 mmHg and $PaCO_2$ 40 mmHg breathing pure oxygen ($FiO_2 = 1.0$). The PB is 747 mmHg and the P_{H_2O} 47 mmHg. The a/A is:

$$PAO_2 = (747 - 47)1.0 - 40/0.8$$
$$PAO_2 = 700 - 50$$
$$PAO_2 = 650 \text{ mmHg}$$

$$a/A = 310/650$$
$$a/A = 0.48 \text{ (normal greater than 0.75)}$$

Mixed Venous PO$_2$

The mixed venous PO$_2$ is determined by the cardiac output and tissue oxygen consumption. In the presence of unchanging tissue oxygen consumption, the mixed venous PO$_2$ varies directly with changes in cardiac output. For example, when the cardiac output is decreased, less blood flow is available for tissue oxygen extraction. Therefore, the continued extraction of the same amount of oxygen from a decreased blood flow must result in a reduced mixed venous PO$_2$. Tissue hypoxemia is likely when the mixed venous PO$_2$ is less than 30 mmHg. Disease states associated with arterial to venous admixture (sepsis, portal hypertension) may result in a high mixed venous PO$_2$ despite inadequate tissue oxygenation.

Arterial and Mixed Venous Content of Oxygen

The difference between the arterial and mixed venous content of oxygen is an estimate of the adequacy of cardiac output relative to tissue oxygen consumption (Table 17-7). The normal difference in oxygen content of arterial and mixed venous blood is 4 ml·dl^{-1} to 6 ml·dl^{-1} of blood. When tissue oxygen consumption is constant, a decreased cardiac output is accompanied by an increased oxygen content difference between arterial and mixed venous blood.

Oxyhemoglobin Dissociation Curve

The oxyhemoglobin dissociation curve describes the saturation of hemoglobin with oxygen relative to the PO$_2$ (Fig. 17-6). Alternatively, this curve may be viewed as depicting the loading and unloading of oxygen from hemoglobin at a varying PO$_2$. The benefit of the sigmoid shape of the curve is ease of oxygen-loading onto hemoglobin over a wide range of minimally changing PO$_2$ values (flat upper portion of the curve) and ease of release of oxygen from hemoglobin with small changes in PO$_2$ values (steep lower portion of curve). A normal oxyhemoglobin dissociation curve is characterized by 50 percent saturation of hemoglobin with oxygen at a PO$_2$ of 26 mmHg. The PO$_2$ that results in 50 percent saturation is referred to as the P$_{50}$. Events that shift the oxyhemoglobin dis-

Table 17-7. Calculation of Arterial and/or Venous Content of Oxygen

CaO$_2$ = (Hb × 1.39)Sat + PaO$_2$(0.003)
CaO$_2$ = oxygen content of arterial blood, ml·dl^{-1}
C$\bar{v}$O$_2$ = oxygen content of mixed venous blood, ml·dl^{-1}
Hb = hemoglobin, g·dl^{-1}
1.39 = oxygen bound to hemoglobin, ml·g^{-1}
Sat = percent saturation of hemoglobin with oxygen
PaO$_2$ = arterial partial pressure of oxygen, mmHg
P$\bar{v}$O$_2$ = mixed venous partial pressure of oxygen, mmHg
0.003 = dissolved oxygen, ml·mmHg^{-1}

Example. Hb = 15 g·dl^{-1} and PaO$_2$ 100 mmHg resulting in nearly 100% saturation, P$\bar{v}$O$_2$ 40 mmHg resulting in 75% saturation.

$$CaO_2 = (15 \times 1.39)100 + 100(0.003)$$
$$= 20.85 + 0.03$$
$$= 21.15 \text{ ml·dl}^{-1}$$

$$C\bar{v}O_2 = (15 \times 1.39)75 + 40(0.003)$$
$$= 15.63 + 0.12$$
$$= 15.75 \text{ ml·dl}^{-1}$$

$$CaO_2 - C\bar{v}O_2 = 5.4 \text{ ml·dl}^{-1}$$

sociation curve to the left (P$_{50}$ less than 26 mmHg) may jeopardize tissue oxygenation as oxygen is more tightly bound to hemoglobin, and the PaO$_2$ must fall to a lower than normal level before oxygen is released from hemoglobin and becomes available to tissues (Table 17-8). Events that shift the oxyhemoglobin dissociation curve to the right (P$_{50}$ greater than 26 mmHg) facilitate tissue oxygen availability by permitting the unloading of oxygen from hemoglobin at an increased PaO$_2$ (Table 17-8).

Compensation for Arterial Hypoxemia

Increased cardiac output is the most important compensatory mechanism for correction of arterial hypoxemia. For example, if cardiac output increases and tissue oxygen consumption is unchanged, the result is decreased extraction of oxygen from venous blood. The effect of this

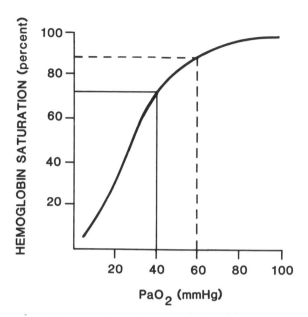

Fig. 17-6. The oxyhemoglobin dissociation curve describes the relation of hemoglobin saturation with oxygen (percent) to the PaO_2. The P_{50} is the PaO_2, which results in 50 percent saturation of hemoglobin with oxygen. In the presence of a normal pHa (7.4) and body temperature (37° Celsius) hemoglobin is 50 percent saturated with oxygen at a PaO_2 of 26 mmHg (P_{50}). Events that shift the oxyhemoglobin dissociation curve to the left (P_{50} less than 26 mmHg) may jeopardize tissue oxygenation since the PaO_2 must decrease further to permit release of oxygen from hemoglobin. Conversely, a shift of the oxyhemoglobin dissociation curve to the right (P_{50} greater than 26 mmHg) permits unloading of oxygen from hemoglobin at a higher PaO_2 and thus favors tissue oxygenation. The mixed venous PO_2 is near 40 mmHg and the associated hemoglobin saturation with oxygen is about 75 percent. Saturation of hemoglobin with oxygen is about 90 percent when the PaO_2 is 60 mmHg. The saturation of hemoglobin with oxygen can be considered to be 100 percent when the PaO_2 exceeds 150 mmHg.

decreased oxygen extraction is an increased mixed venous PO_2 that produces less dilution when arterial and shunted venous blood mix. A less efficient compensatory mechanism to offset arterial hypoxemia is hyperventilation. For example, the resulting alveolar PCO_2 decrease is paralleled by

Table 17-8. Events that Shift the Oxyhemoglobin Dissociation Curve

Left Shift (P_{50} less than 26 mmHg)	Right Shift (P_{50} greater than 26 mmHg)
Alkalosis	Acidosis
Hypothermia	Hyperthermia
Decreased 2,3-diphosphoglycerate	Increased 2,3-diphosphoglycerate due to chronic arterial hypoxemia or anemia

a similar increase in the PaO_2. Nevertheless, an accompanying increased oxygen consumption of the respiratory muscles is likely to offset any gain in available oxygen produced by hyperventilation.

Ventilation

The $PaCO_2$ reflects the adequacy of the lung for removing carbon dioxide from pulmonary capillary blood. In the steady state, $PaCO_2$ is directly proportional to the metabolic production of carbon dioxide and inversely proportional to alveolar ventilation. The production of carbon dioxide depends on the metabolic state of the individual and parallels tissue oxygen consumption. Under normal conditions, only 80 percent as much carbon

Table 17-9. Calculation of the Deadspace-to-Tidal-Volume Ratio

$$V_D/V_T = \frac{PaCO_2 - P_ECO_2}{PaCO_2}$$

V_D/V_T = ratio of dead space to tidal volume
$PaCO_2$ = arterial partial pressure of carbon dioxide, mmHg
P_ECO_2 = mixed exhaled partial pressure of carbon dioxide, mmHg

Example. The $PaCO_2$ is 40 mmHg and P_ECO_2 20 mmHg during controlled ventilation of the lungs. The V_D/V_T is:

$$V_D/V_T = \frac{40 - 20}{40}$$

$V_D/V_T = 20/40$
$V_D/V_T = 0.5$ (normal less than 0.3)

dioxide is produced as oxygen is consumed (respiratory quotient = 0.8). Assuming a tissue oxygen consumption of 250 ml·min^{-1}, the production of carbon dioxide would be 200 ml·min^{-1}. When the $PaCO_2$ is above 44 mmHg, the patient is hypoventilating relative to carbon dioxide production, whereas a $PaCO_2$ below 36 mmHg is defined as hyperventilation. Wasted ventilation or increased physiologic deadspace may result in an elevated $PaCO_2$ even when minute ventilation is increased. The V_D/V_T ratio, which depicts areas in the lung that receive adequate ventilation but inadequate or no pulmonary blood flow, should not exceed 0.3 (Table 17-9). In contrast to PaO_2, venous admixture has little to no impact on $PaCO_2$, reflecting the extreme diffusibility of carbon dioxide.

REFERENCES

1. Narins RG, Emmett M. Simple and mixed acid base disorders: A practical approach. Medicine 1980;59:161–87.
2. Siggard-Anderson O. Blood acid-base alignment nomogram. Scan J Clin Lab Invest 1963;15:211–7.
3. Mitchell RA, Singer MM. Respiration and cerebrospinal fluid pH in metabolic acidosis and alkalosis. J Appl Physiol 1965;20:905–11.
4. Edelist G, Osorio A. Postanesthetic initiation of spontaneous ventilation after passive hyperventilation. Anesthesiology 1969;31:222–7.
5. Barcenas CG, Fuller TJ, Knochel JP. Metabolic alkalosis after massive blood transfusion. JAMA 1976;236:953–4.
6. Ream AK, Reitz BA, Silverberg G. Temperature correction of PCO_2 and pH in estimating acid-base status: An example of the emperor's new clothes? Anesthesiology 1982;56:41–4.
7. Clark LC. Monitor and control of blood and tissue oxygen tensions. Trans Am Soc Artif Intern Organs 1956;2:41–8.
8. Severinghaus JW, Bradley AF. Electrodes for blood PO_2 and PCO_2 determination. J Appl Physiol 1958;13:515–20.
9. Williamson DC, Munson ES. Correlation of peripheral venous and arterial blood gas values during general anesthesia. Anesth Analg 1982;61:950–2.
10. Doyle JD. Arterial/alveolar oxygen tension ratio: A critical appraisal. Can Anaesth Soc J 1986;33:471–4.
11. Stoelting RK, Dierdorf SF, McCammon RL. Acid-base disturbances. In: Stoelting RK, Dierdorf SF, McCammon RL, eds. Anesthesia and Co-Existing Disease. New York, Churchill Livingstone, 1983;251–62.

Chapter 18

Fluid and Blood Therapy

Perioperative management of a patient's fluid balance includes preoperative evaluation and intraoperative maintenance and replacement of fluid losses. Preoperative treatment of hypovolemia is helpful because circulatory changes induced by anesthetics and surgery are augmented by co-existing reductions of intravascular fluid volume. Intraoperatively, in addition to blood loss, fluids can shift into various body compartments. Knowledge of these shifts can aid in predicting fluid requirements. Maintaining normal intravascular fluid volume is dependent on knowledge of these compartmental fluid changes, quantitation of blood loss, and selection of the appropriate fluid for infusion.

BODY FLUID COMPARTMENTS

Total body water can be divided into extracellular fluid (ECF) and intracellular fluid (ICF) (Fig. 18-1). Approximately 20 percent of the body weight (kg) is represented by ECF and 30 percent by ICF. The ECF is further divided into plasma volume (PV) and interstitial fluid (ISF). These latter two compartments are separated by the walls of the blood vessels, with the PV being defined as that fluid contained within the vascular system, but external to the erythrocytes, whereas ISF is confined to the compartment external to the blood

vessels and cells. PV represents about 5 percent of the body weight and ISF constitutes about 15 percent of body weight. If erythrocytes are added to the PV, a total blood volume equal to approximately 7.5 percent of body weight results.

Total body water content varies with age, sex, and body habitus. Fifty-five percent of the body weight is constituted by body water in adult men, whereas 45 percent of the body weight is represented by total body water in adult women. Because fat contains little water, obese adults have less total body water per kg than lean adults. Total body water constitutes about 80 percent of the total body weight in infants.

Preoperative Evaluation

The patient's mental status, history of input and output, blood pressure in both supine and sitting positions, heart rate, skin turgor, and urinary output should be evaluated with respect to alterations in these parameters produced by changes in intravascular fluid volume and/or concentration of electrolytes. Serum electrolytes should be measured along with, in some situations, serum osmolarity. Volume, concentration, and composition of the ECF are the three steps by which the intraoperative fluid and electrolyte status are evaluated.

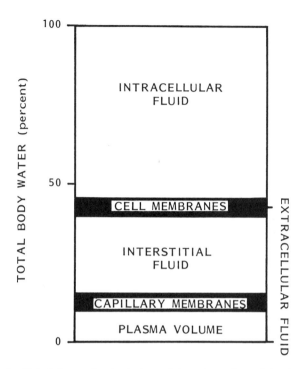

Fig. 18-1. Schematic depiction of location of total body water.

Steps for Evaluation of Fluid and Electrolyte Status

Volume
    Blood pressure sitting and supine
    Heart rate
    Mucous membrane moisture
    Skin turgor
    Urine output

Concentration
    Serum sodium
    Serum osmolarity

Composition
    Serum electrolytes
    Blood urea nitrogen
    Blood glucose
    Arterial blood gases and pH

Volume

ECF volume is best determined at the bedside. This volume should be accurately assessed because most anesthetic techniques and drugs can lead to marked circulatory depression in patients who have a deficit of ECF volume. Tachycardia and dry mucous membranes may indicate a mild volume deficit, even though the blood pressure is normal. This type of deficit can be seen in patients who have had extensive preoperative evaluation that required restricted oral intake, enemas for diagnostic radiologic procedures, and blood withdrawal for various laboratory tests.

Determining whether orthostatic hypotension is present is extremely useful in detecting more severe forms of intravascular fluid volume deficits. If the systolic blood pressure decreases more than 20 mmHg when the patient changes from the supine to standing or sitting position, there is a deficit of 6 percent to 8 percent of body weight as fluid. In this regard, observation of the heart rate is important in differentiating orthostatic hypotension due to autonomic drugs (antihypertensives) from an intravascular fluid volume deficit. If orthostatic hypotension occurs, the heart rate should increase in a compensatory manner. If this does occur, most likely the decrease in blood pressure is due to an intravascular fluid volume deficit. If, however, the blood pressure decreases and the heart rate does not increase, a defect in autonomic nervous system function, which could reflect antihypertensives the patient is receiving, should be suspected (see Chapter 3).

In severe cases of ECF deficits, the bladder probably should be catheterized to accurately quantitate urinary output. A decrease or absence of urinary output obviously indicates a severe deficit in ECF volume.

Conversely, an intravascular volume excess may be present in surgical patients, either from iatrogenic causes (excessive fluid administration), or pathologic causes (cirrhosis of the liver). Soft tissue edema and diuresis (>100 ml·hr^{-1}) are usually signs of excessive intravenous fluid administration. Blood pressure will initially increase but will subsequently decrease if the intravascular fluid overload induces cardiac failure. In this situation, patients will exhibit edema, which may manifest initially in the scleral conjunctiva. In severe cases, peripheral edema and even pulmonary edema will result. Treatment of congestive heart failure should be undertaken before proceeding with elective anesthesia and surgery.

Concentration

The concentration of constituents in ECF is determined to a large extent by total body water content. Although some bedside clues may be present, laboratory diagnosis is helpful for diagnosing abnormalities in body fluid concentrations. Valuable laboratory tests are the serum sodium concentration and, if available, the serum osmolarity. The definition of osmolarity is often confusing to physicians. One osmole is defined as one mole of nondissociating substance in one liter of solution. The term milliosmole (mOsm) is 1/1000 of an osmole of a substance in solution. Osmolarity is the number of osmoles·L^{-1} of solution, whereas osmolality is the number of osmoles·100 g^{-1} of solvent. In dilute solutions, as exist in the human body, osmolality is approximately equal to osmolarity. The normal osmolarity of ECF is 285 mOsm·L^{-1} to 295 mOsm·L^{-1}. When electrolyte-free water is lost from the body, the serum sodium and serum osmolarity increase. Usually, these increases are due to inadequate water intake or can occur in pathologic situations such as fever and loss of fluid from denuded tissues (burns).

When water is present in body fluids in excess of the normal ratio, the serum sodium concentration and osmolarity are reduced. Also, patients can develop a hypovolemic/hyponatremic condition in which electrolyte-rich fluids (such as vomitus, diarrhea, or fistula drainage) are lost and are replaced with water. Obviously, proper treatment consists of replacement with crystalloid solutions that are rich in electrolytes, such as lactated Ringer's solution. A normovolemic/hyponatremic condition results from failure of the kidneys to conserve sodium when the intake of sodium is reduced, but volume intake has been adequate. A hypervolemic/hyponatremic condition results from excessive water intake or retention, which, during anesthesia, is most commonly seen after

transurethral resection of the prostate (see Chapter 22), and when 5 percent dextrose in water is used to correct intravascular fluid volume deficits.

Composition

The composition of ECF is determined by the presence of various electrolytes. The distribution of electrolytes differs among the fluid compartments of the body (Table 18-1). The major cation in the blood is sodium, whereas the major cation of ICF is potassium. The electrophysiology of excitable cells depends on the intracellular and extracellular concentrations of sodium, potassium, and calcium.

Hypernatremia. Hypernatremia (serum sodium concentration exceeds 145 mEq·L^{-1}) is most often due to a deficit of total body content of water and not to an excess of total body sodium. Total body sodium can increase, however, when renal function is impaired, as occurs in patients with kidney disease, cirrhosis of the liver, or congestive heart failure. Peripheral edema is the hallmark of hypernatremia. An expanded intravascular fluid volume may manifest as hypertension. Treatment of hypernatremia due to excess total body sodium content is with renal tubular diuretics.

Hyponatremia. Hyponatremia (serum sodium concentration below 135 mEq·L^{-1}) is most often due to an excess of total body water and not to a deficiency of total body sodium. Total body sodium can decrease, however, with vomiting, diarrhea, and third-degree burns. Hyponatremia due to sodium loss is characterized by a decreased intravascular fluid volume, which manifests as hypotension, tachycardia, oliguria, and hemoconcentra-

Table 18-1. Approximate Distribution of Electrolytes

	Extracellular (Plasma) Fluid (mEq·L^{-1})	Intracellular Fluid (mEq·L^{-1})
Sodium	140	10
Potassium	4.5	150
Calcium	5	1
Magnesium	2	40

tion. Central nervous system signs of hyponatremia do not usually occur until the serum sodium concentration decreases below 110 mEq·L^{-1}. Treatment of hyponatremia rarely requires the intravenous administration of hypertonic saline.

Hyperkalemia. Hyperkalemia (serum potassium concentration above 5.5 mEq·L^{-1}) can be due to an increased total body potassium content (renal failure) or altered distribution of potassium between intracellular and extracellular sites (respiratory acidosis or metabolic acidosis, succinylcholine). Adverse effects of hyperkalemia are likely to accompany acute increases in serum potassium concentrations. In contrast, chronic hyperkalemia is more likely to be associated with normal gradients between extracellular and intracellular concentrations of potassium. That patients with chronic elevations of potassium are often asymptomatic suggests that potassium gradients across cell membranes are more important than the absolute serum concentrations of potassium.

The most detrimental effect of hyperkalemia is on the cardiac conduction system, manifesting on the electrocardiogram (ECG) as prolongation of the P-R interval, widening of the QRS complex, and peaking of the T wave. Treatment of acute hyperkalemia is designed to shift potassium from the serum into the cells so as to antagonize the effects of potassium on the heart. Therefore, the most rapidly acting therapeutic approach for reversal of cardiac effects of hyperkalemia is intravenous administration of calcium. Potassium can also be shifted into cells by production of systemic alkalosis (iatrogenic hyperventilation, intravenous administration of sodium bicarbonate), or intravenous injection of glucose (25 grams) combined with regular insulin (10 units to 15 units). Insulin is given to ensure that glucose enters the cell and carries potassium with it. All these treatments represent temporizing measures to be taken until elimination of excess potassium from the body can be accomplished.

Ideally, serum potassium concentrations should be below 5.5 mEq·L^{-1} before proceeding with elective surgery. Emergency surgery in the presence of hyperkalemia requires careful monitoring of the ECG to detect adverse effects of potassium on the heart. Avoidance of systemic acidosis due to hypoventilation or arterial hypoxemia is important, as this change would accentuate hyperkalemia.

Hypokalemia. Hypokalemia (serum potassium concentration below 3.5 mEq·L^{-1}) can be due to a decreased total body potassium content (vomiting, diarrhea, nasogastric suction) or an alteration in the distribution of potassium between intracellular and extracellular sites (respiratory alkalosis, metabolic alkalosis, beta-adrenergic stimulation). Adverse effects of chronic hypokalemia include decreased myocardial contractility and skeletal muscle weakness. There is increased automaticity of the atria and ventricles, manifesting as cardiac dysrhythmias. Alterations in cardiac conduction manifest on the ECG as prolongation of the P-R interval and Q-T interval and flattening of the T wave. Treatment of chronic hypokalemia is with potassium chloride supplementation given orally, remembering that several days will be necessary to replete potassium stores. Intravenous administration of potassium chloride (0.2 mEq·kg^{-1}·hr^{-1} to 0.4 mEq·kg^{-1}·hr^{-1}) is recommended when hypokalemia is associated with adverse cardiac changes.

The advisability of proceeding with elective surgery in the presence of serum potassium concentrations below 3.5 mEq·L^{-1} is controversial.[1] Nevertheless, in the absence of skeletal muscle weakness or abnormal findings on the ECG, elective operations can most likely be safely performed in the presence of moderate hypokalemia. Indeed the incidence of intraoperative cardiac dysrhythmias is not increased in otherwise asymptomatic patients with chronic hypokalemia (2.6 mEq·L^{-1} to 3.5 mEq·L^{-1}) undergoing elective operations.[2,3] Certainly, events known to acutely lower serum potassium concentration, such as iatrogenic hyperventilation, should be avoided.

Hypercalcemia. Hypercalcemia (serum calcium concentration above 5.5 mEq·L^{-1}) is typically due to hyperparathyroidism and neoplastic disorders with bone metastases (see Chapter 23). When serum calcium exceeds 8 mEq·L^{-1}, cardiac conduction disturbances manifest on the ECG as a prolonged P-R interval, wide QRS complex, and shortened Q-T interval. During anesthesia, it is important to maintain hydration and urine output to minimize further increases in the serum calcium concentration.

Hypocalcemia. Hypocalcemia (serum concentration below 4.5 mEq·L^{-1}) can be due to reduced serum albumin concentrations, hypoparathyroidism, pancreatitis, and renal failure (see Chapter 23). Impaired neuromuscular function in the presence of hypocalcemia reflects decreased presynaptic release of acetylcholine. Decreased myocardial contractility with elevated central venous pressure and hypotension are typical. Skeletal muscle spasm, including laryngospasm, may accompany hypocalcemia. During anesthesia, it is important to remember that respiratory alkalosis due to iatrogenic hyperventilation can rapidly reduce the serum ionized calcium concentration.

INTRAOPERATIVE FLUID THERAPY WITHOUT BLOOD LOSS

Solutions administered intravenously are required for maintenance of normal body fluid composition. Available solutions are classified either as crystalloids or colloids (see the section *Other Intravenous Solutions*). Colloids are frequently recommended for specific situations, such as fluid loss from fistulae, oozing from raw surfaces, and ascitic fluid. Crystalloid solutions are sufficient to maintain normal body fluid composition in the majority of patients (Table 18-2).

Independent of the type of surgery, all patients have insensible losses, which include evaporation of water from the respiratory tract, sweat, feces, and urinary excretion, all of which need to be replaced. This requires administration of about 2 ml·kg^{-1}·hr^{-1} intravenously of crystalloid solutions. Febrile patients or children may have larger insensible losses. As most patients have had no caloric intake for several hours, it may be useful to include some glucose in the crystalloid solutions.

In addition to replacing insensible losses, the extent to which surgery is traumatic will dictate how much additional crystalloid solution should be given intravenously. This reflects isotonic transfer of ECF from functional body fluid compartments to nonfunctional ones termed the *third space* (i.e., an acute sequestered edema space). This loss of fluid from the functional ECF to the third space needs to be replaced intraoperatively.

Guidelines for Intraoperative Crystalloid Therapy

Step 1: Administer isotonic electrolyte containing solutions (2 ml·kg^{-1}·hr^{-1}) to replace insensible losses.

Step 2: Administer additional electrolyte containing solutions at a rate based on estimated surgical trauma.
minimal trauma 3–4 ml·kg^{-1}·hr^{-1}
moderate trauma 5–6 ml·kg^{-1}·hr^{-1}
severe trauma 7–8 ml·kg^{-1}·hr^{-1}

Step 3: Replace every 1 ml of blood loss with 3 ml of crystalloid solution.

Step 4: Monitor vital signs and maintain urine output (0.5–1 ml·kg^{-1}·hr^{-1})

INTRAOPERATIVE FLUID THERAPY WITH BLOOD LOSS

If blood loss is sufficiently large, erythrocytes in the form of whole blood or packed red blood cells should be administered. Whole blood is probably preferable to packed red blood cells when replacing blood losses greater than 1500 ml. Compensatory changes in response to blood loss include vasoconstriction of the splanchnic system and the venous capacitance vessels. This vasoconstriction can conceal the signs of acute blood loss until at least 10 percent of the blood volume is lost. Healthy patients may lose up to 20 percent of their blood volume before signs occur, such as a reduction in central venous pressure, hypotension, or tachycardia. Anesthetics reduce the ability of the body to compensate for changes in blood loss and attenuate the classic signs of hypovolemia, such as tachycardia.

With acute blood loss, ISF and extravascular protein are transferred to the intravascular space, which tends to maintain PV. For this reason, when

Table 18.2. Comparison of Crystalloid Solutions

	Dextrose (mg·dl^{-1})	Na (mEq·L^{-1})	Cl (mEq·L^{-1})	K (mEq·L^{-1})	Mg (mEq·L^{-1})	Ca (mEq·L^{-1})	Lactate (mEq·L^{-1})	Approximate pH	mOsm·L^{-1} (calculated)
ECF	90-110	140	108	4.5	2.0	5.0	5.0	7.4	290
5% dextrose in water	50							5.0	253
5% dextrose in 0.45% NaCl	50	77	77					4.2	407
5% dextrose in 0.9% NaCl	50	154	154					4.2	407
0.9% NaCl		154	154					4.2	561
Lactated Ringer's solution		130	109	4.0		3.0	28	5.7	308
5% dextrose in lactated Ringer's solution	50	130	109	4.0		3.0	28	6.7	273
Normosol-R		140	98	5.0	3.0		a	5.3	527
5% NaCl		855	855					7.4	295
								5.6	1171

a Contains acetate 27 mEq·L^{-1} and gluconate 23 mEq·L^{-1}.

crystalloid solutions are used to replace blood loss, they must be given in amounts equal to about three times the amount of blood loss not only to replenish intravascular fluid volume, but also to replenish the fluid lost from interstitial spaces. Dextran and hetastarch are examples of artificial solutions that are useful for acute expansion of the intravascular fluid volume. In contrast to crystalloid solutions, dextran and hetastarch are more likely to remain in the intravascular space for prolonged periods of time. These solutions avoid complications associated with blood-containing products but obviously do not improve oxygen carrying capacity of the blood and in large volumes (greater than 20 ml·kg^{-1}) may cause coagulation defects. In the case of dextran, anaphylactoid reactions can result.

Arterial blood pressure, heart rate, and central venous pressure should be monitored to determine whether intravascular fluid volume is being adequately maintained. Although intravascular fluid volume can be maintained with crystalloid solutions, the underlying question is when should whole blood be administered. Serial determinations of the hematocrit may be helpful in this regard. Even though the hematocrit is not a reliable guide for assessing adequacy of intravascular fluid volume, it is useful for determining whether the ratio between crystalloid and blood therapy has been appropriate. To maximize oxygen carrying capacity and, conversely, to ensure that the viscosity of blood is such that capillary flow will be adequate, a hematocrit of 30 percent is often adequate. Therefore, when intravascular fluid volume is replaced, the hematocrit should be determined to assess whether the appropriate amount of blood has been given. For example, if the hematocrit is 35 percent to 40 percent, it would be appropriate to continue replacing blood loss with crystalloid solutions alone. If the hematocrit is 25 percent to 30 percent, it would be appropriate to administer blood as part of the replacement solutions.

BLOOD THERAPY

Determination of the blood type of the recipient and donor is the first step in selecting blood for transfusion therapy. Routine typing of blood is performed to identify the antigens (A, B, Rh) on the membrane of erythrocytes (Table 18-3). Naturally occurring antibodies (anti-B, anti-A) are formed whenever erythrocyte membranes lack A and/or B antigens. These antibodies are capable of causing rapid intravascular destruction of erythrocytes that contain the corresponding antigens.

Crossmatch

The major crossmatch occurs when the donor's erythrocytes are incubated with the recipient's plasma. Incubation of the donor's plasma with the recipient's erythrocytes is a minor crossmatch. Agglutination occurs if either the major or minor crossmatch is incompatible. The major crossmatch also checks for immunoglobulin G antibodies (Kell, Kidd). Type-specific blood means only the ABO-Rh type has been determined. The chances of a significant hemolytic reaction related to transfusion of type-specific blood is about 1 in 1000. If the recipient has a history of pregnancy or receipt of blood transfusions, the incidence, although undefined, may be higher with the use of type-specific blood.

Type and Screen

Type and screen denotes blood that has been typed for A, B, and Rh antigens and screened for common antibodies. This approach is used when the scheduled surgical procedure is unlikely to require transfusion of blood (hysterectomy, cholecystectomy) but is one in which blood should be available. Use of type and screen permits more efficient use of stored blood because it is available to more than one patient. The chances of a significant hemolytic reaction related to use of type and screen blood is 1 in 10,000. As indicated with type-specific blood, a history of pregnancy or receipt of blood transfusions, may be associated with a higher incidence of hemolytic reactions.

Predeposited Autologous Blood

Patients scheduled for elective surgery that may require transfusion of blood may elect to predonate (predeposit) blood for possible transfusion in the perioperative blood. This approach eliminates the chances of hemolytic reactions or transmission of viral diseases. Most patients can donate a unit

Table 18-3. Blood Groups and Crossmatch

Blood Group	Antigen on Erythrocyte	Plasma Antibodies	Incidence (%) Whites	Incidence (%) Blacks
A	A	Anti-B	40	27
B	B	Anti-A	11	20
AB	AB	None	4	4
O	None	Anti-A Anti-B	45	49
Rh	Rh		42	17

of blood every 7 days to 10 (maximum of 3 units) days, with the last unit collected 72 hours or more before surgery to permit restoration of plasma volume.

Blood Storage

Blood is stored either in citrate-phosphate-dextrose (CPD) or citrate-phosphate-dextrose-adenine (CPD-A_1) preservative at temperatures of 1° Celsius to 6° Celsius. Storage time (70 percent viability of transfused erythrocytes 24 hours after transfusion) is 21 days for CPD blood and 35 days for CPD-A_1 blood. Adenine increases erythrocyte survival by allowing these cells to resynthesize adenosine triphosphate needed to fuel metabolic reactions. Changes that occur in blood during storage reflect the length of storage and the type of preservative used (Table 18-4). A unit of blood contains about 450 ml of blood and 65 ml of citrate-containing preservative.

Component Therapy

A unit of blood can be divided into several components that allow prolonged storage and specific treatment of underlying abnormalities without simultaneous infusion of unnecessary fractions such as plasma, which may contain antigens or antibodies.[4]

Packed Red Blood Cells

Packed red blood cells (volume 250 ml to 300 ml and hematocrit 70 percent to 80 percent) are used for treatment of anemia not associated with acute hemorrhage. Nevertheless, it is recommended that packed erythrocytes be used to replace blood loss in adults less than 1500 ml.[5] The goal is to increase the oxygen carrying capacity of blood. A single unit of packed red blood cells will increase adult hemoglobin concentrations about 1 g·dl^{-1}.

Administration of packed red blood cells is

Table 18-4. Changes that Occur During Storage of Whole Blood in Citrate-Phosphate-Dextrose

	Days of Storage at 4° Celsius 1	7	14	21
pH	7.1	7.0	7.0	6.9
PCO_2 (mmHg)	48	80	110	140
Potassium (mEq·L^{-1})	3.9	12	17	21
2,3-Diphosphoglycerate (μM·ml^{-1})	4.8	1.2	1	1
Viable platelets (%)	10	0	0	0
Factors V and VIII (%)	70	50	40	20

Components Derived from Whole Blood

Packed red blood cells
Platelet concentrates
Fresh frozen plasma
Cryoprecipitate
Albumin
Plasma protein fraction
Leukocyte poor blood
Factor VIII
Antibody concentrates

---

facilitated by reconstituting them in crystalloid solutions such as 50 ml to 100 ml of saline. Use of hypotonic glucose solutions may cause hemolysis, whereas calcium, as present in lactated Ringer's solution, may cause clotting if mixed with packed red blood cells.

Complications associated with packed red blood cells are similar to those of whole blood. An exception would be the chance of developing citrate intoxication, which would be less with packed red blood cells than whole blood because less citrate is infused. Infusion of less plasma reduces the likelihood of allergic reactions accompanying the administration of packed red blood cells. Conversely, removal of plasma also reduces the concentration of factors V and VIII. No data document a decreased risk of post-transfusion hepatitis when packed red blood cells are used instead of whole blood.[4]

Platelet Concentrates

Platelet concentrates allow specific treatment of thrombocytopenia without infusion of unnecessary blood components. One unit of platelet concentrate will increase the platelet count 5000 mm^3 to 10,000 mm^3 as documented by platelet counts obtained 1 hour after infusion. Risks of platelet concentrate infusions are (1) sensitization reactions due to HLA antigens on cell membranes of platelets, and (2) transmission of viral diseases, especially if pooled donor products are administered.

Fresh Frozen Plasma

Fresh frozen plasma is the fluid portion obtained from a single unit of whole blood that is frozen within 6 hours of collection. All coagulation factors, except platelets, are present in fresh frozen plasma, explaining the use of this component for treatment of hemorrhage due to presumed coagulation factor deficiencies. Nevertheless, there is no evidence that fresh frozen plasma is superior to specific factor concentrates or that its use is indicated in hemorrhaging patients in the absence of a documented procoagulant defect.[4,6] Risks of fresh frozen plasma include transmission of viral diseases and allergic reactions.

Cryoprecipitate

Cryoprecipitate is that fraction of plasma that precipitates when fresh frozen plasma is thawed. This component is useful for treating hemophilia A because it contains high concentrations of factor VIII in a small volume.

Albumin

Albumin is available as 5 percent and 25 percent solutions. The 5 percent solution is isotonic with pooled plasma and is most often used when rapid expansion of the intravascular fluid volume is indicated. Hypoalbuminemia is the most frequent indication for administration of 25 percent albumin. It must be recognized that albumin solutions do not provide coagulation factors. Plasma protein fractions (Plasmanate) are 5 percent solutions of plasma proteins in saline. The risk of transmission of hepatitis with all these protein solutions is eliminated by heat treatment to 60° Celsius for 10 hours.

COMPLICATIONS OF BLOOD THERAPY

Complications of blood therapy, like an adverse effect of any therapy, must be considered when evaluating the risk-to-benefit ratio for treatment of individual patients with blood products. Anesthesiologists are among the most likely physicians to administer blood products to patients; therefore, it is imperative that complications of this therapy be fully appreciated.

Complications of Blood Therapy

Transfusion reactions
   Febrile
   Allergic
   Hemolytic

Metabolic abnormalities
   Acidosis
   Accumulation of potassium
   Decreased 2,3-diphosphoglycerate

Citrate intoxication
   Alkalosis
   Hypocalcemia

Transmission of viral diseases

Microaggregates

Hypothermia

Coagulation disorders
   Dilutional thrombocytopenia
   Dilution of factors V and VIII
   Disseminated intravascular coagulation

Transfusion Reactions

Transfusion reactions are categorized as febrile, allergic, and hemolytic.

Febrile Reactions

Febrile reactions are the most common adverse nonhemolytic responses to transfusion of blood accompanying 0.5 percent to 1 percent of transfusions.[4] The most likely explanation for febrile reactions is an interaction between recipient antibodies and antigens present on the leukocytes and/or platelets of the donor. Temperature rarely increases above 38° Celsius and treatment is by slowing the infusion and administration of antipyretics. Severe febrile reactions accompanied by chills and shivering may require discontinuation of the blood infusion.

Allergic Reactions

Allergic reactions to properly typed and cross-matched blood manifest as body temperature elevations, pruritus, and urticaria. Treatment often includes administration of antihistamines and, in severe cases, discontinuation of the blood infusion. Examination of the plasma and urine for free hemoglobin is useful to rule out hemolytic reactions.

Hemolytic Reactions

Hemolytic reactions occur when the wrong blood type is administered to a patient. The common factor in the production of intravascular hemolysis and development of spontaneous hemorrhage is activation of the complement system. With the exception of hypotension, the immediate signs (lumbar and substernal pain, fever, chills, dyspnea, skin flushing) of hemolytic reactions are masked by general anesthesia. Appearance of free hemoglobin in the plasma or urine is presumptive evidence of a hemolytic reaction. Acute renal failure reflects precipitation of stromal and lipid contents (not free hemoglobin) of hemolyzed erythrocytes in distal renal tubules. Disseminated intravascular coagulation is initiated by material released from hemolyzed erythrocytes (see the section *Disseminated Intravascular Coagulation*).

Treatment of acute hemolytic reactions is immediate discontinuation of the incompatible blood infusion and maintenance of urine output by infusion of crystalloid solutions and administration of mannitol or furosemide. Sodium bicarbonate to alkalinize the urine and improve solubility of hemoglobin degradation products in the renal tubules is of unproven value as is the administration of corticosteroids.

Metabolic Abnormalities

Metabolic abnormalities that accompany the storage of whole blood include accumulation of hydrogen ions and potassium, and decreased 2,3-diphosphoglycerate (2,3-DPG) concentrations (Table 18-4). Citrate present in the blood preservative may produce changes in the recipient.

Hydrogen Ions

Addition of CPD preservative (pH 5 to 5.6) immediately increases the hydrogen ion content of stored whole blood. Continued metabolic function of erythrocytes results in additional production of hydrogen ions. Despite these changes, metabolic acidosis is not a consistent occurrence, even with rapid infusion of large volumes of stored blood. Therefore, intravenous administration of sodium bicarbonate to patients receiving transfusions of whole blood should be determined by measurement of pH and not based on arbitrary regimens.

Potassium

Potassium content of stored blood increases progressively with storage, but even massive transfusions rarely increase plasma potassium concentrations. Failure of potassium concentrations to increase most likely reflects the small amount of potassium actually present in a unit of stored blood. For example, since a unit of whole blood contains only 300 ml of plasma, a measured plasma potassium concentration of 21 $mEq \cdot L^{-1}$ would represent less than 7 mEq of potassium.

Decreased 2,3-Diphosphoglycerate (2,3-DPG)

Storage of blood is associated with progressive reductions in concentrations of 2,3-DPG in erythrocytes, resulting in increased affinity of hemoglobin for oxygen (decreased P_{50} values). Conceivably, this change could jeopardize tissue oxygen delivery. Nevertheless, the clinical significance of 2,3-DPG changes remains unconfirmed.

Citrate

Citrate metabolism to bicarbonate may contribute to metabolic alkalosis, whereas binding of calcium by citrate could result in hypocalcemia. Indeed, metabolic alkalosis, rather than metabolic acidosis, is a common accompaniment of massive blood transfusions. Hypocalcemia due to citrate binding of calcium is rare, reflecting mobilization of calcium stores in bone and the ability of the liver to metabolize rapidly citrate to bicarbonate. Therefore, arbitrary administration of calcium in the absence of objective evidence of hypocalcemia

(prolonged Q-T intervals on the ECG; measured reductions in plasma ionized calcium concentrations) is not indicated. Supplemental calcium may be needed when (1) the rate of blood infusion exceeds 50 $ml \cdot min^{-1}$ (as may be required during liver transplantation), (2) hypothermia or liver disease interferes with metabolism of citrate, or (3) the patient is a neonate (Fig. 18-2).[7]

Transmission of Viral Diseases

Transmission of viral diseases (acquired immunodeficiency syndrome [AIDS], hepatitis, cytomegalovirus) is a risk of administration of blood or its components. Despite careful screening of blood, before 1985, the incidence of non-A non-B hepatitis was 5 percent to 10 percent of patients receiving five or more blood transfusions, and several thousand patients had received blood containing the virus responsible for AIDS.[8] Since the institution of elimination of donors in high risk groups for AIDS and testing donor blood for antibodies to the AIDS virus in 1985, only 13 cases of transfusion-transmitted AIDS have been reported, and the incidence of hepatitis has been reduced by 50 percent. Nevertheless, possible transmission of diseases should assume a prominent place in the evaluation of the risk-to-benefit ratio associated with treatment of individual patients with blood. In many instances, nonblood solutions become more acceptable treatment when the risk of transmission of disease is considered.

Microaggregates

Microaggregates consisting of platelets and leukocytes form during storage of whole blood (Fig. 18-3).[9] Infusion of these microaggregates may be undesirable (pulmonary dysfunction), and micropore filters have been developed to remove particles with diameters in the 10 micron to 40 micron range. Nevertheless, use of these filters has not been documented to be beneficial.[10] Resistance to flow is increased and hemolysis can occur when blood more than 14 days old is forced through micropore filters. It must be recognized, however, that stored blood should always be administered through 170 micron filters.

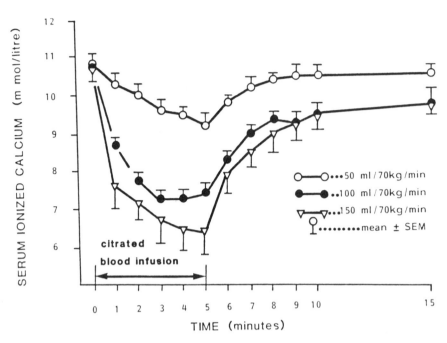

Fig. 18-2. Serum ionized calcium concentrations were measured at three different rates of infusion over a 5-minute period. (From Denlinger et al.,[7] with permission.)

Hypothermia

Administration of blood stored at less than 6° Celsius can result in decreases in the patient's body temperature, with the possible development of cardiac irritability. Even a decrease of body temperature as small as 0.5° Celsius to 1° Celsius may induce shivering postoperatively, which in turn may increase oxygen consumption by as much as 400 percent. To meet the demands of an elevated oxygen consumption, cardiac output must be increased. This may be too much stress for patients with marginal cardiac reserves. Passage of blood through specially designed warmers greatly reduces the likelihood of transfusion related hypothermia. Use of a blood warmer, however, does not alter the concentration of potassium in stored blood.[11]

Coagulation Disorders

Massive blood transfusions (10 units or more) can result in coagulation disorders due to dilutional thrombocytopenia and/or dilution of plasma con-

centrations of factors V and VIII. Disseminated intravascular coagulation due to hemolytic transfusion reactions must also be considered when intraoperative bleeding due to unknown causes occurs.

Dilutional Thrombocytopenia

Dilutional thrombocytopenia reflects the virtual absence of viable platelets in blood stored at 4° Celsius for more than 24 hours (Table 18-4). It is likely that platelet counts will decline below 100,000 mm^3 in adult patients receiving 10 units to 15 units of whole blood (Fig. 18-4).[12] Bleeding may be associated with acute reductions in the platelet count to less than 100,000 mm^3. Treatment of dilutional thrombocytopenia is with infusion of platelet concentrates (see the section *Platelet Concentrates*).

Dilution of Factors V and VIII

Levels of factors V and VIII decrease in stored whole blood (all other clotting factors remain stable), but dilution of these factors in the patient's

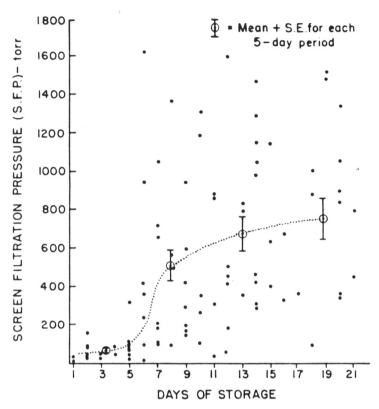

Fig. 18-3. Screen filtration pressures as a reflection of accumulation of microaggregates with increasing duration of storage of blood. (From Harp et al.,[9] with permission.)

plasma from massive blood transfusions is rarely sufficient to cause bleeding (Table 18-4). Indeed, only 5 percent to 20 percent of the normal amount of factor V and 30 percent of factor VIII are necessary for hemostasis during surgery. Abnormalities due to dilution of clotting factors are more likely to occur with infusion of erythrocytes that include minimal plasma volume. Fresh frozen plasma is the indicated treatment when specific measurements (prothrombin time, plasma thromboplastin time) confirm reduced plasma concentrations of these factors.

Disseminated Intravascular Coagulation

Disseminated intravascular coagulation is characterized by uncontrolled activation of the coagulation system, with consumption of platelets and coagulants. Thrombocytopenia, prolongation of the prothrombin time and thromboplastin time, and increased circulating concentrations of fibrin degradation products in the presence of diffuse hemorrhage (as around catheter placement sites) suggest the diagnosis. Treatment is removal of the underlying cause (hemolytic transfusion reaction, low cardiac output, hypovolemia, sepsis) and administration of platelet concentrates and fresh frozen plasma.

Immunosuppression

Blood transfusions exert a nonspecific immunosuppressive action that may be therapeutic for renal transplant recipients and detrimental for patients with cancer.[13] Packed erythrocytes, which contain less plasma than whole blood, may produce less immunosuppression, suggesting that plasma contains an undefined immunosuppressive factor.

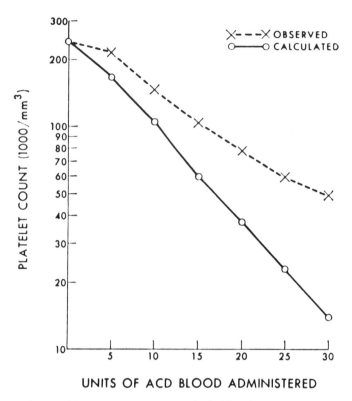

Fig. 18-4. Platelet counts observed in patients receiving whole blood stored longer than 24 hours are compared with predicted platelet counts if platelet-free solutions had been administered. (From Miller et al.,[12] with permission.)

INDICATIONS FOR BLOOD TRANSFUSIONS

The increased concern relating to the infectivity of blood transfusions (i.e., AIDS, hepatitis) has resulted in anesthesiologists becoming especially conservative with respect to the indications for administration of homologous blood to patients. A general rule of thumb is that perioperative blood transfusions are probably not indicated for patients with hematocrit values above 30 percent.

REFERENCES

1. Harrington JT, Isner JM, Kassirer JP. Our national obsession with potassium. Am J Med 1982;73:155–9.
2. Vitez TS, Soper LE, Wong KC, Soper P. Chronic hypokalemia and intraoperative dysrhythmias. Anesthesiology 1985;63:130–3.
3. Hirsh IA, Tomlinson DL, Slogoff S, Keats AS. The overstated risk of preoperative hypokalemia. Anesth Analg 1988;67:131–6.
4. Stehling LC. Recent advances in transfusion therapy. In: Stoelting RK, Barash PG, Gallagher TJ, eds. Advances in Anesthesia. Chicago, Year Book Medical Publishers, 1987;4:213–52.
5. Grindon AJ, Tomasulo PS, Bergen JJ, et al. The hospital transfusion committee: Guidelines for improving practice. JAMA 1985;253:540–3.
6. Bove JR. Fresh frozen plasma: Too few indications—too much use. Anesth Analg 1985;64:849–50.
7. Denlinger JK, Nahrwold ML, Gibbs PS, Lecky JH. Hypocalcemia during rapid blood transfusion in anesthetized man. Br J Anaesth 1976;48:995–1000.
8. Dienstag JL. Non-A, non-B hepatitis. I. Recognition, epidemiology, and clinical features. Gastroenterology 1983;439–62.
9. Harp JR, Wyche MQ, Marshall BE, Wurzel HA. Some factors determining rate of microaggregate formation in stored blood. Anesthesiology 1974;40:398–400.
10. Snyder EL, Hazzey A, Barash PG, Palmero G. Microaggregate blood filtration in patients with com-

promised pulmonary function. Transfusion 1982;22:21–5.

11. Eurenius S, Smith RM. The effect of warming on the serum potassium content of stored blood. Anesthesiology 1973;38:482–4.

12. Miller RD, Robbins TO, Tong MJ. Coagulation de-fects associated with massive blood transfusions. Ann Surg 1971;174:798–801.

13. Schriemer PA, Longnecker DE, Mintz PD. The possible immunosuppressive effects of perioperative blood transfusion in cancer patients. Anesthesiology 1988;68:422–8.

Special Anesthetic Considerations

Chapter 19

Cardiac Disease

Management of anesthesia for patients with cardiovascular disease requires an understanding of the pathophysiology of the disease process and a careful selection of anesthetics, muscle relaxants, and monitors to match the unique needs introduced by each individual patient.

CORONARY ARTERY DISEASE

Coronary artery disease is estimated to be present in 10 million adults, and it is likely that 5 percent to 10 percent of patients who undergo anesthesia and surgery have associated coronary artery disease. The presence of coronary artery disease in patients who undergo anesthesia for noncardiac surgery is associated with increased morbidity and mortality. Patient history, physical examination, and evaluation of the electrocardiogram (ECG) are important components of the routine preoperative cardiac evaluation.[1] More specialized procedures, such as the ambulatory ECG (Holter monitoring), exercise electrocardiography, echocardiography, radioisotope imaging, cardiac catheterization, and angiography, are performed on selected patients. Ultimately, data should determine whether patients are in the best medical condition possible before elective cardiac or noncardiac surgery.

Patient History

Important aspects of the history taken from patients with coronary artery disease before noncardiac surgery include cardiac reserve, characteristics

of angina pectoris, and the presence of a prior myocardial infarction. Potential interactions of medications used in the treatment of coronary artery disease with drugs used to produce anesthesia must also be considered. Co-existing noncardiac diseases that often present in these patients include peripheral vascular disease, chronic obstructive airways disease from cigarette smoking, renal dysfunction associated with chronic hypertension, and diabetes mellitus. A thorough evaluation is especially important because patients can remain asymptomatic despite 50 percent to 70 percent stenosis of a major coronary artery.

Cardiac Reserve

Limited exercise tolerance in the absence of significant pulmonary disease is the most striking evidence of reduced cardiac reserve. If a patient can climb two flights to three flights of stairs without symptoms, cardiac reserve is probably adequate.

Angina Pectoris

Angina pectoris is considered to be stable when no change has occurred for at least 60 days in precipitating factors, frequency, and duration. Chest pain produced with less than normal activity or lasting for increasingly longer periods of time is considered to be characteristic of unstable angina pectoris and may signal an impending myocardial infarction. Dyspnea following the onset of angina pectoris is indicative of acute left ventricular dysfunction due to myocardial ischemia. Angina pectoris due to spasm of the coronary arteries (variant or Prinzmetal's angina) differs from classic angina pectoris in that it may occur at rest but not during vigorous exertion.

Knowledge of the heart rate and/or systolic blood pressure at which angina pectoris or evidence of myocardial ischemia occurs on the ECG is important preoperative information. These values should not be exceeded intraoperatively. An increased heart rate is more likely than hypertension to produce signs of myocardial ischemia. This is predictable because a rapid heart rate increases myocardial oxygen requirements and reduces the time during diastole for coronary blood flow and thus delivery of oxygen to occur. Conversely, elevated myocardial oxygen requirements produced by increased systolic blood pressure are offset by improved perfusion through pressure-dependent atherosclerotic coronary arteries.

Prior Myocardial Infarction

The incidence of myocardial reinfarction in the perioperative period is related to the time elapsed since the previous myocardial infarction (Table 19-1).[2,3] The incidence of perioperative myocardial reinfarctions does not stabilize at 5 percent to 6 percent until 6 months after the prior myocardial infarction. Thus, a common recommendation is to delay elective surgery especially thoracic and upper abdominal procedures for about 6 months after a

myocardial infarction. Even after 6 months, the 5 percent to 6 percent incidence of myocardial reinfarction is about 50 times greater than the 0.13 percent incidence of perioperative myocardial infarction in patients undergoing similar operations but in the absence of a prior myocardial infarction. None of the myocardial reinfarctions observed in these studies occurred intraoperatively. Indeed, the greatest incidence of myocardial reinfarction is observed on the third postoperative day.

Several factors influence the incidence of myocardial reinfarction in the perioperative period. For example, the incidence of myocardial reinfarction is increased in patients undergoing intrathoracic or intra-abdominal operations lasting longer than 3 hours. Factors that have not been shown to predispose to a myocardial reinfarction include the (1) site of the previous myocardial infarction, (2) history of prior aortocoronary bypass graft surgery, (3) site of the operative procedure if the duration of the surgery is less than 3 hours, and (4) drugs and/or techniques used to produce anesthesia. Finally, close hemodynamic monitoring using intra-arterial and pulmonary artery catheters and prompt pharmacologic intervention or fluid infusions to treat hemodynamic alterations from a normal range may reduce the risk of perioperative myocardial reinfarctions in high risk patients (Table 19-1).[4]

Current Medications

Drugs most likely to be encountered in patients with coronary artery disease are beta antagonists, nitrates, and calcium channel blockers. In addition, patients with coronary artery disease may be receiving drugs classified as antihypertensives and diuretics. A knowledge of the pharmacology of these drugs and potential adverse interactions with anesthetics is an important preoperative consideration (see Chapters 3 and 22). Despite the potential for adverse drug interactions, cardiac medications being taken preoperatively probably should be continued without interruption through the perioperative period.

Electrocardiogram

The preoperative ECG should be examined for evidence of (1) myocardial ischemia, (2) prior myocardial infarction, (3) cardiac hypertrophy, (4)

Table 19-1. Incidence of Perioperative Myocardial Infarction

Time Elapsed Since Prior Myocardial Infarction	Tarhan et al.[2]	Steen et al.[3]	Rao et al.[4]
Less than 3 months	37%	27%	5.7%
3 months to 6 months	16%	11%	2.3%
Greater than 6 months	5%	6%	

Values for Rao et al. are 0 to 3 months and 4 months to 6 months respectively.

Table 19-2. Area of Myocardial Ischemia as Reflected by the Electrocardiogram

Electro-cardiogram Lead	Coronary Artery Responsible for Myocardial Ischemia	Area of Myocardium that may be Involved
II, III, aVF	Right coronary artery	Right atrium Sinus node Atrioventricular node Right ventricle
$V_3 - V_5$	Left anterior descending coronary artery	Anterolateral aspects of the left ventricle
I, aVL	Circumflex coronary artery	Lateral aspects of the left ventricle

abnormal cardiac rhythm and/or conduction disturbances, and (5) electrolyte abnormalities. The resting ECG in the absence of angina pectoris may be normal despite extensive coronary artery disease. Nevertheless, an ECG demonstrating S-T segment depression greater than 1 mm, particularly during angina pectoris, confirms the presence of myocardial ischemia. Furthermore, the ECG lead demonstrating changes of myocardial ischemia can help determine the specific diseased coronary artery (Table 19-2). It should be remembered that prior myocardial infarctions, especially if subendocardial, may not be accompanied by persistent changes on the ECG. The preoperative presence of premature ventricular beats may signal their likely occurrence intraoperatively. A P-R interval on the electrocardiogram greater than 0.2 second is most often related to digitalis therapy. Conversely, blocks of conduction of cardiac impulses that occur below the atrioventricular node most likely reflect pathologic changes rather than drug effect.

Management of Anesthesia

Management of anesthesia in patients with coronary artery disease is based on a preoperative evaluation of left ventricular function and the maintenance of a favorable balance between myocardial oxygen requirements and myocardial oxygen delivery so as to prevent myocardial ischemia

(Table 19-3). Any perioperative event associated with persistent tachycardia, systolic hypertension, arterial hypoxemia, or diastolic hypotension can adversely influence this delicate balance. The maintenance of this balance is more important than the specific technique and/or drugs selected to produce anesthesia and skeletal muscle paralysis. It is critical that persistent and excessive changes in heart rate and blood pressure be avoided. Heart rate and blood pressure probably should be maintained within 20 percent of the awake values. Nevertheless, an estimated one-half of all new perioperative ischemic episodes are not preceded by or associated with significant changes in heart rate or blood pressure.[5] These episodes of silent myocardial ischemia are likely due to regional reductions in myocardial perfusion and oxygenation that are of questionable significance and identical to episodes that occur in these same patients during their daily activities unassociated with angina pectoris.

Induction of Anesthesia

Preoperative medication should produce reliable sedation so as to allay anxiety, which if unopposed could lead to secretion of catecholamines and an increase in myocardial oxygen requirements due to an elevation of blood pressure and heart rate. A frequent approach is intramuscular administration of morphine plus scopolamine with or without benzodiazepines. Scopolamine is valuable because of its profound sedative and amnesic effects without producing undesirable changes in heart rate. It may also be appropriate to apply a transdermal preparation of nitroglycerin at the time the preoperative medication is administered. Furthermore, a continuous intravenous infusion of nitroglycerin (0.25 $\mu g \cdot kg^{-1} \cdot min^{-1}$ to 0.5 $\mu g \cdot kg^{-1} \cdot min^{-1}$) during the perioperative period should also be considered in patients with known coronary artery disease.

Induction of anesthesia is acceptably accomplished with the intravenous administration of barbiturates, benzodiazepines, opioids or etomidate, or by inhalation via a mask. Ketamine increases heart rate and blood pressure and would likely increase myocardial oxygen requirements. Intubation of the trachea is facilitated by the

Table 19-3. Evaluation of Left Ventricular Function

	Good Function	Impaired Function
Prior myocardial infarction	No	Yes
Evidence of congestive heart failure	No	Yes
Ejection fraction	>0.55	<0.4
Left ventricular end-diastolic pressure	<12 mmHg	>18 mmHg
Cardiac index	>2.5 $L \cdot min^{-1} \cdot m^{-2}$	<2 $L \cdot min^{-1} \cdot m^{-2}$
Areas of ventricular dyskinesia	No	Yes

administration of succinylcholine or nondepolarizing muscle relaxants.

Myocardial ischemia may accompany the hypertension and tachycardia that result from the stimulation of direct laryngoscopy necessary for intubation of the trachea. A short duration of direct laryngoscopy (ideally less than 15 seconds) is important in minimizing the magnitude of these circulatory changes. When the duration of direct laryngoscopy is not likely to be short or when hypertension co-exists, the addition of other drugs to minimize the pressor response produced by intubation of the trachea should be considered. For example, laryngotracheal lidocaine (2 $mg \cdot kg^{-1}$) administered just before inserting the tube into the trachea minimizes the magnitude and duration of the blood pressure increase. Likewise, lidocaine 1.5 $mg \cdot kg^{-1}$, administered intravenously about 90 seconds before beginning direct laryngoscopy, is efficacious. An alternative to lidocaine is nitroprusside 1 $\mu g \cdot kg^{-1}$ to 2 $\mu g \cdot kg^{-1}$ administered intravenously about 15 seconds before beginning direct laryngoscopy or short acting opioids such as fentanyl (1 $\mu g \cdot kg^{-1}$ to 3 $\mu g \cdot kg^{-1}$) or sufentanil (0.1 $\mu g \cdot kg^{-1}$ to 0.3 $\mu g \cdot kg^{-1}$) injected 2 minutes to 4 minutes before beginning direct laryngoscopy. None of these pharmacologic interventions, however, reliably prevent heart rate increases produced by direct laryngoscopy. Continuous intravenous infusions of esmolol, a short acting beta antagonist, are effective in attenuating heart rate increases associated with painful stimulation including direct laryngoscopy.

Maintenance of Anesthesia

Choice of anesthesia is often based on the patient's left ventricular function. For example, patients with coronary artery disease but normal left ven-

---

Determinants of Myocardial Oxygen Requirements and Delivery

Myocardial oxygen requirements
  Heart rate
  Systemic blood pressure
  Myocardial contractility
  Ventricular volume

Myocardial oxygen delivery
  Coronary blood flow
  Oxygen content of arterial blood

---

tricular function are likely to develop tachycardia and hypertension in response to intense stimulation. Controlled myocardial depression produced by volatile anesthetics with or without nitrous oxide may be appropriate if the primary goal is to prevent increased myocardial oxygen requirements. Equally acceptable for the maintenance of anesthesia is the use of a nitrous oxide-opioid technique, with the addition of volatile anesthetics as necessary to treat hypertension. When hypertension is treated with a volatile anesthetic, isoflurane lowers blood pressure by decreasing systemic vascular resistance whereas halothane tends to lower blood pressure by reducing cardiac output (see Chapter 4).

Isoflurane is a more potent coronary arteriole vasodilator than halothane.[6] Conceivably, isoflurane-induced coronary arteriole vasodilation could result in diversion of blood flow from ischemic areas of myocardium (blood vessels already fully dilated) to nonischemic areas of myocardium supplied by vessels capable of vasodilation. Regional myocardial ischemia associated with drug-induced vasodilation is known as *coronary artery steal.*[7] Evidence of isoflurane-induced coronary artery steal is the appearance of ischemic changes on the ECG. Nevertheless, most patients with coronary artery disease do not develop evidence of myocardial ischemia during administration of isoflurane, and evidence of myocardial ischemia on the ECG may disappear when isoflurane is used to normalize blood pressure in anesthetized hypertensive patients.[8] All factors considered, isoflurane, enflurane, and halothane may be (1) beneficial in patients with coronary artery disease because they reduce myocardial oxygen requirements, or (2) detrimental because they lower blood pressure and coronary perfusion pressure or produce coronary artery steal (isoflurane).

Patients with impaired left ventricular function, as associated with a prior myocardial infarction, may not tolerate direct myocardial depression produced by volatile anesthetics. In these patients, the use of short-acting opioids with nitrous oxide may be more appropriate. It must be remembered that nitrous oxide, when administered to patients who have received opioids for anesthesia, may produce undesirable reductions in blood pressure and cardiac output. High dose fentanyl (50 $\mu g \cdot kg^{-1}$ to 100 $\mu g \cdot kg^{-1}$) or equivalent doses of sufentanil as the sole anesthetic has been advocated for patients who cannot tolerate even minimal anesthetic induced myocardial depression.

A regional anesthetic is an acceptable technique in patients with coronary artery disease. It is important to realize, however, that flow through coronary arteries narrowed by atherosclerosis is pressure dependent. Therefore, reductions in blood pressure associated with a regional anesthetic that exceed about 20 percent of the preblock value probably should be treated with an intravenous infusion of crystalloid solutions and/or sympathomimetics such as ephedrine.

Muscle Relaxant

The choice of nondepolarizing muscle relaxant during maintenance of anesthesia for patients with coronary artery disease is influenced by the circulatory effects of these drugs and the likely impact of these changes on myocardial oxygen require-

ments and myocardial oxygen delivery (see Chapter 8). Metocurine, atracurium, and vecuronium are useful choices in patients with coronary artery disease, as these drugs do not produce significant changes in heart rate or blood pressure and are, therefore, unlikely to alter myocardial oxygen requirements. Pancuronium increases heart rate and blood pressure, but these changes are usually less than 10 percent to 15 percent above predrug values, making this drug a possible choice for administration to patients with coronary artery disease. Furthermore, circulatory changes produced by pancuronium can be used to offset negative inotropic and/or chronotropic effects of drugs being used for anesthesia. Atracurium or vecuronium, in contrast to pancuronium, would not be expected to offset reductions in blood pressure or heart rate. Indeed, bradycardia associated with administration of high doses of opioids may be particularly prominent in patients receiving intermediate acting muscle relaxants.[9] Reductions in blood pressure produced by d-tubocurarine could jeopardize myocardial oxygen delivery by decreasing coronary blood flow, making this drug an unlikely choice.

Reversal of nondepolarizing neuromuscular blockade with anticholinesterase-anticholinergic combinations can be safely accomplished in patients with coronary artery disease. Glycopyrrolate apparently has less of a chronotropic effect than atropine and may be the anticholinergic of choice. Nevertheless, marked increases in heart rate rarely occur with reversal of nondepolarizing muscle relaxants and, therefore, atropine seems as acceptable as glycopyrrolate for combination with anticholinesterases.

Monitoring

The intensity of monitoring in the perioperative period is influenced by the complexity of the operative procedure and severity of the coronary artery disease. The ECG is the only practical way to monitor the balance between myocardial oxygen requirements and myocardial oxygen delivery in unconscious patients (see Chapter 16). When this balance is unfavorably altered, myocardial ischemia occurs as evidenced on the ECG by at least 1 mm downsloping of the S-T segment from the base line. A precordial V5 lead is a useful selection for detecting S-T segment changes characteristic of myocardial ischemia of the left ventricle during anesthesia. A pulmonary artery catheter is helpful for monitoring responses to intravenous fluid replacement and the therapeutic effects of drugs on left ventricular function. Right atrial pressure may not reliably reflect left heart filling pressure in the presence of left ventricular dysfunction due to coronary artery disease. Conversely, right atrial pressure correlates with pulmonary artery occlusion pressure in patients with coronary artery disease when the ejection fraction is above 0.5 and there is no evidence of left ventricular dysfunction.[10]

The appearance of signs of myocardial ischemia on the ECG supports the aggressive treatment of adverse changes in heart rate and/or blood pressure. Tachycardia is treated with the intravenous administration of propranolol or esmolol, whereas excessive increases in blood pressure respond to nitroprusside. Nitroglycerin is a more appropriate choice than nitroprusside when myocardial ischemia is associated with a normal blood pressure. Hypotension should be treated with sympathomimetics so as to rapidly restore pressure-dependent perfusion through atherosclerotic coronary arteries. In addition to drugs, the intravenous infusion of fluids to restore blood pressure is useful because myocardial oxygen requirements for volume work of the heart are less than those for pressure work. A disadvantage of this approach is the time necessary for fluid treatment to be effective.

Reductions in body temperature that occur intraoperatively may predispose to shivering on awakening, leading to abrupt increases in myocardial oxygen requirements. Attempts to minimize reductions in body temperature and provision of supplemental oxygen are of obvious importance. Postoperative pain relief is important as pain-induced activation of the sympathetic nervous system can increase myocardial oxygen requirements.

VALVULAR HEART DISEASE

The most frequently encountered forms of valvular heart disease produce pressure overload (mitral stenosis, aortic stenosis) or volume overload (mitral regurgitation, aortic regurgitation) of the left ventricle. The net effect of valvular heart disease is interference with forward flow of blood from the heart into the systemic circulation. Selection of anesthetic drugs and muscle relaxants for patients with valvular heart disease are based on the likely effects that drug-induced changes in cardiac rhythm, heart rate, blood pressure, systemic vascular resistance, and pulmonary vascular resistance will have relative to maintenance of cardiac output in these patients. When cardiac reserve is minimal, high doses of short-acting opioids may be used as the sole anesthetic. Patients with valvular heart disease should receive antibiotics in the perioperative period for protection against infective endocarditis.

Mitral Stenosis

Mitral stenosis is characterized by mechanical obstruction to left ventricular diastolic filling secondary to a progressive decrease in the orifice of the mitral valve. The obstruction produces an increase in left atrial and pulmonary venous pressure. Increased pulmonary vascular resistance is likely when the left atrial pressure is chronically elevated above 25 mmHg. Distension of the left atrium predisposes to atrial fibrillation, whereas stasis of blood in this chamber favors the formation of thrombi, which can be displaced as systemic emboli. Mitral stenosis is almost always due to the fusion of the mitral valve leaflets during the healing process of acute rheumatic carditis. Symptoms of mitral stenosis do not usually develop until about 20 years after the initial episode of rheumatic fever. A sudden increase in the demand for cardiac output as produced by pregnancy or sepsis, however, may unmask previously asymptomatic mitral stenosis.

Patients taking digitalis preoperatively for the control of heart rate should continue to take this drug until surgery. Adequate digitalis effect for heart rate control is reflected by a ventricular rate of less than 80 beats·min^{-1}. Because diuretic therapy is common, the serum potassium concentration should be measured preoperatively. Also, patients with mitral stenosis can be more susceptible than normal individuals to the ventilatory depressant effects of sedative drugs used for preoperative medication. When anticholinergics are included in the preoperative medication, scopolamine, or glycopyrrolate, have fewer chronotropic effects than atropine.

Management of Anesthesia

Induction of anesthesia in the presence of mitral stenosis can be safely achieved with intravenous administration of barbiturates, benzodiazepines, or etomidate followed by succinylcholine or nondepolarizing muscle relaxants to facilitate intubation of the trachea. Ketamine is probably not a good choice for induction of anesthesia because of its propensity to increase heart rate. Drugs used for maintenance of anesthesia should cause minimal changes in heart rate and in systemic and pulmonary vascular resistance. Furthermore, these drugs should not greatly reduce myocardial contractility. These goals can be achieved with combinations of nitrous oxide and opioids or low concentrations of volatile anesthetics. Although nitrous oxide can increase pulmonary vascular resistance, it is not of sufficient magnitude to justify avoiding this drug in all patients with mitral stenosis (Fig. 19-1).[11] The effect of nitrous oxide on pulmonary vascular resistance, however, seems to be accentuated when co-existing pulmonary hypertension is severe.

Nondepolarizing muscle relaxants with minimal circulatory effects (metocurine, atracurium, vecuronium) are useful in patients with mitral stenosis. Pancuronium is less appropriate because of its ability to increase the speed of transmission of cardiac impulses through the atrioventricular node, which could lead to excessive increases in heart rate. Such increases would seem particularly likely in the presence of atrial fibrillation because the ventricular response to atrial impulses is determined by the degree of atrioventricular conduction. There is no reason to avoid pharmacologic reversal of nondepolarizing muscle relaxants, but the adverse effects of drug-induced tachycardia should be anticipated. Intraoperative fluid therapy must be carefully titrated as these patients are susceptible to intravascular volume overload and to the development of left ventricular failure and pulmonary edema. Likewise, the head-down position is not well tolerated because the pulmonary

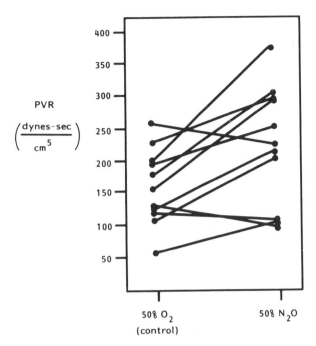

Fig. 19-1. Compared with control values for calculated pulmonary vascular resistance (PVR), the inhalation of 50 percent nitrous oxide increased PVR in 8 of 11 patients. Nevertheless, the magnitude of increase in PVR is not sufficient to recommend the routine avoidance of nitrous oxide in patients with co-existing pulmonary hypertension. (From Hilgenberg et al.,[11] with permission.)

blood volume is already increased. Monitoring right atrial pressure is a helpful guide to the adequacy of intravascular fluid replacement. An increase in right atrial pressure could also reflect nitrous oxide-induced pulmonary vasoconstriction, suggesting the need to discontinue this drug.

Postoperatively, patients with mitral stenosis are at high risk for developing pulmonary edema and right heart failure. Mechanical support of ventilation of the lungs is often necessary, particularly after major thoracic or abdominal surgery.

Mitral Regurgitation

Mitral regurgitation is characterized by left atrial volume overload and decreased left ventricular forward stroke volume due to passage of part of each stroke volume through the incompetent mitral valve back into the left atrium. This regurgitant flow is responsible for the characteristic V waves seen on the recording of the pulmonary artery occlusion pressure (Fig. 19-2).[12] Mitral regurgitation is usually due to rheumatic fever and is almost always associated with mitral stenosis. Isolated mitral regurgitation is often acute, reflecting papillary muscle dysfunction after a myocardial infarction or rupture of a chordae tendinae secondary to infective endocarditis.

Management of Anesthesia

Management of anesthesia in patients with mitral regurgitation should be designed to reduce the likelihood of reductions in heart rate or increases in systemic vascular resistance that would lead to decreases in the forward left ventricular stroke volume. Conversely, cardiac output can be improved by mild increases in heart rate and mild reductions in systemic vascular resistance.

A general anesthetic is the usual choice for patients with mitral regurgitation. Although reductions in systemic vascular resistance are theoretically beneficial, the uncontrolled nature of this response with a regional anesthetic detracts from the use of this technique for other than surgery on peripheral sites. Maintenance of anesthesia can be provided with nitrous oxide plus volatile drugs, the concentration of which can be adjusted to attenuate undesirable increases in blood pressure and systemic vascular resistance that can accompany surgical stimulation. Nondepolarizing muscle relaxants, such as metocurine, atracurium, and

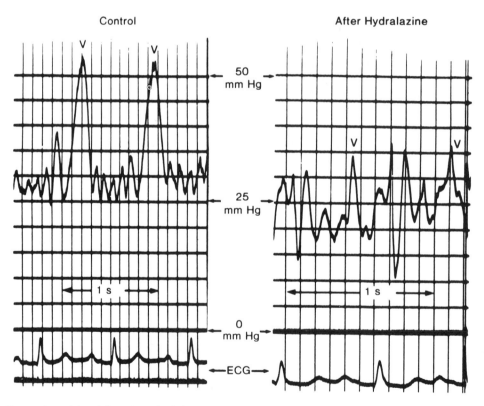

Fig. 19-2. Regurgitant blood flow into the left atrium via an incompetent mitral valve produces a V wave on the trace of the pulmonary artery occlusion pressure. Vasodilation produced by hydralazine reduces impedance to forward ejection of blood from the left ventricle such that regurgitant flow into the left atrium is less and the size of the V wave is decreased. (From Greenberg and Rahimtoola,[12] with permission.)

vecuronium, that lack significant circulatory effects are useful. Pancuronium is also acceptable as the increases in heart rate produced by this drug could increase forward left ventricular stroke volume. Although d-tubocurarine reduces systemic vascular resistance, the magnitude of this response is not predictable, making this an unlikely drug choice for patients with mitral regurgitation. Intravascular fluid volume must be maintained by the prompt replacement of blood loss so as to assure adequate cardiac filling and ejection of an optimal forward left ventricular stroke volume.

Aortic Stenosis

Aortic stenosis is characterized by increased left ventricular systolic pressure so as to maintain the forward stroke volume through a narrowed aortic valve. The magnitude of the pressure gradient serves as an estimate of the severity of valvular stenosis. Hemodynamically significant aortic stenosis is associated with pressure gradients greater than 50 mmHg. Increased intraventricular pressures are accompanied by compensatory increases in the thickness of the left ventricular wall. Angina pectoris occurs often in these patients in the absence of coronary artery disease, reflecting increased myocardial oxygen needs due to the increased amounts of ventricular muscle associated with myocardial hypertrophy. Furthermore, myocardial oxygen delivery is decreased due to compression of subendocardial coronary blood vessels by increased left ventricular systolic pressures.

Isolated nonrheumatic aortic stenosis usually results from progressive calcification and stenosis of a congenitally abnormal (usually bicuspid) valve. Aortic stenosis due to rheumatic fever almost always occurs in association with mitral valve disease. Likewise, aortic stenosis is usually accompanied by some degree of aortic regurgitation. Regardless of the etiology of aortic stenosis, the natural history of the disease includes a long latent period, often 30 years or more, before symptoms occur. Because many patients with aortic stenosis are asymptomatic, it is important to listen for this cardiac murmur (systolic murmur in the second right intercostal space) in all patients scheduled for surgery. Indeed, the incidence of sudden death is increased in patients with aortic stenosis.

Management of Anesthesia

Goals during management of anesthesia in patients with aortic stenosis are maintenance of normal sinus rhythm and avoidance of extreme and prolonged alterations in heart rate, systemic vascular resistance, and intravascular fluid volume. Preservation of normal sinus rhythm is critical because the left ventricle is dependent on properly timed atrial contractions to assure an optimal left ventricular filling and stroke volume. Marked increases in heart rate (above 100 beats·min^{-1}) can reduce the time for left ventricular filling and ejection, whereas bradycardia (below 60 beats·min^{-1}) can lead to acute overdistension of the left ventricle. In view of the obstruction to left ventricular ejection, it must be appreciated that decreases in systemic vascular resistance may be associated with large reductions in blood pressure and coronary blood flow.

A general anesthetic is usually preferred to a regional anesthetic because sympathetic nervous system blockade can lead to undesirable decreases in systemic vascular resistance. Maintenance of anesthesia can be with nitrous oxide plus opioids or low concentrations of volatile drugs. A potential disadvantage of volatile drugs (especially halothane) is depression of sinus node automaticity, which may lead to junctional rhythm and decreased left ventricular filling due to loss of properly timed atrial contractions.

Intravascular fluid volume must be maintained by prompt replacement of blood loss and liberal administration of intravenous fluids. If a pulmonary artery catheter is used, it should be remembered that the occlusion pressure may underestimate the left ventricular end-diastolic pressure because of the decreased compliance of the left ventricle that accompanies chronic aortic stenosis. An electric defibrillator should be immediately available when anesthesia is administered to patients with aortic stenosis since external cardiac massage is unlikely to be effective in creating an adequate stroke volume across a stenosed valve.

Aortic Regurgitation

Aortic regurgitation is characterized by decreased forward left ventricular stroke volume due to regurgitation of part of the ejected stroke volume from the aorta back into the left ventricle through an incompetent aortic valve. A gradual onset of aortic regurgitation results in marked left ventricular hypertrophy. Increased myocardial oxygen requirements secondary to left ventricular hypertrophy, plus a characteristic decrease in aortic diastolic pressure that reduces coronary blood flow, can manifest as angina pectoris in the absence of coronary artery disease. Acute aortic regurgitation is most often due to infective endocarditis, trauma, or dissection of a thoracic aneurysm. Chronic aortic regurgitation is usually due to prior rheumatic fever. In contrast to aortic stenosis, the occurrence of sudden death with aortic regurgitation is rare. Management of anesthesia for noncardiac surgery in patients with aortic regurgitation is as described for patients with mitral regurgitation.

Mitral Valve Prolapse

Mitral valve prolapse (click-murmur syndrome, Barlow syndrome) is characterized by an abnormality of the mitral valve support structure that permits prolapse of the valve into the left atrium during contraction of the left ventricle. Based on the presence of a characteristic systolic murmur best heard at the apex, it is estimated that about 5 percent of the adult population exhibits this valve abnormality. Echocardiography is helpful in confirming the diagnosis of mitral valve prolapse, particularly in the absence of the characteristic systolic murmur. There seems to be an increased incidence of mitral valve prolapse in patients with musculoskeletal abnormalities, including Marfan syndrome, pectus excavatum, and kyphoscoliosis.

Despite the prevalence of mitral valve prolapse, the majority of patients are asymptomatic, emphasizing the usual benign course of this abnormality. Nevertheless, serious complications may accompany mitral valve prolapse. For example, mitral valve prolapse is probably the most common cause of pure mitral regurgitation, which may progress to the need for surgical intervention. Infective

---

Complications Associated with Mitral Valve Prolapse

Mitral regurgitation
Infective endocarditis
Transient ischemic events
Cardiac dysrhythmias
Sudden death (extremely rare)

---

endocarditis is a potential complication, and transient ischemic attacks in patients less than 45 years of age are often associated with mitral valve prolapse. Sudden death is an extremely rare complication that is presumed to be due to ventricular cardiac dysrhythmias.

Management of Anesthesia

The important principle in the management of anesthesia in patients with mitral valve prolapse is the avoidance of events that can increase cardiac emptying and accentuate prolapse of the mitral valve into the left atrium.[13] Perioperative events that can increase cardiac emptying include (1) sympathetic nervous system stimulation, (2) decreased systemic vascular resistance, and (3) performance of surgery with patients in the head-up or sitting position. With this in mind, it is important to optimize intravascular fluid volume in the preoperative period. Induction of anesthesia is acceptably accomplished with intravenous administration of barbiturates, benzodiazepines, or etomidate. Ketamine or pancuronium are not recommended because of their ability to increase cardiac contractility and heart rate. Maintenance of anesthesia is most often with nitrous oxide plus volatile anesthetics so as to minimize sympathetic nervous system activation due to noxious intraoperative stimulation. The dose of volatile anesthetics must be titrated to avoid excessive reductions in systemic vascular resistance. A regional anesthetic could also produce undesirable reductions in systemic vascular resistance. Prompt replacement of blood loss and generous administration of intravenous fluids will contribute to maintenance of an optimal intravascular fluid volume and reduce potential adverse effects of positive pressure ventilation of the lungs. Lidocaine and propranolol should be immediately available to treat cardiac dysrhythmias. If sympathomimetics are needed to treat hypotension, an alpha agonist, such as phenylephrine, is useful.

CONGENITAL HEART DISEASE

Approximately 8 of every 1000 live births are associated with some form of congenital heart disease. Although more than 100 different congenital heart lesions are known, nearly 90 percent of all cardiac defects can be placed in 1 of 10 categories (Table 19-4). From the standpoint of management of anesthesia, it is helpful to categorize congenital heart defects as those lesions that result in a left-to-right intracardiac shunt and those that result in a right-to-left intracardiac shunt. Patients with congenital heart disease should receive antibiotics in the perioperative period for protection against infective endocarditis.

Left-to-Right Intracardiac Shunt

A left-to-right intracardiac shunt may be due to an atrial septal defect or ventricular septal defect. Patent ductus arteriosus is an example of a left-to-right shunt at the level of the aorta. The result of these shunts is increased pulmonary blood flow with pulmonary hypertension, right ventricular hypertrophy, and eventually congestive heart failure.

Table 19-4. Common Congenital Heart Defects

Defect	Percent of Total Defects
Ventricular septal defect	28
Secundum atrial septal defect	10
Patent ductus arteriosus	10
Tetralogy of Fallot	10
Pulmonary stenosis	10
Aortic stenosis	7
Coarctation of the aorta	5
Transposition of the great vessels	5
Other	15

Atrial Septal Defect

An atrial septal defect is often first suspected when there is a history of frequent pulmonary infections or when a systolic murmur is noted over the area of the pulmonary valve during a routine physical examination. Surgical closure of an atrial septal defect is indicated when the pulmonary blood flow is at least twice the systemic blood flow.

Management of Anesthesia. The presence of an atrial septal defect has only minor implications for the management of anesthesia. For example, as long as systemic blood flow remains normal, the pharmacokinetics of inhaled drugs will probably not be altered despite increased pulmonary blood flow. Increased pulmonary blood flow means that hemodynamic effects of positive intrathoracic pressure during controlled ventilation of the lungs are well tolerated. Drugs or events that increase systemic blood pressure and/or systemic vascular resistance should be avoided as this change will favor an increase in the magnitude of the left-to-right shunt at the atrial level. Conversely, decreases in these parameters as produced by volatile anesthetics or increases in pulmonary vascular resistance due to positive pressure ventilation of the lungs will tend to decrease the magnitude of the shunt. Finally, it is imperative to avoid the entrance of air into the right atrium as can occur via the tubing used to deliver intravenous solutions. This air could bypass the lungs and cross directly into the systemic circulation to enter coronary and/or cerebral arteries.

Ventricular Septal Defect

Patients with small ventricular septal defects (ratio of pulmonary-to-systemic blood flow less than 1.5 to 1) are usually asymptomatic with the only evidence of the cardiac abnormality being a pansystolic murmur that is of maximum intensity along the left sternal border. A large ventricular septal defect is characterized by a left-to-right intracardiac shunt that results in a pulmonary blood flow that exceeds systemic blood flow by three times to five times. Recurrent pulmonary infections and eventually congestive heart failure are typical complications in patients with large ventricular septal defects. Management of anesthesia is as described for atrial septal defect.

Patent Ductus Arteriosus

Failure of the ductus arteriosus to close after birth results in passage of oxygenated blood from the aorta into the pulmonary artery. Most patients are asymptomatic with the only manifestation being a continuous systolic and diastolic murmur. Management of anesthesia is as described for atrial septal defect.

Right-to-Left Intracardiac Shunt

A right-to-left intracardiac shunt is characterized by decreased pulmonary blood flow and arterial hypoxemia. Tetralogy of Fallot is the most common of the congenital cardiac defects that result in a right-to-left intracardiac shunt.

Tetralogy of Fallot

Tetralogy of Fallot is characterized by the presence of a ventricular septal defect, an aorta that overrides the pulmonary artery outflow tract, obstruction to blood flow through the pulmonary artery outflow tract and right ventricular hypertrophy. Arterial blood gases and pH are likely to reveal a normal $PaCO_2$ and pH and a markedly reduced PaO_2 (usually below 50 mmHg) even when breathing oxygen. Squatting is a common feature of children with tetralogy of Fallot. Presumably, squatting increases systemic blood pressure and systemic vascular resistance by kinking the large arteries in the inguinal area. These circulatory changes reduce the magnitude of the right-to-left intracardiac shunt leading to increased pulmonary blood flow and improved arterial oxygenation.

Hypercyanotic attacks ("tet spells") can occur without provocation but are often associated with crying or exercise. The most likely explanation for these attacks is a sudden reduction in pulmonary blood flow due either to a decrease in systemic vascular resistance or spasm of cardiac muscle in the region of the pulmonary artery outflow (infundibular) tract. Phenylephrine is an effective treatment presumably because this drug increases systemic vascular resistance and forces more blood through the lungs. Sympathomimetics, such as ephedrine with beta agonist properties, are not

selected because sympathetic stimulation could accentuate spasm of the infundibular cardiac muscle. Propranolol is effective when hypercyanotic attacks are due to cardiac muscle spasm in the region of the pulmonary artery outflow tract.

Management of Anesthesia. Management of anesthesia for patients with tetralogy of Fallot requires a thorough understanding of those events or drugs that can alter the magnitude of the right-to-left intracardiac shunt. For example, drug-induced responses that decrease systemic vascular resistance and blood pressure (volatile anesthetics, histamine release) will increase the magnitude of the right-to-left shunt and decrease the PaO_2. Pulmonary blood flow can also be reduced by increases in pulmonary vascular resistance that accompany positive pressure ventilation of the lungs or application of positive end-expiratory pressure. Nevertheless, the advantages of controlled ventilation of the lungs offset the potential hazards as evidenced by the fact that the PaO_2 usually improves.

Preoperatively, it is important to avoid dehydration by maintaining oral feedings in the very young or by providing intravenous fluids before arriving in the operating room. Crying associated with intramuscular administration of drugs used for preoperative medication can lead to hypercyanotic attacks. For this reason, it may be prudent to avoid intramuscular administration of drugs until the patient is in a highly supervised environment and alpha agonists, such as phenylephrine, are immediately available for treatment of hypercyanotic attacks.

Induction of anesthesia in patients with tetralogy of Fallot is often accomplished with intramuscular (4 mg·kg^{-1} to 6 mg·kg^{-1}) or intravenous (1 mg·kg^{-1} to 2 mg·kg^{-1}) administration of ketamine. Indeed, the onset of anesthesia after the injection of ketamine is often associated with an improvement in the PaO_2, which presumably reflects increased pulmonary blood flow due to ketamine-induced elevations in systemic vascular resistance that leads to a decrease in the magnitude of the right-to-left intracardiac shunt.

Maintenance of anesthesia is often achieved with ketamine plus nitrous oxide. Disadvantages of nitrous oxide include possible increases in pulmonary vascular resistance evoked by this drug and reductions in inspired concentrations of oxygen that are necessitated by use of this anesthetic. Therefore, it would seem prudent to limit inspired concentrations of nitrous oxide to no more than 50 percent. Volatile anesthetics are not recommended for induction or maintenance of anesthesia because of the propensity of these drugs to increase the magnitude of right-to-left intracardiac shunt by decreasing systemic vascular resistance and blood pressure.

Pancuronium is a useful muscle relaxant selection, as this drug maintains systemic blood pressure. d-Tubocurarine would not be a logical choice because this muscle relaxant could increase the magnitude of the right-to-left intracardiac shunt by virtue of its ability to decrease systemic vascular resistance secondary to histamine release and blockade of impulse transmission through autonomic ganglia.

Ventilation of the lungs should be controlled, but it must be appreciated that excessive positive airway pressures may adversely increase resistance to blood flow through the lungs. Intravascular fluid volume must be maintained with intravenous fluid administration because acute hypovolemia will tend to increase the magnitude of the right-to-left intracardiac shunt. In view of co-existing polycythemia, it is probably not necessary to replace blood loss that is less than 20 percent of the estimated blood volume. It is crucial that care be taken to avoid infusion of air via the tubing used to deliver intravenous solutions as this could lead to direct air embolization to coronary and/or cerebral arteries. Finally, phenylephrine should be immediately available to treat undesirable reductions in systemic vascular resistance and blood pressure.

DISTURBANCES OF CARDIAC CONDUCTION AND RHYTHM

The ECG is the most valuable tool for diagnosing and treating disturbances of cardiac conduction and rhythm. The following questions should be asked when interpreting the ECG:

1. What is the heart rate?

2. Are P waves present and what is their relationship to the QRS complex?
3. What is the duration of the P-R interval (normal 0.12 second to 0.2 second)?
4. What is the duration of the QRS complex (normal 0.05 second to 0.1 second)?
5. Is the ventricular rhythm regular?
6. Are there early cardiac beats or abnormal pauses after a preceding QRS complex?

Heart Block

Disturbances of conduction of cardiac impulses can be classified according to the site of the conduction block relative to the atrioventricular node. Heart block occurring above the atrioventricular node is usually benign and transient. Heart block occurring below the atrioventricular node tends to be progressive and permanent.

A theoretical concern in patients with bifasicular heart block is that perioperative events, such as alterations in blood pressure, arterial oxygenation,

---

Classification of Heart Block

First-degree atrioventricular heart block

Second-degree atrioventricular heart block
  Mobitz type I (Wenckebach)
  Mobitz type II

Unifasicular heart block
  Left anterior hemiblock
  Left posterior hemiblock

Right bundle branch block

Left bundle branch block

Bifasicular heart block

  Right bundle branch block plus left anterior hemiblock
  Right bundle branch block plus left posterior hemiblock

Third-degree (trifasicular, complete) atrioventricular heart block

or electrolyte concentrations, might compromise conduction in the one remaining intact fasicle, leading to the acute onset intraoperatively of third-degree atrioventricular heart block. There is no evidence, however, that surgery performed during a general or regional anesthetic predisposes to the development of third-degree atrioventricular heart block in patients with co-existing bifasicular block. Therefore, placement of a prophylactic artificial cardiac pacemaker is not recommended before anesthesia and surgery.

Treatment of third-degree atrioventricular heart block is with a permanently implanted artificial cardiac pacemaker. A temporary transvenous artificial cardiac pacemaker should be placed before induction of anesthesia for placement of a permanent artificial pacemaker. This recommendation is based on the clinical impression that the incidence of cardiac arrest is increased during induction of anesthesia in patients with third-degree atrioventricular heart block. It must be remembered that the presence of a transvenous artificial cardiac pacemaker creates a direct connection between external electrical sources and the endocardium. This predisposes the patients to the hazards of ventricular fibrillation from microshock levels of electrical current. Continuous intravenous infusions of isoproterenol acting as a pharmacologic cardiac pacemaker may be necessary to maintain an adequate heart rate until the artificial cardiac pacemaker can be placed.

Sick Sinus Syndrome

Sick sinus syndrome is characterized by inappropriate sinus bradycardia associated with degenerative changes in the sinoatrial node. Frequently, bradycardia due to this syndrome is complicated by episodes of supraventricular tachycardia. Artificial cardiac pacemakers are indicated only when therapeutic plasma concentrations of drugs necessary to control tachycardia result in bradycardia. The high incidence of pulmonary embolism in these patients is the rationale for anticoagulation.

Ventricular Premature Beats

Ventricular premature beats are recognized on the ECG by virtue of (1) premature occurrence, (2) absence of a P wave preceding the QRS complex, (3) wide and often bizarre QRS complex, (4) inverted T wave, and (5) compensatory pause that follows the premature beat. Ventricular premature beats should be treated with the intravenous administration of lidocaine 1 mg·kg^{-1} to 2 mg·kg^{-1} when they are (1) frequent (more than 6 beats·min^{-1}), (2) multifocal, (3) occur in salvos of three or more, or (4) take place during the ascending limb of the T wave (R on T phenomenon) that corresponds to the relative refractory period of the ventricle. At the same time the underlying cause (arterial hypoxemia, hypercarbia, hypertension, hypokalemia, mechanical irritation of the ventricles) should be eliminated.

Ventricular Tachycardia

Ventricular tachycardia is defined as the appearance of at least three consecutive wide QRS complexes on the ECG (duration at least 0.12 second) occurring at an effective heart rate greater than 120 beats·min^{-1}. Ventricular tachycardia not associated with hypotension is initially treated with the intravenous administration of lidocaine. Symptomatic ventricular tachycardia is best treated with external electrical cardioversion (see Chapter 34).

Pre-excitation Syndromes

Pre-excitation syndromes are characterized by activation of a portion of the ventricles by cardiac impulses that travel from the atria via accessory (anomalous) conduction pathways.[14] These pathways bypass the atrioventricular node such that activation of the ventricles occurs earlier than it would if impulses reached the ventricles by normal pathways.

Wolff-Parkinson-White Syndrome

The Wolff-Parkinson-White syndrome is the most frequently occurring of the pre-excitation syndromes, with an incidence that may approach 0.3 percent of the general population. The lack of a physiologic delay in transmission of cardiac impulses along the Kent fibers results in the characteristic short P-R interval (less than 0.12 second) on the ECG. The wide QRS complex and delta wave on the ECG reflect the composite of cardiac impulses conducted by normal and accessory pathways. Paroxysmal atrial tachycardia is the most frequent cardiac dysrhythmia associated with this syndrome. An increasing number of patients with Wolff-Parkinson-White syndrome are being treated by surgical division of accessory pathways as identified by intraoperative endocardial mapping.

Management of Anesthesia

The goal during management of anesthesia in the presence of pre-excitation syndromes is to avoid events (anxiety) or drugs (anticholinergics, ketamine, pancuronium) that might increase sympathetic nervous system activity and predispose to tachydysrhythmias.[14] All antidysrhythmics should be continued throughout the perioperative period. Large doses of droperidol (0.2 mg·kg^{-1} to 0.6 mg·kg^{-1}) may be protective in preventing tachydysrhythmias in these patients. Induction of anesthesia can be safely accomplished with the intravenous administration of barbiturates, benzodiazepines, or etomidate. Intubation of the trachea should be performed only after a sufficient depth of anesthesia has been achieved with nitrous oxide plus volatile anesthetics or opioids. Nondepolarizing muscle relaxants with minimal effects on heart rate (metocurine, atracurium, vecuronium) or succinylcholine are useful to facilitate intubation of the trachea or to provide skeletal muscle paralysis during surgery.

The onset of paroxysmal atrial tachycardia or fibrillation in the perioperative period can be treated with the intravenous administration of drugs that abruptly prolong the refractory period of the atrioventricular node (verapamil, propranolol) or lengthen the refractory period of accessory pathways (procainamide). Digitalis and verapamil may decrease the refractory period of accessory pathways responsible for atrial fibrillation, resulting in an increase in ventricular response during this dysrhythmia. Electrical cardioversion is indicated when tachydysrhythmias are life-threatening.

Prolonged Q-T Interval Syndrome

Prolonged Q-T interval (greater than 0.44 second on the electrocardiogram) syndrome is associated with ventricular dysrhythmias, syncope, and sudden death. Treatment of these patients is with beta antagonists or left stellate ganglion block. The effectiveness of a left stellate ganglion block supports the hypothesis that this syndrome results from a congenital imbalance of autonomic innervation to the heart produced by decreases in right cardiac sympathetic nerve activity. Management of anesthesia includes avoidance of events or drugs that are likely to activate the sympathetic nervous system and immediate availability of beta-antagonists and/or electrical cardioversion to treat life-threatening ventricular dysrhythmias.[15]

ARTIFICIAL CARDIAC PACEMAKERS

Preoperatively the adequacy of artificial cardiac pacemaker function must be confirmed. The rate of discharge of an artificial atrial or ventricular asynchronous (fixed rate) pacemaker is the most important indicator of pulse generator function.[16] A 10 percent decrease in heart rate from the initial fixed discharge rate is a sign of battery failure. Proper function of artificial ventricular synchronous and sequential cardiac pacemakers can be confirmed by demonstrating the appearance of captured beats on the electrocardiogram when the artificial cardiac pacemaker is converted to the asynchronous mode by an externally applied converter magnet.

Intraoperative monitoring of patients with artificial cardiac pacemakers includes the ECG so as to detect promptly the appearance of asystole. Atropine and isoproterenol should be immediately available should artificial cardiac pacemaker function cease. If electrocautery interferes with the ECG, monitoring a palpable peripheral pulse and/or auscultation through an esophageal stethoscope confirms continued cardiac activity. Inhibition of pulse generator activity by electromagnetic interference, which is interpreted as spontaneous cardiac activity by the artificial cardiac pacemaker, is most likely when the ground plate for electrocautery is placed too near the pulse generator. For this reason, the ground plate should be placed as far as possible from the pulse generator. Despite these concerns, it is alleged that improved shielding and circuit design of pulse generators results in conversion of artificial ventricular synchronous pacemakers to the asynchronous mode during continuous use of electrocautery, thus eliminating the hazard of electromagnetic inhibition or the need for an external converter magnet. Finally, selection of drugs or techniques for anesthesia is not influenced by the presence of artificial cardiac pacemakers as there is no evidence that the threshold and subsequent response of these devices is altered by drugs administered in the perioperative period. Insertion of pulmonary artery catheters will not disturb epicardial electrodes but might dislodge recently placed (less than 2 weeks) transvenous endocardial electrodes.[16]

ESSENTIAL HYPERTENSION

Essential hypertension is defined as sustained elevations of arterial blood pressure (systolic blood pressure above 160 mmHg and/or a diastolic blood pressure greater than 95 mmHg) independent of any known cause. It is estimated that 35 million adults in the United States have essential hypertension, but only about one-third of these individuals are being treated with antihypertensives. Appropriate drug therapy reduces the incidence of stroke and congestive heart failure, but there is no convincing evidence that adverse events associated with coronary artery disease are altered.

Management of Anesthesia

Management of anesthesia for patients with essential hypertension includes preoperative evaluation of the treatment and extent of the disease plus a consideration of the implications of exaggerated blood pressure elevations intraoperatively in response to noxious stimulation.[17]

Preoperative Evaluation

Preoperative evaluation of patients with essential hypertension begins with a determination of the adequacy of blood pressure control and a review of the pharmacology of the antihypertensives being used for therapy (see Chapter 3). It is important to maintain current therapy with antihypertensives throughout the perioperative period. Evidence of major organ dysfunction (congestive heart failure, coronary artery disease, cerebral ischemia, renal dysfunction) must be sought. Patients with essential hypertension are

---

Management of Anesthesia for the Patient with Essential Hypertension

Preoperative evaluation
  Determine adequacy of blood pressure control
  Review pharmacology of antihypertensives
  Evaluate associated organ dysfunction (cardiac, CNS, renal)

Induction of anesthesia and intubation of the trachea
  Anticipate exaggerated blood pressure changes
  Minimize pressor response during intubation of the trachea by limiting duration of laryngoscopy to less than 15 seconds

Maintenance of anesthesia
  Use volatile anesthetic to control blood pressure
  Monitor electrocardiogram for evidence of myocardial ischemia

Postoperative management
  Anticipate excessive increases in blood pressure

---

assumed to have coronary artery disease until proven otherwise. Evidence of peripheral vascular disease must be recognized, particularly when placement of an intra-arterial catheter in the perioperative period is anticipated. It can be assumed that nearly one-half of patients with evidence of peripheral vascular disease will have 50 percent or greater stenosis of one or more coronary arteries even in the absence of angina pectoris and the presence of a normal resting ECG. Essential hypertension is associated with a shift to the right of the curve for the autoregulation of cerebral blood flow, emphasizing that these patients are more vulnerable to cerebral ischemia should perfusion pressures decrease. Detection of renal dysfunction due to chronic hypertension may influence the selection of drugs (possibly avoid enflurane and decrease doses of nondepolarizing muscle relaxants) used during anesthesia.

The value of treating essential hypertension before elective operation is suggested by the observation that the incidence of hypotension and evidence of myocardial ischemia on the ECG during the maintenance of anesthesia is increased in patients who remain hypertensive before induction of anesthesia.[17] Nevertheless, blood pressure elevations during the intraoperative period are more likely to occur in patients with a history of essential hypertension regardless of the degree of blood pressure control established preoperatively. Furthermore, there is no evidence that the incidence of postoperative cardiac complications is increased when hypertensive patients undergo elective operations as long as the preoperative diastolic blood pressure does not exceed 110 mmHg. In the future, pretreatment with alpha-2 agonists, such as clonidine, may be useful in blunting exaggerated sympathetic nervous system responses in these types of patients.

Induction of Anesthesia

Induction of anesthesia with the intravenous administration of barbiturates, benzodiazepines, or etomidate is acceptable, remembering that an exaggerated reduction in blood pressure may occur particularly if hypertension is present preoperatively. This response most likely reflects unmasking of a reduced intravascular fluid volume due to chronic hypertension. Ketamine is rarely selected for induction of anesthesia as its circulatory effects could adversely increase blood pressure, especially in patients with co-existing hypertension.

Exaggerated blood pressure increases during direct laryngoscopy for intubation of the trachea are predictable in patients with the preoperative diagnosis of essential hypertension. Evidence of myocardial ischemia on the ECG may appear at this time. It would seem logical to assure maximal attenuation of sympathetic nervous system responses evoked by direct laryngoscopy by administering volatile anesthetics or intravenous opioids before intubation of the trachea is attempted. Regardless of the drugs administered before intubation of the trachea, however, it must be recognized that an excessive depth of anesthesia can produce reductions in blood pressure that are as undesirable as hypertension. An important concept for limiting pressor responses elicited by intubation of the trachea is to minimize the duration of direct laryngoscopy to 15 seconds or less. In addition, the administration of laryngotracheal lidocaine immediately before placement of the tube in the trachea will minimize any additional pressor response.

Maintenance of Anesthesia

The goal during maintenance of anesthesia is to adjust the depth of anesthesia in appropriate directions so as to minimize wide fluctuations in blood pressure. In this regard, a technique using nitrous oxide plus a volatile anesthetic is useful for permitting rapid adjustments in depth of anesthesia in response to elevations or decreases in blood pressure. Indeed, the management of intraoperative blood pressure lability by adjusting the concentrations of volatile anesthetics is probably more important than preoperative control of hypertension.

The most likely intraoperative changes in blood pressure are hypertensive episodes produced by surgical stimulation. Volatile anesthetics are useful for attenuating activity of the sympathetic nervous system, which is responsible for these pressor responses. Halothane, enflurane, and isoflurane produce dose-dependent reductions in blood pressure by different primary mechanisms (see Chapter 4). A nitrous oxide-opioid technique is also acceptable for the maintenance of anesthesia, but the addition of volatile anesthetics is often necessary to control undesirable elevations in blood pressure, particularly during periods of maximal surgical stimulation. Continuous intravenous infusions of nitroprusside are alternatives to the use of volatile anesthetics for maintaining normotension during the intraoperative period. Hypotension that occurs during maintenance of anesthesia is often treated by reducing the concentrations of volatile anesthetics plus infusing fluids intravenously to increase intravascular fluid volume. Sympathomimetics, such as ephedrine, may be necessary to restore perfusion pressures until the underlying cause of hypotension can be corrected.

Intraoperative monitors for patients with co-existing essential hypertension are influenced by the complexity of the surgery. The ECG is monitored with the goal of recognizing changes suggestive of myocardial ischemia. Invasive monitoring using an intra-arterial and pulmonary artery catheter is indicated if major surgery is planned and there is evidence preoperatively of left ventricular dysfunction.

There is no evidence that a specific muscle relaxant is the best selection in patients with essential hypertension. Although pancuronium can increase the blood pressure, no data suggest that this mild pressor response is exaggerated by co-existing hypertension.

A regional anesthetic is a questionable choice when high levels of sympathetic nervous system blockade would be associated with the sensory level necessary for the planned surgery. This caution is based on the possibility of excessive reductions in blood pressure when vasodilation unmasks a decreased intravascular fluid volume associated with chronic hypertension.

Postoperative Management

Hypertension in the early postoperative period is a frequent response in patients with a preoperative diagnosis of essential hypertension. If hypertension persists despite adequate analgesia, it may be necessary to administer a peripheral vasodilator such as hydralazine (5 mg to 10 mg intravenously every 10 minutes to 20 minutes) or a continuous intravenous infusion of nitroprusside. Intermittent intravenous injections of labetalol, a combined alpha and beta antagonist, may be a useful alternative to these drugs.

CONGESTIVE HEART FAILURE

Elective surgery should not be performed in patients who manifest evidence of congestive heart failure. Indeed, the presence of congestive heart failure has been reported to be the single most important factor for predicting postoperative morbidity. When surgery cannot be delayed, however, the drugs and techniques chosen to provide anesthesia must be selected with the goal of optimizing cardiac output. Ketamine is useful for the induction of anesthesia in the presence of congestive heart failure (see Chapter 6). Use of volatile an-

esthetics for maintenance of anesthesia is not recommended because of the potential for cardiac depression. In the presence of severe congestive heart failure, the use of opioids in high doses as the sole anesthetic may be justified. Positive pressure ventilation of the lungs may be beneficial by decreasing pulmonary congestion and improving arterial oxygenation. Invasive monitoring of arterial pressure, as well as cardiac filling pressures, is justified when major surgery is necessary. Maintenance of myocardial contractility with continuous infusions of dopamine or dobutamine may be necessary in the perioperative period.

A regional anesthetic is a consideration for patients with congestive heart failure requiring peripheral surgery. The mild reduction in systemic vascular resistance secondary to peripheral sympathetic nervous system blockade could facilitate an increased left ventricular stroke volume. Nevertheless, a regional anesthetic should probably not be selected in preference to a general anesthetic if the only reason is the belief that a regional block will reliably improve cardiac output.

HYPERTROPHIC CARDIOMYOPATHY

Hypertrophic cardiomyopathy (idiopathic hypertrophic subaortic stenosis, IHSS) is characterized by obstruction to left ventricular outflow produced by asymmetric hypertrophy of the intraventricular septal muscle. Associated left ventricular hypertrophy in an attempt to overcome the obstruction may be so massive that the volume of the left ventricular chamber is reduced. Despite these adverse changes, the stroke volume remains normal or increased due to the hypercontractile state of the myocardium.

Management of Anesthesia

The goal during management of anesthesia for patients with hypertrophic cardiomyopathy is to decrease the pressure gradient across the left ventricular outflow obstruction. Reductions in myocardial contractility and increases in preload (ventricular volume) and afterload will decrease the magnitude of left ventricular outflow obstruction. With this in mind, halothane is useful for maintenance of anesthesia providing mild myo-

---

Events that Decrease Left Ventricular Outflow Obstruction in the Presence of Hypertrophic Cardiomyopathy

Decreased myocardial contractility
  Beta-adrenergic blockade (propranolol)
  Volatile anesthetics (halothane)

Increased preload
  Increased intravascular fluid volume
  Bradycardia

Increased afterload
  Alpha-adrenergic stimulation (phenylephrine)
  Increased intravascular fluid volume

---

cardial depression. Theoretically, enflurane and isoflurane would be less ideal choices than halothane as these drugs decrease systemic vascular resistance more than does halothane (see Chapter 4). Opioids are not likely choices, as they do not produce myocardial depression and can reduce systemic vascular resistance. Pancuronium is not a good muscle relaxant selection because of its ability to increase heart rate and myocardial contractility.

Intraoperative hypotension is best treated with intravenous fluids and/or alpha agonists such as phenylephrine. Drugs with beta agonist activity are not likely to be used to treat hypotension, as any increase in cardiac contractility or heart rate could increase left ventricular outflow obstruction. When hypertension occurs, an increased delivered concentration of halothane is a useful treatment. Vasodilators, such as nitroprusside or nitroglycerin, are not good choices for lowering blood pressure because reductions in systemic vascular resistance can increase left ventricular outflow obstruction.

COR PULMONALE

Cor pulmonale is the designation for right ventricular hypertrophy and eventual cardiac dysfunction that occurs secondary to chronic pulmonary hypertension. Elective operations in patients with cor pulmonale should not be performed until any reversible component of the co-existing pulmonary disease has been treated.

Goals during management of anesthesia in patients with cor pulmonale are to avoid events or drugs that could increase pulmonary vascular resistance. Volatile anesthetics are useful for relaxing vascular smooth muscle and attenuating airway responsiveness to stimuli produced by a tracheal tube. Nitrous oxide has been shown to increase pulmonary vascular resistance in the presence of large doses of opioids.[11] Another disadvantage of nitrous oxide is the associated reduction in the inspired concentrations of oxygen necessitated by the administration of this drug. Therefore, delivered concentrations of nitrous oxide are usually limited to 50 percent, and right atrial pressure is monitored to detect any adverse drug-induced effect on pulmonary vascular resistance.

CARDIAC TAMPONADE

Cardiac tamponade is characterized by reductions in the (1) diastolic filling of the ventricles, (2) stroke volume, and (3) blood pressure due to increased intrapericardial pressure from accumulation of fluid in the pericardial space. Decreased stroke volume results in activation of the sympathetic nervous system (tachycardia, vasoconstriction) in attempts to maintain the cardiac output. Cardiac output and blood pressure are maintained as long as the pressure in the central veins exceeds the right ventricular end-diastolic pressure. Institution of general anesthesia and positive pressure ventilation of the lungs in the presence of cardiac tamponade can lead to profound hypotension reflecting anesthetic-induced peripheral vasodilation, direct myocardial depression, and decreased venous return. When percutaneous pericardiocentesis cannot be performed using local anesthesia, the induction and maintenance of general anesthesia is often achieved with ketamine. Potential adverse effects of increased intrathoracic pressure on venous return must be considered. Perhaps positive pressure ventilation of the lungs should be avoided until drainage of the pericardial space is imminent. With this in mind, it may be prudent to perform intubation of the trachea using topical anesthesia before the induction of anesthesia. Continuous intravenous infusions of catecholamines (isoproterenol, dopamine, dobutamine) may be necessary to maintain myocardial contractility.

ANEURYSMS OF THE AORTA

Aneurysms of the aorta most often involve the abdominal aorta. A majority of patients are hypertensive and many have associated atherosclerosis. A dissecting aneurysm denotes a tear in the intima of the aorta that allows blood to enter and penetrate between the walls of the vessel producing a false lumen. Ultimately, the dissection may re-enter the lumen through another tear in the intima or rupture through the adventitia.

Elective resection of an abdominal aneurysm is indicated when the estimated diameter of the aneurysm exceeds 5 cm. The incidence of spontaneous rupture increases dramatically when the diameter of the aneurysm exceeds 5 cm. Extension of the abdominal aneurysm to include the renal arteries occurs in about 5 percent of patients.

Management of Anesthesia

Management of anesthesia for resection of an abdominal aortic aneurysm includes monitoring of arterial and left atrial filling pressures. Patients with co-existing coronary artery disease are likely to develop increases in the pulmonary artery occlusion pressure and evidence of myocardial ischemia during cross-clamping of the abdominal aorta. Treatment of intraoperative myocardial ischemia is by reducing blood pressure and filling pressures to acceptable levels by pharmacologic interventions, which may include continuous intravenous infusions of nitroprusside or nitroglycerin. Urine output should be maintained with intravenous infusions of crystalloid solutions and administration of diuretics so as to minimize the likelihood of postoperative renal failure.

Hypotension can accompany unclamping of the abdominal aorta, presumably reflecting sudden increases in venous capacitance. In addition, the release of acid metabolites that have accumulated in the ischemic extremities can produce myocardial depression and peripheral vasodilation. Blood pressure decreases can be minimized by infusing intravenous fluids to maintain the pulmonary artery occlusion pressure between 10 mmHg to 20 mmHg before removal of the aortic cross-clamp. Gradual removal of the aortic cross-clamp minimizes reductions in blood pressure by allowing time for return of pooled venous blood to the circulation. Intravenous administration of sodium bicarbonate is indicated if the arterial pH is below 7.2 after unclamping of the abdominal aorta.

CARDIOPULMONARY BYPASS

Cardiopulmonary bypass (extracorporeal circulation) is characterized by gravity drainage of blood from the vena cavae into an oxygenator followed by its return to the arterial system, usually the ascending aorta, by means of a roller pump (Fig. 19-3). In the presence of a competent aortic valve, the heart is excluded from the patient's circulation by tightening occlusive ligatures that have been placed around the superior and inferior vena cava so that all returning blood enters the large cannulae in these vessels. If the aortic valve is not competent, it is also necessary to cross-clamp the aorta distal to the aortic valve and proximal to the inflow cannula. Otherwise, retrograde blood flow through the incompetent aortic valve would prevent exclusion of the heart from the circulation. When the heart is isolated from the circulation, total cardiopulmonary bypass is present and ventilation of the lungs is no longer necessary to maintain oxygenation. Elevating the patient above the level of the cardiopulmonary bypass machine facilitates the gravity-dependent venous return.

The roller pump produces nonpulsatile flow into the patient's aorta by compression of the fluid-containing tubing between the roller and curved metal back plate. The required cardiac index delivered by the roller pump depends on the patient's body temperature and oxygen consumption. For normothermia or mild hypothermia, a cardiac index of 2 $L \cdot min^{-1} \cdot m^{-2}$ to 2.4 $L \cdot min^{-1} \cdot m^{-2}$ is satisfactory, although flows of approximately half these levels have been used successfully. Low flows have the advantage of (1) less blood trauma, and (2) less noncoronary collateral blood flow, which might result in better myocardial protection.

Blood is oxygenated in either a bubble or mem-

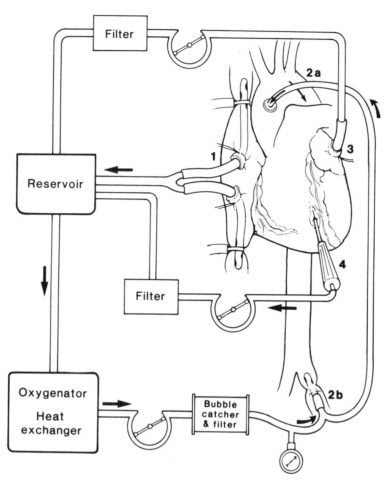

Fig. 19-3. Schematic diagram of a cardiopulmonary bypass circuit. Blood from cannulae (1) placed in the superior and inferior vena cava drains by gravity into a reservoir and then to an oxygenator and heat exchanger. A roller pump returns oxygenated blood to the ascending aorta (2a) or rarely the femoral artery (2b). In addition, blood is returned to the reservoir from the left ventricular vent (3) and cardiotomy suction (4). (From Nosé,[18] with permission.)

brane oxygenator. The bubble oxygenator is most popular, consisting of an oxygenating column, a defoaming section to remove air bubbles, and an arterial reservoir. The PaO$_2$ is maintained between 100 mmHg to 150 mmHg by adjusting the flow of oxygen into the oxygenator. Addition of carbon dioxide to maintain a PaCO$_2$ and pH at levels considered normal for 37° Celsius may not be necessary during hypothermic cardiopulmonary bypass. Membrane oxygenators do not use a blood-gas interface and produce less trauma to the blood compared with bubble oxygenators. Nevertheless,

these more complex and expensive oxygenators have not proven to be more advantageous than bubble oxygenators.

Heat exchangers are incorporated into oxygenators to control the patient's body temperature by heating or cooling blood as it circulates. Hot or cold water entering the unit at one end with blood entering at the other provides an efficient countercurrent flow system.

Blood from the pericardial cavity and the opened heart as during a valve replacement is returned to a cardiotomy reservoir where it is filtered, defoamed, and returned to the oxygenator for recirculation. The cardiotomy suction is a major cause of hemolysis during cardiopulmonary bypass. When the heart is not opened, as during aortocoronary bypass graft operations, it may be necessary to insert a catheter (vent) into the left ventricle (either through the apex of the left ventricle or via the right superior pulmonary vein) to prevent distension of the left ventricle with blood returning via thebesian veins or bronchial veins. Filters are incorporated in the oxygen delivery line and arterial delivery system to act as traps for cellular debris.

The tubing used for the cardiopulmonary bypass system is filled with blood and fluid (prime) in a predetermined ratio that is calculated to produce a specific hematocrit with institution of total cardiopulmonary bypass. Because whole body hypothermia (22° Celsius to 28° Celsius) is commonly used, the pump prime usually contains little or no blood such that the hematocrit of blood during bypass is reduced. Hemodilution is important to lessen viscosity during hypothermia. It is mandatory that all air be cleared from the arterial side of the circuit before institution of cardiopulmonary bypass. Indeed, pumping of air into the patient by the cardiopulmonary bypass machine is an ever present hazard.

Heparin-induced anticoagulation of the patient is mandatory before placement of the venous and aortic cannulae used for cardiopulmonary bypass. The usual initial dose of heparin administered intravenously is 300 units·kg^{-1}. The adequacy of anticoagulation is subsequently confirmed by determination of the activated coagulation time (ACT), which should remain above 400 seconds (normal 90 seconds to 120 seconds) during cardiopulmonary bypass.

Monitoring During Cardiopulmonary Bypass

Institution of cardiopulmonary bypass is often associated with declines in mean arterial pressure, presumably reflecting the dramatic decreases in viscosity that result from infusion of prime solutions. In addition, peripheral vasodilation may accompany decreased oxygen delivery that occurs in the early period of hemodilution. Administration of alpha agonists, such as phenylephrine, to increase perfusion pressures above 50 mmHg in the early period after institution of cardiopulmonary bypass has been a common practice assuming elevated perfusion pressures are important for maintenance of cerebral blood flow. Supportive evidence for this practice is not available and many now feel that drug support of mean arterial pressure that remains above 30 mmHg is not necessary if hypothermia is being simultaneously produced.

After the initial decline, blood pressure often begins to increase spontaneously, perhaps reflecting activation of the renin-angiotensin system or sympathetic nervous system. Mean arterial pressures above 100 mmHg can lead to impairment of tissue perfusion as well as the risk of intracranial hemorrhage. Furthermore, noncoronary collateral flow is likely to be increased as mean arterial pressures rise resulting in perfusion of the heart with blood at higher temperatures than desired for optimal cellular protection. For this reason, some recommend aggressive attempts to lower mean arterial pressures that exceed 65 mmHg. Hypertension is ideally treated by reducing systemic vascular resistance with the continuous intravenous administration of nitroprusside. Alternatively, the vapors of volatile anesthetics can be introduced from vaporizers incorporated into the cardiopulmonary bypass circuit.

A rising central venous pressure with or without facial edema (eyelids and sclera) may reflect improper placement of the vena cava cannulae with obstruction to venous drainage. For example, insertion of a cannula too far into the superior vena cava can obstruct the right innominate vein leading to an increase of venous pressure in the head with associated cerebral edema. Placement of a cannula too far into the inferior vena cava results in abdominal distension. Confirmatory evidence of misplacement of a vena cava cannula is inadequate venous return from the patient to the cardiopulmonary bypass machine. Prompt withdrawal of the vena cava cannula to a more proximal position should immediately improve venous drainage.

A pulmonary artery catheter detects increases in pulmonary artery pressures due to malfunction of the left ventricular vent and the associated inadequate decompression of the left ventricle. Persistent left ventricular distension can result in damage to the contractile elements of the myocardium.

Blood gases and pH are monitored frequently during cardiopulmonary bypass. A mixed venous PO_2 less than 30 mmHg associated with metabolic acidosis suggests inadequate tissue perfusion. Temperature correction of $PaCO_2$ and pH is probably not necessary (see Chapter 17). Urine output serves as a guide to the adequacy of renal perfusion, with an output of $1 \ ml \cdot kg^{-1} \cdot hr^{-1}$ being a reasonable expectation.

During total cardiopulmonary bypass the lungs are left quiescent with or without moderate continuous positive airway pressure. The best composition of gases in the lungs during this time is unsettled, although it seems unnecessary to expose unperfused alveoli to high concentrations of oxygen. Continued ventilation of the lungs with oxygen is appropriate when there is some pulmonary blood flow as evidenced by a pulsatile pulmonary artery trace (e.g., partial cardiopulmonary bypass).

Esophageal and rectal temperatures are monitored routinely. Drug-induced vasodilation as produced by isoflurane or nitroprusside may speed the rewarming process as reflected by a more rapid approach of the rectal (core) to esophageal (blood) temperature. Measurement of urinary bladder temperature is an alternative to monitoring rectal temperature, although high urine flow rates during rewarming may cause bladder temperature to more closely parallel blood than core temperature.

Myocardial Preservation

The goal of myocardial preservation is to reduce myocardial damage introduced by the period of ischemia associated with cardiopulmonary bypass. This goal is achieved by reducing myocardial oxygen consumption by infusing cold (4° Celsius) cardioplegia solutions containing potassium (about $20 \ mEq \cdot L^{-1}$) into the aortic root, which in the presence of a distally cross-clamped aorta and competent aortic valve assures diversion of the solution into the coronary arteries. Potassium blocks the initial phase of myocardial depolarization, resulting in cessation of electrical and mechanical activity. The cold solution produces selective hypothermia of the cardiac muscle. At 37° Celsius, the normally contracting heart muscle consumes oxygen at a rate of $8 \ ml \cdot 100 \ g^{-1} \cdot min^{-1}$ to $10 \ ml \cdot 100 \ g^{-1} \cdot min^{-1}$. This consumption in the fibrillating heart at 22° Celsius is $2 \ ml \cdot 100 \ g^{-1} \cdot min^{-1}$. The electromechanically quiet heart at 22° Celsius consumes oxygen at a rate of $0.3 \ ml \cdot 100 \ g^{-1} \cdot min^{-1}$. The effectiveness of cold cardioplegia is monitored by measuring heart temperature with a temperature probe placed into the left ventricular muscle plus the absence of any visible electrical activity on the electrocardiogram. Cold cardioplegia infusions are supplemented by total body hypothermia and localized epicardial surface cooling using ice or cold irrigation solutions placed into the pericardial space. Adequate myocardial preservation is suggested by good myocardial contractility without the use of inotropic drugs at the conclusion of cardiopulmonary bypass.

A side effect of cardioplegia solutions is an increased incidence of atrioventricular heart block due to intramyocardial hyperkalemia. This heart block usually resolves in 1 hour to 2 hours and can be treated temporarily by use of an artificial cardiac pacemaker. Intramyocardial hyperkalemia also produces decreased myocardial contractility. Systemic hyperkalemia is likely to occur when coronary sinus blood containing cardioplegia solutions is returned to the oxygenator for subsequent circulation. Decreased renal function during cardiopulmonary bypass will also contribute to hyperkalemia. If hyperkalemia persists at the conclusion of cardiopulmonary bypass, it may be necessary to administer glucose (25 grams) plus regular insulin (10 units to 15 units) intravenously in attempts to shift potassium into the cells.

Maintenance of Anesthesia

Drugs selected for maintenance of anesthesia in patients undergoing cardiopulmonary bypass are determined by the patient's cardiac disease. Institution of cardiopulmonary bypass, however, produces a sudden dilution of circulating drug concentrations that can acutely reduce the depth of anesthesia. For this reason, supplemental anesthetics, such as benzodiazepines or opioids, may be administered intravenously at this time. Likewise, skeletal muscle paralysis may be supplemented with additional nondepolarizing muscle relaxants. Anesthetic depth can also be increased by volatile anesthetics from vaporizers incorporated into the cardiopulmonary bypass circuit. It must be appreciated that the impact of hemodilution on drug concentrations is likely to be offset by decreased drug needs during hypothermia. For reasons that are not clear, anesthetic requirements seem to be minimal following rewarming to a normal body temperature at the conclusion of cardiopulmonary bypass. Therefore, additional anesthesia is not routinely required during rewarming or the early period after the conclusion of cardiopulmonary bypass.

Discontinuation of Cardiopulmonary Bypass

Cardiopulmonary bypass is discontinued when the patient is hemodynamically stable and normothermia has been re-established. In the absence of adequate rewarming before discontinuing cardiopulmonary bypass, body temperature is likely to decline rapidly, resulting in metabolic acidosis and poor myocardial contractility. When the left side of the heart has been opened as during valve replacement surgery, it is mandatory to remove all air from the cardiac chambers and pulmonary veins before permitting the heart to eject blood into the aorta. Otherwise, systemic air emboli can occur, with disastrous cardiac and central nervous system effects. Unrecognized air in the coronary arteries may be a cause of poor myocardial contractility after discontinuation of cardiopulmonary bypass. Measurement of cardiac filling pressures, determination of thermodilution cardiac outputs, and calculation of systemic and pulmonary vascular resistance is necessary to guide intravenous fluid replacement and the appropriate selection of drugs in the early postcardiopulmonary bypass period. On occasion, a continuous intravenous infusion of vasodilators, such as nitroprusside or nitroglycerin, or inotropes, such as dopamine, dobutamine, or epinephrine are necessary to maintain optimal cardiac output. Posterior papillary muscle dysfunction at the conclusion of cardiopulmonary bypass may result in mitral regurgitation as evidenced by the presence of prominent V waves on the pulmonary artery occlusion pressure tracing. This dysfunction may reflect less than optimal cardioplegic protection of the posterior myocardium, which is most vulnerable to warming effects from blood in the adjacent descending thoracic aorta, as well as perfusion with warm blood representing noncoronary collateral circulation.

A mechanical alternative to inotropic support of cardiac output is the intra-aortic balloon pump. The intra-aortic balloon pump (a 25 cm long balloon mounted on a 90 cm stiff plastic catheter) is typically inserted percutaneously through the femoral artery and advanced so that the tip is just distal to the left subclavian artery. The balloon is timed to deflate immediately before systole, thus reducing end-diastolic pressure (afterload reduction) so as to enhance forward left ventricular stroke volume and to reduce myocardial oxygen requirements. Balloon inflation during diastole elevates diastolic blood pressure (diastolic augmentation) and increases the gradient for coronary perfusion. Rapid heart rates and cardiac dysrhythmias interfere with proper balloon timing and optimal augmentation of cardiac output.

When an adequate blood pressure and cardiac output have been maintained for several minutes, the aortic and vena cava cannulae are removed and protamine is administered intravenously usually over 3 minutes to 5 minutes to reverse heparin anticoagulation. Occasionally, infusion of protamine is accompanied by hypotension and pulmonary hypertension, possibly reflecting the release of histamine. Administration of nitrous oxide after cardiopulmonary bypass is questionable because this gas would unmask the presence of air in the heart or coronary arteries. For this reason, anesthesia is most often supplemented when necessary by the intravenous administration of opioids or low inhaled concentrations of volatile anesthetics. The blood and fluid that remains in the cardiopulmonary bypass circuit is washed and collected into plastic bags as packed cells for possible reinfusion to the patient. Vasoconstriction in the early period after cardiopulmonary bypass may result in false low blood pressure readings from the radial artery. The gradient between central aortic and radial artery blood pressure usually disappears within 20 minutes to 40 minutes.

Cerebral protection during cardiopulmonary bypass is enhanced by institution of hypothermia and use of filters in the arterial delivery system so as to remove debris that could become emboli. In addition, administration of sufficient barbiturates to maintain an isoelectric electroencephalogram may be effective in decreasing the incidence of neurologic dysfunction after cardiopulmonary bypass, although associated adverse cardiac effects and delayed awakening detract from this approach.[19]

REFERENCES

1. Foex P. Preoperative assessment of patients with cardiac disease. Br J Anaesth 1978;50:15–23.
2. Tarhan S, Moffitt EA, Taylor WF, Guiliani ER. Myocardial infarction after general anesthesia. JAMA 1972;220:1451–4.
3. Steen PA, Tinker JH, Tarhan S. Myocardial reinfarction after anesthesia and surgery. An update: Incidence, mortality, and predisposing factors. JAMA 1978;239:2566–70.
4. Rao TLK, Jacobs KH, El-Etr AA. Reinfarction following anesthesia in patients with myocardial infarction. Anesthesiology 1983;59:499–505.
5. Slogoff S, Keats AS. Further observations on perioperative myocardial ischemia. Anesthesiology 1986;65:539–42.
6. Reiz S, Balfors E, Sorensen MD, Ariola S, Friedman A, Truedsson H. Isoflurane-a powerful coronary vasodilator in patients with ischemic disease. Anesthesiology 1983;59:91–7.
7. Sill JC, Bove AA, Nugent M, Blaise GA, Dewey JD, Grabau C. Effects of isoflurane on coronary arterioles in the intact dog. Anesthesiology 1987;66:273–9.
8. O'Young J, Mastrocostopoulos G, Hilgenberg A, Palacios I, Kyristis A, Lappas DG. Myocardial circulatory and metabolic effects of isoflurane and sufentanil during coronary artery surgery. Anesthesiology 1987;666:653–8.
9. Starr NJ, Sethna DH, Estafanous FG. Bradycardia and asystole following rapid administration of sufentanil with vecuronium. Anesthesiology 1986;64:521–3.
10. Mangano DT. Monitoring pulmonary artery pressure in coronary-artery disease. Anesthesiology 1980;53:364–70.
11. Hilgenberg JC, McCammon RL, Stoelting RK. Pulmonary and systemic vascular responses to nitrous oxide in patients with mitral stenosis and pulmonary hypertension. Anesth Analg 1980;59:323–6.
12. Greenberg BH, Rahmitoola SH. Vasodilator therapy for valvular heart disease. JAMA 1981;246:269–72.
13. Kowalski SE. Mitral valve prolapse. Can Anaesth Soc J 1985;32:138–41.
14. Wellens HJJ, Brugada P, Penn OC. The management of preexcitation syndromes. JAMA 1987;257:2325–33.
15. Galloway PA, Glass PSA. Anesthetic implications of prolonged QT interval syndromes. Anesth Analg 1985;64:612–20.
16. Zaidan JR. Pacemakers. Anesthesiology 1984;60:319–34.
17. Prys-Roberts C. Anaesthesia and hypertension. Br J Anaesth 1984;56:711–24.
18. Nosé Y. Manual on Artificial Organs. Vol. 2. The Oxygenator. St. Louis, CV Mosby, 1973.
19. Nussmeier NA, Arlund C, Slogoff S. Neuropsychiatric complications after cardiopulmonary bypass: Cerebral protection by barbiturates. Anesthesiology 1986;64:165–70.

Chapter 20

Chronic Pulmonary Disease

Patients with chronic pulmonary disease present a challenge for management during the intraoperative and especially the postoperative period regardless of the operative site. Nevertheless, thoracic and upper abdominal operations are a particular risk for patients with chronic pulmonary disease. Furthermore, patients with chronic pulmonary disease often manifest co-existing coronary artery disease and/or essential hypertension (see Chapter 19).

OBSTRUCTIVE AIRWAYS DISEASE

Obstructive airways disease is the most frequent cause of pulmonary dysfunction. The common pathophysiologic characteristic of all of the obstructive airways disorders is an increased resistance to the flow of gases in the airways. Regional differences in airway resistance lead to areas of mismatching of ventilation to perfusion. As a result, arterial hypoxemia is likely to develop while breathing room air. Retention of carbon dioxide with the development of respiratory acidosis can also occur when regional hypoventilation is severe. All obstructive airways diseases are characterized by dyspnea, reflecting the increased work of breathing introduced by the elevated airway resistance.

Auscultation of the chest will likely reveal wheezing during exhalation, reflecting turbulent gas flow through narrowed airways. Radiographs of the chest show hyperinflated lungs with increased radiolucency due to decreased pulmonary blood flow. The diaphragm is likely to be depressed. Pulmonary function studies reveal reductions in expiratory flow rates due to increased airway resistance. For example, the forced exhaled volume in 1 second (FEV_1) is typically less than 80 percent of the vital capacity in the presence of obstructive airways disease (Fig. 20-1). Measurement of the FEV_1 alone can be misleading as the value may be low if the vital capacity is also reduced.

Bronchial asthma is the classic example of obstructive airways disease that is characterized by acute and reversible elevations of airway resistance. Pulmonary emphysema and chronic bronchitis are examples of obstructive airways diseases characterized by progressive and persistent increases in airway resistance despite treatment.

Bronchial Asthma

Bronchial asthma is estimated to be present in 3 percent to 5 percent of the population of the United States.[1] The majority of individuals develop symptoms of asthma before 5 years of age, and male patients outnumber female patients by about two to one. Bronchial asthma is usually, but not always, an inherited disorder in which inhalation of antigens elicits the elaboration of antibodies of the immunoglobulin E class. The sub-

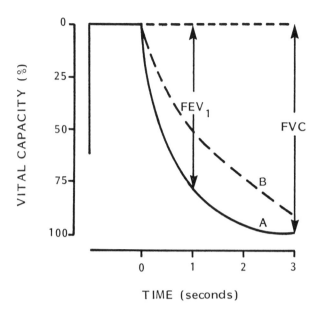

Fig. 20-1. Schematic diagram of the forced exhaled volume in 1 second (FEV₁) and forced vital capacity (FVC). The total volume of air exhaled in the first second should be equivalent to at least 80 percent of the FVC(A). In the presence of obstructive airways disease, the FEV₁ is less than 80 percent of the FVC(B).

sequent antigen-antibody interactions cause the release of vasoactive substances, including histamine, from mast cells in the lungs. These vasoactive substances result in bronchoconstriction, edema of the bronchial mucosa, and secretion of viscous mucus.

Diagnosis

Active bronchial asthma is recognized by the presence of audible wheezing during auscultation of the chest. The ratio of the FEV_1 to the vital capacity is likely to be decreased to less than 80 percent. Administration of bronchodilators can be expected to improve expiratory flow rates at least 20 percent, emphasizing the reversible aspect of the airway narrowing that is associated with bronchial asthma. The blood eosinophil count is almost invariably elevated above 300 mm³ in the presence of active immunoglobulin E-mediated bronchial asthma. An adequately treated patient with bronchial asthma will usually have a total blood eosinophil count less

than 50 mm³, whereas a rising count often signals the acceleration of bronchial asthma even before the onset of clinical symptoms. Mild bronchial asthma is usually accompanied by a normal PaO_2 and $PaCO_2$. Further progression of bronchial asthma is associated with reductions in PaO_2, whereas the $PaCO_2$ begins to increase. Elevation of the $PaCO_2$ above 50 mmHg in the presence of an acute bronchial asthma attack signals the likely need for intubation of the trachea and mechanical ventilation of the lungs.

Treatment

Drug therapy for bronchial asthma most often includes beta agonists, corticosteroids, and cromolyn. Aerosol administration of beta-2 agonists, such as albuterol or terbutaline, is an effective way to deliver high drug concentrations to the airways to produce bronchodilation with minimal likelihood of systemic effects (see Chapter 3). Aminophylline, administered as a continuous intravenous infusion, is a frequent treatment for acute bronchial asthma. Corticosteroids are presumably effective in the management of acute exacerbations of bronchial asthma as well as in the maintenance of a stable asymptomatic state by virtue of their anti-inflammatory effects plus their membrane stabilizing actions, which may reduce the release of vasoactive substances (histamine) from mast cells. Cromolyn is a membrane stabilizer that prevents the degranulation of mast cells and the subsequent release of vasoactive substances responsible for bronchoconstriction. As such, this drug is effective for prophylaxis but is of no value in the management of acute exacerbations of bronchial asthma.

Management of Anesthesia

Preoperatively, the absence of wheezing during quiet breathing and a total blood eosinophil count below 50 mm³ suggests that the patient is not experiencing an acute exacerbation of bronchial asthma. Bronchodilator drugs should be continued until the induction of anesthesia. Supplementation with cortisol may be indicated before major surgery if adrenal cortex suppression from corticosteroids used to treat asthma is a possibility (see Chapter 23). The use of anticholinergics should be individualized, remembering that although these drugs can decrease airway resistance, they can also increase the viscosity of secretions, making it difficult to remove them from the airway. Administration of H_2 antagonists is questionable because antagonism of H_2-mediated bronchodilation could unmask histamine-mediated H_1-receptor bronchoconstriction.

Regional anesthesia is an excellent choice when the surgery is superficial or on the extremities. Otherwise, the goal during induction and maintenance of general anesthesia in patients with bronchial asthma is to depress airway reflexes so as to avoid bronchoconstriction of hyper-reactive airways in response to mechanical stimulation. Induction of anesthesia is with the intravenous administration of barbiturates, benzodiazepines, or etomidate. These drugs, however, are unlikely to adequately depress airway reflexes, allowing the precipitation of bronchospasm should intubation of the trachea be attempted. Ketamine, because of its sympathomimetic effects on bronchial smooth muscle, is an alternative selection for induction of anesthesia. Increased secretions associated with administration of ketamine, however, may detract from use of this drug in patients with bronchial asthma. Before intubation of the trachea, a sufficient depth of anesthesia should be established so as to depress hyper-reactive airway reflexes and minimize the likelihood of bronchoconstriction with stimulation of the upper airway. Halothane is a popular drug for administration to patients with bronchial asthma, although enflurane and isoflurane are as effective as halothane in reversing allergic bronchoconstriction in a dog model (see Fig. 4-5).[2] Furthermore, enflurane and isoflurane, unlike halothane, do not sensitize the heart to the cardiac dysrhythmic effects of beta stimulation as produced by beta agonists including aminophylline. Intravenous administration of lidocaine 1 mg·kg^{-1} to 2 mg·kg^{-1} before intubation of the trachea is also useful for preventing reflex bronchoconstriction provoked by instrumentation of the airway.[3] Intubation of the trachea is often facilitated by the administration of succinylcholine. Although histamine release has been attributed to succinylcholine, there is no evidence that this drug is associated with the onset of increased airway resistance in patients with bronchial asthma. Skeletal muscle relaxation during maintenance of anesthesia is often provided with nondepolarizing muscle relaxants such as pancuronium or vecuronium that have minimal ability to elicit the release of histamine. Indeed, d-tubocurarine, which can stimulate the release of histamine, has been shown to increase airway resistance.[4]

Intraoperatively, the PaO_2 and $PaCO_2$ can be maintained at normal levels by mechanical ventilation of the lungs using a slow inspiratory flow rate to optimize distribution of inhaled gases. A slow breathing rate (6 breaths·min^{-1} to 10 breaths·min^{-1}) allows sufficient time for passive exhalation to occur in the presence of increased airway resistance. Positive end-expiratory pressure (PEEP) may not be ideal because adequate exhalation may be impaired in the presence of narrowed airways. Liberal intravenous administration of crystalloid solutions during the perioperative period is important for maintaining adequate hydration and assuring the presence of less viscous secretions that can be more easily expelled from the airway. At the conclusion of elective surgery, the trachea should be extubated while the depth of anesthesia is still sufficient to suppress hyper-reactive airway reflexes. The fact that bronchospasm does not predictably follow administration of anticholinesterases to reverse the effects of nondepolarizing muscle relaxants may reflect protective effects (decreased airway resistance) of simultaneously administered anticholinergics. When it is considered unsafe to extubate the trachea until the patient is awake because of the presumed presence of gastric contents, intravenous administration of lidocaine may minimize the likelihood of airway stimulation due to the continued presence of the tracheal tube.

Intraoperative Bronchospasm

Bronchospasm that occurs intraoperatively is rarely due to bronchial asthma but rather reflects other causes such as obstruction of the tracheal tube with secretions or by kinking, endobronchial intubation, pulmonary edema, inhalation of gastric fluid, or pneumothorax. In the rare instance that bronchospasm is due to bronchial asthma, the cornerstone of treatment is the intravenous administration of aminophylline (5 mg·kg^{-1} to 7 mg·kg^{-1}) administered over 15 minutes to 30 minutes followed by a continuous infusion (0.5 $mg \cdot kg^{-1} \cdot hr^{-1}$ to 1 $mg \cdot kg^{-1} \cdot hr^{-1}$). Alternatively, administration of a beta-2 agonist, such as albuterol, can be achieved by placement of a device in the inspiratory limb of the anesthetic breathing system (see Chapter 31).

Pulmonary Emphysema

Pulmonary emphysema is characterized by loss of elastic recoil of the lungs, which results in collapse of airways during exhalation leading to increased airway resistance (Table 20-1). Severe dyspnea is typical of emphysema, reflecting increased work of breathing due to loss of elastic recoil of the lungs. Preoperative evaluation of patients with emphysema should determine the severity of the disease and elucidate any reversible components such as infection or bronchospasm.

The presence of dyspnea, cough, sputum production, and decreased exercise tolerance suggests the need for preoperative pulmonary function studies. The risk of postoperative respiratory failure is increased if the preoperative ratio of FEV_1 to vital capacity is less than 50 percent. Arterial blood gases are usually normal ("pink puffers"), reflecting a high minute ventilation in an attempt to overcome increased airway resistance. The presence of a $PaCO_2$ above 50 mmHg cautions against performance of elective surgery as the risk of postoperative respiratory failure is increased. Finally, preoperative detection and treatment of cor pulmonale with supplemental oxygen is essential.

Table 20-1. Comparative Features of Chronic Obstructive Airways Disease

	Pulmonary Emphysema	Chronic Bronchitis
FEV_1	Decreased	Decreased
Total lung capacity	Increased	Increased
Dyspnea	Severe	Moderate
Arterial hypoxemia	Late	Early
Hypercarbia	Late	Early
Cor pulmonale	Late	Early
Prognosis	Good	Poor

Management of Anesthesia

The presence of pulmonary emphysema does not dictate the use of specific drugs (inhaled or injected) or techniques (regional or general) for the management of anesthesia. More important than the drugs or techniques selected is the realization that these patients are susceptible to the development of acute respiratory failure in the postoperative period.

If general anesthesia is selected, a volatile anesthetic using humidification of the inhaled gases and mechanical ventilation of the lungs is useful. The need to support ventilation of the lungs is emphasized by the observation that patients with chronic obstructive airways disease who did not retain carbon dioxide awake, hypoventilated to a greater degree than normal patients during halothane anesthesia.[5] Nitrous oxide is frequently administered in combination with volatile anesthetics. Potential disadvantages of nitrous oxide include limitation of the inhaled concentrations of oxygen and passage of this gas into bullae that result from emphysema. Conceivably, nitrous oxide could lead to enlargement and rupture of bullae, resulting in the development of a tension pneumothorax. Opioids, although acceptable, are less ideal for maintenance of anesthesia due to the frequent need for high inhaled concentrations of nitrous oxide (and associated reductions in inhaled concentrations of oxygen) to assure amnesia. Furthermore, opioids can be associated with prolonged depression of ventilation postoperatively.

Humidification of inspired gases during anesthesia is important to prevent drying of secretions in the airways. It must be appreciated that systemic dehydration due to inadequate fluid administration during the perioperative period can result in excessive drying of secretions in the airways despite humidification of inhaled gases.

Controlled ventilation of the lungs using large tidal volumes (10 $ml \cdot kg^{-1}$ to 15 $ml \cdot kg^{-1}$) combined with a slow inspiratory flow rate is useful for optimizing arterial oxygenation. A slow breathing rate (6 $breaths \cdot min^{-1}$ to 10 $breaths \cdot min^{-1}$) allows sufficient time for venous return to the heart and is less likely to be associated with undesirable degrees of hyperventilation. Continued intubation of the trachea and mechanical ventilation of the lungs in the postoperative period is likely to be necessary following major surgery in patients with severe emphysema (see Chapter 32).

Chronic Bronchitis

Chronic bronchitis is characterized by chronic or recurrent secretion of excess mucus into the bronchi resulting in increased resistance to gas flow through these airways. Patients with chronic broncitis tend to develop arterial hypoxemia ("blue bloaters"), hypercarbia, and cor pulmonale early in contrast to the delayed onset of these changes with emphysema (Table 20-1). Because the small airways account for only a minor proportion of total airway resistance, chronic bronchitis must be advanced before dyspnea becomes apparent. Cigarette smoking is the major predisposing factor to the development of chronic bronchitis. Preoperative evaluation and management of anesthesia are as described for patients with pulmonary emphysema.

RESTRICTIVE PULMONARY DISEASE

Restrictive pulmonary disease is characterized by reductions in lung compliance that result in decreased lung volumes (Fig. 20-2). A reduction in vital capacity (normal 50 ml·kg^{-1} to 70 ml·kg^{-1}) in the presence of a normal FEV$_1$ is the classic evidence of restrictive pulmonary disease.

Patients with restrictive pulmonary disease complain of dyspnea, reflecting the increased work of breathing necessary to expand poorly compliant lungs. A rapid and shallow pattern of breathing is characteristic because it minimizes the work of breathing in the presence of decreased lung compliance. A reduction in the PaCO$_2$ reflects hyperventilation produced by the rapid and shallow pattern of breathing. Indeed, the PaCO$_2$ is usually maintained at a decreased to normal value until restrictive pulmonary disease is far advanced.

Acute restrictive pulmonary disease is most often due to leakage of intravascular fluid into the interstitium of the lungs and into the alveoli,

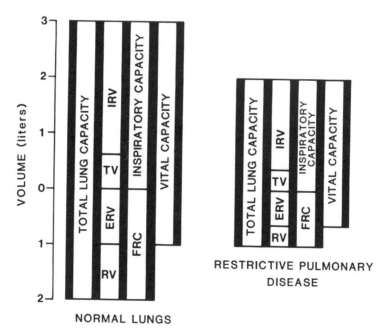

Fig. 20-2. Compared with normal lungs, restrictive pulmonary disease is characterized by a decrease in total lung capacity and all the components that comprise this capacity, especially vital capacity. IRV = inspiratory reserve volume, TV = tidal volume, ERV = expiratory reserve volume, RV = residual volume, FRC = functional residual capacity.

manifesting as pulmonary edema. Examples of acute restrictive pulmonary disease include adult respiratory distress syndrome, aspiration pneumonitis, neurogenic pulmonary edema, opioid-induced pulmonary edema, and high-altitude pulmonary edema. Chronic restrictive pulmonary disease is characterized by the presence of pulmonary fibrosis (sarcoidosis) or processes that interfere with expansion of the lungs (effusions, kyphoscoliosis, obesity, ascites, pregnancy).

Management of Anesthesia

Regional anesthesia is appropriate for peripheral surgery, but it must be appreciated that sensory levels above T10 can be associated with impairment of respiratory muscle activity necessary for patients with restrictive pulmonary disease to maintain acceptable ventilation. Restrictive pulmonary disease does not influence the choice of drugs used for the induction or maintenance of general anesthesia. The need to minimize depression of ventilation that may persist into the postoperative period should be considered when selecting these drugs. Mechanical ventilation of the lungs is useful, but high inflation pressures may be necessary to inflate the poorly compliant lungs and/or thorax. Continued ventilation of the lungs in the postoperative period is likely to be necessary when the vital capacity is less than 15 ml·kg^{-1} or the PaCO$_2$ is above 50 mmHg preoperatively. It should be appreciated that restrictive pulmonary disease contributes to decreased lung volumes, making it difficult to generate an effective cough for removal of secretions from the airways in the postoperative period.

ANESTHESIA FOR THORACIC SURGERY

Anesthesia for thoracic surgery begins with the preoperative performance of pulmonary function tests and evaluation of the adequacy of medical management of chronic pulmonary disease. Choice of drugs to produce anesthesia, selection of monitors, the impact of the lateral decubitus position on pulmonary physiology, and indications and techniques for one-lung anesthesia are considerations in planning the management of anesthesia for thoracic surgery. Postoperatively, a high index

of suspicion must be maintained for life-threatening complications (hemorrhage, bronchopleural fistula) associated with thoracic surgery. It may be necessary to continue mechanical ventilation of the lungs into the postoperative period. Finally, methods to provide postoperative analgesia should receive high priority because pain is intense after thoracic surgery.

Preoperative Preparation

Patients undergoing thoracic surgery are at high risk for developing postoperative pulmonary complications, particularly if there is co-existing chronic pulmonary disease. Specific preoperative findings that make postoperative pulmonary complications likely include dyspnea, cough and sputum production, wheezing, history of cigarette smoking, obesity, and old age. In addition, a recent upper respiratory infection may be associated with increased airway resistance that persists for as long as 5 weeks. Respiratory defense mechanisms against bacteria may also be impaired after viral respiratory infections.

The main purpose of preoperative testing is to identify patients at risk for complications and to institute appropriate perioperative therapy. Indeed, the incidence of postoperative pulmonary complications can be reduced by preoperative prophylactic measures (Table 20-2).

Discontinuation of Smoking

Smoke free intervals of 12 hours to 18 hours result in substantial declines in carboxyhemoglobin levels and normalization of the oxyhemoglobin dissociation curve as evidenced by an increase in the P$_{50}$ (arterial partial pressure of oxygen at which 50 percent of hemoglobin is saturated with oxygen).[6] Carbon monoxide may also exert negative inotropic effects. In contrast to these favorable effects, improvement in ciliary and small airway function and decreases in sputum production require prolonged abstinence from smoking. For example, the incidence of postoperative pulmonary complications after coronary artery surgery decreases only when abstinence from cigarette smoking exceeds 8 weeks (Fig. 20-3).[7]

Table 20-2. Preoperative Prophylactic Measures

Measures	Results
Discontinue smoking	Carboxyhemoglobin levels decrease within 12 hours to 18 hours so as to increase available hemoglobin
Treat pulmonary infection	Select antibiotics on basis of culture and sensitivity
Treat reversible component of increased airway resistance	Beta-2 agonists by aerosol with or without aminiphylline
Thin and mobilize secretions	Hydration and chest percussion
Teach deep breathing and coughing exercises	

Pulmonary Function Tests

Pulmolnary function tests are helpful for identifying patients at increased risk for developing pulmonary complications and for evaluating responses to preoperative pulmonary therapy. Patients with findings suggestive of the presence of chronic pulmonary disease on the history, physical examination, or chest radiograph who are scheduled for upper abdominal or thoracic surgery should undergo preoperative pulmonary function tests. In addition, elderly patients and morbidly obese patients are candidates for preoperative pulmonary function tests. Measurement of arterial blood gases and pH should be performed in patients with complaints of severe dyspnea and reduced exercise tolerance.

Numerous pulmonary function tests can be used to quantitate pulmonary disease preoperatively. The simplest and often most informative tests are measurements of flow rates during exhalation (see the section *Obstructive Airways Disease*), vital capacity (see the section *Restrictive Pulmonary Disease*), and maximum breathing capacity. The risk of postoperative pulmonary morbidity is predictably increased when preoperatively (1) the FEV_1 is less than 2 liters, (2) the ratio of the FEV_1 to forced vital capacity is less than 0.5, (3) the vital capacity is less than 15 ml·kg^{-1}, or (4) maximum breathing capacity is less than 50 percent of the predicted value. It is unusual for the $PaCO_2$ to increase before the ratio of FEV_1 to forced vital capacity is less than about 0.5. Pulmonary function studies and arterial blood gases should be repeated after antibiotic and bronchodilator therapy to confirm a beneficial response to therapy.

Prophylactic Digitalis

Resection of pulmonary tissue reduces the available pulmonary vascular bed and can cause postoperative right atrial and ventricular enlargement

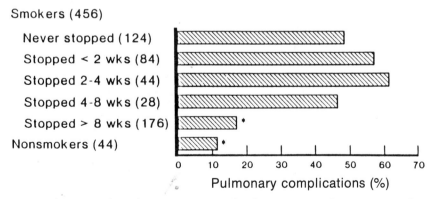

Fig. 20-3. Preoperative duration of smoking cessation and pulmonary complication rates after cardiac surgery. The incidence of pulmonary complications begins to decrease only when abstinence from cigarette smoking is greater than 8 weeks. (From Warner et al.,[7] with permission.)

with associated cardiac dysrhythmias, especially atrial fibrillation. For this reason, prophylactic use of digitalis (oral digoxin 0.75 mg in divided doses the day before surgery and 0.25 mg before the induction of anesthesia) has been recommended, particularly in elderly patients undergoing resection of large amounts of lung tissue.[8] A disadvantage of prophylactic digitalis is confusion with digitalis toxicity should cardiac dysrythmias develop postoperatively. Indeed, events such as alterations in renal function, decreases in serum potassium concentrations due to hyperventilation of the lungs, and increases in sympathetic nervous system activity are likely to occur intraoperatively and thus increase the likelihood of increased pharmacologic effects from circulating digitalis.[9]

Management of Anesthesia

General anesthesia with controlled ventilation of the lungs is appropriate for thoracic surgery. Use of volatile anesthetics with or without nitrous oxide is common, as these potent drugs reduce irritability of the airways and can be rapidly eliminated at the conclusion of surgery. In addition, volatile anesthetics do not seem to inhibit hypoxic pulmonary vasoconstriction, thus contributing to maintenance of arterial oxygenation during one-lung anesthesia (Fig. 20-4).[10] If nitrous oxide is administered, the inhaled concentrations should be limited to 50 percent until the adequacy of oxygenation can be confirmed by pulse oximetry or measurement of the PaO_2. Nondepolarizing muscle relaxants are usually administered to facilitate controlled ventilation of the lungs, to improve surgical exposure by maximizing mechanical separation of the ribs, and to decrease requirements for volatile anesthetics. Ketamine is useful for induction of anesthesia for emergency thoracotomy associated with hypovolemia (blunt trauma, gun shot, stab wound). Most patients undergoing thoracotomy should have an intra-arterial catheter in place to permit continuous monitoring of blood pressure and frequent measurement of blood gases and pH. A central venous pressure catheter is helpful for guiding intravenous fluid replacement. Alternatively, a pulmonary artery catheter should be considered if co-existing coronary artery disease or cardiac valvular dysfunction is present. A cath-

eter should be inserted into the bladder of patients who are expected to undergo long operations associated with alterations in blood volume, necessitating infusions of large amounts of intravenous fluids.

Lateral Decubitus Position

The lateral decubitus position necessary for thoracic surgery plus the need for mechanical ventilation of the lungs results in an altered distribution of ventilation relative to perfusion (see Chapter 15).

One-Lung Anesthesia

One-lung anesthesia using a double lumen tracheal tube is indicated when one lung can contaminate the other lung with either infected material or blood or when the distribution of ventilation between the two lungs must be separated as in the presence of a bronchopleural fistula. A relative indication for one-lung anesthesia is to provide a quiet lung and improved operating conditions as during lobectomy (especially upper lobectomy, which is technically most difficult), pneumonectomy, resection of a thoracic aneurysm, or operations on the esophagus.

A clear plastic disposable Robertshaw tube with a low pressure cuff is the most frequently used double-lumen tracheal tube (Fig. 20-5). Inflation of the proximal cuff on this tube provides a seal with the tracheal mucosa. Inflation of the cuff on the distal portion of the tube that is present in the left or right mainstem bronchus provides a seal to isolate that lung from the contralateral lung. A left Robertshaw tube is used for operations requiring isolation of the right lung and ventilation of the left lung. When isolation of the left lung is required, either a left or right Robertshaw tube may be used. The nearness of the right upper lobe bronchus to the carina introduces the risk of inadequate ventilation of the right upper lobe when a right tube is used. To avoid this complication, it is acceptable to use a left Robertshaw tube for all one-lung anesthetics.[11] Should clamping of the left mainstem bronchus be necessary, the left Robertshaw endobronchial cuff is deflated and the tube is withdrawn into the trachea at the appropriate time, thus effectively converting this

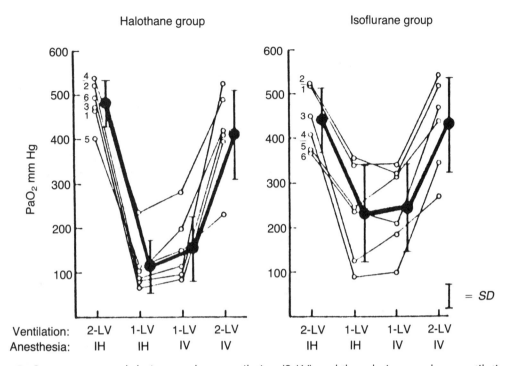

Fig. 20-4. PaO₂ was measured during two-lung ventilation (2-LV) and then during one-lung ventilation (1-LV) during inhalation (IH) or intravenous (IV) anesthesia. Addition of halothane or isoflurane (about 1.0 MAC) did not greatly alter PaO₂, suggesting that these anesthetics do not significantly inhibit hypoxic pulmonary vasoconstriction. Clear circles indicate individual patient data and closed circles indicate mean ± SD for each group. (From Benumof et al.,[10] with permission.)

double lumen tube to a single lumen tube for ventilation of the right lung. Proper placement of the Robertshaw tube is confirmed by auscultation of the chest during positive pressure ventilation of the lungs with both the tracheal and endobronchial cuffs inflated. Then one connecting tube should be clamped and the disappearance of breath sounds on that side and continuance of breath sounds on the other side should be confirmed to ensure proper positioning of the tube. Auscultation of the lungs in the axilla minimizes possible confusion from transmitted breath sounds. In addition to auscultation it is useful to confirm the position of the tube with a fiberoptic laryngoscope (see Chapter 12). Looking down the right lumen, the endoscopist should see the carina and the upper surface of the left endobronchial cuff. The left endobronchial cuff must not herniate over the carina. When it is not possible

to pass or correctly position a double lumen tube the same result may be achieved by passing a Fogarty catheter through a single lumen tube into either the right or left mainstem bronchus.

The major disadvantage of one-lung anesthesia is the introduction of an iatrogenic right-to-left intrapulmonary shunt by virtue of continued perfusion to both lungs while only the dependent lung is ventilated. An unpredictable degree of variability in the magnitude of this shunt between patients reflects multiple factors involved in determining the amount of perfusion to the upper nonventilated lung. In addition to gravity, the amount of perfusion to the nonventilated lung is influenced by (1) hypoxic pulmonary vasoconstriction, (2) surgical compression, and (3) the method used to ventilate the dependent lung. Arterial hypoxemia may also be due to unrecognized blockade of the tracheal tube lumen with secretions.

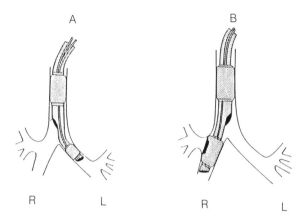

Fig. 20-5. The Robertshaw double-lumen tracheal tube is available as a left (A) or right (B) design. Placed in the trachea, the distal end of the double lumen tube is directed into the left (L) or right (R) mainstem bronchus. The distal end of the right Robertshaw tube incorporates a slotted cuff to permit ventilation of the right upper lobe.

For all these reasons, use of high inspired concentrations of oxygen, continuous monitoring of arterial oxygen saturations by pulse oximetry, and frequent measurements of the PaO_2 are indicated during one-lung anesthesia. If arterial hypoxemia persists despite inhalation of high concentrations of oxygen, the selective application of a low level of PEEP (2.5 cm H_2O to 10 cm H_2O) to the ventilated and dependent lung can be instituted in an attempt to divert more ventilation to this lung. Although selective dependent lung PEEP may improve arterial oxygenation, it may also increase pulmonary vascular resistance in the ventilated lung, resulting in further intrapulmonary shunt. In fact, selective continuous positive airway pressure (CPAP, 2.5 cm H_2O to 10 cm H_2O) applied to the nonventilated and nondependent lung is the most efficacious maneuver for improving arterial oxygenation during one-lung anesthesia. Presumably, this selective CPAP causes some oxygenation of blood perfusing the nondependent lung while also increasing pulmonary vascular resistance in this lung, thus diverting more blood flow to the ventilated and dependent lung. Ligation of the pulmonary artery during one-lung anesthesia for a pneumonectomy improves oxygenation by removing perfusion to the unventilated lung. Elimination of carbon dioxide is not usually a problem during one-lung anesthesia. An alternative to one-lung anesthesia using a double-lumen tracheal tube is the use of high frequency positive pressure ventilation.

Conclusion of Surgery

Hyperinflation of the lungs is important to exclude air from the pleural space at the conclusion of thoracic surgery. Furthermore, alveoli incised during segmental resection of the lungs continue to leak air into the pleural space necessitating the placement of drainage tubes (chest tubes) to assure removal of this air and continued expansion of the lung. These drainage tubes are connected to a sterile disposable plastic unit, which incorporates a one-way valve that permits continuous suction. Chest tubes must not be allowed to kink because sudden increases in intrathoracic pressure, as with coughing, may accentuate the leak and cause a tension pneumothorax if air cannot escape.

Placement of drainage tubes is not necessary after a pneumonectomy. Instead, intrapleural pressure on the operated side is adjusted by aspirating air to slightly below atmospheric pressure. Excessive negative pressure can cause hypotension by shifting the mediastinum and compromising cardiac output.

The trachea may be extubated when the adequacy of spontaneous ventilation is confirmed and protective upper airway reflexes have returned. In otherwise healthy patients, extubation of the trachea may be performed at the conclusion of surgery. Often, however, continued mechanical ventilation of the lungs via a tracheal tube is indicated in the postoperative period (see Chapter 32).

Postoperative Pulmonary Complications

Postoperative pulmonary complications after thoracic surgery (other forms of surgery too, especially upper abdominal operations) are most often characterized as atelectasis followed by pneumonia and arterial hypoxemia. The severity of these complications parallels the magnitude of reductions in vital capacity and functional residual capacity (see Chapter 31). Presumably, reductions in these lung volumes interfere with generation of an effective cough, as well as contributing to atelectasis. The net effect is decreased clearance of secretions from the airways and atelectasis, leading to pneumonia and arterial hypoxemia.

Treatment of Postoperative Pain

Adequate analgesia after thoracic surgery permits patients to breathe deeply and cough effectively so as to minimize the likelihood of postoperative atelectasis and/or pneumonia. Intermittent administration of parenteral opioids is a frequent approach, adjusting the dose to achieve maximal analgesia without excessive sedation or depression of ventilation. In the early postoperative period, the intravenous administration of morphine (1 mg to 2 mg increments) until adequate analgesia is achieved can be used. Intravenous infusion devices that permit the patient to self-dose with opioids when pain intensity increases (patient controlled analgesia) are useful after patients awaken from anesthesia (see Chapters 30 and 33). Intercostal nerve blocks with long-acting local anesthetics such as bupivacaine are an alternative to parenteral opioids for providing analgesia. Intercostal nerve blocks can be performed under direct vision (intrathoracic) by the surgeon before closing the chest or postoperatively by the anesthesiologist. Transient hypotension has been associated with intrathoracic performance of these blocks, presumably reflecting thoracic sympathectomy.[12] Total spinal block has also followed intrathoracic performance of intercostal nerve blocks.[13] Assuming this latter complication represents unrecognized dural puncture or perineural spread of local anesthetics, it is recommended that intercostal nerve blocks be performed at least 8 cm lateral to the intervertebral foramen. Thoracic epidural placement of local anesthetics is an effective but often an impractical method for providing analgesia after a thoracotomy. Alternatively, placement of opioids in the lumbar epidural or subarachoid space has been shown to provide long-lasting analgesia after thoracotomy without associated sympathetic and proprioceptive nerve blockade. Finally, transcutaneous electrical stimulation provides weak analgesic effects but is devoid of undesirable depressant effects.

MEDIASTINOSCOPY

Mediastinoscopy is often performed before thoracotomy to establish the diagnosis and/or resectability of carcinoma of the lung. Hemorrhage and pneumothorax are the most frequently encountered complications of this procedure. If a thoracotomy is not subsequently performed, it is important to maintain a high index of suspicion for pneumothorax in the immediate postoperative period. Radiographs of the chest in the recovery room are helpful in detecting the presence of a pneumothorax.

Positive pressure ventilation of the lungs during mediastinoscopy is recommended so as to minimize the risk of venous air embolism. The mediastinoscope can also exert pressure against the right subclavian artery, causing the loss of a pulse distal to the site of compression and an erroneous diagnosis of cardiac arrest. Likewise, unrecognized compression of the right carotid artery has been proposed as an explanation for postoperative neurologic deficits that may occur after this procedure. Bradycardia during mediastinoscopy may be due to stretching of the vagus nerve or trachea by the mediastinoscope. Treatment is by repositioning of the mediastinoscope followed by intravenous administration of atropine if bradycardia persists.

REFERENCES

1. Kingston HGG, Hirshman CA. Perioperative management of the patient with asthma. Anesth Analg 1984;63:844–55.
2. Hirshman CA, Edelstein G, Peetz S, Wayne R, Downes H. Mechanism of action of inhalational anesthesia on airways. Anesthesiology 1982;56:107–11.
3. Downes H, Gerber N, Hirshman CA. I.V. lignocaine in reflex and allergic bronchoconstriction. Br J Anaesth 1980;52:873–8.
4. Crago RR, Bryan AC, Laws AIC, Winestock AE. Respiratory flow resistance after curare and pancuronium measured by forced oscillations. Can Anaesth Soc J 1972;19:607–14.
5. Pietak S, Weenig CS, Hickey RF, Fairley HB. Anesthetic effects on ventilation in patients with chronic obstructive pulmonary disease. Anesthesiology 1975;42:160–6.
6. Kambam JR, Chen LH, Hyman SA. Effect of short-term smoking halt on carboxyhemoglobin levels and P_{50} values. Anesth Analg 1986;65:1186–8.

7. Warner MA, Divertie MB, Tinker JH. Preoperative cessation of smoking and pulmonary complications in coronary artery bypass patients. Anesthesiology 1984;60:380–3.

8. Chee TP, Prakash NS, Desser KB, Benchimol A. Postoperative supraventricular arrhythmias and the role of prophylactic digoxin in cardiac surgery. Am Heart J 1982;104:974–7.

9. Chung DC. Anesthetic problems associated with the treatment of cardiovascular disease: I. Digitalis toxicity. Can Anaesth Soc J 1981;28:6–16.

10. Benumof JL, Augustine SD, Gibbons JA. Halothane and isoflurane only slightly impair arterial oxygenation during one-lung ventilation in patients undergoing thoracotomy. Anesthesiology 1987;67:910–5.

11. Benumof JL, Partridge BL, Salvatierra C, Keating J. Margin of safety in positioning double-lumen endotracheal tubes. Anesthesiology 1987;67:729–38.

12. Cottrell WM, Schick LM, Perkins HM, Modell JH. Hemodynamic changes after intercostal nerve block with bupivacaine-epinephrine solution. Anesth Analg 1978;57:492–5.

13. Benumof JL, Semenza J. Total spinal anesthesia following intrathoracic intercostal nerve blocks. Anesthesiology 1975;43:124–5.

Chapter 21

Hepatic Disease

Management of anesthesia in the presence of liver disease requires an understanding of the physiologic functions of the liver. In addition, the impact of anesthesia and surgery on hepatic blood flow has important implications for the management of anesthesia. Liver function tests are useful for detecting unsuspected liver disease preoperatively and for establishing the diagnosis when postoperative liver dysfunction occurs. Liver transplantation represents one of the most demanding and intense anesthetic challenges with which anesthesiologists are confronted.

PHYSIOLOGIC FUNCTIONS OF THE LIVER

Physiologic functions of the liver that may be altered by co-existing liver disease include glucose homeostasis, protein synthesis, drug metabolism, and bilirubin formation and excretion. Hepatic sinuses are lined by Kupffer's cells that are capable of phagocytizing bacteria absorbed from the gastrointestinal tract into the portal vein. The response of patients during the perioperative period may be influenced by disease-induced alterations in these important functions of the liver.

Glucose Homeostasis

The liver is responsible for the storage and release of glucose. Glucose enters hepatocytes, where it is stored as glycogen. Breakdown of glycogen (glycogenolysis) releases glucose back into the systemic circulation to maintain normal blood glucose concentrations. The liver can store only about 75 g of glycogen, which can be depleted by 24 hours to 48 hours of starvation. Glucose homeostasis depends primarily on conversion of lactate, glycerol, and amino acids to glucose (gluconeogenesis) when liver glycogen stores are depleted. Exogenous sources of glucose during the fasting period associated with surgery become important when glycogen stores are depleted due to poor preoperative nutrition and when gluconeogenesis is inhibited by anesthesia.[1] Indeed, patients with cirrhosis of the liver may be vulnerable to the development of hypoglycemia in the perioperative period.

Protein Synthesis

All proteins except gamma globulins and antihemophilic factor (factor VIII) are synthesized in the rough endoplasmic reticulum of hepatocytes. Approximately 10 g to 15 g of albumin are produced daily to maintain plasma concentrations of this protein between 3.5 g·dl^{-1} to 5.5 g·dl^{-1}. Plasma albumin concentrations less than 3.5 g·dl^{-1} signify significant liver disease. The half-time for albumin, however, is about 23 days, emphasizing that acute liver dysfunction will not be reflected by decreased plasma concentrations of this protein.

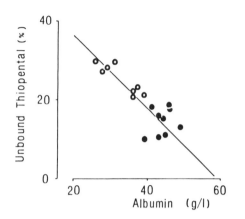

Fig. 21-1. Unbound thiopental concentrations parallel serum concentrations of albumin in patients with cirrhosis of the liver (clear circles) and normal patients (solid circles). Reduced serum albumin concentrations in patients with cirrhosis result in higher unbound serum concentrations of thiopental. (From Pandele et al.,[2] with permission.)

Protein synthesis in the liver is important for drug binding, coagulation, and production of enzymes necessary for hydrolysis of ester linkages.

Drug Binding

When liver disease results in decreased albumin production, fewer sites will be available for drug binding. As a result, the unbound, pharmacologically active fractions of drugs, such as thiopental, increase (Fig. 21-1).[2] Increased drug sensitivities due to decreased protein binding are most likely to manifest when plasma albumin concentrations are less than 2.5 g·dl^{-1}.

Coagulation

Clotting abnormalities must be suspected in patients with liver disease because hepatocytes are responsible for the synthesis of most procoagulants. The adequacy of clotting factor levels is evaluated by measuring the prothrombin time, partial thromboplastin time, and bleeding time. Liver function must be dramatically depressed before impaired coagulation manifests because many coagulation factors require only 20 percent to 30 percent of their normal levels to prevent bleeding. Nevertheless, the plasma half-time of hepatic-produced clotting factors, such as prothrombin and fibrinogen, is short and acute liver dysfunction is likely to be associated with clotting abnormalities.

Liver disease associated with splenomegaly can alter the normal coagulation mechanism independent of procoagulant synthesis by virtue of trapping platelets in the spleen. Another factor predisposing to a bleeding diathesis is the failure of a diseased liver to clear plasma activators of the fibrinolytic system.

Hydrolysis of Ester Linkages

Severe liver disease may decrease the production of cholinesterase (pseudocholinesterase) enzyme that is necessary for the hydrolysis of ester linkages in drugs such as succinylcholine and ester local anesthetics. As a result, the duration of apnea after the administration of succinylcholine may be prolonged in the presence of liver disease (Fig. 21-2).[3] The plasma half-time for plasma cholinesterase is about 14 days, emphasizing that acute liver failure is unlikely to be associated with a slowed rate of succinylcholine hydrolysis.

Drug Metabolism

Drug metabolism, characterized by the conversion of lipid soluble drugs to a more water soluble and pharmacologically less active substances, is under the control of microsomal enzymes, which are present in the smooth endoplasmic reticulum of hepatocytes. Chronic liver disease may interfere with metabolism of drugs by virtue of reduced numbers of enzyme-containing hepatocytes and/or decreased hepatic blood flow that typically accompanies cirrhosis of the liver. Indeed, prolonged elimination half-times for morphine, alfentanil, diazepam, lidocaine, pancuronium, and, to a lesser extent, vecuronium have been demonstrated in patients with cirrhosis of the liver (Fig. 21-3).[4–6] Repeated injections of these drugs would be likely to produce cumulative effects in patients with severe liver disease. Conversely, cirrhosis of the liver does not greatly influence elimination half-times of thiopental or fentanyl compared with normal patients. Despite further reductions in

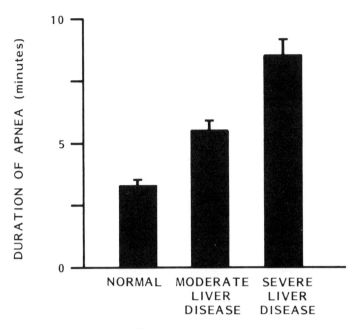

Fig. 21-2. The duration of apnea (mean ± SE) after intravenous administration of succinylcholine (0.6 mg·kg^{-1}) is prolonged in the presence of moderate and severe liver disease, reflecting decreased hepatic production of plasma cholinesterase necessary for the hydrolysis of the muscle relaxant. (Data from Foldes et al.,[3] with permission.)

hepatic blood flow during anesthesia, reduced clearance of drugs seems to be principally due to inhibition of microsomal enzymes.[7]

It is conceivable that accelerated drug metabolism could accompany cirrhosis of the liver. For example, in the presence of reduced numbers of hepatocytes, the amount of drug presented to each cell is increased. This may stimulate microsomal enzyme activity (enzyme induction). Enzyme induction may also be a response to chronic drug therapy or alcohol abuse. In addition, there seems to be cross-tolerance between substances known to produce liver disease (alcohol) and other depressant drugs, including inhaled and injected anesthetics.

Bilirubin Formation and Excretion

Bilirubin is produced in the reticuloendothelial system from the breakdown of hemoglobin. This bilirubin is bound to albumin for transport to the liver. Because protein-bound bilirubin (unconju-gated) is not water soluble, urinary excretion is minimal. Conjugation of bilirubin with glucuronic acid in the liver renders bilirubin water soluble. This conjugation is under the control of the enzyme, glucuronyl transferase, which is susceptible to enzyme induction. A small amount of conjugated bilirubin enters the circulation and undergoes renal excretion. The remainder is excreted into the biliary canaliculi and eventually into the small intestine.

HEPATIC BLOOD FLOW

The liver is unique in that it receives a dual afferent blood supply equivalent to about 25 percent of the cardiac output (Fig. 21-4). The majority of hepatic blood flow (70 percent) is via the portal vein and the remainder is derived from the hepatic artery. Oxygen delivery to the liver may be marginal because most of the blood flow is with desaturated hemoglobin delivered via the portal vein.

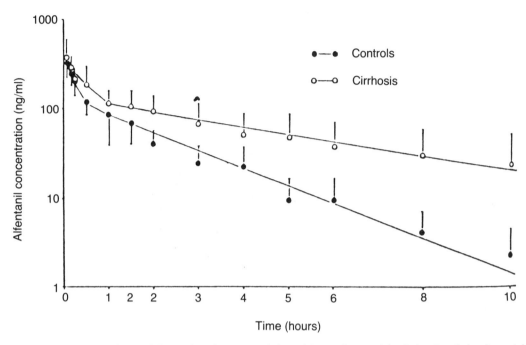

Fig. 21-3. Clearance of alfentanil from the plasma is delayed in patients with cirrhosis of the liver (clear circles) compared with normal (control) patients (solid circles). Mean ± SD. (From Ferrier et al.,[5] with permission.)

Determinants of Hepatic Blood Flow

Hepatic blood flow is determined by perfusion pressure (mean arterial or portal vein pressure minus hepatic vein pressure) and splanchnic vascular resistance. The splanchnic vessels are innervated by vasoconstrictor nerve fibers from the sympathetic nervous system. Splanchnic nerve stimulation, as produced by arterial hypoxemia, hypercapnia, or increased circulating concentrations of catecholamines, results in increased splanchnic vascular resistance and decreased hepatic blood flow. The hepatic circulation is also supplied with beta receptors, and blockade of these receptors as produced by propranolol is associated with reductions in hepatic blood flow. Positive pressure ventilation of the lungs or congestive heart failure can decrease hepatic blood flow, presumably by increasing central venous pressure (hepatic vein pressure) and thus decreasing hepatic perfusion pressure. Autoregulation of hepatic blood flow is not prominent, emphasizing that

drug-induced decreases in blood pressure, as occur during anesthesia, are likely to be associated with similar reductions in hepatic blood flow. Cirrhosis of the liver that is associated with increased resistance to flow through the liver is predictably accompanied by reductions in hepatic blood flow (see the section *Cirrhosis of the Liver*).

Impact of Anesthetic Drugs on Hepatic Blood Flow

Inhaled anesthetics, as well as regional anesthesia, typically reduced hepatic blood flow 20 percent to 30 percent in the absence of surgical stimulation. These changes reflect drug- or technique-induced effects on perfusion pressure and/or splanchnic vascular resistance. For example, reductions in hepatic blood flow associated with volatile anesthetics as well as regional anesthesia (T5 sensory level) are most likely due to decreased perfusion pressure. Positive pressure ventilation of the lungs may reduce perfusion pressure across the liver by elevating venous pressure. Isoflurane, adminis-

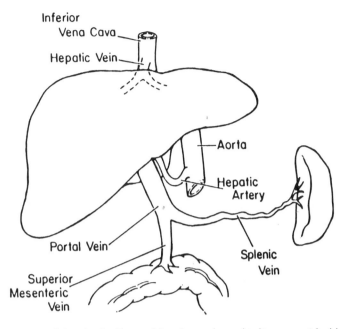

Fig. 21-4. Schematic depiction of the dual afferent blood supply to the liver provided by the portal vein and hepatic artery. About 70 percent of hepatic blood flow is via the portal vein with the remainder derived from the hepatic artery. Total hepatic blood flow is directly proportional to perfusion pressure across the liver and inversely related to splanchnic vascular resistance. Cirrhosis of the liver increases resistance to flow thorugh the portal vein and decreases hepatic blood flow.

tered to animals, is less likely to decrease hepatic blood flow than is halothane, thus better maintaining hepatocyte oxygen delivery (Fig. 21-5).[8] Selective hepatic artery constriction due to volatile anesthetics has been observed in occasional patients without liver disease. The mechanism and clinical significance of this selective hepatic artery constriction is not known.

Ideally, reductions in hepatic blood flow would be accompanied by similar reductions in hepatic oxygen consumption. Nevertheless, hepatic blood flow during anesthesia decreases more than does splanchnic oxygen consumption. There is no evidence, however, that these drug-induced reductions in hepatic blood flow are associated with inadequate hepatocyte oxygenation. It is conceivable, however, that cirrhosis of the liver could make hepatocytes more vulnerable to adverse effects from drug-induced reductions in hepatic blood flow.

Impact of Surgical Stimulation on Hepatic Blood Flow

Surgical stimulation and the nearness of the operative site to the liver are important determinants of the magnitude of decrease in hepatic blood flow during general anesthesia. For example, the greatest reductions in hepatic blood flow occur when the operative site is near the liver, as occurs during a cholecystectomy.[9]

LIVER FUNCTION TESTS

Liver function tests are used to detect the presence of liver disease preoperatively and to establish the diagnosis when postoperative liver dysfunction occurs. It is important to remember that liver function tests are rarely specific. Furthermore, the large reserve of the liver means that considerable hepatic damage can be present before liver func-

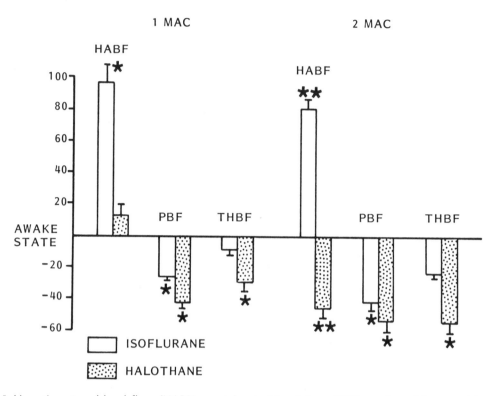

Fig. 21-5. Hepatic artery blood flow (HABF), portal vein blood flow (PBF), and total hepatic blood flow (THBF) were measured in dogs (mean ± SE) as percent changes from awake values. HABF was increased during 1 MAC and 2 MAC isoflurane, and PBF was decreased by both drugs at each dose. THBF and presumably hepatocyte oxygen delivery was better maintained during administration of isoflurane compared with halothane. *$P < 0.05$ vs. awake. **$P < 0.05$ isoflurane vs. halothane. (From Gelman et al.,[8] with permission.)

tion tests are altered. Indeed, cirrhosis of the liver may produce little alteration in liver function, and only when some additional insult, such as anesthesia and surgery, produces further deterioration does the underlying liver disease become obvious.

Postoperatively, the magnitude of liver dysfunction, as reflected by liver function tests, is exaggerated by operations near the liver (Fig. 21-6).[10] The specific anesthetic drug, however, does not influence the magnitude of postoperative liver dysfunction as reflected by liver function tests. It seems likely that surgical stimulation and associated reductions in hepatic blood flow can adversely alter hepatic function independent of the inhaled anesthetic. Indeed, postoperative liver dysfunction is likely to be greater in the presence of co-existing

liver disease (Fig. 21-7).[11] These observations, however, have not been consistently reproducible.[12]

Commonly measured liver function tests include the serum concentrations of albumin, bilirubin, transaminase enzymes, and alkaline phosphatase, and determination of the prothrombin time (Table 21-1). Based on these tests, postoperative liver dysfunction can be categorized as prehepatic, intrahepatic, and posthepatic (Table 21-2).

Prehepatic Dysfunction

Prehepatic dysfunction as a cause of postoperative jaundice most likely reflects delivery of bilirubin overloads to patients. Causes of hyperbilirubinemia include hemolysis, hematoma resorption or whole blood administration. Hemolysis is often

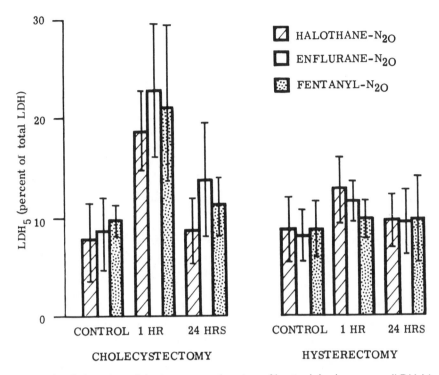

Fig. 21-6. The magnitude of elevation of the isoenzyme fraction of lactic dehydrogenase (LDH₅) is determined by the nearness of the operation to the liver and not the drugs used for maintenance of anesthesia. (From Viegas and Stoelting,[10] with permission.)

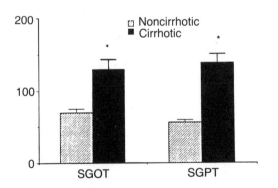

Fig. 21-7. Percent increase (mean ± SE) of liver transaminase enzymes (SGOT and SGPT) in noncirrhotic and cirrhotic rats after exposure to 1.5 percent halothane in 50 percent oxygen for 3 hours. *P < 0.05 compared with noncirrhotic rats. (From Baden et al.,[11] with permission.)

accompanied by decreases in the hematocrit or increases in the reticulocyte count. A 500 ml transfusion of fresh whole blood contains 250 mg of bilirubin. The bilirubin load increases as the age of transfused blood increases. Patients with normal hepatic function can receive large amounts of blood without any appreciable increase in serum bilirubin concentrations. This response can be different in patients with co-existing liver disease.

Overt jaundice is usually present when serum bilirubin concentrations exceed 3 mg·dl⁻¹. The unconjugated fraction of bilirubin is increased more than the conjugated fraction when prehepatic dysfunction is present.

Intrahepatic Dysfunction

Intrahepatic dysfunction reflects direct hepatocellular damage due to toxic effects of drugs, sepsis, arterial hypoxemia, congestive heart failure, or viruses. This form of postoperative dysfunction is

Table 21-1. Liver Function Tests

Test	Normal values[a]
Albumin	$3.5-5.5$ g·dl^{-1}
Bilirubin	$0.3-1.1$ mg·dl^{-1}
Unconjugated bilirubin (indirect-reacting)	$0.2-0.7$ mg·dl^{-1}
Conjugated bilirubin (direct-reacting)	$0.1-0.4$ mg·dl^{-1}
Glutamic oxalacetic transaminase (SGOT, asparatate aminotransferase)	$15-40$ units·ml^{-1}
Glutamic pyruvic transaminase (SGPT, alanine aminotransferase)	$5-35$ units·ml^{-1}
Lactic dehydrogenase (LDH)	$60-100$ units·ml^{-1}
Alkaline phosphatase	$10-30$ units·ml^{-1}
Prothrombin time	$12-14$ sec

[a] Normal values for each individual laboratory should be consulted when interpreting liver function tests.

recognized by hyperbilirubinemia and marked increases in serum transaminase concentrations. Although intrahepatic dysfunction can occasionally cause accumulation of unconjugated bilirubin due to impaired hepatic uptake or conjugation, accumulation of conjugated bilirubin is more common reflecting impaired excretion of bilirubin conjugates into bile. Hepatocytes contain large amounts of transaminase enzymes (glutamic oxalacetic transaminase, glutamic pyruvic transaminase, lac-

tic dehydrogenase) that spill into the circulation when hepatocytes are acutely damaged. Other tissues, however, such as the heart, lung, and skeletal muscles, also contain transaminase enzymes. Indeed, postoperative increases in the serum transaminase concentrations may reflect skeletal muscle damage from intramuscular injections given preoperatively or damage to skeletal muscles during surgery. Nevertheless, marked elevations of the serum transaminase enzyme concentrations to three times normal or greater in the postoperative period should suggest acute hepatocellular damage.

Posthepatic Dysfunction

Posthepatic dysfunction reflects bile duct obstruction and is characterized by hyperbilirubinemia (predominately the conjugated fraction) and elevated serum concentrations of alkaline phosphatase. Alkaline phosphatase is present in bile duct cells such that even slight degrees of biliary obstruction are manifested by threefold or greater elevations of the serum concentrations of this enzyme. It must be remembered, however, that there are also extrahepatic stores of alkaline phosphatase, particularly in skeletal muscles.

Benign postoperative intrahepatic cholestasis may occur postoperatively, especially if surgery is in elderly patients and is complicated by hypotension, arterial hypoxemia, and massive blood transfusion. Jaundice in association with elevated serum

Table 21-2. Classification and Causes of Hepatic Dysfunction

	Prehepatic	Intrahepatic	Posthepatic
Bilirubin	Increased (unconjugated fraction)	Increased (conjugated fraction)	Increased (conjugated fraction)
Transaminases	Normal	Markedly elevated	Normal to slightly elevated
Alkaline phosphatase	Normal	Normal to slightly elevated	Markedly elevated
Causes	Hemolysis Hematoma resorption Bilirubin overload from whole blood	Viral Drugs Sepsis Hypoxemia Cardiac failure Cirrhosis	Stones Cancer Sepsis

concentrations of conjugated bilirubin is typically present within 48 hours postoperatively and may persist for 14 days to 28 days in these patients.

DRUG-INDUCED HEPATITIS

Many drugs including isoniazid, phenytoin, sulfonamides, chlorpromazine, and alpha-methyldopa can cause hepatic cellular changes that are indistinguishable from viral hepatitis. Likewise, administration of halothane, particularly with repeated exposures at short intervals, is occasionally (between 1 in 22,000 to 1 in 35,000 administrations) associated with hepatic dysfunction (see Chapter 5). Certainly, halothane should not be administered to patients who have experienced postoperative hepatic dysfunction for unknown reasons after a previous operation performed with halothane anesthesia.

CIRRHOSIS OF THE LIVER

Cirrhosis of the liver is a chronic disease process that destroys the hepatic parenchyma and subsequently replaces it with collagen. Excessive use of alcohol is the most frequent cause of cirrhosis. Cirrhosis is associated with decreases in the number of hepatocytes, leading to an impairment of all the physiologic functions of the liver (see the section *Physiologic Functions of the Liver*). Another important change associated with cirrhosis is a reduction in hepatic blood flow, due to increased resistance to blood flow through the portal vein. As a result of this increased resistance, the proportion of hepatic blood flow delivered via the portal vein is decreased, and the contribution to total hepatic blood flow from the hepatic artery is increased. Therefore, decreases in systemic perfusion pressure or arterial oxygenation during anesthesia and surgery are more likely to jeopardize the adequacy of hepatic blood flow and delivery of oxygen to the liver in patients with cirrhosis as compared with normal patients.

Portal Vein Hypertension

The most striking finding on physical examination related to portal vein hypertension due to cirrhosis of the liver is hepatomegaly with or without splenomegaly and ascites. Ascites reflects decreased plasma oncotic pressure secondary to low serum albumin concentrations, elevated resistance to blood flow through the portal vein, and increased secretion of antidiuretic hormone. Despite the loss of skeletal muscle mass, body weight is often maintained due to accumulation of ascitic fluid.

Gastroesophageal varices are predictable complications of portal vein hypertension. Varices are massively dilated submucosal veins that develop to allow passage of splanchnic venous blood from the high pressure portal system to the low pressure azygous and hemiazygous thoracic veins. Chronic bleeding from these varices is reflected by moderate reductions in the hematocrit. Hemorrhage may be severe, requiring massive blood replacement, balloon tamponade, or sclerotherapy. Portasystemic shunts represent a surgical treatment for portal hypertension.

Extrahepatic Complications of Cirrhosis

A hyperdynamic circulation characterized by an increased cardiac output is often present in patients with cirrhosis. This increased cardiac output may reflect increased intravascular fluid volume, decreased viscosity of the blood secondary to anemia, and generalized peripheral arteriolar vasodilation. In contrast to a hyperdynamic circulation, patients with alcoholic cirrhosis may also develop congestive heart failure due to cardiomyopathy. Megaloblastic anemia is frequent and is probably due to antagonism of folate by alcohol rather than a dietary deficiency.

Arterial hypoxemia is a common finding in patients with cirrhosis of the liver. Indeed, many of these patients have chronic obstructive airways disease associated with cigarette smoking. Furthermore, right-to-left intrapulmonary shunts may develop in the presence of portal vein hypertension leading to arterial hypoxemia. Ascitic fluid may impair movement of the diaphragm, thus contributing to maldistribution of ventilation to perfusion. Arterial hypoxemia may be due to pneumonia, which is common in alcoholic patients. The vulnerability to developing pneumonia may reflect the ability of alcohol to inhibit phagocytic activity normally present in the lungs. As a result, bacteria inhaled into the respiratory tract are more likely to produce pneumonia. Indeed, the majority of lung abscesses are found in chronic alcoholic patients.

Cirrhosis of the liver is associated with a reduction in renal blood flow and glomerular filtration rate. Hypoglycemia is a constant threat in alcoholic patients. The incidence of gallstones is increased, presumably reflecting an elevated bilirubin load due to hemolysis of erythrocytes in the spleen. Peptic ulcer disease is twice as common in patients with cirrhosis of the liver. Spontaneous bacterial peritonitis develops in nearly 10 percent of patients with alcohlic liver disease and ascites. Hepatic encephalopathy, presumably due to the systemic accumulation of nitrogenous waste products, is evidenced by asterixis (flapping motion of the hands caused by intermittent loss of extensor muscle tone) and mental obtundation. The development of hepatic encephalopathy is associated with a high mortality rate.

Management of Anesthesia in the Sober Alcoholic Patient

It is estimated that 5 percent to 10 percent of patients with cirrhosis of the liver undergo surgery in the last 2 years of their lives. Postoperative morbidity is increased, especially with respect to bleeding, sepsis, and deterioration of hepatic function after surgery (Table 21-3).[13]

Coagulation status should be evaluated preoperatively and parenteral vitamin K administered if the prothrombin time is prolonged. Failure of parenteral vitamin K to improve synthesis of prothrombin suggests the presence of severe hepato-

cellular disease. Conversely, impaired prothrombin production due to biliary obstruction and absence of bile salts to facilitate gastrointestinal absorption of vitamin K is promptly restored by parenteral vitamin K therapy. All jaundiced patients should receive parenteral vitamin K preoperatively, and if prothrombin time does not return to normal, fresh frozen plasma should be available. It is important to remember that hepatic blood flow is predictably decreased in patients with cirrhosis of the liver, and any further reduction due to anesthetic-induced depression of cardiac output or blood pressure could jeopardize hepatocyte oxygenation.

There is evidence that chronic alcohol abuse increases anesthetic requirements (minimum alveolar concentration [MAC]) for volatile anesthetics (Fig. 21-8).[14] The most likely explanation for this increase is a cross-tolerance among depressant drugs. Accelerated metabolism of drugs in the presence of alcohol-induced microsomal enzyme stimulation might alter the amount of inhaled anesthetic needed to achieve a given brain partial pressure but would not alter the partial pressures required to produce anesthesia. In contrast to resistance to depressant drugs, alcohol-induced cardiomyopathy could make these patients unusually sensitive to the cardiac depressant effects of volatile anesthetics. The responsiveness of the cardiovascular system to sympathetic nervous system stimulation and infused catecholamines or sympathomimetics is reduced, perhaps reflecting decreased vascular reactivity owing to elevated plasma concentrations of glucagon that

Table 21-3. Surgical Risk Based on Preoperative Evaluation

	Minimal	Modest	Marked
Bilirubin (mg·dl^{-1})	2	2–3	3
Albumin (g·dl^{-1})	3.5	3–3.5	3
Prothrombin time (seconds prolonged)	1–4	4–6	6
Encephalopathy	None	Moderate	Severe
Nutrition	Excellent	Good	Poor
Ascites	None	Moderate	Marked

(Data from Strunin.[13])

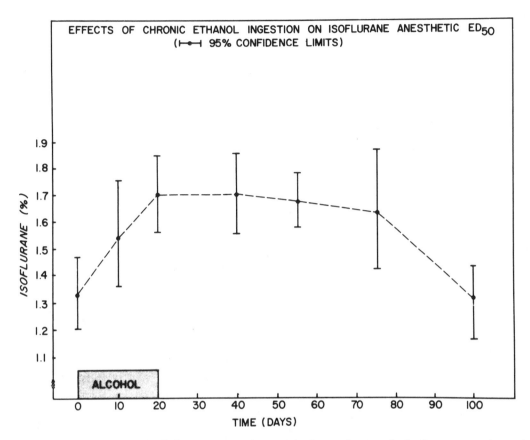

Fig. 21-8. The effect of chronic alcohol ingestion on the anesthetic requirement for isoflurane was determined in mice during and after continuous exposure to ethanol. Isoflurane anesthetic requirements on days 20, 40, 55, and 75 were significantly ($P < 0.05$) elevated above the control value. (From Johnstone et al.,[14] with permission.)

predictably accompany cirrhosis of the liver. Likewise, decreased protein binding of drugs in the presence of reduced serum albumin concentrations would increase the pharmacologically active unbound fractions of injected drugs available to act at peripheral receptors.[2] Finally, severely jaundiced patients (total serum bilirubin concentrations above 8 mg·dl^{-1}) are more likely to develop acute renal failure and sepsis postoperatively, emphasizing the importance of establishing a diuresis with mannitol preoperatively and initiating antibiotic therapy.[1]

It would seem prudent to select drugs for production of anesthesia that do not increase splanchnic vascular resistance and, at the same time,

undergo minimal metabolism. In this regard, nitrous oxide, enflurane, and isoflurane are attractive choices. Among the volatile anesthetics, isoflurane may be associated with the best maintenance of hepatic blood flow and hepatocyte oxygenation (Fig. 21-5).[8] There is no evidence, however, that halothane-associated hepatic dysfunction is more likely to occur in patients with co-existing liver disease. It is, nevertheless, undeniable that events likely to favor reductive metabolism of halothane (enzyme induction from alcohol and malnutrition plus hepatocyte hypoxia from decreased hepatic blood flow) are predictably present in patients with cirrhosis of the liver. In view of alternative drugs (isoflurane, enflurane, opioids, benzodiazepines), it would seem logical to avoid administering halothane to patients with known liver disease. When opioids or benzodiazepines are used, it must be remembered that cumulative drug effects are likely if liver disease is severe enough to slow metabolism.

The role of the liver in the clearance of muscle relaxants must be considered when selecting these drugs for administration to patients with cirrhosis of the liver. Succinylcholine is an acceptable muscle relaxant, but the dose should be adjusted if liver disease is sufficiently advanced so as to decrease cholinesterase activity (Fig. 21-2).[3] Hepatic dysfunction does not influence clearance of atracurium, and the elimination half-time of vecuronium is not prolonged unless doses larger than 0.15 $mg \cdot kg^{-1}$ are administered, making these drugs attractive selections for patients with cirrhosis.[6] Resistance to the neuromuscular blocking effects of long-acting nondepolarizing muscle relaxants, such as d-tubocurarine and pancuronium, may reflect alcohol-induced changes in the distribution volume of these drugs. Indeed, the distribution volume of pancuronium is increased and the plasma clearance decreased in patients with alcoholic cirrhosis, as compared with normal patients.[15] Based on these observations, the initial dose of pancuronium necessary to produce skeletal muscle relaxation in alcoholic patients might be increased, reflecting dilution of the drug in a larger distribution volume. Conversely, the duration of paralysis might be prolonged due to slowed plasma clearance. Resistance to effects of long-acting nondepolarizing muscle relaxants based on altered protein binding is not supported by a study failing to show altered binding of d-tubocurarine in the presence of hepatic disease.[16]

Monitoring of intraoperative blood gases, pH, and urine output plus provision of exogenous glucose are important principles. Arterial hypoxemia may be exaggerated intraoperatively if drugs used for anesthesia produce vasodilation of coexisting portasystemic and intrapulmonary shunts. When blood replacement is necessary, it is logical to administer the stored blood as slowly as possible to compensate for decreased clearance of citrate by the diseased liver. A practical point is the avoidance of unnecessary esophageal instrumentation (stethoscope, gastric tube) in patients with known esophageal varices.

Manifestations of a severe alcohol withdrawal syndrome (delerium tremens) usually appear 48 hours to 72 hours after the cessation of drinking. This syndrome represents a medical emergency, as mortality may approach 15 percent. Postoperatively, patients will manifest tremulousness and hallucinations. There is increased activity of the sympathetic nervous system with catecholamine release, leading to diaphoresis, hyperpyrexia, tachycardia, and hypertension. In some patients grand mal seizures may be the first indication of the alcohol withdrawal syndrome. When seizures occur, hypoglycemia must be ruled out as a possible cause. Initial treatment of delerium tremens consists of sedation with intravenous administration of diazepam (10 mg initially, followed by 5 mg every 5 minutes until the patient is calm), propranolol to reduce sympathetic nervous system activity, vitamin replacement including thiamin, and correction of fluid and electrolyte (magnesium, potassium) disorders.

Management of Anesthesia in the Intoxicated Alcoholic Patient

In contrast to the chronic but sober alcoholic, acutely intoxicated patients require less anesthesia because there is an additive depressant effect between alcohol and anesthetics. Acutely intoxicated patients also withstand stress and blood loss poorly. Furthermore, intoxicated patients are more vulnerable to regurgitation of gastric contents, as alcohol slows gastric emptying and reduces the tone of the lower esophageal sphincter.

LIVER TRANSPLANTATION

Liver transplantation is the only curative therapy for patients in hepatic failure.[17] The impact of liver transplantation on not only anesthesia resources (two or more people are usually required) but also hospital and blood resources are profound and require careful planning. Because of the predictable need for massive blood and fluid replacement during surgery, maintenance of intravascular fluid volume and myocardial contractility are especially challenging. Impaired myocardial contractility may reflect citrate-induced hypocalcemia due to the inability of the liver to metabolize this anticoagulant, especially when massive blood transfusions are required. This is one of the rare clinical situations in which intravenous administration of calcium is indicated. Arterial and venous catheters are placed above the diaphragm, as it may be necessary to clamp the abdominal aorta and/or inferior vena cava. Marked cardiovascular changes can result, ranging from decreased venous return to the heart with clamping of the inferior vena cava to a marked increase in intravascular volume when the infradiaphragmatic inferior vena cava is opened to the donor liver. Nitrous oxide is sometimes discontinued after induction of anesthesia because of the risk of air embolization at the time of revascularization of the liver, reflecting air previously trapped in the liver. Hepatic and renal routes of elimination must be considered in selection of all drugs. Venoveno bypass or partial cardiopulmonary bypass is useful for reducing blood loss and minimizing circulatory changes that may otherwise require administration of inotropes when the inferior vena cava is clamped. Multiple types of coagulopathies can occur, including thrombocytopenia (from massive blood transfusions), low levels of coagulation factors, hemodilution, heparin activity, fibrinolysis, and possible release from the donor liver of inhibitors of coagulation.[17] These multiple coagulopathies require immediate and complex monitoring. Metabolic

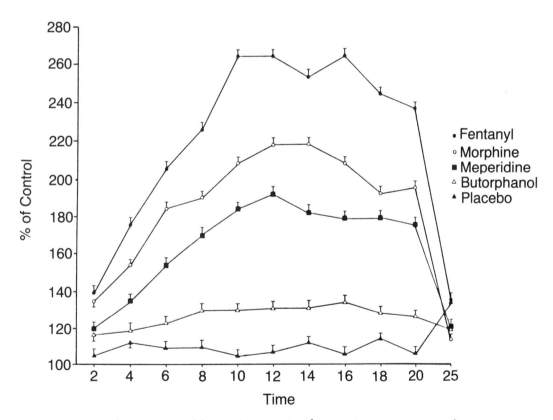

Fig. 21-9. Intravenous administration of fentanyl (1.5 μg·kg^{-1}), morphine (0.15 mg·kg^{-1}), and meperidine (1 mg·kg^{-1}) results in increased common bile duct pressures (percent of control) in patients anesthetized with nitrous oxide-enflurane. Changes in common bile duct pressures after intravenous administration of butorphanol (0.03 mg·kg^{-1}) are modest. Intravenous administration of naloxone (5 μg·kg^{-1}) 20 minutes after injection of the opioids results in prompt decreases in common bile duct pressures. Mean ± SD. (From Radnay et al.,[18] with permission.)

acidosis and hypoglycemia can occur. Hypotension and hyperkalemia may accompany unclamping of previously clamped vessels. Mechanical support of ventilation via a tracheal tube is likely to be necessary for several hours postoperatively.

DISEASES OF THE BILIARY TRACT

Gallstones are reported to be present in 10 percent of men and 20 percent of women between 55 years and 65 years of age. Patients who experience repeated attacks of acute cholecystitis eventually develop a fibrotic gallbladder. Liver function tests are usually normal, but elevated serum bilirubin or alkaline phosphatase concentrations suggest the presence of choledocholithiasis (common bile duct stone) or chronic cholangitis.

Management of Anesthesia

Management of anesthesia for cholecystectomy and/or common bile duct exploration is influenced by the effects of drugs used for anesthesia on intraluminal pressures in the biliary tract. Specifically, opioids (morphine, meperidine, fentanyl) can produce spasm of the choledochoduodenal sphincter, which elevates common bile duct pressures (Fig. 21-9).[18] This spasm could impair passage of contrast media into the duodenum, erroneously suggesting the need for a sphincteroplasty or the presence of common bile duct stones. Nevertheless, opioids have been used in many instances without adverse effects, emphasizing that not all patients respond to opioids with choledochoduodenal sphincter spasm. Indeed, some believe that the incidence of opioid-induced sphincter spasm during cholecystectomy is so low (3 percent or less) that the possibility of this response should not influence the use of opioids during anesthesia for this operation. The alternative to opioids for maintenance of anesthesia is the use of volatile anesthetics, although the possible presence of liver disease is often a concern when selecting volatile anesthetics for patients undergoing cholecystectomy. Nevertheless, there is no evidence that hepatic dysfunction after a cholecystectomy is differ-

ent in patients anesthetized with nitrous oxide plus fentanyl, halothane, or enflurane (Fig. 21-6).[10]

REFERENCES

1. Biebuyck JK. Effects of anesthetic agents on metabolic pathways: Fuel utilization and supply during anaesthesia. Br J Anaesth 1973;45:263–8.
2. Pandele G, Chaux F, Salvadori C, Farinott M, Duvaldestin P. Thiopental pharmacokinetics in patients with cirrhosis. Anesthesiology 1983;59:123–6.
3. Foldes FF, Swerdlow M, Lipschitz E, Van Hees GR, Shanor SP. Comparison of the respiratory effects of suxamethonium and suxethonium in man. Anesthesiology 1956;17:559–68.
4. Majoit J-X, Sandouk P, Zetlaoui P, Scherrmann J-M. Pharmacokinetics of unchanged morphine in normal and cirrhotic subjects. Anesth Analg 1987;66:293–8.
5. Ferrier C, Marty J, Bouffard Y, Haberer JP, Levron JC, Duvaldestin P. Alfentanil pharmacokinetics in patients with cirrhosis. Anesthesiology 1985;62:480–4.
6. Arden JR, Lynam DP, Castagnoli KP, Canfell PC, Cannon JC, Miller RD. Vecuronium in alcoholic liver disease: A pharmacokinetic and pharmacodynamic analysis. Anesthesiology 1988;68:771–6.
7. Reilly CS, Wood AJJ, Koshakjr RP, Wood M. The effect of halothane on drug disposition: Contribution of changes in intrinsic drug metabolizing capacity and hepatic blood flow. Anesthesiology 1985;63:70–6.
8. Gelman S, Fowler KC, Smith LR. Liver circulation and function during isoflurane and halothane anesthesia. Anesthesiology 1984;61:726–30.
9. Gelman SI. Disturbances in hepatic blood flow during anesthesia and surgery. Arch Surg 1976;111:881–3.
10. Viegas OJ, Stoelting RK. LDH5 changes after cholecystectomy or hysterectomy in patients receiving halothane, enflurane, or fentanyl. Anesthesiology 1979;51:556–8.
11. Baden JM, Serra M, Fujinaga M, Mazze RI. Halothane metabolism in cirrhotic rats. Anesthesiology 1987;67:600–4.
12. Maze M, Smith CM, Baden JM. Halothane anesthesia does not exacerbate hepatic dysfunction in cirrhotic rats. Anesthesiology 1985;62:1–5.
13. Strunin L. Preoperative assessment of the patient with liver dysfunction. Br J Anaesth 1978;50:25–34.
14. Johnstone RE, Kulp RA, Smith TC. Effects of acute and chronic ethanol administration on isoflurane requirement in mice. Anesth Analg 1975;54:177–81.
15. Duvaldestin P, Agoston S, Henzel D, Kersten UW, Desmonts JM. Pancuronium pharmacokinetics in patients with liver cirrhosis. Br J Anaesth 1978; 50:1131–6.

16. Martyn JAJ, Matteo RS, Greenblatt DJ, Lebowitz PW, Savarese JJ. Pharmacokinetics of d-tubocurarine in patients with thermal injury. Anesth Analg 1982;241–6.

17. Borland LM, Cook DR. Anesthesia for organ transplantation. In: Stoelting RK, Barash PG, Gallagher TJ, eds. Advances in Anesthesia. Chicago, Year Book Medical Publishers, 1986:1–28.

18. Radnay PA, Duncalf D, Novakovic M, Lesser ML. Common bile duct pressure changes after fentanyl, morphine, meperidine, butorphanol, and naloxone. Anesth Analg 1984;63:441–4.

Chapter 22

Renal Disease

Essential physiologic functions of the kidneys include (1) excretion of end products of metabolism (urea) while retaining nutrients (amino acids, glucose), and (2) control of electrolyte and hydrogen ion concentration of body fluids. In addition to these physiologic functions, the kidneys secrete hormones (renin, erythropoietin) and metabolize hormones such as insulin. Therefore, impaired renal function is associated with characteristic changes (see the section *Changes Characteristic of Chronic Renal Disease*). Co-existing renal disease can predispose patients to perioperative morbidity and mortality. Furthermore, the possibility of impaired renal function during the perioperative period should be considered in otherwise healthy patients undergoing major operations.

ANATOMY AND PHYSIOLOGY OF THE KIDNEY

The functional unit of the kidneys is the nephron (Fig. 22-1).[1] Each kidney contains about 1.2 million nephrons, and this number does not change after birth. The two components of the nephron are the glomerulus and renal tubule. Physiologic function of the kidneys is dependent on renal blood flow, glomerular filtration rate, and responses evoked by nonrenal (parathormone and antidiuretic hormone) and renal (renin and prostaglandins) humoral substances.

Glomerulus

The glomerulus is formed by the invagination of a tuft of capillaries into the dilated and blind end of the nephron, known as Bowman's capsule. Each tuft of capillaries arises from a single afferent arteriole and is drained by an efferent arteriole. The hydrostatic pressure inside these capillaries can be varied by changing the tone of their afferent or efferent arterioles. It is the pressure in glomerular capillaries that causes water and low molecular weight substances to filter through the tuft of capillaries known as Bowman's capsule, which is in direct continuity with the proximal convoluted tubule (see the section *Glomerular Filtration Rate*).

Renal Tubule

The renal tubule consists of the proximal convoluted tubule, the loop of Henle, and the distal convoluted tubule. Several distal convoluted tubules join to form the collecting ducts, which subsequently drain into the renal pelvis. As glomerular filtrate travels along the renal tubule, most of its water and varying amounts of its solutes are reabsorbed from the renal tubular lumen into peritubular capillaries. In addition, small amounts of other solutes are secreted into the lumen of the renal tubule. The resulting glomerular filtrate and solute becomes urine.

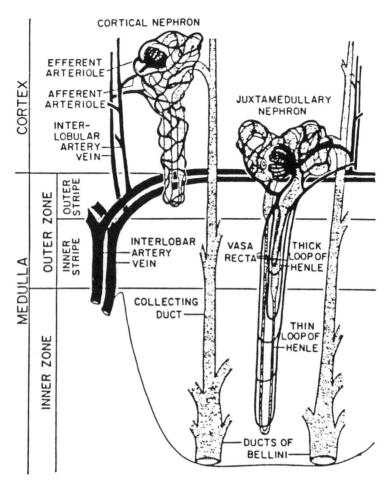

Fig. 22-1. Schematic depiction of the nephron and accompanying blood supply. (From Pitts,[1] with permission.)

Renal Blood Flow

Renal blood flow is equivalent to about 20 percent of the cardiac output despite the fact the kidneys represent only 0.5 percent of total body weight. Approximately two-thirds of the renal blood flow is to the renal cortex. The impact, if any, of anesthetic drugs on distribution of blood flow between the renal cortex and medulla is not known. It is known, however, that the positive pressure ventilation of the lungs is associated with a decrease in renal cortical blood flow. Renal blood flow and glomerular filtration rate remains constant at mean arterial pressures ranging from 60

mmHg to 160 mmHg. This ability to maintain renal blood flow constant despite changes in perfusion pressure is known as autoregulation. Autoregulation is achieved by adjustment of the afferent arteriolar tone and subsequent resistance imparted to blood flow. Impaired autoregulation occurs in denervated and isolated-perfused kidneys and, therefore, perfusion pressure is under the control of an intrinsic mechanism. Autoregulation is important because it protects glomerular capillaries from large increases in arterial blood pressure during acute hypertensive episodes and maintains glomerular filtration rate and renal tubule function during modest decreases in blood pressure. Outside the range of mean arterial pressure associated with autoregulation, renal blood flow becomes pressure-dependent.

Autoregulation does not preclude changes in renal blood flow due to other mechanisms. For example, renal blood flow is influenced by activity of the sympathetic nervous system and the release of renin. Indeed, the kidneys are richly innervated by the sympathetic nervous system (T4-L4). Sympathetic nervous system stimulation produces renal vascular vasoconstriction with marked reductions in renal blood flow even if blood pressure is maintained in the range associated with autoregulation. Any reduction in renal blood flow will initiate release of renin which can further reduce renal blood flow (see the section *Humoral Substances*). Release of prostaglandins from the kidneys produces vasodilation and can offset renal artery vasoconstriction that results from release of renin (see the section *Humoral Substances*). Prostaglandins may also be important for optimal effects of antidiuretic hormone on collecting ducts.

Glomerular Filtration Rate

Hydrostatic pressure in the glomerular capillaries is about 50 mmHg. This pressure acts to force water and other low molecular weight substances such as electrolytes through the glomerular capillaries into Bowman's space. The outward filtration force produced by hydrostatic pressure is opposed by the plasma oncotic pressure. Plasma oncotic pressure is about 25 mmHg at the afferent arteriole and with the filtration of electrolytes increases to about 35 mmHg at the efferent arteriole. Despite the relatively low net filtration pressure, the glomerular capillaries are able to filter plasma at a rate equivalent to about 125 ml·min^{-1}. Glomerular filtration rate is reduced by decreased mean arterial pressure or reductions in renal blood flow. Ultimately, about 90 percent of the fluid resulting from glomerular filtration is reabsorbed from renal tubules into peritubular capillaries and thus returned to the circulation.

Humoral Substances

Renin is a proteolytic enzyme secreted by the juxtaglomerular apparatus of the kidneys in response to (1) sympathetic nervous system stimu-

---

Tests Used for Evaluation of Renal Function

Glomerular filtration rate
  Blood urea nitrogen
  Serum creatinine
  Creatinine clearance
  Proteinuria

Renal tubular function
  Urine specific gravity
  Urine osmolarity
  Urine sodium

---

lation, (2) decreased renal perfusion pressure, and (3) reductions in the delivery of sodium to the distal convoluted tubules. Renin acts on an alpha-2 globulin in the plasma to form angiotensin I. Angiotensin I is then split by converting enzyme in the lungs to form angiotensin II. Angiotensin II is a potent vasoconstrictor and an important stimulus for the release of aldosterone from the adrenal cortex.

Prostaglandins are produced in the renal medulla and released in response to sympathetic nervous system stimulation and elevated levels of angiotensin II. Prostaglandins designated as PGE$_2$ and PGI$_2$ are vasodilators that tend to offset the reductions in renal blood flow produced by vasoconstrictive stimuli.

TESTS USED FOR EVALUATION OF RENAL FUNCTION

Renal function can be evaluated preoperatively by laboratory tests that reflect glomerular filtration rate and renal tubule function. These tests are not sensitive measurements and significant renal disease can exist despite normal laboratory values. Furthermore, trends are more useful than a single laboratory measurement for evaluating renal function.

Blood Urea Nitrogen

Blood urea nitrogen concentrations (normal 10 mg·dl^{-1} to 20 mg·dl^{-1}) vary with the glomerular filtration rate. Nevertheless, the influence of dietary intake, associated illnesses, and intravascular fluid volume on blood urea nitrogen concentrations make this a potentially misleading test of renal function. For example, production of urea is increased by high protein diets or gastrointestinal bleeding resulting in elevated blood urea nitrogen concentrations despite a normal glomerular filtration rate. Other causes for increased blood urea nitrogen concentrations despite a normal glomerular filtration rate include increased catabolism during febrile illnesses and dehydration. Increased blood urea nitrogen concentrations in the presence of dehydration most likely reflect increased urea absorption due to slow movement of fluid through the renal tubules. When slow movement of fluid through the renal tubules is responsible for elevation of the blood urea nitrogen concentrations, the serum creatinine levels remain normal. Blood urea nitrogen concentrations can remain normal in the presence of low protein diets (hemodialysis patients) despite reductions in glomerular filtration rate. Finally, low blood urea nitrogen concentrations (less than 10 mg·dl^{-1}) can reflect an excess total body water content. Despite these extraneous influences, blood urea nitrogen concentrations above 50 mg·dl^{-1} almost always reflect a decreased glomerular filtration rate.

Serum Creatinine

Serum creatinine concentrations are specific indicators of the glomerular filtration rate. In contrast to blood urea nitrogen concentrations, the serum creatinine levels are not influenced by protein metabolism or the rate of fluid flow through renal tubules. As a guide, a 50 percent increase in serum creatinine concentration reflects a similar decrease in the glomerular filtration rate. Creatinine is a product of skeletal muscle metabolism and its release into the circulation is believed to be relatively constant. Serum creatinine concentrations are influenced by skeletal muscle mass in that normal levels (0.7 mg·dl^{-1} to 1.5 mg·dl^{-1}) tend to be higher in muscular males than less muscular females. Conversely, the maintenance of normal serum creatinine concentrations in elderly patients with known reductions in glomerular filtration rates reflects decreased creatinine production due

to reduced skeletal muscle mass that accompanies aging. Indeed, mild elevations in serum creatinine concentrations in elderly patients suggest significant renal disease. Likewise, in patients with chronic renal failure, serum creatinine concentrations may not accurately reflect the glomerular filtration rate because of decreased creatinine production in the presence of reduced skeletal muscle mass or nonrenal (gastrointestinal tract) excretion of creatinine. Finally, serum creatinine concentrations may not be elevated in the presence of acute renal failure because at least 8 hours are required for serum creatinine concentrations to rise from normal levels to that suggestive of acute renal failure.

Creatinine Clearance

Creatinine clearance (normal 110 ml·min^{-1} to 150 ml·min^{-1}) measures the ability of the glomeruli to excrete creatinine into the urine for a given serum creatinine concentration. This measurement does not depend on corrections for age or the presence of a steady state. As such, creatinine clearance is the most reliable measurement of the glomerular filtration rate. The major disadvantage of this test is the need for timed (2 hours as acceptable as 24 hours) urine collections (Fig. 22-2).[2] Preoperatively, patients with creatinine clearances between 10 ml·min^{-1} and 25 ml·min^{-1} must be considered at risk for developing prolonged or adverse responses to drugs, such as nondepolarizing muscle relaxants, that depend on renal excretion. In these patients, the doses of such drugs should be reduced and intravenous fluid and electrolyte replacement carefully monitored.

Proteinuria

Small amounts of protein are normally filtered through glomerular capillaries and then reabsorbed in the proximal convoluted tubules. Proteinura (excretion of greater than 150 mg·day^{-1} of protein) is most likely due to abnormally high filtration rather than impaired reabsorption by the renal tubules. At a constant rate of loss, the concentrations of protein in the urine will be inversely related to urine volumes. Thus, a 2 plus protein in dilute urine signifies a greater excretion rate

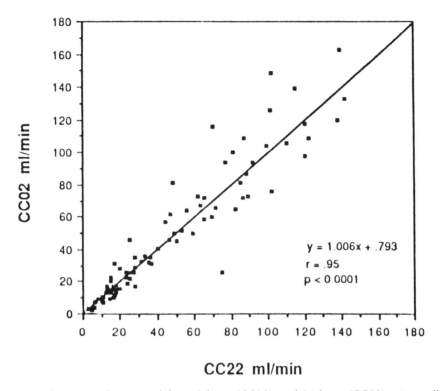

Fig. 22-2. Creatinine clearance determined from 2-hour (CC02) and 24-hour (CC22) urine collections are similar. (From Sladen et al.,[5] with permission.)

than 2 plus protein in highly concentrated urine. Intermittent proteinuria occasionally occurs in healthy individuals when standing and disappears when supine. Other nonrenal causes of proteinuria include exercise, fever, and congestive heart failure. Severe proteinuria may result in hypoalbuminemia with associated reductions in plasma oncotic pressures and decreased protein binding of drugs.

Urine Concentrating Ability

The diagnosis of renal tubule dysfunction is established by demonstrating that the kidneys do not produce appropriately concentrated urine in the presence of a physiologic stimulus for the release of antidiuretic hormone. In the absence of diuretic therapy or glycosuria, a urine specific gravity above 1.018 after an overnight fast, as precedes elective surgery, suggests that the ability of renal tubules to concentrate urine is adequate. High output renal failure following anesthesia with drugs, such as methoxyflurane and rarely enflurane, reflects the inability of renal tubules to concentrate urine in the presence of high serum concentrations of fluoride (see Chapter 5). Other causes of inability of the renal tubules to adequately concentrate urine include (1) hypokalemia, (2) hypercalcemia, (3) chronic pyelonephritis, and (4) treatment with diuretics or lithium.

Sodium Excretion

Urinary excretion of greater than 40 $mEq \cdot L^{-1}$ of sodium reflects a decreased ability of the renal tubules to conserve sodium. Examples of sodium wasting by the renal tubules include (1) drug-induced diuresis (see the section *Pharmacology of Diuretics*), (2) adrenal insufficiency, and (3) hypoaldosteronism.

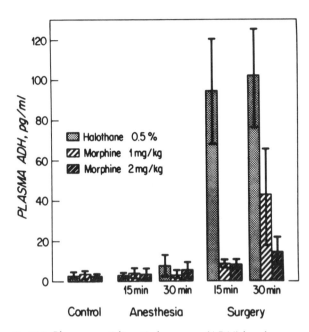

Fig. 22-3. Plasma antidiuretic hormone (ADH) levels mean ± SE) in adult patients are not altered from control measurements during anesthesia. Surgical stimulation increases ADH concentrations, particularly in patients receiving halothane. (From Philbin and Coggins,[2] with permission.)

EFFECTS OF ANESTHETICS ON RENAL FUNCTION

Anesthetics can alter renal function by their effects on the systemic circulation and the sympathetic nervous system. In rare instances, drugs used for anesthesia produce direct nephrotoxicity (see Chapter 5).

Decreased urine output during anesthesia suggests the release of antidiuretic hormone. However, serum concentrations of antidiuretic hormone are not increased during halothane or morphine anesthesia (Fig. 22-3).[3] Instead, painful stimulation associated with the onset of surgery produces significant increases in circulating levels of antidiuretic hormone. Positive pressure ventilation of the lungs, as well as positive end-expiratory pressure, can also stimulate the release of antidiuretic hormone by altering left atrial pressure leading to activation of baroreceptors.[4] Hydration before the induction of anesthesia attenuates the rise in serum antidiuretic hormone

concentrations produced by surgical stimulation. Like antidiuretic hormone, there is no evidence that anesthetics in the absence of surgical stimulation evoke the release of renin.[5]

Systemic Circulation

Volatile anesthetics most likely depress renal function by producing dose-dependent decreases in cardiac output and reductions in blood pressure. The net effect is a decrease in renal blood flow, glomerular filtration rate, and urine output during anesthesia. These reductions in renal blood flow and glomerular filtration rate are likely to be attenuated by preoperative hydration and administration of low concentrations of the anesthetic.

Alterations in the autoregulation of renal blood flow due to effects produced by volatile anesthetics could exaggerate the changes in renal function that occur in response to blood pressure reductions produced by the anesthetics. Animal studies, however, suggest that halothane, with or without thiopental or nitrous oxide, does not alter autoregulation of renal blood flow (Fig. 22-4).[6] The impact, if any, of enflurane or isoflurane on autoregulation of renal blood flow has not been determined.

Changes in renal function during barbiturate-opioid-nitrous oxide anesthesia are similar to those observed during administration of low concentrations of volatile anesthetics. Epidural or spinal block result in minimal changes in renal blood flow and glomerular filtration rate. When alterations in renal hemodynamics occur during regional anesthesia, the most likely explanation is a decrease in the systemic blood pressure.

Sympathetic Nervous System

The renal vasculature is richly innervated by the sympathetic nervous system such that drug-induced changes in systemic vascular resistance can lead to alterations in renal blood flow and glomerular filtration rate. For example, ketamine is associated with decreased renal blood flow and glomerular filtration rate despite increases in cardiac output and mean arterial pressure. Presumably, these changes reflect constriction of renal vasculature by ketamine-induced increases in sympathetic nervous system activity. Conversely, volatile anesthetics that reduce sympathetic nervous

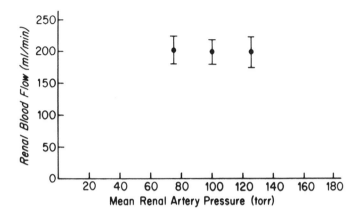

Fig. 22-4. Halothane administered to dogs does not alter autoregulation as evidenced by an unchanging renal blood flow despite changes in mean renal artery pressure. (From Bastron et al.,[6] with permission.)

system activity might reduce renal vascular resistance. Indeed, low concentrations of halothane partially restore renal blood flow when administered to animals in hemorrhagic shock.[7] Perhaps this change reflects halothane-reduced reductions in sympathetic nervous system activity with subsequent reductions in renal vascular resistance.

Direct Nephrotoxicity

It could be argued that all anesthetics are direct nephrotoxins because these drugs produce generalized depression of measurable renal function. This depression, however, is transient and usually clinically insignificant. The exception to this generalization is nephrotoxicity produced by fluoride resulting from metabolism of certain volatile anesthetics (see Chapter 5).

CHRONIC RENAL DISEASE

Changes Characteristic of Chronic Renal Disease

Chronic renal disease is characterized by progressive decreases in the number of functioning nephrons, leading to irreversible reductions in the glomerular filtration rate. Rational management of anesthesia in patients with chronic renal disease requires an understanding of those pathologic changes that accompany renal disease. Furthermore, the management of anesthesia is influenced by whether the renal disease is sufficient to require hemodialysis.

Anemia

Hemoglobin concentrations in the range of 5 $g \cdot dl^{-1}$ to 8 $g \cdot dl^{-1}$ (hematocrit 15 percent to 25 percent) are hallmarks of chronic renal disease. Decreased production of erythropoietin in the presence of elevated blood urea nitrogen levels is the most likely explanation for the reduced pro-

---

Changes Characteristic of Chronic Renal Disease

Anemia

Increased cardiac output

Decreased platelet adhesiveness

Hyperkalemia

Unpredictable intravascular fluid volume

Metabolic acidosis

Systemic hypertension

Decreased sympathetic nervous system activity

Increased susceptibility to sepsis

duction of erythrocytes. Furthermore, survival time for erythrocytes is shortened about 50 percent in the presence of chronic uremia, reflecting erythrocyte membrane fragility. This anemia is well tolerated because of its slow onset, which permits time for compensatory increases in cardiac output and to a lesser extent 2,3-diphosphoglycerate concentrations to occur. The greatest hazard of anemia is decreased oxygen carrying capacity, which can result in tissue hypoxia. The importance of increased tissue blood flow in offsetting the effects of anemia emphasizes the need to minimize changes in cardiac output produced by volatile anesthetics (use low concentrations) and positive pressure ventilation of the lungs (use slow breathing rate to assure time for venous return between breaths).

Attempts to correct chronic anemia preoperatively are not recommended unless there is a history of cardiopulmonary dysfunction that limits daily activity. In these patients, the preoperative administration of erythrocytes should be considered. Whole blood is not a logical selection as the excess volume may contribute to fluid overload.

Coagulopathies

Coagulopathies must be suspected in patients with chronic renal disease. The most likely coagulation defect is decreased platelet adhesiveness as reflected by prolonged bleeding times. Hemodialysis is usually effective in reversing this platelet dysfunction. The possibility of impaired coagulation probably should be considered when selecting a regional anesthetic technique in patients with chronic renal disease.

Electrolyte and Hydration Status

Hyperkalemia is the most serious electrolyte abnormality associated with chronic renal disease (see Chapter 18). Even when hemodialysis has been performed in the previous 6 hours to 8 hours, the serum potassium concentration should be measured before induction of anesthesia since unexpected hyperkalemia can occur rapidly. If surgery cannot be delayed, the serum potassium concentration can be lowered by hyperventilation of the lungs (a 10 mmHg decrease in $PaCO_2$ or 0.1 unit increase in pH lowers serum potassium

about 0.5 mEq$\cdot$L^{-1}) and/or intravenous infusion of a glucose-insulin mixture (25 g glucose plus 10 units to 15 units of regular insulin). Intravenous administration of calcium is effective in restoring normal cardiac conduction in the presence of hyperkalemia. Sodium bicarbonate is indicated if metabolic acidosis accompanies hyperkalemia.

Regardless of hydration status, patients with chronic renal disease often respond to induction of anesthesia as if they are hypovolemic. The likelihood of hypotension during induction of anesthesia may be increased if sympathetic nervous system function is attenuated by antihypertensives. Attenuated sympathetic nervous system activity produced by these drugs impairs compensatory peripheral vasoconstriction, such that a small decrease in blood volume, positive pressure ventilation of the lungs or sudden changes in body position can result in exaggerated reductions in blood pressure.

Metabolic Acidosis

Chronic renal disease interferes with the normal renal excretion of hydrogen ions leading to the appearance of metabolic acidosis. Hemodialysis is effective in restoring the pH to nearly normal values. Acidosis in renal patients is particularly undesirable because a low pH favors an extracellular rather than intracellular distribution of potassium.

Systemic Hypertension

Hypertension is a frequent complication of chronic renal disease. Preoperative hypertension is often due to fluid overload and is best treated by hemodialysis. Refractory hypertension occurs in 10 percent to 15 percent of patients despite hemodialysis and requires treatment with antihypertensives. Management of hypertension in the perioperative period is with vasodilators such as hydralazine, labetalol, or nitroprusside. Cyanide toxicity from nitroprusside is unlikely because excretion of thiosulfate, which is necessary for conversion of cyanide to thiosulfate, is decreased in the presence of renal dysfunction.

Sepsis

The most common cause of death in patients with chronic renal disease is sepsis, often originating from pulmonary infections. A high incidence of viral hepatitis most likely reflects the frequent use of blood products, as well as the effects of immunosuppression. Strict attention to asepsis is important when placing vascular cannulae and tracheal tubes in these patients.

Management of Anesthesia

Patients on hemodialysis scheduled for elective surgery should undergo hemodialysis before surgery. Knowledge of the serum potassium concentration before induction of anesthesia is important because cardiac dysrhythmias may accompany hyperkalemia. Antihypertensive therapy is usually continued. Signs of digitalis toxicity should be sought in treated patients, emphasizing the role of renal clearance of this drug.

Induction of anesthesia and intubation of the trachea can be safely accomplished with intravenous drugs, including barbiturates, benzodiazepines, or etomidate. An alternative to succinylcholine would be intermediate-acting muscle relaxants, such as, atracurium or vecuronium. None of these anesthetia induction drugs or muscle relaxants depend significantly on renal excretion for clearance from the plasma. Potassium release after administration of succinylcholine is not exaggerated in normokalemic patients with chronic renal disease.[8] Caution is necessary, however, because preoperative serum potassium concentrations in a high range (near 5.5 mEq·L^{-1}) combined with a high normal increase of serum potassium concentrations (0.5 mEq·L^{-1} to 1 mEq·L^{-1}) after administration of succinylcholine could theoretically result in dangerous hyperkalemia. A possible but undocumented concern is the potential for exaggerated potassium release after administration of succinylcholine to patients with neuropathies associated with chronic uremia. Exaggerated pharmacologic effects produced by drugs used for induction of anesthesia could reflect reduced protein binding resulting in more unbound drug to act at receptors. Furthermore, the blood-brain barrier may not be intact in the presence of uremia. Exaggerated decreases in arterial blood pressure after induction of anesthesia may also reflect autonomic nervous system dysfunction and impaired baroreceptor-mediated reflex responses.

Maintenance of anesthesia is often achieved with nitrous oxide combined with volatile anesthetics or short-acting opioids. Some avoid nitrous oxide so as to permit administration of higher inspired concentrations of oxygen. Potent volatile anesthetics are useful in controlling intraoperative hypertension and reducing the dose of muscle relaxants needed for adequate surgical relaxation. The use of halothane is sometimes questioned in patients requiring hemodialysis, in view of the high incidence of co-existing liver disease due to viral hepatitis in these patients. Likewise, enflurane, because of its modest metabolism to fluoride, may be avoided in patients with chronic renal disease. Anemia reduces blood solubility of volatile anesthetics, which could speed the rate at which the alveolar concentration can be increased or decreased. Excessive depression of cardiac output is a potential hazard of volatile anesthetics. Opioids decrease the likelihood of cardiovascular depression and avoid the concern of hepatotoxicity, but have the disadvantage of being unreliable for controlling intraoperative hypertension. Furthermore, occasional prolonged central nervous system and ventilatory depression from even small doses of opioids may reflect accumulation of pharmacologically active metabolites of opioids when renal function is absent. Excessive serum fluoride elevations do not occur in anephric patients after administration of enflurane because storage of fluoride in bone is able to offset the lack of its renal excretion.[9]

Meticulous attention must be given to management of ventilation and intravenous fluid replacement. Normocapnia is ideal, as hyperventilation of the lungs with associated respiratory alkalosis adversely affects the position of the oxyhemoglobin dissociation curve, whereas respiratory acidosis from hypoventilation could result in acute increases in serum potassium concentrations. Patients dependent on hemodialysis have a narrow margin of safety between insufficient and excessive fluid administration. Replacement of insensible water losses with 5 percent glucose in water is appropriate, whereas any urine output is replaced with 0.45 percent sodium chloride. Lactated Ringer's solution (4 mEq of potassium in each liter) or other potassium-containing fluids probably should not be administered to anuric patients. Measurement of central venous pressure is useful in guiding fluid replacement. Monitoring of the electrocardiogram is important for recognizing signs of hyperkalemia. Finally, arteriovenous shunts must be carefully protected to assure continued patency during the perioperative period.

Blockade of the brachial plexus with local anesthetic is useful for the placement of vascular shunts in the arm as are necessary for hemodialysis. The duration of brachial plexus block produced by local anesthetics is shortened by nearly 40 percent in patients with chronic renal disease.[10] It is presumed that increased tissue blood flow due to elevated cardiac output results in a more rapid clearance of local anesthetics from active sites, leading to a shorter duration of block. Adequacy of coagulation should be confirmed and the presence of uremic neuropathies ascertained before regional anesthesia is selected for these patients. Whether regional anesthesia should be selected in patients with uremic neuropathy is controversial. Some anesthesiologists fear that the regional anesthetic may be blamed for any subsequent progression of the pre-existing neuropathy. Co-existing metabolic acidosis may also decrease the seizure threshold for local anesthetics.

A perplexing problem regarding altered drug responses in patients with chronic renal disease relates to the use of nondepolarizing muscle relaxants as many of these drugs undergo extensive renal excretion (see Chapter 8). In this regard, intermediate-acting muscle relaxants are often selected since atracurium, and to a somewhat lesser extent vecuronium, are not principally dependent on renal function for their clearance from the plasma. Therefore, the duration of action of atracurium is not prolonged and that of vecuronium is only slightly prolonged.[11,12] Excretion of laudanosine, which is the major metabolite of atracurium, however, is prolonged in the presence of renal failure. Laudanosine lacks effects at the neuromuscular junction but at high serum concentrations may produce stimulation of the central nervous system. Regardless of the muscle relaxant selected, it would seem prudent to reduce the initial dose of drug and to administer subsequent doses based on the response observed using a peripheral nerve stimulator.

A diagnosis of residual neuromuscular blockade after apparent reversal of nondepolarizing neuromuscular blockade with anticholinesterases should be considered in anephric patients who manifest signs of skeletal muscle weakness in the early postoperative period. In normal patients who are adequately reversed with anticholinesterases, reappearance of neuromuscular blockade does not occur because continued renal elimination of the muscle relaxant offsets waning effects of the anticholinesterase. Even in anephric patients, there is some protection because renal elimination of anticholinesterases is delayed as long as, if not longer than, the nondepolarizing muscle relaxants. Indeed, other explanations (antibiotics, acidosis, electrolyte imbalance, diuretics) should be considered when neuromuscular blockade persists or reappears in patients with renal dysfunction. Finally, caution must be exercised in the use of opioids for postoperative analgesia in these patients in view of the possibility of exaggerated central nervous system and ventilatory depression after even small doses of opioids. Hypertension is a frequent problem in the postoperative period and hemodialysis is the best treatment if fluid excess is the cause.

DIFFERENTIAL DIAGNOSIS OF PERIOPERATIVE OLIGURIA

Perioperative oliguria (less than $0.5 \ ml\cdot kg^{-1}\cdot hr^{-1}$) is classified as prerenal oliguria or acute tubular necrosis (Table 22-1).

Prerenal Oliguria

Prerenal oliguria is characterized by excretion of concentrated urine (greater than 400 $mOsm\cdot L^{-1}$) containing minimal (less than 40 $mEq\cdot L^{-1}$) amounts of sodium. Excretion of a highly concentrated and sodium-poor urine confirms that renal tubule function is intact and reflects an attempt by the kidneys to conserve sodium and restore intravascular fluid volume in response to decreased renal blood flow. Decreased renal blood flow most likely reflects an acute reduction in intravascular fluid volume or a decreased cardiac output.

Table 22-1. Differential Diagnosis and Causes of Perioperative Oliguria

	Prerenal Oliguria	Acute Tubular Necrosis
Urinary sodium ($mEq \cdot L^{-1}$)	Below 40	Above 40
Urine osmolarity ($mOsm \cdot L^{-1}$)	Above 400	Below 400
Causes	Hypovolemia Decreased renal blood flow due to low cardiac output	Renal ischemia Nephrotoxins Free hemoglobin or myoglobin

Treatment

The key strategy in reducing the likelihood of oliguria progressing to acute renal failure is limiting the duration and magnitude of reductions in renal blood flow. A brisk diuresis in response to rapid infusions of 3 $ml \cdot kg^{-1}$ to 6 $ml \cdot kg^{-1}$ of crystalloid, such as lactated Ringer's solution (fluid challenge), suggests that an acute reduction in intravascular fluid volume is the cause of prerenal oliguria. When fluid replacement does not result in an improved urine output, the possibility of decreased renal blood flow due to a low cardiac output should be considered. Dopamine (3 $\mu g \cdot kg^{-1} \cdot min^{-1}$ to 5 $\mu g \cdot kg^{-1} \cdot min^{-1}$) is a useful drug to administer when oliguria is caused by a reduced cardiac output. A small dose of furosemide (0.1 $mg \cdot kg^{-1}$) may re-establish urine output in the presence of oliguria due to pain-induced release of antidiuretic hormone. Conversely, this small dose of diuretic is unlikely to reverse oliguria due to decreased renal blood flow. Finally, if a urinary catheter is in place, it is important to confirm its patency.

Use of diuretics to maintain or stimulate urine flow in the perioperative period is controversial. Some believe that prevention of renal tubule urine stasis with diuretics, such as furosemide, can prevent prerenal oliguria from progressing to acute tubular necrosis. Nevertheless, supportive evidence for this conclusion is not available.[13] Under any circumstance, it is crucial to restore intravascular fluid volume before administration of di-

uretics as drug-induced diuresis could exaggerate hypovolemia and further reduce cardiac output and renal blood flow. Measurement of central venous or pulmonary artery occlusion pressures is helpful in evaluating the adequacy of volume replacement before administration of diuretics. Another disadvantage of diuretics is the impairment of sodium reabsorption for at least 6 hours to 12 hours, making the urine of prerenal oliguria indistinguishable from the urine excreted in the presence of acute tubular necrosis.

Acute Tubular Necrosis

Acute tubular necrosis is another cause of perioperative oliguria. In contrast to oliguria due to hypovolemia, the urine of patients developing acute tubular necrosis contains excessive amounts of sodium (greater than 40 $mEq \cdot L^{-1}$) and is poorly concentrated. Hyperkalemia can accompany acute tubular necrosis reflecting the release of potassium from surgically damaged tissues. In the absence of renal function, the serum potassium concentration increases at a rate of 0.3 $mEq \cdot L^{-1} \cdot day^{-1}$ to 0.5 $mEq \cdot L^{-1} \cdot day^{-1}$. After surgery, however, the increase may be 1 $mEq \cdot L^{-1} \cdot day^{-1}$ to 2 $mEq \cdot L^{-1} \cdot day^{-1}$. Furthermore, in patients with extensive tissue injury, the rate of increase in the serum potassium concentration may be as high as 1 $mEq \cdot L^{-1} \cdot hr^{-1}$ to 2 $mEq \cdot L^{-1} \cdot hr^{-1}$. For this reason, the serum concentrations of potassium should be monitored frequently when acute tublar necrosis is suspected.

PHARMACOLOGY OF DIURETICS

Frequent administration of diuretics to patients undergoing anesthesia and operation emphasizes the need to appreciate the pharmacology of these drugs.

Thiazide Diuretics

Thiazide diuretics are administered orally for treatment of essential hypertension and mobilization of edema fluid associated with renal, hepatic, or cardiac dysfunction. Diuresis occurs as a result of inhibition of reabsorption of sodium and chloride from the renal tubules. Hypochloremic, hypokalemic metabolic alkalosis is a consequence of prolonged administration of thiazide diuretics. Side effects associated with hypokalemia may include (1) skeletal muscle weakness, (2) increased likelihood of developing digitalis toxicity, and (3) potentiation of nondepolarizing muscle relaxants (see Chapter 8). Preoperative detection of orthostatic hypotension should arouse suspicion of diuretic-induced reductions in intravascular fluid volume.

Loop Diuretics

Loop diuretics (ethacrynic acid, furosemide) inhibit reabsorption of sodium and chloride and augment secretion of potassium primarily in the loop of Henle (hence the designation as loop diuretics). Intravenous administration of these drugs produces a diuretic response in 2 minutes to 10 minutes. Contraction of the intravascular fluid volume (manifesting as orthostatic hypotension) may occur. Chronic administration of loop diuretics may result in hypochloremic, hypokalemic metabolic alkalosis, and in rare instances deafness occurs. Furosemide is used to (1) treat acute pulmonary edema, (2) reduce intracranial pressure, and (3) to aid in the differential diagnosis of acute renal failure.

Osmotic Diuretics

The most frequently administered osmotic diuretic is the six-carbon sugar, mannitol. Mannitol produces diuresis because it is filtered by the glomeruli and not reabsorbed from the renal tubules, leading to increased osmolarity of renal tubule fluid and associated excretion of water. In addition, mannitol increases plasma osmolarity, which will then draw fluid from intracellular spaces into extracellular spaces and thus expand, acutely, the intravascular fluid volume. This redistribution of fluid from intracellular to extracellular compartments decreases brain size and intracranial pressure and may increase renal blood flow so as to protect the kidneys from acute tubular necrosis. In patients who are oliguric secondary to congestive heart failure, however, mannitol-induced increases in intravascular fluid volume may precipitate pulmonary edema.

Preoperative and intraoperative administration of mannitol seems to be particularly beneficial in preventing postoperative renal failure in jaundiced patients (see Chapter 21) or patients undergoing resection of abdominal aortic aneurysms. However, the value of mannitol after oliguria has developed is not well established.

TRANSURETHRAL SURGERY

Transurethral resection of the prostate (TURP) or bladder tumors entails the excision of tissue and coagulation of bleeding vessels through a modified cystoscope. The use of continuous irrigation with fluid is necessary to improve visibility through the cystoscope, distend the prostatic urethra or bladder, and maintain the operative field free of blood and dissected tissue. Complications of transurethral surgery include (1) intravascular absorption of irrigating fluid, (2) hemorrhage, and (3) perforation of the bladder or urethra.

Intravascular Absorption of Irrigating Fluid

The opening of venous sinuses in association with transurethral surgery leads to intravascular absorption of irrigating fluid. The amount of irrigating fluid absorbed depends on the (1) hydrostatic pressure of the fluid (determined by the height of the fluid container above the patient), (2) number and size of the venous sinuses opened, and (3) duration of the resection.

Fluids suitable for irrigation must be nonelectrolytic to prevent the dispersion of high frequency electrical current from the operative area. These fluids should also be transparent and nontoxic to tissues. In the past, distilled water was a popular irrigating fluid because of superior visibility. Nevertheless, distilled water cannot be recommended, as intravascular absorption of this hypotonic fluid produces hemolysis. Commonly used irrigating fluids that are nonhemolytic and nearly isotonic include glycine and Cytal. Glycine is an amino acid that normally occurs in the body. A metabolite of glycine is ammonia, but complications from this substance are rarely observed clinically. Nevertheless, prolonged central nervous system depression after use of glycine as the irrigating fluid should suggest the possibility of ammonia toxicity.[14] Glycine may also act as an inhibitory neurotransmitter in the retina and transient blindness after TURP has been attributed to intravascular absorption of this irrigating fluid.[15] Cytal is the trade name for the irrigating solution that consists of two sugars, mannitol, and sorbitol. The major problem associated with Cytal is the possibility of bacterial contamination, as the sugars provide excellent culture medium.

Absorption of large volumes of isotonic irrigating fluids produces symptoms of acute increases in intravascular fluid volume and dilution of electrolytes, especially sodium. Serum osmolarity parallels reductions in sodium concentrations. Early signs of increasing intravascular fluid volume include hypertension and reflex bradycardia. If the transurethral resection continues, pulmonary edema and congestive heart failure eventually occur. Cerebral edema and increased intracranial pressure manifest as headache, restlessness, confusion, and eventually mental obtundation. Seizures are likely when the volume of intravascular fluid absorption is sufficiently large to abruptly reduce serum sodium concentrations below 100 $mEq \cdot L^{-1}$.

Management of Anesthesia

Management of anesthesia for transurethral surgery is with a regional or general anesthetic. Because patients are often elderly, they are likely to have co-existing medical diseases, especially cardiopulmonary disorders. A T10 sensory level is necessary when a regional anesthetic is selected for transurethral surgery that includes distension of the bladder. Cited advantages of a regional anesthetic include the ability of awake patients to voice symptoms suggestive of bladder perforation and/or excessive intravascular absorption of irrigating fluid. For example, bladder perforation is often accompanied by complaints of shoulder discomfort that reflects referred pain due to subdiaphragmatic irritation by extravasated irrigating fluid. Despite the alleged advantages of a regional anesthetic, there is no evidence of differences in morbidity or mortality when a general anesthetic is selected. Regardless of the technique of anesthesia selected, it is important to monitor these patients carefully for signs and symptoms of excessive intravascular absorption of irrigating fluid. In addition to monitoring blood pressure, heart rate, and the electrocardiogram, it may be prudent to measure central venous pressure and to obtain periodic blood samples for determination of serum osmolarity and sodium concentration. Resection time should be limited to as brief a time as possible. Based on an estimated intravascular absorption of irrigating fluid equal to 20 $ml \cdot min^{-1}$, the usual recommended resection time is 1 hour. It must be appreciated, however, that resection times as short as 15 minutes have resulted in symptoms of excessive intravascular absorption of irrigating fluid.[16]

EXTRACORPOREAL SHOCK WAVE LITHOTRIPSY

Extracorporeal shock wave lithotripsy is a noninvasive treatment of renal stones that produces destruction of stones by shock waves. Patients undergoing lithotripsy are placed in a hydraulically operated chair-lift support device and then submerged in water from the clavicles down in a large immersion tub. The impact of the shock waves at the flank entry site is painful and necessitates anesthesia. Immobilization is also important as any movement may displace stones from the predetermined focus sites for shock waves. General anesthesia or regional anesthesia including epidural and intercostal nerve blocks with local infiltration have been used to provide anesthesia. The head-up position during anesthesia can be associated with peripheral pooling of blood, but this effect is usually offset by the hydrostatic pressure of water

on submerged portions of the body. This same
hydrostatic pressure can displace blood centrally,
causing acute congestive heart failure in patients
with limited cardiac reserves. Likewise, hydrostatic
forces on the thorax may decrease functional
residual capacity and aggravate mismatching of
ventilation to perfusion. The immersion bath is
warmed to avoid hypothermia. Monitors and vascular access sites must be placed to avoid immersion.

RENAL TRANSPLANTATION

Regional and general anesthesia have been successfully used during renal transplantation. Advantages of regional anesthesia include elimination
of the need for intubation of the trachea in immunosuppressed patients as well as elimination of
the need for muscle relaxants. These advantages
are negated, however, if regional anesthesia must
be supplemented with depressant drugs. Furthermore, blockade of the peripheral sympathetic nervous system as produced by regional anesthesia
can make control of blood pressure difficult, especially considering the unpredictable intravascular fluid volume status of these patients. Use of
regional anesthesia is also controversial in the
presence of abnormal coagulation.

When general anesthesia is chosen, the selection
of anesthetic drugs, muscle relaxants, fluid replacement, and monitors follows the same principles as detailed for patients with chronic renal
disease (see the section *Changes Characteristic of
Chronic Renal Disease, Management of Anesthesia*). Reversal of neuromuscular blockade should pose no
unusual problems because excretion of muscle
relaxants and anticholinesterases are similarly influenced by impaired renal function and, furthermore, the newly transplanted kidney should begin
to excrete drugs promptly.[17] Mannitol is often
administered to facilitate urine formation by the
newly transplanted kidney.

REFERENCES

1. Pitts RF. Physiology of the Kidney and Body Fluids,
   3rd ed. Chicago, Year Book Medical Publishers, 1974.
2. Philbin DM, Coggins CH. Plasma antidiuretic hormone levels in cardiac surgical patients during morphine and halothane anesthesia. Anesthesiology
1974;40:95–8.
3. Fewell J, Bond, GC. Role of sinoaortic baroreceptors
in initiating the renal response to continuous positive-
pressure ventilation in the dog. Anesthesiology
1980;52:408–13.
4. Miller ED, Gianfagra W, Ackerly JA, Peach MJ.
Converting enzyme activity and pressure responses
to angiotensin I and II in the rat awake and during
anesthesia. Anesthesiology 1979;50:88–102.
5. Sladen RN, Endo E, Harrison T. Two-hour versus
22-hour creatinine clearance in critically ill patients.
Anesthesiology 1987;67:1013–6.
6. Bastron RD, Perkins FM, Pyne JL. Autoregulation
of renal blood flow during halothane anesthesia.
Anesthesiology 1977;46:142–4.
7. Macdonald AG. The effect of halothane on renal
cortical blood flow in normotensive or hypotensive
dogs. Br J Anaesth 1969;41:644–54.
8. Powell DR, Miller RD. The effect of repeated doses
of succinylcholine on serum potassium in patients
with renal failure. Anesth Analg 1975;54:746–8.
9. Carter R, Heerdt M, Acchiardo S. Fluoride kinetics
after enflurane anesthesia in healthy and anephric
patients and in patients with poor renal function.
Clin Pharmacol Ther 1977;20:565–70.
10. Bromage PR, Gertel M. Brachial plexus anesthesia
in chronic renal failure. Anesthesiology 1972;
36:488–93.
11. Fahey MR, Rupp SM, Fisher DM, et al. The pharmacokinetics and pharmacodynamics of atracurium
in patients with and without renal failure. Anesthesiology 1984;61:699–702.
12. Lynam DP, Cronnelly R, Arden J, Castagnoli K,
Canfell C, Miller RD. The pharmacokinetics and
pharmacoydnamics of vecuronium in patients with
and without renal failure. Anesthesiology 1986;
65:A296.
13. Brown RS. Renal dysfunction in the surgical patient-
maintenance of the high output state with furosemide. Crit Care Med 1979;7:63–8.
14. Roesch R, Stoelting RK, Lingeman JE, Kahnoski RJ,
Backes DJ, Gephardt SA. Ammonia toxicity due to
glycine absorption during a transurethral resection
of the prostate. Anesthesiology 1983;58:577–9.
15. Ovassapian A, Joshi CW, Brunner EA. Visual disturbance: An unusual symptom of transurethral prostatic resection reaction. Anesthesiology 1982;57:332–
4.
16. Hurlbert BJ, Wingard DW. Water intoxication after
15 minutes of transurethral resection of the prostate.
Anesthesiology 1979;50:355–6.
17. Morris RB, Cronnelly R, Miller RD, Stanski DR,
Fahey MR. Pharmacokinetics of edrophonium in
anephric and renal transplant patients. Br J Anaesth
1981;53:1311–3.

Chapter 23

Endocrine, Metabolic, and Nutritional Diseases

An understanding of the pathophysiology of endocrine gland function, disorders of metabolism, and abnormalities of nutrition is essential for the management of patients in the perioperative period who manifest diseases related to these systems. These disorders may be the primary reason for surgery or may co-exist in patients requiring operations unrelated to these disorders.

THYROID GLAND

Thyroid gland dysfunction reflects overproduction or underproduction of the two physiologically active thyroid gland hormones, triiodothyronine, and thyroxine (tetraiodothyronine). These hormones produce changes in the speed of biochemical reactions, total body oxygen consumption, and heat production. Calcitonin (thyrocalcitonin) is a third hormone released by the thyroid gland in response to elevations of the serum calcium concentration.

Synthesis and Secretion

Synthesis and secretion of triiodothyronine and thyroxine is regulated by thyroid stimulating hormone released from the anterior pituitary. Thyroid stimulating hormone release is controlled by thyrotropin-releasing hormone from the hypothalamus, as well as the circulating concentrations of thyroid gland hormones. Therefore, thyroid gland dysfunction can reflect disease processes involving the hypothalamus, the anterior pituitary, or the thyroid gland itself.

Laboratory Tests

Total serum thyroxine concentration is the standard screening test for evaluation of thyroid gland function. This value will be elevated in about 90 percent of patients who are hypothyroid. Serum triiodothyronine concentration is a sensitive test for detection of hyperthyroidism but not hypothyroidism. Measurement of the serum concentration of thyroid stimulating hormone is the most sensitive screening test for the detection of hypothyroidism.

Hyperthyroidism

Hyperthyroidism typically occurs in women between 20 years and 40 years of age. It is estimated that hyperthyroidism occurs in 0.2 percent of parturients.[1] The majority of patients demonstrate the presence of long-acting thyroid stimulator in the plasma, which mimics the effects of thyroid stimulating hormone producing effects lasting as long as 12 hours.

Signs and symptoms of hyperthyroidism (fatigue, weight loss, skeletal muscle weakness, heat intolerance, tachycardia, cardiac dysrhythmias, and congestive heart failure) reflect the impact of excess (5 times to 15 times normal) circulating thyroid gland hormones. Excess sympathetic nervous system activity, as well as attempts to eliminate excess heat are suggested by a hyperdynamic circulation manifesting as tachycardia, tachydysrhythmias, and increased cardiac output. The responsiveness of beta receptors to catecholamines may increase in hyperthyroid patients. Adrenal cortex hyperplasia reflects increased production and use of cortisol.

Management of Anesthesia

Elective surgery should not be considered until the patient has been rendered euthyroid with antithyroid drugs and the hyperdynamic circulation has been controlled with beta antagonists as evidenced by a resting heart rate less than 90 beats·min^{-1}. The combined use of beta antagonists and potassium iodide is effective in rendering most patients euthyroid in 10 days. Alternatively, treatment for 6 weeks to 8 weeks with antithyroid drugs, plus an oral iodide solution for 7 days to 10 days before surgery, will produce a euthyroid state and reduce the vascularity of the thyroid gland. When surgery cannot be delayed, the management of anesthesia in hyperthyroid patients is designed to minimize the effects of excess sympathetic nervous system activity.

Induction of anesthesia can be accomplished with the intravenous administration of thiopental. The chemical structure of thiopental is similar to antithyroid drugs, but it is unlikely that a significant antithyroid effect is produced by an induction dose of thiopental. Ketamine is not a good selection for induction of anesthesia because of the ability of this drug to stimulate the sympathetic nervous system.

The possibility of organ toxicity due to altered or accelerated drug metabolism in the presence of hyperthyroidism must be considered when selecting drugs for the maintenance of anesthesia. In animals pretreated with triiodothyronine and exposed to isoflurane, enflurane, or halothane the incidence of hepatic centrilobular necrosis after exposure to the anesthetic was 28 percent, 24 percent, and 92 percent respectively.[2] Isoflurane, which provides sufficient potency to offset adverse sympathetic nervous system responses to surgical stimulation and at the same time does not sensitize the myocardium to catecholamines or undergo significant metabolism, would seem a useful selection to combine with nitrous oxide. In view of the increased oxygen consumption characteristic of these patients, it would seem prudent to limit the inhaled concentration of nitrous oxide to 50 percent. Nitrous oxide combined with opioids is an alternative to the use of volatile drugs but has the disadvantage of not providing inhibition of sympathetic nervous system activity. Before intubation of the trachea, it is important to produce a depth of anesthesia sufficient to minimize sympathetic nervous system responses elicited by direct laryngoscopy. Administration of succinylcholine or nondepolarizing muscle relaxants (metocurine, atracurium, vecuronium), which rarely evoke undesirable cardiovascular effects is indicated to facilitate intubation of the trachea.

Controlled studies in animals do not support the clinical impression that anesthetic requirements for inhaled drugs (MAC) are increased in the presence of hyperthyroidism (Fig. 23-1).[3] The discrepancy between clinical impression and objective data is presumed to reflect the increased cardiac output characteristic of hyperthyroidism. For example, increased cardiac output accelerates uptake of inhaled anesthetics, resulting in the need to raise the inspired concentration of the drug so as to achieve a brain partial pressure similar to that achieved with a lower inspired concentration in the euthyroid patient. It should be appreciated that accelerated metabolism of the anesthetic does not alter the partial pressure of the drug necessary in the brain to produce the desired pharmacologic effect. Finally, any elevation in body temperature due to hyperthyroidism would be expected to increase anesthetic requirements about 5 percent for every degree the body temperature exceeds 37° Celsius.

In view of the likely presence of skeletal muscle weakness, it is important to monitor the responses produced by muscle relaxants with a peripheral nerve stimulator. When reversal of nondepolarizing neuromuscular blockade is indicated, it may be wise to combine glycopyrrolate rather than

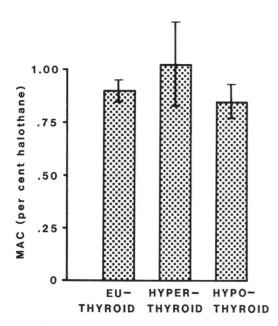

Fig. 23-1. The minimum alveolar concentration of halothane (MAC, mean ± SD) measured in dogs is not influenced by the level of activity of the thyroid gland. (Data from Babad and Eger,[3].)

atropine with anticholinesterases so as to minimize the possibility of excessive increases in heart rate.

Regional anesthesia with its associated blockade of the sympathetic nervous system is an attractive selection for hyperthyroid patients requiring surgery on the extremities or lower abdomen. Advantages of regional anesthetic techniques are somewhat offset by the possible need to treat hypotension. Considering the possible sensitivity of these patients to sympathomimetics, it is best to treat hypotension with reduced doses of direct-acting drugs, such as phenylephrine, if intravenous infusion of fluids is not effective. Epinephrine should not be added to local anesthetic solutions as systemic absorption of the catecholamine could produce exaggerated circulatory responses.

Constant monitoring of body temperature is important and means to lower body temperature, including cold solutions for intravenous infusion, must be available. The electrocardiogram (ECG) may reveal tachycardia and/or cardiac dysrhythmias, indicating the need for the intravenous administration of propranolol or lidocaine.

Thyroid Storm

Thyroid storm associated with surgery in hyperthyroid patients can occur intraoperatively but is most likely to manifest in the first 6 hours to 18 hours after surgery, emphasizing the need to maintain close monitoring of these patients in the early postoperative period. Symptoms of thyroid storm are due to the sudden and excessive release of thyroid gland hormones, leading to hyperthermia, tachycardia, cardiac dysrhythmias, congestive heart failure, dehydration, and shock. Thyroid storm can mimic the onset of malignant hyperthermia.

Treatment of thyroid storm includes intravenous infusion of cold crystalloid solutions some of which contain glucose plus administration of drugs to treat specific manifestations of excessive thyroid gland hormone concentrations. Sodium iodide is effective for acutely reducing the release of active hormones from the thyroid gland. Cortisol is indicated to offset the increased endogenous use of corticosteroids that could result in acute primary adrenal insufficiency. Propranolol is necessary to alleviate the peripheral effects of thyroid gland hormones on the cardiovascular system. Propylthiouracil is necessary to reduce the synthesis of new thyroid gland hormones, including those that result from the administration of sodium iodide.

Complications After Total or Partial Thyroidectomy

Damage to the laryngeal nerves, tracheal compression, and inadvertent removal of the parathyroid glands are early complications that can follow thyroid surgery.

Laryngeal Nerves. The entire sensory and motor supply to the larynx is from the two superior and two recurrent laryngeal nerves. The superior laryngeal nerves provide the motor supply to the cricothyroid muscles and sensation above the level of the vocal cords. The recurrent nerves supply motor innervation to all the muscles of the larynx except the cricothyroid muscles plus sensation below the level of the vocal cords. Function of the vocal cords after thyroid surgery can be evaluated by asking patients to say "e". The most common nerve injury after thyroid surgery is damage to the recurrent laryngeal nerve manifesting as hoarseness and a paralyzed vocal cord, which assumes an intermediate position. Bilateral recurrent nerve injury results in aphonia and paralyzed vocal cords that can flap together during inspiration to produce airway obstruction. Superior laryngeal nerve paralysis manifests as hoarseness and loss of sensation above the cords, making patients vulnerable to inhalation of any material present in the pharynx.

Compression of the Trachea. Compression of the trachea leading to airway obstruction may reflect a hematoma at the operative site or tracheomalacia due to weakening of the tracheal rings by chronic pressure from a goiter. Airway obstruction after extubation of the trachea and in the presence of normal vocal cord function should suggest the diagnosis of tracheomalacia.

Inadvertent Removal of the Parathyroid Glands. Hypoparathyroidism due to inadvertent removal of the parathyroid glands occurs in about 1 percent of patients who undergo a total thyroidectomy. In these patients, signs of hypocalcemia can manifest as early as 1 hour to 3 hours after surgery but typically do not appear until 24 hours to 72 hours postoperatively. Laryngeal muscles are very sensitive to hypocalcemia, and inspiratory stridor progressing to laryngospasm may be the first suggestion that surgically induced hypoparathyroidism is present.

Hypothyroidism

Subclinical hypothyroidism manifested solely by elevated plasma concentrations of thyroid stimulating hormone is present in about 5 percent of the population with a prevalence of greater than 13 percent in elderly patients.[4] Medical or surgical treatment of hyperthyroidism may become a cause of iatrogenic hypothyroidism. The development of hypothyroidism in adulthood is insidious and gradual and may go unrecognized in part because of the associated apathy that minimizes complaints by the patient. Characteristically, there is a generalized reduction in metabolic activity. Lethargy is prominent and intolerance to cold is present. Bradycardia and decreased stroke volume contrib-

ute to significant reductions (up to 40 percent) in cardiac output. Overt congestive heart failure, however, is unlikely and if present may indicate heart disease unrelated to thyroid gland dysfunction. Peripheral vasoconstriction, presumably in attempts to offset heat loss, leads to the characteristic cool and dry skin in these patients. There is often atrophy of the adrenal cortex and an associated decrease in the production of cortisol.

Treatment of hypothyroidism is with exogenous replacement of thyroid gland hormones by oral administration of levo-thyroxine or desiccated thyroid. Intravenous administration of triiodothyronine exerts physiologic effects within 6 hours, making it the treatment of choice when a rapid response is necessary. Thyroxine requires 10 days to exert a physiologic effect and is, therefore, not effective for emergency treatment of hypothyroidism.

Management of Anesthesia

Elective surgery should not be performed until patients have been rendered euthyroid.[5] When surgery cannot be delayed in known hypothyroid patients, it is important to consider changes characteristic of this disease that have a potential significant impact on management of anesthesia.

Induction of anesthesia can be accomplished with ketamine. Maintenance of anesthesia is often achieved by inhalation of nitrous oxide plus supplementation if necessary with minimal doses of ketamine, opioids, or benzodiazepines. Volatile anesthetics are not recommended because of the exquisite sensitivity of hypothyroid patients to drug-induced myocardial depression. The failure of decreases in thyroid activity to reduce anesthetic requirements (MAC) may reflect the maintenance of cerebral metabolic requirements for oxygen that are independent of thyroid activity (Fig. 23-1).[3,5] Reduced skeletal muscle activity associated with hypothyroidism suggests the possibility of prolonged responses should traditional doses of muscle relaxants be administered to these patients. Pancuronium, because of its mild sympathomimetic effects, would seem a useful selection for production of skeletal muscle paralysis. Reduced production of carbon dioxide associated with the decreased metabolic rate makes the hypothyroid

---

Characteristics of Hypothyroidism Relevant to Management of Anesthesia

Exquisite sensitivity to depressant drugs

Decreased cardiac output due to poor myocardial contractility and bradycardia

Slowed metabolism of drugs

Unresponsive baroreceptor reflexes

Skeletal muscle weakness

Hypovolemia

Prolonged gastric emptying time

Hyponatremia due to impaired clearance of free water

Hypothermia

Anemia

Hypoglycemia

Adrenal insufficiency

---

patient vulnerable to excessive reductions in the $PaCO_2$ during controlled ventilation of the lungs.

Monitoring of hypothyroid patients is directed towards early recognition of congestive heart failure and detection of the onset of hypothermia. Continuous recording of arterial blood pressure and cardiac filling pressures are indicated for invasive operations. In addition to glucose, intravenous solutions should contain sodium so as to prevent the development of hyponatremia. The possibility of acute primary adrenal insufficiency should be remembered when hypotension persists despite intravenous infusion of fluids and/or administration of sympathomimetics. Maintenance of body temperature is facilitated by increasing the temperature of the operating room and passing intravenous fluid solutions through warming devices.

Recovery from the sedative effects of anesthetics may be delayed in hypothyroid patients. Support of ventilation of the lungs may be required postoperatively, especially if body temperature is reduced. Indeed, prolonged postoperative lethargy

and inability to wean from mechanical support of ventilation may reflect previously unrecognized hypothyroidism.[6] Postoperative analgesia must be provided with minimal doses of drugs, as these patients are susceptible to the ventilatory depressant effects of opioids.

Regional anesthesia is acceptable for management of anesthesia in hypothyroid patients. Although supporting evidence is not available, it is possible the doses of local anesthetics necessary for peripheral nerve blocks might be reduced.

Adrenal Cortex

The adrenal cortex is responsible for the synthesis of three groups of hormones classified as glucocorticoids (cortisol), mineralocorticoids (aldosterone), and androgens (estradiol and testosterone) (Table 23-1). Synthesis and release of glucocorticoids and androgens from the adrenal cortex is regulated by adrenocorticotrophic hormone (ACTH) that is produced in the anterior pituitary. ACTH release is determined by corticotropin-releasing factor from the hypothalamus and a negative feedback mechanism regulated by the serum concentration of cortisol.

Cortisol

Cortisol is the only hormone produced by the adrenal cortex that is essential for life. In addition to its well known anti-inflammatory effects, cortisol is important for facilitating the (1) conversion of norepinephrine to epinephrine and the subsequent maintenance of blood pressure, (2) retention of sodium and secretion of water and potassium, and (3) breakdown of proteins and subsequent formation of glucose from amino acids by gluconeogenesis. Hyperglycemia in response to cortisol reflects both gluconeogenesis and inhibition by cortisol of peripheral use of glucose by cells.

Treatment of hypoadrenocorticism associated with circulatory collapse is with the intravenous administration of cortisol 100 mg followed by the continuous infusion of 50 mg every 4 hours to 6 hours during the first 48 hours after the crisis. Restoration of intravascular fluid volume requires intravenous infusion of glucose in saline.

Table 23-1. Endogenous and Synthetic Corticosteroids

	Glucocorticoid Potency[a] (Anti-Inflammatory Effect)	Mineralocorticoid Potency[a] (Salt-Retaining Effect)	Equivalent Oral or IV Dose (mg)[a]
Cortisol	1	1	20[b]
Cortisone	0.8	0.8	25
Prednisolone	4	0.8	25
Prednisone	4	0.8	5
Methylprednisolone	5	0	4
Dexamethasone	25	0	0.75
Aldosterone		3000	

[a] Potencies and equivalent doses are as compared with cortisol.
[b] Assumed daily endogenous cortisol production.

Aldosterone

Secretion and synthesis of aldosterone by the adrenal cortex are regulated by the renin-angiotensin system and the serum concentrations of potassium. For example, angiotensin II is a potent stimulus for the release of aldosterone from the adrenal cortex. The mineralocorticoid effects of aldosterone at the renal tubules are reflected by reabsorption of sodium and excretion of potassium. Reabsorption of sodium induced by aldosterone is an important mechanism for regulating the extracellular fluid volume. Indeed, renin release in response to hypovolemia ultimately leads to release of aldosterone and increased reabsorption of sodium in attempts to restore extracellular fluid volume.

Corticosteroid Therapy Before Surgery

Corticosteroid supplementation should be increased whenever patients being treated for chronic hypoadrenocorticism undergo surgical procedures. This recommendation is based on the concern that these patients are susceptible to cardiovascular collapse because they cannot release additional endogenous cortisol in response to the stress of surgery. More controversial is the management of patients who may manifest suppression of the pituitary-adrenal axis due to current or previous administration of corticosteroids for treatment of diseases unrelated to pathology in the anterior pituitary or adrenal cortex. The dose of corticosteroids or duration of therapy with corticosteroids that produces suppression of the pituitary-adrenal axis is not known. Suppression, however, may persist as long as 12 months after discontinuation of therapy. Therefore, the tendency empirically is to administer supplemental corticosteroids in the perioperative period when surgery is planned in patients who are being treated with corticosteroids or who have been treated for more than 1 month in the past 6 months to 12 months. Nevertheless, it should be appreciated that cause and effect relationships between intraoperative hypotension and acute hypoadrenocorticism in patients previously treated with corticosteroids has never been documented.

A useful empiric regimen is the administration of intravenous cortisol 25 mg at the time of induction of anesthesia followed by a continuous intravenous infusion of cortisol 100 mg during the next 24 hours.[7] This regimen maintains plasma concentrations of cortisol above normal during major surgery in patients receiving chronic treatment with corticosteroids and manifesting subnormal responses to preoperative infusions of ACTH (Fig. 23-2).[7] Use of this regimen should provide adequate plasma concentrations of cortisol in patients considered to be at risk from the presence of a suppressed pituitary-adrenal axis and in whom

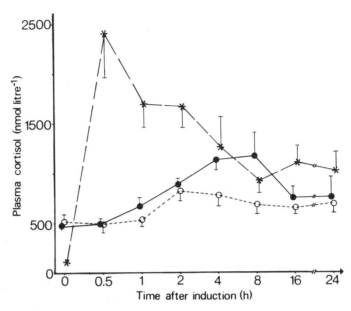

Fig. 23-2. Plasma cortisol concentrations (mean ± SE) were measured in patients who had never been treated with cortisol (solid circles), patients receiving long-term corticosteroid treatment but manifesting normal increases in the plasma concentrations of cortisol in response to preoperative administration of adrenocorticotrophic hormone (open circles), and patients receiving long-term corticosteroid treatment who manifested subnormal changes in the plasma concentrations of cortisol in response to preoperative administration of adrenocorticotrophic hormone (asterisks). Only these latter patients received additional exogenous corticosteroids consisting of intravenous administration of cortisol 25 mg after the induction of anesthesia plus a continuous infusion of cortisol 100 mg during the next 24 hours. Plasma concentrations of cortisol were not different among patient groups after the 2 hour measurement. (From Symreng et al.,[7] with permission.)

major surgery is necessary. It is likely that patients undergoing minor operations will need minimal to no additional corticosteroid coverage during the perioperative period.

In addition to low dose intravenous cortisol supplementation, patients receiving daily maintenance doses of corticosteroids should also receive this dose with the preoperative medication on the day of surgery. This maintenance dose should be continued after surgery. No objective evidence supports increasing maintenance doses of corticosteroids preoperatively and then gradually decreasing the doses back to maintenance levels during the first few days postoperatively. When postoperative events (sepsis, burns) could exaggerate needs for exogenous corticosteroid supple-

mentation, the continuous infusion of cortisol 100 mg every 12 hours to 24 hours is sufficient.

ADRENAL MEDULLA

The adrenal medulla is a specialized part of the sympathetic nervous system capable of synthesizing norepinephrine and epinephrine. The majority of norepinephrine synthesized in the adrenal medulla is methylated to epinephrine by the action of the enzyme phenylethanolamine N-methyltransferase. The activity of this enzyme is stimulated by cortisol that flows through the adrenal medulla from the adrenal cortex. Thus, cortisol ultimately regulates production of epinephrine.

Pheochromocytoma

Pheochromocytoma is a catecholamine-secreting tumor that originates in the adrenal medulla or aberrant tissue along the paravertebral sympathetic chain. The hallmark of pheochromocytoma is paroxysmal or sustained hypertension. Less than 0.1 percent of all cases of hypertension, however, are due to pheochromocytoma. The triad of diaphoresis, tachycardia, and headaches in hypertensive patients is highly suggestive of pheochromocytoma. Other manifestations of pheochromocytoma include weight loss and orthostatic hypotension. Orthostatic hypotension, along with an increased hematocrit, reflects the decrease in intravascular fluid volume associated with sustained hypertension. Myocarditis due to the chronic excess of circulating catecholamines may manifest as ST-T changes on the ECG. Hyperglycemia reflects inhibition of insulin release secondary to catecholamine-produced alpha stimulation.

Definitive diagnosis of pheochromocytoma requires biochemical confirmation of excessive catecholamine production. Measurement of urinary excretion of catecholamines or metabolites of catecholamines, such as metanephrines or vanillylmandelic acid, can be used as an index of catecholamine production. Measurement of total plasma concentrations of catecholamines, however, is the most reliable measurement for the diagnosis of a pheochromocytoma (Fig. 23-3).[8] Total plasma concentrations of catecholamines above 2000 pg·ml^{-1} are considered diagnostic of pheochromocytoma. When the diagnosis of pheochromocytoma is equivocal on the basis of plasma concentrations of catecholamines (1000 pg·ml^{-1} to 2000 pg·ml^{-1}) the administration of a single oral dose of clonidine (0.3 mg) will reduce plasma catecholamine concentrations below 500 pg·ml^{-1} only in hypertensive patients who do not have a pheochromocytoma.

Treatment of pheochromocytoma is surgical excision of the catecholamine-secreting tumor or tumors. Before surgical excision, however, it is mandatory to produce alpha blockade with drugs, such as phenoxybenzamine or prazosin, which lead to reductions in blood pressure and normalization of the blood volume. Prazosin may be preferable, as it is a relatively selective alpha-1 antagonist in contrast to phenoxybenzamine, which acts at alpha-1 and alpha-2 receptors. By sparing alpha-2 receptors, prazosin allows released norepinephrine to continue exerting a negative feedback effect on additional release of the neurotransmitter.[9] Alpha blockade also reduces the risk of intraoperative hypertension during the manipulation of the tumor. The persistence of tachycardia and/or cardiac dysrhythmias despite alpha blockade is an indication for the administration of drugs, such as propranolol, to produce beta blockade. The recommendation that beta blockade not be instituted in the absence of alpha blockade is based on the theoretical concern that a heart depressed by beta antagonists could not maintain an adequate cardiac output should unopposed alpha mediated vasoconstriction from the release of catecholamines result in abrupt increases in the systemic vascular resistance. In this regard, labetalol, which produces alpha and beta blockade, may be useful in preoperative preparation of these patients.[9] Preoperative preparation also includes attempts to localize the anatomic position of the tumor most often with computed tomography and/or arteriography.

Management of Anesthesia

Management of anesthesia for patients requiring excision of pheochromocytoma is based on avoidance of drugs or events that might activate the sympathetic nervous system and use of invasive monitoring techniques (arterial and pulmonary artery catheters) that permit early and appropriate interventions when catecholamine-induced changes in cardiovascular function occur.[9] Continuation of alpha and beta antagonists until the induction of anesthesia is recommended. The goal of preoperative medication is to reduce the likelihood of apprehension-induced activation of the sympathetic nervous system. A catheter should be placed in a peripheral artery to provide continuous monitoring of blood pressure before the induction of anesthesia. Induction of anesthesia can be accomplished with the intravenous administration of barbiturates, benzodiazepines, or etomidate. After the onset of unconsciousness and before direct laryngoscopy for intubation of the trachea, the

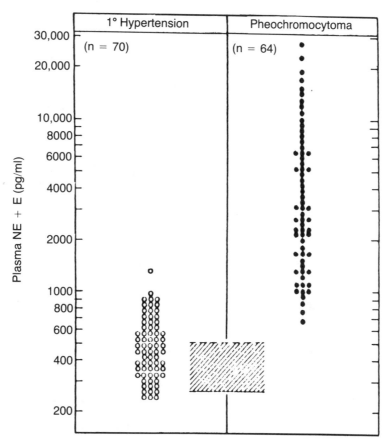

Fig. 23-3. Plasma concentrations of norepinephrine (NE) and epinephrine (E) as measured in patients with essential hypertension and patients with pheochromocytoma. The cross-hatched area represents the mean $\pm$ 2 SD of values in a control group of normotensive patients. Pheochromocytoma was present in every patient with total plasma catecholamine concentrations exceeding 2000 pg·ml^{-1}. (From Bravo and Gifford,[8] with permission.)

depth of anesthesia should be increased by ventilation of the lungs with nitrous oxide plus enflurane or isoflurane. Selection of enflurane or isoflurane for maintenance of anesthesia is based on the ability of these drugs to reduce sympathetic nervous system activity. Furthermore, these drugs are unlikely to sensitize the heart to the dysrhythmic effects of catecholamines. Halothane is not recommended because of the likelihood of cardiac dysrhythmias in the presence of catecholamine release from the pheochromocytoma. Likewise, maintenance of anesthesia with nitrous oxide and opioids is not ideal as this drug combination does not suppress activity of the sympathetic ner-

vous system and hypertensive responses are likely. The use of Innovar (fentanyl plus droperidol) is questionable because droperidol has been reported to provoke hypertension in the presence of a pheochromocytoma.

Intubation of the trachea is facilitated by the administration of succinylcholine or nondepolarizing muscle relaxants with minimal cardiovascular effects (metocurine, atracurium, vecuronium). The histamine-releasing effects of d-tubocurarine and the vagolytic and possibly mild sympathomimetic effects of pancuronium would make these drugs unlikely selections. Establishment of an adequate depth of anesthesia before intubation of the trachea is recommended to minimize the pressor effects evoked by direct laryngoscopy. Intravenous administration of lidocaine or opioids 1 minute to 3 minutes before induction of anesthesia may be useful for attenuating pressor responses evoked by intubation of the trachea. It must also be remembered that a short duration of direct laryngoscopy (less than 15 seconds) is important for attenuating sympathetic nervous system stimulation associated with intubation of the trachea.

A continuous intravenous infusion of nitroprusside during surgery will be necessary if hypertension persists despite maximum concentrations (about 1.5 MAC to 2 MAC) of enflurane or isoflurane. Subsequent reductions in blood pressure may accompany decreases in plasma concentrations of catecholamines that occur as the veins draining the pheochromocytoma are surgically ligated. This hypotension is treated by decreasing the delivered concentrations of volatile anesthetics; intravenous infusion of crystalloid and/or colloid solutions; and, in some patients with persistent reductions in blood pressure, a continuous infusion of norepinephrine, dopamine, or dobutamine. A pulmonary artery catheter is helpful in evaluating the responses of these patients to therapeutic interventions. Monitoring serum glucose concentrations is indicated, as hypoglycemia may occur when plasma catecholamine concentrations decrease after removal of the tumor.

Regional anesthesia for excision of a pheochromocytoma has the attractive features of blocking the sympathetic nervous system and not sensitizing the heart to catecholamines. Nevertheless, postsynaptic alpha receptors can still respond to the direct effects of circulating catecholamines. Furthermore, hypotension that accompanies ligation of the veins draining a pheochromocytoma cannot be offset by sympathetic nervous system activation in the presence of a regional block. Finally, selection of a regional technique is practical only if the surgical procedure is performed in a supine position.

DIABETES MELLITUS

Diabetes mellitus is a chronic systemic disease due to a relative or absolute lack of insulin that is estimated to affect 2 percent to 5 percent of the

Table 23-2. Classification of Diabetes Mellitus

	Juvenile Onset	Maturity Onset
Age of onset (years)	Before 16	After 35
Require exogenous insulin	Yes	Not always
Ketoacidosis prone	Yes	No
Blood glucose concentration	Wide fluctuations	Less marked fluctuations
Nutrition	Thin	Obese
Vascular complications	Rare	Common

population. Classically, diabetes manifests as hyperglycemia and degeneration of small blood vessels. Diabetes may be considered as juvenile onset (insulin-dependent) or adult onset (noninsulin-dependent, nonketoacidosis prone) (Table 23-2). Adult onset diabetes composes over 90 percent of all diabetics and is almost always associated with obesity.

Complications of Diabetes Mellitus

Complications of diabetes include ketoacidosis, neuropathies, atherosclerosis (coronary artery disease, cerebral vascular disease, peripheral vascular disease), microangiopathy (retinopathy, renal dysfunction), and an increased incidence of infection and decreased postoperative wound tensile strength.

Ketoacidosis

Ketoacidosis is the most serious metabolic complication of diabetes. The finding of metabolic acidosis in the presence of hyperglycemia plus the history of diabetes is sufficient to establish the diagnosis of ketoacidosis. Infection is often responsible for resistance to insulin that leads to the development of ketoacidosis.

Ketoacids have a low renal threshold and about one-half the acid load is excreted in combination with sodium, resulting in hyponatremia. In the presence of acidosis potassium leaves the cells such that serum potassium concentrations are likely to be elevated despite the presence of total body potassium deficits. Myocardial contractility and peripheral vascular tone are diminished by ketoacidosis. Hyperglycemia associated with acidosis causes increased serum osmolarity such that water is transferred from cells to extracellular fluid producing intracellular dehydration. Concomitantly, osmotic diuresis induced by hyperglycemia results in urinary loss of electrolytes particularly potassium and depletion of intravascular fluid volume, which may be so severe that cardiovascular collapse occurs. Compensatory responses to ketoacidosis are chloride loss via the kidneys and hyperventilation.

Definitive treatment of ketoacidosis is the intravenous administration of insulin. Supplemental potassium infusion may be necessary when acidosis is corrected and potassium re-enters the cells.

Neuropathies

Segmental demyelination associated with diabetes leads to the development of neuropathies. Autonomic nervous system neuropathy that can accompany diabetes is characterized by orthostatic hypotension, resting tachycardia and prolonged gastric emptying time (gastroparesis diabeticorum). Compared with nondiabetic patients, diabetic patients with autonomic nervous system neuropathy manifest minimal heart rate responses after the intravenous administration of atropine or propranolol. Bradycardia that does not respond to treatment with atropine has been observed in these patients after pharmacologic reversal of nondepolarizing muscle relaxants.[10] Painless myocardial infarction and unexplained cardiorespiratory arrest have been reported in diabetic patients with autonomic nervous system neuropathy. Involvement of somatic nerves may manifest as nocturnal sensory discomfort. Further expression of neuropathy is the increased incidence of carpal tunnel syndrome among diabetics.

Management of Anesthesia

The two goals in the management of anesthesia for the patient with diabetes are to prevent hypoglycemia by providing exogenous glucose and to prevent ketoacidosis by assuring an adequate supply of exogenous insulin. The preoperative evaluation should include the adequacy of blood glucose control. The absence of ketoacidosis must be confirmed before undertaking any elective surgery. Manifestations of coronary artery disease, cerebral vascular disease, renal dysfunction, and signs of peripheral and autonomic nervous system neuropathy should be noted. Choice of drugs for induction and maintenance of general anesthesia is less important than monitoring blood glucose concentrations and treating the potential physiologic derangements associated with diabetes. Volatile anesthetics tend to inhibit the endogenous release of insulin but this is probably clinically insignificant with respect to the total management of anesthesia in the diabetic patient. Intubation of the trachea with a cuffed tube seems prudent in view of the prolonged gastric emptying times associated with autonomic nervous system neuropathy. The high incidence of peripheral neuropathy must be considered and documented in the patient's medical record if regional anesthetic techniques are selected so as to avoid the erroneous assumption postoperatively that the anesthetic caused the co-existing neurologic deficit.

Management of the Daily Insulin Dose

Traditionally, one-fourth to one-half the usual daily dose of lente or NPH insulin is administered subcutaneously on the morning of surgery with the preoperative medication. It is usually recommended that an intravenous infusion of glucose be started at the same time to replace the carbohydrate content of missed meals. An appropriate fluid selection and infusion rate is 5 percent dextrose in lactated Ringer's solution delivered at 100 ml·hr^{-1} (5 g glucose·hr^{-1} to 7 g glucose·hr^{-1}).

An acceptable alternative to routine administration of preoperative insulin is to withhold insulin and measure blood glucose concentrations every hour during the intraoperative period (Fig. 23-4).[11] Based on this measurement, blood glucose concentrations can be maintained between 100 mg·dl^{-1} to 250 mg·dl^{-1} during the intraoperative period by the intravenous infusion of additional glucose or regular insulin (5 units to 10 units).

A third option for management of insulin requirements is continuous intravenous infusion of low doses of regular insulin during the operation. For example, 1 unit to 2 units of regular insulin administered intravenously, followed by continu-

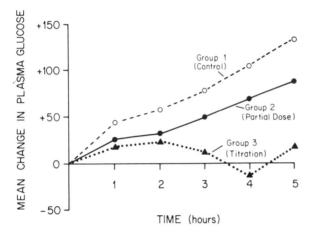

Fig. 23-4. Mean changes in blood glucose concentrations were determined in insulin-dependent adult diabetic patients undergoing elective surgery. Group 1 patients received no preoperative insulin or glucose. Group 2 patients received one-fourth to one-half of their usual dose of insulin on the morning of surgery plus the intravenous infusion of 6.25 g·hr⁻¹ of glucose. Group 3 patients did not receive insulin or glucose preoperatively but were treated with intravenous administration of regular insulin if blood glucose concentrations exceeded 200 mg·dl⁻¹. (From Walts et al.,[11] with permission.)

ous intravenous infusion of 1 unit·hr⁻¹ of regular insulin results in blood glucose concentrations during the operative period similar to blood glucose levels present in diabetic patients receiving a portion of their normal daily insulin dose subcutaneously as part of the preoperative medication.

If oral hypoglycemic drugs are being used, they can be continued until the evening before surgery. It should be remembered, however, that these drugs may produce hypoglycemia as long as 24 hours to 48 hours after their administration.

Determination of blood glucose concentrations before the induction of anesthesia is recommended. Comparison of the glucose concentration in this blood sample as reported from the laboratory with that glucose value estimated by using a Dextrostix or Chemstrip confirms the accuracy of the latter approach. Estimation of blood glucose concentrations using these commercially available devices can then be repeated with confidence as to their accuracy during surgery. Simultaneous estimates of blood glucose concentrations and the presence or absence of ketone bodies in the blood can be determined using a Keto-Diastix.

NONKETOTIC HYPEROSMOLAR HYPERGLYCEMIC COMA

Nonketotic hyperosmolar hyperglycemic coma occurs most often in elderly patients with an impaired thirst mechanism. Two-thirds of patients who develop this syndrome do not have a history of diabetes mellitus. Typical findings of this syndrome include severe hyperglycemia (usually above 600 mg·dl⁻¹) that leads to osmotic diuresis with associated loss of sodium, potassium, and intravascular fluid volume. Plasma osmolarity often exceeds 330 mOsm·L⁻¹. Altered mentation culminating in seizures and coma reflects a decrease in intracellular brain water due to the extreme hyperosmolarity of the plasma. Ketoacidosis does not occur. Treatment is with intravenous regular insulin, potassium supplementation, and restoration of intravascular fluid volume with sodium containing solutions.

MORBID OBESITY

Obesity is the most common nutritional disorder in the United States. Obesity is defined as a body weight of 20 percent above the ideal weight. Morbid obesity is present when body weight is twice the ideal weight. A metabolic defect to explain obesity has not been found. In adults, the final common pathway leading to obesity is a positive caloric intake.

Adverse Changes Associated with Obesity

Obesity increases the risk for developing medical and surgical diseases. Manifestations of adverse changes associated with obesity are metabolic, pulmonary, cardiovascular, and hepatic.

Metabolic

Obese individuals are resistant to the effects of insulin, which is consistent with the several-fold increase in the incidence of adult onset diabetes mellitus in obese patients. Oxygen consumption and carbon dioxide production are increased by obesity.

Pulmonary

Pulmonary function changes in obese patients suggest restrictive pulmonary disease characterized by reductions in expiratory reserve volume, inspiratory capacity, vital capacity, and functional residual capacity. The diaphragm is elevated and its excursion is markedly limited due to the weight of the abdominal wall. The work of breathing is increased and ventilation becomes diaphragmatic and position dependent.

The PaO_2 is predictably decreased by obesity, presumably reflecting overperfusion of underventilated alveoli. Conversely, the $PaCO_2$ and the ventilatory response to carbon dioxide remain normal. The margin of reserve, however, is small and administration of ventilatory depressant drugs or assumption of the head-down position can lead to the accumulation of carbon dioxide in obese patients.

Obesity-Hypoventilation Syndrome. Over 8 percent of morbidly obese patients manifest episodic somnolence and hypoventilation. The elevated $PaCO_2$ is associated with respiratory acidosis, arterial hypoxemia, polycythemia, pulmonary hypertension, and right ventricular failure. The etiology of this syndrome is unknown but may represent a disorder of central nervous system regulation of ventilation.

Cardiovascular

Cardiac output is increased, emphasizing the increased oxygen demand present in obese individuals. There is a positive correlation between increases in blood pressure and weight gain. Increased cardiac output is the presumed cause of increased blood pressure. Pulmonary hypertension is common and most likely reflects the effects of chronic arterial hypoxemia and/or increased pulmonary blood volume. The risk of coronary artery disease is doubled in obese patients. Finally, care should be taken to use a blood pressure cuff of the correct size. As a general rule, the width of the blood pressure cuff should be greater than one-third of the circumference of the arm. When the cuff is too narrow a higher amount of pressure will be required to compress the extra tissues and a false high blood pressure will be recorded.

Hepatic

Abnormal liver function tests and fatty infiltration of the liver occur frequently in obese individuals. There is evidence that fluorinated volatile anesthetics are metabolized to a greater extent in obese patients (see Chapter 5).

Management of Anesthesia

Obese patients should be considered at a greater risk for inhalation of gastric contents in view of the increased incidence of gastroesophageal reflux and hiatal hernia in these patients. Furthermore, gastric acidity, gastric fluid volume, and intragastric pressures are often increased. Preoperative administration of antacid or H_2-receptor antagonists and metoclopramide can be used to increase gastric fluid pH and decrease gastric fluid volume in obese patients. Finally, drug treatment of obesity with amphetamines can influence anesthetic requirements for volatile anesthetics (see Chapter 2).

The massive amount of soft tissue about the head and upper trunk can impair mandibular and cervical mobility, making maintenance of the upper airway and intubation of the trachea difficult. After induction of anesthesia, the low functional residual capacity reduces the mixing time for inhaled gases in the lung. As a result, the rate of increase in the alveolar concentrations of inhaled anesthetics is accelerated. Furthermore, the low functional residual capacity predisposes obese patients to rapid reductions in the PaO_2 during any period of apnea as may accompany direct laryngoscopy for intubation of the trachea.

The impact of obesity on the necessary dose of injected drugs is difficult to access. Blood volume is often increased in obese patients, which would tend to reduce the plasma concentrations achieved with single rapid injections of drugs such as thiopental. Conversely, adipose tissue has a low blood flow such that increased doses calculated on an absolute weight basis in obese patients could result in exposing well perfused tissues to excessive concentrations of drugs. Perhaps the most logical approach is to calculate the initial doses on an ideal rather than actual body weight. Subsequent doses would be based on the patient's response. Repeated injections of drugs, however, could result in cumulative effects and prolonged responses, reflecting storage of lipid soluble drugs in adipose tissue for subsequent release into the circulation as the plasma concentrations of the drugs decline.

Present evidence does not make it possible to recommend specific drugs or drug combinations for maintenance of anesthesia in obese patients. Nevertheless, the high incidence of co-existing liver disease and altered metabolism of fluorinated anesthetics must be considered in selection of volatile drugs. There is no evidence that the high lipid solubility of volatile anesthetics results in delayed postanesthesia awakening in morbidly obese patients (Fig. 23-5).[12] The use of spinal or epidural anesthesia is limited in obese patients because bony landmarks are obscured and predictability of the level of anesthesia that will be produced by a given dose of drug is difficult.

Monitoring of arterial blood gases and pH is helpful in evaluating the adequacy of oxygenation and ventilation. Controlled ventilation of the lungs using large tidal volumes to facilitate the maintenance of the functional residual capacity during the intraoperative period is recommended.

Postoperatively, the semisitting position should be employed so as to optimize the mechanics of breathing and to minimize the development of arterial hypoxemia. Supplemental oxygen should be provided, remembering the maximum reduction in PaO_2 typically occurs 2 days to 3 days postoperatively. The risk of deep vein thrombosis and pulmonary embolism are increased, emphasizing the importance of early ambulation for these patients.

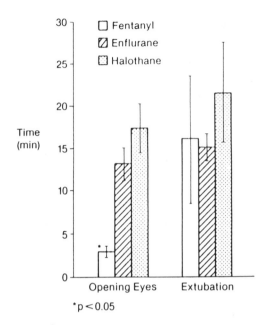

Fig. 23-5. Awakening time (mean ± SE), as defined by the time from the last skin stitch until opening the eyes on command, and by the time from the last skin stitch until extubation of the trachea, was measured in obese patients anesthetized with nitrous oxide plus fentanyl, enflurane, or halothane for gastric stapling operations. Criteria for extubation of the trachea included sustained responses to electrical stimulation delivered from a peripheral nerve stimulator (tetanus) and the ability to maintain head lift for 5 seconds. The time to opening eyes on command was shortest in patients receiving nitrous oxidide-fentanyl. The time to extubation of the trachea, however, was similar, regardless of the anesthetic drugs administered. (From Cork et al.,[12] with permission.)

ENTERAL AND PARENTERAL NUTRITION

Caloric support in the presence of increased energy requirements is best provided by enteral or total parenteral nutrition (hyperalimentation). It is recommended that patients who have lost more than 20 percent of their body weight should be treated nutritionally before surgery.[13]

Enteral Nutrition

The gastrointestinal tract should be the site used for nutritional supplementation whenever possible. Enteral nutrition is delivered by a nasogastric or orogastric tube. Complications of enteral feedings are not common but can include hyperglycemia, leading to osmotic diuresis and hypovolemia. Therefore, blood glucose concentrations should be monitored and exogenous insulin administered when levels exceed 250 mg·dl^{-1}. The high osmolality of elemental diets often causes diarrhea.

Total Parenteral Nutrition

Total parenteral nutrition is indicated when the gastrointestinal tract is not functioning. Most often a catheter is placed in the subclavian vein so as to permit infusion of hypertonic solutions.

The potential complications of total parenteral nutrition include catheter related sepsis, hyperglycemia, nonketotic hyperosmolar hyperglycemic coma, hepatic dysfunction, hypomagnesemia, and hyperchloremic metabolic acidosis due to liberation of hydrochloric acid during the metabolism of amino acids present in the parenteral nutrition solutions. Concern about catheter-related sepsis precludes use of the catheter as a blood withdrawal site or to monitor central venous pressure. Hypophosphatemia from the administration of phosphate-depleted solutions can result in a shift of the oxyhemoglobin dissociation curve to the left and decreased release of oxygen from hemoglobin to tissues. The main reason for slowing or discontinuing infusion of parenteral nutrition solutions before the induction of anesthesia is to avoid intraoperative hyperosmolarity secondary to rapid infusion of the solution. Abrupt discontinuation, however, should be avoided, as persistence of increased circulating levels of endogenous insulin could contribute to hypoglycemia. Preoperatively, it is important to measure blood concentrations of glucose, phosphate, and potassium. Finally, increased production of carbon dioxide resulting from metabolism of large quantities of glucose may result in the need to initiate artificial ventilation of the lungs or in failure to wean patients from long-term ventilatory support.[14]

ENDOCRINE AND METABOLIC CHANGES IN THE PERIOPERATIVE PERIOD

Surgical stimulation produces profound endocrine and metabolic responses that parallel the magnitude of the operative trauma.[15] Conversely, inhaled or injected drugs used to produce anesthesia result in minimal effects on hormone secretion in the absence of surgical stimulation.

The initial endocrine response to surgical stimulation is an increase in the circulating concentrations of cortisol and catecholamines and a decrease in the plasma concentrations of insulin despite hyperglycemia. In view of the latter, excessive infusion of glucose via intravenous solutions could result in intraoperative hyperglycemia.

Surgical trauma evokes protein degradation as reflected by loss of lean body weight and increased urinary excretion of nitrogen postoperatively. Sodium and water retention and excretion of potassium in the postoperative period, presumably reflect release of antidiuretic hormone and activation of the renin-angiotensin-aldosterone system.

Although it is difficult to quantitate total adverse effects produced by endocrine and metabolic responses to surgical stimulation, it would seem prudent to minimize the magnitude and duration of these changes whenever possible. Attenuation or prevention of the endocrine responses to surgery can be produced by afferent neuronal blockade, as with regional anesthesia (T4 sensory level) or by inhibition of hypothalamic function with large doses of opioids. For these reasons, the concept that the administration of the lowest dose of anesthetic is best may not be valid during periods of acute surgical stimulation.[16] It is likely, however, that regional anesthesia merely postpones endocrine responses to surgery until the postoperative period.

REFERENCES

1. Burrow GN. The management of thyrotoxicosis in pregnancy. N Engl J Med 1985;313:562–8.
2. Berman ML, Kuhnert L, Phythyon JM, Holaday DA. Isoflurane and enflurane-induced hepatic necrosis in triiodothyronine-pretreated rats. Anesthesiology 1983;58:1–5.
3. Babad AA, Eger EI II. The effects of hyperthyroidism and hypothyroidism on halothane and oxygen requirements in dogs. Anesthesiology 1968;29:1087–93.
4. Cooper DS. Subclinical hypothyroidism. JAMA 1987;258:246–7.
5. Murkin JM. Anesthesia and hypothyroidism: A review of thyroxine physiology, pharmacology, and anesthetic implications. Anesth Analg 1982;61:371–83.
6. Levelle JP, Jopling MW, Sklar GS. Perioperative hypothyroidism: An unusual postanesthetic diagnosis. Anesthesiology 1985;63:195–7.
7. Symreng T, Karlberg BE, Kagedal B, Schildt B. Physiological cortisol substitution of long-term steroid-treated patients undergoing major surgery. Br J Anaesth 1981;53:949–53.
8. Bravo EL, Gifford RW. Pheochromocytoma: Diagnosis, localization and management. N Engl J Med 1984;311:1298–1303.
9. Hull CJ. Pheochromocytoma. Diagnosis, preopera-

tive preparation and anesthetic management. Br J Anaesth 1986;58:1453–8.

10. Triantafillou AN, Tsuda K, Berg J, Wieman TJ. Refractory bradycardia after reversal of muscle relaxant in a diabetic with vagal neuropathy. Anesth Analg 1986;65:1237–41.

11. Walts LF, Miller J, Davidson MB, Brown J. Perioperative management of diabetes mellitus. Anesthesiology 1981;55:104–9.

12. Cork RC, Vaughn RW, Bentley JB. General anesthesia for morbidly obese patients—an examination of postoperative outcomes. Anesthesiology 1981; 54:310–3.

13. Powell-Tuck J, Goode AW. Principles of enteral and parenteral nutrition. Br J Anaesth 1981;53: 169–80.

14. Askanzi J, Nordenstrom J, Rosenbaum SH, et al. Nutrition for the patient with respiratory failure: glucose vs. fat. Anesthesiology 1981;54:373–7.

15. Traymor C, Hall GM. Endocrine and metabolic changes during surgery: anaesthetic implications. Br J Anaesth 1981;53:153–60.

16. Roizen MF, Horrigan RW, Frazer BM. Anesthetic doses blocking adrenergic (stress) and cardiovascular responses to incision-MAC BAR. Anesthesiology 1981;54:390–8.

Chapter 24

Central Nervous System Disease

Anesthesia for surgical treatment of diseases of the central nervous system requires an understanding of relationships between cerebral blood flow (CBF), cerebral metabolic rate for oxygen ($CMRO_2$) and intracranial pressure (ICP). Physiologic and pharmacologic influences, which are often under the control of the anesthesiologist, may alter the fragile relationship between CBF, $CMRO_2$, and ICP. Indeed, selection of drugs, the technique of ventilation of the lungs and choice of monitors have uniquely important implications in the care of patients with diseases involving the central nervous system.

INTRACRANIAL TUMORS

Intracranial tumors occur most often in patients 40 years to 60 years of age with initial signs and symptoms reflecting increases in ICP. Seizures that appear in adult years suggest the presence of intracranial tumors. Eventually, the presence of intracranial tumors is confirmed by specific diagnostic tests, most often computed tomography.

Management of Anesthesia

Management of anesthesia for removal of intracranial tumors is designed to prevent undesirable changes in CBF or ICP.

Cerebral Blood Flow

Determinants of CBF include (1) $PaCO_2$, (2) PaO_2, (3) cerebral perfusion pressure and autoregulation, and (4) anesthetic drugs (Fig. 24-1). Cerebral blood vessels receive innervation from the autonomic nervous system but the impact on CBF seems to be minimal. The role of $CMRO_2$ is emphasized by reductions in CBF of about 7 percent for every degree Celsius reduction in body temperature below 37° Celsius.

$PaCO_2$. Changes in $PaCO_2$ produce corresponding directional changes in CBF. As a guide, CBF (normal 50 ml·100 g^{-1}·min^{-1}) increases or decreases 1 ml·100 g^{-1}·min^{-1} for every 1 mmHg increase or decrease of $PaCO_2$ from 40 mmHg. These changes in CBF reflect the impact of carbon dioxide mediated alterations in pH leading to dilation or constriction of cerebral arterioles. The ability of reductions in $PaCO_2$ to lower CBF and ICP is the basis of neuroanesthesia.

The influence of $PaCO_2$ on local CBF may be altered by acidosis that often surrounds intracranial tumors. For example, acid metabolites from tumors cause vasomotor paralysis in surrounding vessels, leading to maximal vasodilation and increased local blood flow (luxury perfusion). If $PaCO_2$ increases, normal vessels but not vessels surrounding tumors will dilate, and blood flow could be diverted to normal areas (intracranial

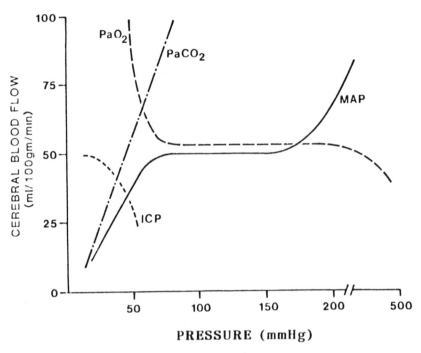

Fig. 24-1. Schematic depiction of the impact of ICP, PaO_2, $PaCO_2$, and mean arterial pressure (MAP) on cerebral blood flow.

steal syndrome). Conversely, hyperventilation of the lungs to lower $PaCO_2$ might constrict normal vessels, thus diverting blood flow to diseased or ischemic areas of the brain (reverse steal syn-

drome). The relative importance of these steal syndromes is not known.

PaO_2. Decreases in PaO_2 do not produce significant increases in CBF until a threshold value of about 50 mmHg is present.

Cerebral Perfusion Pressure and Autoregulation. Cerebral perfusion pressure is the difference between mean arterial pressure and right atrial pressure or ICP, whichever is greater. Nevertheless, CBF remains relatively constant between mean arterial pressures of 60 mmHg to 150 mmHg reflecting autoregulation. Below or above this range of autoregulation, CBF is directly related to mean arterial pressure. Chronic hypertension shifts the autoregulation curve to the right such that higher mean arterial pressures are tolerated before CBF becomes pressure dependent. Autoregulation of CBF is impaired in the presence of intracranial tumors or volatile anesthetics.

Anesthetic Drugs. Volatile anesthetics administered

Symptoms of Increased Intracranial Pressure

Nausea and vomiting

Hypertension

Bradycardia

Personality change

Altered levels of consciousness

Altered patterns of breathing

Papilledema

Seizures

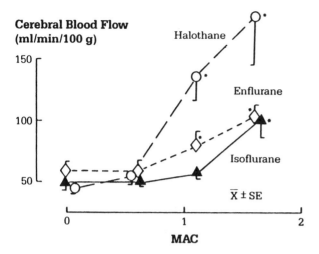

Fig. 24-2. Volatile anesthetics administered during normocapnia in concentrations above 0.6 MAC are potent cerebral vasodilators and produce dose-dependent increases in CBF. These drug-induced increases in cerebral blood flow are greatest with halothane, intermediate with enflurane, and least for isoflurane. (From Eger,[1] with permission.)

during normocapnia in concentrations above 0.6 MAC are potent cerebral vasodilators (halothane greater than enflurane greater than isoflurane) and produce dose-dependent increases in CBF (Fig. 24-2).[1] These increases in CBF occur despite concomitant reductions in $CMRO_2$ (greater with isoflurane than halothane). Nitrous oxide is a cerebral vasodilator, but limitation of its dose to usually less than 0.7 MAC seems to minimize associated increases in CBF. Ketamine is a potent cerebral vasodilator increasing CBF more than 60 percent despite normocapnia. Drug-induced cerebral vasodilation and associated increases in CBF predictably increases ICP in patients with intracranial tumors. In normal patients, compensatory mechanisms, including displacement of cerebrospinal fluid from the cranium, prevent increases in ICP. Opioids, benzodiazepines, and barbiturates are cerebral vasoconstrictors producing reductions in CBF and ICP.

Pressure-Volume Compliance Curves

Pressure-volume compliance curves reflect changes produced by expanding intracranial tumors (Fig. 24-3). Eventually, a point on the curve

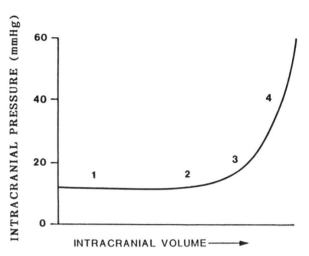

Fig. 24-3. The pressure-volume compliance curve depicts the impact of increasing intracranial volume on ICP. As volume increases from point 1 to point 2 on the curve, the ICP does not increase because cerebrospinal fluid is shifted from the cranium into the spinal subarachnoid space. Patients with intracranial tumors but between points 1 and points 2 on the compliance curve are unlikely to manifest clinical symptoms of increased ICP. Patients who are on the rising portion of the pressure-volume curve[3] can no longer compensate for increases in volume, and ICP begins to increase. Clinical symptoms of elevated ICP are likely. Additional elevations in volume at this point,[3] as produced by increased cerebral blood flow during anesthesia, can precipitate abrupt rises in pressure.[4]

is reached where even small increases in intracranial volume, as produced by drug-induced cerebral vasodilation and increased CBF, result in marked increases in ICP.

Intracranial Pressure

Marked increases in ICP can so reduce cerebral perfusion pressure that CBF is dangerously reduced (see Chapter 32). A normal ICP is below 15 mmHg. In patients with intracranial tumors, ICP is commonly monitored so as to recognize sudden and often unexpected increases in ICP and thus facilitate prompt and aggressive interventions to lower ICP. Methods to decrease ICP include (1) elevation of the head to encourage venous drainage; (2) hyperventilation of the lungs; (3) cerebrospinal fluid drainage; and (4) administration of drugs including osmotic diuretics, renal tubular diuretics, corticosteroids and barbiturates (see Chapter 32).

Preoperative Preparation

Evidence of increased ICP is sought during the preoperative visit. Preoperative medication that produces sedation or depression of ventilation is usually avoided. For example, drug-induced depression of ventilation can lead to increased $PaCO_2$ and subsequent elevations in CBF and ICP. Nevertheless, in otherwise alert patients, small doses of benzodiazepines may provide useful anxiety relief.

Induction of Anesthesia

Induction of anesthesia is achieved with intravenous administration of drugs (thiopental 3 $mg \cdot kg^{-1}$ to 6 $mg \cdot kg^{-1}$, or equivalent doses of etomidate or midazolam) that produce reliable onset of anesthesia and are unlikely to increase ICP. These drugs are followed by nondepolarizing muscle relaxants (vecuronium, atracurium, pancuronium) or succinylcholine (may produce transient increases in ICP) to facilitate mechanical ventilation of the lungs and to produce skeletal muscle relaxation for intubation of the trachea. Intubation of the trachea is performed when intense skeletal muscle paralysis is confirmed by a peripheral nerve stimulator. If paralysis is not intense, reaction to the tracheal tube (attempted coughing) may result in marked increases in ICP. Administration of additional intravenous doses of thiopental, opioids or lidocaine just before beginning direct laryngoscopy may be effective in attenuating increases in blood pressure and ICP that may accompany intubation of the trachea (Fig. 24-4).[2] After intubation of the trachea, the lungs are mechanically ventilated at a rate and tidal volume sufficient to maintain $PaCO_2$ 25 mmHg to 30 mmHg. There is no evidence of additional therapeutic benefit when $PaCO_2$ is reduced below this recommended range. Positive end-expiratory pressure is not encouraged as this could impair cerebral venous drainage and increase ICP.

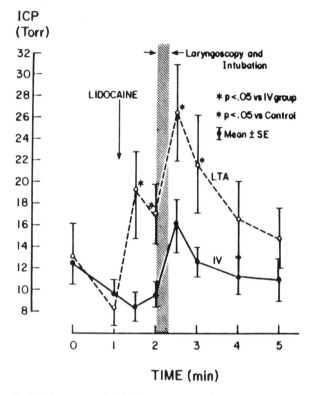

Fig. 24-4. Increases in ICP in response to laryngoscopy and intubation of the trachea are attenuated by administration of intravenous (IV) but not laryngotracheal (LTA) lidocaine. (From Hamill et al.,[2] with permission.)

Maintenance of Anesthesia

Maintenance of anesthesia is often with nitrous oxide plus opioids, benzodiazepines and/or barbiturates. Volatile anesthetics may be avoided because of their ability to increase CBF and to interfere with autoregulation. Nevertheless, low concentrations of volatile anesthetics (less than 0.6 MAC) may be useful for preventing or treating increases in blood pressure evoked by surgical stimulation. Minimal effects of isoflurane on CBF plus the acceptability of initiating hyperventilation of the lungs simultaneously with introduction of this drug (halothane should be preceded by hyperventilation of the lungs) make isoflurane a useful volatile anesthetic in patients undergoing intracranial operations. Peripheral vasodilating drugs (nitroprusside, nitroglycerin, trimethaphan) increase CBF and ICP despite simultaneous reductions in blood pressure. Therefore, use of these drugs before opening the dura is not encouraged in patients with increased ICP.

Skeletal muscle movement is hazardous during intracranial procedures as it can lead to increases in ICP, bleeding in the operative site and a brain that bulges into the operative site making surgical exposure difficult. Therefore, in addition to an adequate depth of anesthesia, it is common to maintain skeletal muscle paralysis during intracranial surgery.

Cerebral Swelling. If cerebral swelling occurs despite hyperventilation of the lungs, it may be useful to administer drugs designed to reduce brain water content. Mannitol, 0.25 $g \cdot kg^{-1}$ to 1 $g \cdot kg^{-1}$ or furosemide 0.5 $mg \cdot kg^{-1}$ to 1 $mg \cdot kg^{-1}$ administered intravenously are effective in reducing cerebral swelling and improving surgical exposure[3] (see Chapter 32). Intermittent intravenous injections of thiopental may also be useful in reducing ICP.

Fluid Therapy

Fluid infusions should be minimal (1 $ml \cdot kg^{-1} \cdot hr^{-1}$ to 3 $ml \cdot kg^{-1} \cdot hr^{-1}$) so as to avoid elevations in brain water content and increased ICP. Glucose and water solutions are not recommended as they are rapidly distributed throughout body water. If blood glucose concentrations decrease more rapidly than brain glucose concentrations, brain water becomes hyperosmolar such that water enters and cerebral edema results. Hypertonic salt solutions such as lactated Ringer's solution are recommended.

Monitors

Continuous monitoring of blood pressure via a catheter in a peripheral artery is recommended as is measurement of exhaled carbon dioxide concentrations. A continuous monitor of ICP is helpful but cannot be considered a routine monitor in every patient undergoing intracranial surgery. A bladder catheter is necessary if drug-induced diuresis is planned during the operation. The electrocardiogram allows prompt detection of cardiac dysrhythmias due to surgical stimulation of vital medullary centers. Neuromuscular blockade is monitored with a peripheral nerve stimulator. A central venous pressure catheter is useful for guiding fluid therapy and aspiration of air from the heart should venous air embolism occur during surgery (see the section *Venous Air Embolism*).

Awakening

On awakening from anesthesia, the patient must avoid coughing or straining, which will increase ICP. For this reason, it may be advisable to extubate the trachea with the patient still anesthetized. Also, prior administration of thiopental and/or lidocaine may further reduce the likelihood of coughing with extubation of the trachea. Delayed return of consciousness postoperatively or neurologic deterioration in the postoperative period is often evaluated with computed tomography. Tension pneumocephalus as a cause for neurologic deterioration is a consideration if nitrous oxide was administered during anesthesia.

Venous Air Embolism

Patients undergoing surgery for resection of intracranial tumors are at increased risk for venous air embolism, not only because the operative site is often above the level of the heart, but also because veins in the cut edge of bone constituting the skull may not collapse when transected. Presumably, air enters the right ventricle, leading to interference with blood flow into the pulmonary artery. Pulmonary edema and reflex bronchoconstriction may result from movement of air into the pulmonary circulation. Death is usually due to cardiovascular collapse and arterial hypoxemia. Air may reach the coronary and cerebral circulations (paradoxical air embolism) by crossing a patent foramen ovale (probe patent foramen ovale is present in up to 25 percent of adults) or traversing the pulmonary circulation.

Detection. A Doppler transducer placed over the right heart (over the second or third intercostal spaces to the right of the sternum) is the most sensitive indicator of intracardiac air.[4] Sudden decreases in end-exhaled concentrations of carbon dioxide reflect increased dead space due to continued ventilation of alveoli no longer perfused because of obstruction of their vascular supply by air. An increase in end-tidal nitrogen concentrations as observed during continuous mass spectrometry monitoring may reflect nitrogen from venous air embolism. During controlled ventilation of the lungs, sudden attempts (gasps) by patients to initiate spontaneous breaths may be the first indication of the occurrence of venous air embolism. Hypotension, tachycardia, cardiac dysrhythmias, cyanosis, and "mill-wheel" murmur are late signs of venous air embolism.

Treatment. Treatment of venous air embolism is by (1) aspiration of air through a right atrial catheter, and (2) irrigation of the operative site with fluid and by applying occlusive material to all bone edges so as to occlude sites of venous air entry. A right atrial catheter with the tip positioned at the junction of the superior vena cava with the right atrium seems to provide the most rapid aspiration of air.[5] A pulmonary artery catheter, because of its small lumen size and slow speed of blood return, is not uniquely useful for aspirating air but may provide additional evidence that venous air embolism has occurred by virtue to increases in pulmonary artery pressure. Nitrous oxide is immediately discontinued to avoid increasing the size of venous air bubbles. Despite the logic of positive end-expiratory pressure to reduce entrainment of air, the efficacy of this maneuver has not been confirmed. Furthermore, positive end-expiratory pressure could reverse the interatrial pressure gradient and predispose to passage of air across a patent foramen ovale. Cardiovascular collapse may require treatment with positive inotropes (see Chapter 3).

CAROTID ENDARTERECTOMY

Carotid endarterectomy is the most commonly performed surgical procedure for treatment of patients with histories of transient ischemic attacks or an occlusive lesion of greater than 80 percent in the carotid artery. The goal during management of anesthesia for carotid endarterectomy surgery is to maintain cerebral perfusion pressure and CBF. The critical period during surgery is cross-clamping of the diseased carotid artery when the patient is dependent on collateral circulation for perfusion of the ipsilateral brain. Rather than rely on collateral circulation, some surgeons routinely place an intraluminal shunt across the surgically clamped carotid artery. Alternatively, a shunt may be placed only when monitors (electroencephalogram, somatosensory evoked potentials, stump pressure) suggest the likelihood of cerebral ischemia (see Chapter 16). Stump pressure is the pressure in the carotid artery distal to the surgical clamp. Therefore, stump pressure reflects transmitted pressure via the circle of Willis and implies adequate (above 60 mmHg) or inadequate collateral circulation (Fig. 24-5).[6] It must be appreciated that variations in cerebral vascular resistance (increased by barbiturates and decreased by volatile drugs) influence interpretation of stump pressure.

Choice of Anesthesia

Anesthesia for carotid endarterectomy surgery can be performed with local or general anesthesia. Choice of local or general anesthesia has not been confirmed to alter morbidity or mortality after this operation.

Local Anesthesia

Local anesthesia includes a cervical plexus block combined with regional infiltration of local anesthetic (see Chapter 14). This approach provides the advantage of being able to monitor cerebral function of the patient by voice contact when the carotid artery is occluded. Nevertheless, strokes still can occur postoperatively despite the apparent maintenance of normal cerebral function intraoperatively.

General Anesthesia

General anesthesia is acceptably produced by intravenous injection of barbiturates, benzodiazepines, or etomidate followed by administration of nitrous oxide plus volatile drugs or opioids for maintenance of anesthesia. Skeletal muscle paralysis is often produced to allow reductions in the depth of anesthesia in response to hypotension without introducing the possibility of unwanted patient movement. Although differences among volatile anesthetics as regards neurologic outcome after carotid endarterectomy surgery are not detectable, it seems likely that isoflurane offers some

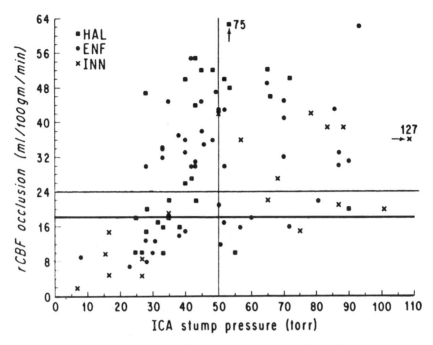

Fig. 24-5. Stump pressures in the internal carotid artery (ICA) above 60 mmHg (torr) are associated with regional cerebral blood flows (rCBF) greater than 18 ml·100 g^{-1}·min^{-1} in the majority of patients anesthetized with nitrous oxide plus halothane (HAL), enflurane (ENF), or Innovar (INN). (From McKay et al.,[6] with permission.)

brain protection if volatile anesthetics are selected for maintenance of anesthesia (Fig. 24-6).[7] Nevertheless, thiopental remains the appropriate drug to select in specific circumstances where pharmacologic brain protection is indicated. In this regard, it may be reasonable to administer thiopental (3 mg·kg^{-1} to 6 mg·kg^{-1}) immediately before clamping the carotid artery. Despite this practice, no data show that barbiturates used in this manner reduce morbidity after carotid endarterectomy.[8]

Regardless of the drugs selected for anesthesia, the goal must be to maintain arterial blood pressure in a normal range for that patient. When reductions in blood pressure below the normal range do not respond to decreases in concentrations of anesthetic drugs, it may be necessary to return blood pressure to a normal level by continuous infusions of sympathomimetics such as phenylephrine. Sustained elevations of blood pressure above normal levels are undesirable as hypertension may contribute to cerebral edema, particularly in dis-

eased areas of the brain with altered ability to autoregulate cerebral blood flow. Furthermore, hypertension increases myocardial oxygen requirements and may contribute to myocardial ischemia in patients with coronary artery disease.

Ventilation of the lungs during carotid endarterectomy surgery is with a tidal volume and respiratory rate that maintains $PaCO_2$ near 35 mmHg. Manipulation of $PaCO_2$ in attempts to alter CBF by vasodilation or vasoconstriction is not recommended (see the section *Cerebral Blood Flow*).

Postoperative Problems

Postoperative problems after carotid endarterectomy surgery include (1) lability of blood pressure, (2) airway compression due to hematoma formation at the operative site, (3) loss of carotid body function, (4) myocardial infarction, and (5) stroke.[8] Hypertension occurs commonly, especially in previously hypertensive patients, and may require

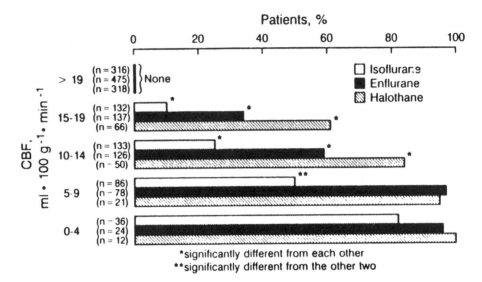

Fig. 24-6. Patients (percent) developing evidence of cerebral ischemia on the electroencephalogram (EEG) at different CBFs during inhalation of three difference anesthetics. Critical CBF (the CBF below which the majority of patients develop EEG signs of ischemia within 3 minutes of carotid occlusion) is lowest with isoflurane (implies brain protection), intermediate with enflurane, and highest during inhalation of halothane. (From Michenfelder et al.,[7] with permission.)

treatment with peripheral vasodilators such as nitroprusside. The mechanism for hypertension is not known but may reflect altered activity of the carotid sinus or loss of carotid sinus function due to denervation at the time of surgery. Likewise, hypotension may be due to increased nerve activity perceived by a carotid sinus previously shielded by an atheromatous plaque. Unilateral loss of carotid body function is not likely to alter the patient's ventilatory response to hypoxemia.

INTRACRANIAL ANEURYSMS

Intracranial aneurysms that rupture are the most common cause of intracranial hemorrhage. Cerebral vasospasm that frequently accompanies rupture of these aneurysms may be reduced by treatment with nimodipine, a calcium channel blocker.

Management of Anesthesia

Management of anesthesia for resection of intracranial aneurysms is designed to (1) prevent elevations in blood pressure and (2) facilitate surgical

exposure and control of the aneurysm. Preoperative medication is desirable to reduce anxiety but must be titrated to prevent hypoventilation and associated increases in CBF. Induction of anesthesia and maintenance of anesthesia must be designed to minimize blood pressure elevations evoked by noxious stimulation, especially during direct laryngoscopy for intubation of the trachea.

Controlled Hypotension

Surgical exposure and control of intracranial aneurysms are facilitated by production of controlled hypotension. The duration of controlled hypotension may be brief, corresponding to isolation and clamping of the aneurysm. In the presence of adequate anesthesia, as provided by volatile anesthetics, the addition of a continuous infusion of nitroprusside (seldom greater than 3 $\mu g \cdot kg^{-1} \cdot min^{-1}$) is usually adequate to lower blood pressure to the desired hypotensive level. The hypotensive effect of nitroprusside is easily reversed by slowing or discontinuing the drug infusion. Nitroprusside is converted to cyanide, and arterial pH should be monitored to detect metabolic acidosis due to cyanide toxicity when high doses of nitroprusside (greater than 8 $\mu g \cdot kg^{-1} \cdot min^{-1}$) are required for longer than 1 hour to 3 hours. Alternative drugs to nitroprusside are nitroglycerin, trimethaphan, and labetalol. Compensatory tachycardia may offset the blood pressure lowering effects of vasodilators used to produce controlled hypotension. Beta antagonists, such as propranolol or esmolol, are useful for slowing this reflex mediated tachycardia. Oxygenation should be monitored during controlled hypotension as peripheral vasodilators may accentuate mismatching of ventilation to perfusion.

As a guideline, mean arterial pressure can be reduced to about 50 mmHg in previously normotensive patients. It should also be appreciated that patients will safely tolerate even lower pressures for short periods of time as may be needed to place a clip on an intracranial aneurysm. The need to monitor blood pressure accurately requires attention to calibration of the transducer used to measure blood pressure and recognition that proper positioning of the height of the transducer relative to heart level is crucial. For example, cerebral perfusion pressure decreases about 0.7 mmHg for every centimeter that the head is above heart level. Therefore, if the head is elevated 20 cm above heart level, cerebral perfusion pressure will be about 14 mmHg less than mean arterial pressure at heart level. In this regard, a useful approach is to place the transducer at brain level (external auditory canal reflects level of circle of Willis) when controlled hypotension is planned and the head is elevated.

SPINAL CORD TRANSECTION

Spinal cord transection is the damage to the spinal cord that manifests as paralysis of the lower extremities (paraplegia) or all the extremities (quadriplegia). Anatomically, the spinal cord is not divided, but the effect physiologically is the same as if it were transected. The most common cause of spinal cord transection is trauma.

Patients with acute spinal cord transection who require surgery present unique problems during the management of anesthesia. For example, further damage to the spinal cord could result from extension of the head in the presence of a cervical fracture. The absence of sympathetic nervous system activity below the level of spinal cord transection makes these patients vulnerable to hypotension, particularly in response to acute changes in body posture, blood loss, or introduction of positive airway pressure. Hypothermia is a hazard, as these patients tend to become poikilothermic below the spinal cord transection. Breathing is best managed by mechanical ventilation of the lungs because abdominal and intercostal muscle paralysis, combined with general anesthesia, makes maintenance of adequate spontaneous ventilation unlikely. Succinylcholine must not be administered, since drug-induced hyperkalemia is a hazard (see Chapter 8). Minimal concentrations of anesthetics are required, as patients are often anesthetic in the operative area.

The most important goal during management of anesthesia for patients with chronic transection of the spinal cord is prevention of autonomic hyperreflexia. Autonomic hyperreflexia manifests as abrupt arterial hypertension with an associated compensatory bradycardia due to activation of the carotid sinus (Fig. 24-7). Spinal cord transection above T6 is most likely to be associated with autonomic hyperreflexia with up to 85 percent of patients manifesting this response. Autonomic hyperreflexia is initiated by cutaneous or visceral stimulation below the level of the spinal cord transection. Distension of a hollow viscus, such as the bladder, during cystoscopy is a common initiating event. Stimulation elicits reflex sympathetic activity and vasoconstriction below the level of the spinal cord transection resulting in hypertension. Vasoconstriction and hypertension persist because vasodilatory impulses from the central nervous system cannot traverse the spinal cord to reach the area below the cord transection. Spinal anesthesia is particularly effective in preventing autonomic hyperreflexia. General anesthesia with volatile drugs or epidural block are also effective but less so than a spinal block. Treatment of hypertension with nitroprusside is necessary if autonomic hyperreflexia occurs despite preventive steps.

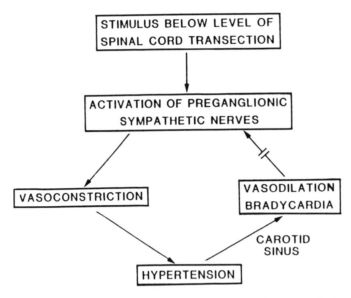

Fig. 24-7. Sequence of events associated with clinical manifestations of autonomic hyperreflexia. Impulses that produce vasodilation cannot reach the neurologically isolated portion of the spinal cord such that vasoconstriction and hypertension persist.

NEURORADIOLOGY

General anesthesia in the neuroradiology area is often fraught with difficulties because the radiology suite has not been designed with anesthesia function in mind. This makes it essential that careful preparation be taken and appropriate anesthetic apparatus and monitoring equipment be available. Other problems may include anesthetizing patients who are comatose from an unknown etiology. The darkened environment of the radiology suite makes it difficult to assess color, ventilation of the lungs, and even to read the dials on the anesthesia machine. Maintenance of the airway may be complicated by numerous changes in position of the patient and poor access to the head. Finally, these procedures are often long and performed in a poorly ventilated room, leading the anesthesiologists to experience fatigue, boredom, and exposure to trace anesthetics.

Because contrast media are often injected into arteries, veins, or cerebrospinal fluid, allergic and toxic reactions can occur. When a history of a previous reaction to iodine compounds is present,

corticosteroids, diphenhydramine, and possibly H_2-receptor antagonists should be administered before the procedure.

Pneumoencephalography is performed by the slow, incremental injections of air or oxygen into the lumbar subarachnoid space with the patient in the sitting position. When general anesthesia is required, a number of problems result. Due to the high solubility of nitrous oxide in blood, relative to nitrogen, it will rapidly equilibrate into an air-filled ventricle, thereby adding to the intracranial volume, with a resulting increase in intracranial pressure (see Chapter 2). Probably, nitrous oxide should not be used for air encephalography. Because the intraventricular air may last as long as 7 days after the procedure, its presence should be ruled out by a skull radiograph before the subsequent anesthetic administration of nitrous oxide.

REFERENCES

1. Eger EI II, Isoflurane (Forane). A compendium and reference. Anaquest, a division of BOC, Inc., Madison, WI, 1986;1–160.

2. Hamill JF, Bedford RF, Weave DC, Colohan AR. Lidocaine before endotracheal intubation: Intravenous or laryngotracheal? Anesthesiology 1981;55:578–81.

3. Cottrell JE, Robustelli A, Post K, Turndorf H. Furosemide- and mannitol-induced changes in intracranial pressure and serum osmolality and electrolytes. Anesthesiology 1977;47:28–30.

4. English JB, Westenskow D, Hodges MR, Stanley TH. Comparison of venous air embolism monitoring methods in supine dogs. Anesthesiology 1978;48:425–9.

5. Bunegin L, Albin MS, Helsel PE, Hoffman A, Hung T-K. Positioning the right atrial catheter: A model for reappraisal. Anesthesiology 1981;55:343–8.

6. McKay RD, Sundt TM, Michenfelder JD, et al. Internal carotid artery stump pressure and cerebral blood flow during carotid endarterectomy: Modification by halothane, enflurane and Innovar. Anesthesiology 1976;45:390–9.

7. Michenfelder JD, Sundt TM, Fode N, Sharbrough FW. Isoflurane when compared to enflurane and halothane decreases the frequency of cerebral ischemia during carotid endarterectomy. Anesthesiology 1987;67:336–40.

8. Keats AS. Anesthesia for carotid endarterectomy. Cleve Clin 1981;48:68–71.

Chapter 25

Ophthalmology and Otolaryngology

Anesthesia for surgery related to ophthalmology or otolaryngology requires an appreciation of the anatomy and physiology of structures present in the operative area, as well as the unique requirements of specific operative procedures. Most of the operative procedures are elective and often the patients represent extremes of age, being very young or elderly.

OPHTHALMOLOGY

Management of anesthesia for patients undergoing ophthalmic surgery requires an understanding of factors that influence intraocular pressure (IOP), a consideration of adverse drug interactions between ophthalmic drugs and drugs administered perioperatively, and an appreciation of the oculocardiac reflex.

Intraocular Pressure

Normal IOP is between 10 mmHg and 22 mmHg, reflecting the balance between aqueous humor formation in the ciliary body and its elimination via the canal of Schlemm. The greatest increase in IOP (as much as 35 mmHg to 50 mmHg) occurs when venous pressure is acutely elevated as during vomiting or coughing. Direct laryngoscopy for intubation of the trachea can increase IOP even in the absence of coughing or hypertension.[1] Nevertheless, an increase in IOP is most likely when coughing accompanies intubation of the trachea. Overhydration leading to elevated venous pressure may increase IOP. Succinylcholine increases IOP an average of 6 mmHg to 8 mmHg, with a return to predrug levels within 5 minutes to 7 minutes.[2] This ocular hypertensive response occurs whether succinylcholine is given as a single intravenous injection, as a continuous infusion, or intramuscularly. In contrast to intravenous administration of succinylcholine, it appears that intramuscular injection of succinylcholine results in a longer duration of increased IOP, necessitating at least a 15-minute wait before the globe is opened. Prolonged tonic contraction of the extraocular muscles produced by succinylcholine is the most likely mechanism for the increase in IOP. Administration of nonparalyzing doses of nondepolarizing muscle relaxants (pretreatment) before the injection of succinylcholine probably attenuates but does not reliably prevent this drug-induced increase in IOP.[3] Conversely, paralyzing doses of nondepolarizing muscle relaxants in the absence of succinylcholine reduce IOP, presumably via their relaxant effects on the extraocular muscles. Inhaled anesthetics are alleged to produce dose-dependent reductions in IOP. Barbiturates, benzodiazepines, and opioids, tend to lower IOP. The effect of ketamine on IOP is controversial, but even if it lowers IOP its use may be considered objectionable for ophthalmic anesthesia for other reasons such as blepharospasm and nystagmus. Changes in arterial blood pressure or the $PaCO_2$ within a normal physiologic range have minimal effect on IOP.

Carbonic anhydrase inhibitors (acetazolamide) and osmotic diuretics (mannitol, urea, glycerin) are used in the perioperative period to acutely reduce IOP. Acetazolamide lowers IOP by interfering with the secretion of aqueous humor. Glycerin is effective orally but introduces the hazard of an increased gastric fluid volume in the perioperative period.

Adverse Drug Interactions

Ophthalmic medications applied topically to the cornea may undergo sufficient absorption to produce systemic effects. Unexpected drug interactions during and after surgery may reflect systemic effects of these drugs. For example, topical application of a beta antagonist, timolol, to treat glaucoma has been associated with bradycardia and bronchospasm.[4] Timolol has been implicated in the exacerbation of myasthenia gravis and the production of postoperative apnea in neonates.[5] Rarely, a long-acting anticholinesterase, echothiophate, is used to treat glaucoma. Systemic absorption of this drug reduces cholinesterase activity, resulting in marked prolongation of the duration of action of succinylcholine should usual doses of this muscle relaxant be administered. At least 3 weeks is required after cessation of echothiophate therapy for cholinesterase activity to return to 50 percent of predrug levels. Topical application of phenylephrine to produce capillary decongestion and mydriasis can result in hypertension if systemic absorption is sufficient. A 2.5 percent phenylephrine solution will minimize the adverse effects should systemic absorption occur. Cyclopentolate is a popular mydriatic that may produce central nervous system toxicity, manifesting as dysarthria, disorientation, and psychotic reactions. Epinephrine applied topically to the cornea to produce mydriasis introduces the possibility of systemic absorption and potential sensitization of the heart in the presence of halothane. Nevertheless, systemic absorption of epinephrine seems to be minimal. Chronic treatment with acetazolamide can be associated with renal loss of bicarbonate ions and potassium, leading to metabolic acidosis with hypokalemia.

Oculocardiac Reflex

The oculocardiac reflex consists of a trigeminal-vagal reflex arc that is characterized by a 10 percent to 50 percent reduction in heart rate. Pressure on the globe and surgical traction (stretch) of extraocular muscles, particularly the medial rectus muscle, are the most likely stimuli to elicit this reflex. Hypercarbia or arterial hypoxemia may also increase the incidence and severity of this reflex. In addition to bradycardia, other manifestations of this reflex include junctional rhythm and premature ventricular contractions. Cardiac arrest has been attributed to the oculocardiac reflex, but the evidence to support this is not convincing. Indeed, the importance of this reflex is controversial, with the most important principle being continuous monitoring of the electrocardiogram so as to detect the appearance of bradycardia or cardiac dysrhythmias. Removal of the surgical stimulus is usually sufficient treatment. Furthermore, this reflex tends to fatigue such that the subsequent stimulation is likely to elicit the same response. Premedication with intramuscular injection of atropine is of little or no value in preventing this reflex. Prophylactic use of atropine administered intravenously, however, may be justified in pediatric patients having strabismus correction because of the more active vagal reflexes in children. Should bradycardia persist after removal of the surgical stimulus, the appropriate treatment is the intravenous administration of atropine, 3 to 6 $\mu g \cdot kg^{-1}$.

Management of Anesthesia

Management of anesthesia for ophthalmic surgery requires maintenance of an unchanging IOP, early recognition of the oculocardiac reflex, the presence of a motionless eye (akinesia), and recovery from anesthesia that is not associated with reaction to the tracheal tube, nausea, or vomiting. Intubation of the trachea to assure control of the airway is necessary because of the proximity of the surgical field and draping. Co-existing disease may influence the management of anesthesia independent of the ophthalmic surgery. For example, elderly patients requiring ophthalmic surgery often have associated illnesses such as diabetes mellitus, coronary artery disease, essential hypertension, or chronic obstructive airways disease. Finally, selection of drugs used for anesthesia must consider potential adverse interactions with medications being used to treat ocular disease, particularly glaucoma.

During operations in which the globe is not opened, there can be more flexibility in surgical conditions, but for intraocular procedures, perfection is required. For example, when the globe is open any uncontrolled elevation of IOP can lead to an extrusion of ocular contents and permanent damage. Certainly, the intraoperative use of succinylcholine should be avoided while the eye is open or in patients who have undergone recent eye surgery. Otherwise, increases in IOP produced by succinylcholine are transient, allowing this drug to be safely administered to most patients undergoing ophthalmic surgery.

Available data have not demonstrated a significant difference in ocular morbidity between local and general anesthesia. Nevertheless, an impressive record of safety is associated with local anesthesia for ophthalmic surgery in patients with heart disease. Retrobulbar block provides local anesthesia and akinesia of the globe. Akinesia of the eyelids, if needed, is obtained by blocking the branches of the facial nerve supplying the obicularis muscle. Complications associated with retrobulbar block include elicitation of the oculocardiac reflex, hemorrhage, and local anesthetic toxicity due to accidental intravascular injection of the drug. Accidental brain stem anesthesia after retrobulbar block manifests as unconsciousness and apnea.[6] Intravenous administration of barbiturates, such as methohexital 10 mg to 30 mg, is often recommended just before performance of the retrobulbar block so as to optimize patient comfort. When local anesthesia is selected, the ophthalmologist is responsible for the management of the patient, although the anesthesiologist may be asked to monitor the patient receiving a local anesthetic (monitored anesthesia care).

When general anesthesia is selected, it is mandatory that the patient avoid coughing during intubation of the trachea, as any elevation in venous pressure will increase IOP. Short duration laryngoscopy in the presence of adequate anesthesia and skeletal muscle relaxation plus the use of topical tracheal lidocaine or intravenous lidocaine are helpful for assuring minimal changes in IOP in response to intubation of the trachea. Likewise, emergence from anesthesia should not be associated with any reaction to the tracheal tube. Maintenance of anesthesia with volatile drugs with or without nitrous oxide is ideal to provide an adequate depth of anesthesia plus rapid awakening and a low incidence of postoperative nausea and vomiting. Nitrous oxide must be used with caution if an intravitreal injection of sulfa hexafluoride is planned (see the section *Retinal Detachment Surgery*). The eye is a highly innervated, pain-sensitive organ and ophthalmic surgery requires surgical levels of anesthesia. Monitoring the electrocardiogram is essential for early recognition of the oculocardiac reflex. Administration of non-depolarizing muscle relaxants to maintain nearly complete suppression of the twitch response elicited by a peripheral nerve stimulator may be used to prevent unexpected patient movement. Large doses of atropine used in conjunction with anticholinesterases to reverse neuromuscular blockade do not alter IOP. Intravenous administration of antiemetics, such as droperidol, near the end of general anesthesia in an attempt to minimize the incidence of postoperative nausea and vomiting may be indicated. This may be more important if opioids have been included in the preoperative medication. Indeed, a surgical repair may be jeopardized by acute elevations in IOP produced by vomiting. Passage of an orogastric tube to decompress the stomach before awakening from anesthesia may also be helpful in reducing the incidence of postoperative vomiting. A catheter placed in the bladder may be indicated if an osmotic diuretic is administered to lower IOP.

Strabismus Surgery

Strabismus surgery is the most common pediatric ocular operation performed. Special considerations in the management of anesthesia for strabismus surgery include the (1) questionable use of succinylcholine, (2) increased incidence of the oculocardia reflex, (3) increased incidence of postoperative nausea and vomiting, and (4) possible susceptibility to malignant hyperthermia. For example, succinylcholine may produce sustained contraction of the extraocular muscles, making interpretation of the forced duction test unreliable for 20 minutes to 30 minutes.[7] Intravenous administration of atropine (7 $\mu g \cdot kg^{-1}$) or local infiltration of the extraocular muscle with lidocaine may be useful in preventing or treating the oculocardiac reflex. Prophylactic intravenous administration of droperidol reduces but does not eliminate the incidence of postoperative vomiting after strabismus surgery.[8] Malignant hyperthermia has been reported in patients undergoing strabismus surgery, suggesting a possible generalized skeletal muscle system disturbance in these patients.

Glaucoma

Special considerations in the management of anesthesia for the patient with glaucoma include (1) maintenance of drug-induced miosis throughout the perioperative period, (2) avoidance of venous congestion, and (3) awareness of potential adverse interactions between drugs used to treat glaucoma and those administered during anesthesia (see the section *Adverse Drug Interactions*). Continuation of the application of topical miotic eye drops on the morning of surgery is appropriate. Inclusion of anticholinergics in the preoperative medication is acceptable because the amount of drug reaching the eye is too small to dilate the pupil. For example, an estimated 0.0001 mg of atropine is absorbed by the eye after parenteral administration of 0.4 mg as preoperative medication. Nevertheless, scopolamine has a greater mydriatic effect than atropine, suggesting the need for caution in consideration of its administration to patients with glaucoma.[9] Likewise, the use of anticholinergics in combination with anticholinesterases to reverse nondepolarizing muscle relaxants is safe because only small amounts of drug reach the eye. The implications of transient elevations in IOP produced when succinylcholine is administered to patients with glaucoma are not known. Presumably, patients with adequate medical control of glaucoma are not jeopardized by this transient drug-induced elevation in IOP. Finally, prolonged

hypotension may predispose to retinal artery thrombosis in these patients.

Cataract Extraction

Special considerations in the management of anesthesia for cataract extraction include the (1) likely presence of co-existing diseases in elderly patients, (2) need for absolute immobility during the operative procedure, and (3) steps to minimize the occurrence of postoperative nausea and vomiting. Sudden movement or attempts to cough when the globe is open can result in extrusion of ocular contents and permanent damage. For these reasons, when general anesthesia is selected for cataract surgery, it is essential to maintain an adequate depth of anesthesia. In addition, skeletal muscle paralysis is often included to minimize the chance of sudden unexpected patient movement. Succinylcholine, to facilitate intubation of the trachea, is acceptable because IOP has returned to normal by the time surgery begins. Modest hyperventilation of the lungs to produce hypocarbia and a 10 degree to 15 degree head-up tilt to promote venous drainage will likely reduce intraocular pressure during intraocular surgery. Steps to reduce the likelihood of postoperative nausea and vomiting may include avoidance of opioids in the preoperative medication and/or intravenous administration of an antiemetic, such as droperidol, near the end of surgery.

Retinal Detachment Surgery

Retinal detachment surgery requires reduction of IOP as often provided by intravenous administration of acetazolamide or mannitol. Rotation of the globe with traction on the extraocular muscles may elicit the oculocardiac reflex. Nitrous oxide must be used with caution when an intravitreal injection of air and sulfur hexafluoride is performed to compensate for loss of vitreous volume during surgery. Sulfur hexafluoride is included with air because the low water solubility of this gas ensures persistence of the intraocular bubble for several days postoperatively. Nitrous oxide, which is 34 times more soluble than nitrogen, can diffuse into the intraocular bubble more rapidly than nitrogen can leave, resulting in an enlargement of the bubble and increased IOP.[10] This increased IOP may be sufficient to compromise retinal blood flow, particularly if systemic blood pressure is reduced. When nitrous oxide is discontinued, IOP falls to below awake levels, which presumably reflects loss of aqueous humor while the IOP was elevated. This rapid fall in IOP may jeopardize the surgical repair, as for a retinal detachment. For these reasons, it may be prudent to discontinue the inhalation of nitrous oxide about 15 minutes before the creation of an intraocular bubble. Furthermore, nitrous oxide should be avoided for up to 10 days after intravitreal injection of sulfur hexafluoride.[10]

Special anesthetic considerations are introduced when the laser is used for repair of retinal detachment and treatment of diabetic retinopathy (see the section *Laser Surgery*).

Open Eye Injury

Special considerations in the management of anesthesia for open eye injury include the (1) possibility of recent ingestion of food, and the (2) need to avoid even minimal increases in IOP if the injured eye is considered salvageable. Therefore, rapid intubation of the trachea facilitated by succinylcholine must be balanced against the possible hazards of elevations in IOP. Nevertheless, administration of succinylcholine (preceded by d-tubocurarine 3 mg to 6 mg or gallamine 10 mg to 15 mg to prevent fasiculations) to patients with open eye injuries has not been associated with vitreous loss.[11] Despite this evidence, many anesthesiologists would not use succinylcholine for induction of anesthesia in patients with open eye injuries. An awake intubation of the trachea, although attractive from the standpoint of airway protection, would be unacceptable because patient reaction to placement of the tube in the trachea would elevate IOP. An alternative to the administration of succinylcholine is the injection of an intubating dose of nondepolarizing muscle relaxants. The disadvantage of this approach is a prolonged duration of skeletal muscle paralysis for what may be a short operation. Regardless of the muscle relaxant selection, it is mandatory to confirm the presence of skeletal muscle paralysis by the use of a peripheral nerve stimulator before initiating direct laryngoscopy for intubation of the trachea. Prema-

ture placement of the tube in the trachea will provoke a cough response and defeat all the prior attempts to minimize the occurrence of vomiting or elevations in IOP.

Corneal Abrasion

Corneal abrasion is the most common ocular complication associated with general anesthesia. Abrasions typically occur in the inferior one-third of the cornea corresponding to the area exposed when the eyes are not mechanically closed. Reduction in tear production by general anesthetics plus the loss of protective eyelid closure renders patients susceptible to corneal abrasions during anesthesia. For these reasons, ophthalmic ointment is often applied to the cornea after induction of anesthesia. Disadvantages of ointments include occasional allergic reactions; flammability, which may make their use undesirable during surgery around the face; and blurred vision in the early postoperative period.[12] Alternatively, mechanical closure of the eyelids by gentle application of adhesive strips protects the cornea and avoids the disadvantages of ophthalmic ointment.

The patient who sustains a corneal abrasion will complain of the sensation of a foreign body, tearing, photophobia, and pain. When a corneal abrasion is suspected, it is desirable to obtain an ophthalmology consultation while the patient is still in the recovery room. After gross examination, a local anesthetic should be instilled and the eye examined with fluorescein to demonstrate the injured area. Corneal abrasions are usually treated by patching the injured eye and applying a prophylactic antibiotic ointment such as erythromycin. Repeated instillation of local anesthetics to control pain is not recommended as these drugs inhibit corneal healing. Healing normally occurs within 48 hours.

OTOLARYNGOLOGY

Optimal management of anesthesia for otolaryngologic surgery is based on reliable control of the upper airway. These patients may present with compromised airways before surgery because of edema, infection, or tumor invasion of the upper airway. After intubation of the trachea, monitoring with a precordial or esophageal stethoscope is essential because the anesthesiologist is often situated away from direct access to the airway. Pulse oximetry is useful for early detection of decreases in arterial oxygen saturation; and monitoring the electrocardiogram is necessary to detect cardiac dysrhythmias that frequently accompany surgical manipulation in the larynx, pharynx, and neck. Blood loss during major otolaryngologic surgery can be substantial and is often underestimated due to hidden losses onto drapes or into the patient's stomach. Extubation of the trachea may be hazardous after otolaryngologic surgery, especially when the airway is compromised, as due to edema or bleeding after endoscopy or upper airway surgery.

Ear Surgery

Special considerations in the management of anesthesia for ear surgery include (1) facial nerve preservation, (2) the use of epinephrine by the surgeon, and (3) the effect of nitrous oxide on middle ear pressure.

Facial Nerve Preservation

Surgical identification and preservation of the facial nerve is essential during ear surgery and many other otolaryngologic operations. This requirement necessitates maintenance of some skeletal muscle activity if muscle relaxants are administered. Ideally, the twitch response produced by stimulation of the ulnar nerve using a peripheral nerve stimulator should remain 10 percent to 20 percent of control when muscle relaxants are administered. A volatile anesthetic is useful because muscle relaxants to prevent unexpected patient movement are not routinely required, thus preserving the ability to easily identify the facial nerve by virtue of skeletal muscle responses to electrical stimulation of tissue presumed to be nerve. Furthermore, if nitrous oxide must be discontinued, the patient remains adequately anesthetized by increasing the inhaled concentration of the volatile anesthetic. Another advantage of volatile anesthetics is the ability to maintain systolic blood pressure between 80 mmHg to 85 mmHg

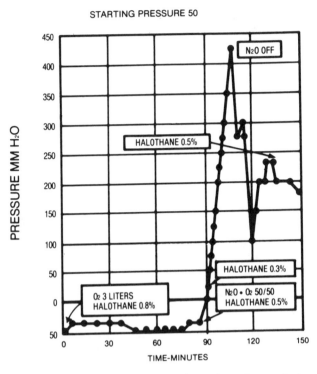

Fig. 25-1. Measurements in a single patient demonstrate an abrupt increase in middle ear pressure (mm H_2O) when nitrous oxide is added to the inhaled gases. (From Patterson, and Bartlett,[13] with permission.)

so as to minimize intraoperative blood loss if this is deemed important for the success of the surgery.

Use of Epinephrine

Epinephrine is often infiltrated in the operative area by the surgeon to produce vasoconstriction and thus decrease blood loss. Halothane is more likely than enflurane or isoflurane to evoke cardiac dysrhythmias in the presence of exogenous epinephrine.

Nitrous Oxide and Middle Ear Pressure

Nitrous oxide, which is 34 times more soluble than nitrogen, enters air-filled cavities such as the middle ear more rapidly than air can leave, resulting in an elevation of middle ear pressures (Fig. 25-1).[13] Under normal conditions, any pressure elevation in the middle ear is passively vented via the eustachian tube into the nasopharynx. Narrowing of the eustachian tube by acute inflammation or the presence of scar tissue, as is likely after an adenoidectomy, impairs the ability of the middle ear to vent passively any pressure increases produced by nitrous oxide. Tympanic membrane rupture, manifesting as bright red blood in the external auditory canal, has been attributed to pressure increases produced by nitrous oxide.[14] Disruption of previous middle ear reconstructive surgery has been reported when nitrous oxide is administered at a later date for operative procedures not involving the ear.[15] During tympanoplasty surgery, the effect of nitrous oxide on middle ear pressures may cause displacement of the tympanic membrane graft. Therefore, inhaled nitrous oxide concentrations should be limited to 50 percent, with discontinuance at least 5 minutes before placement of the graft. The speculation that postoperative nausea and vomiting could be due to increased middle ear pressures that persists after the administration of nitrous oxide remains unproven.

Rapid absorption of nitrous oxide when administration of this gas is discontinued can produce negative pressures in the middle ear, manifesting as serous otitis or transient postoperative hearing loss (Fig. 25-2).[13]

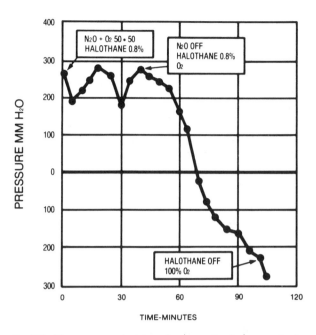

Fig. 25-2. Measurements in a single patient demonstrate an abrupt decrease in middle ear pressures (mm H_2O) to below normal when inhalation of nitrous oxide is discontinued. (From Patterson and Bartlett,[13] with permission.)

Nasal and Sinus Surgery

Special considerations in the management of anesthesia for nasal and sinus surgery include the (1) intraoperative application of topical cocaine to produce maximal vasoconstriction in the operative area, (2) use of a posterior pharyngeal pack, (3) possibility of large intraoperative blood loss, and (4) the need for extubation of the trachea only when protective upper airway reflexes have returned. Systemic absorption of cocaine may manifest as tachycardia and hypertension. The maximum safe dose of topical cocaine is about 3 $mg \cdot kg^{-1}$. The use of a combination of topical cocaine and epinephrine does not increase the vasoconstrictive effectiveness of cocaine. Furthermore, topically applied epinephrine does not retard the systemic absorption nor prolong the anesthetic action of cocaine. Maintenance of anesthesia is acceptably provided by using volatile anesthetics, which offer the advantage of providing better control of the blood pressure than opioid techniques. Alternatively, a nitrous oxide-opioid technique may be selected with intermittent administration of volatile anesthetics to control blood pressure. Although nasal sinuses represent air-filled cavities, there is no evidence that nitrous oxide produces adverse increases in pressures in these structures (see the section *Nitrous Oxide and Middle Ear*). Before extubation of the trachea, the pharynx should be suctioned, the posterior pharyngeal pack removed, and the return of protective upper airway reflexes confirmed.

Endoscopy

Special considerations in the management of anesthesia for endoscopy (laryngoscopy, laser surgery, bronchoscopy, esophagoscopy) include the (1) possibility of co-existing airway pathology, (2) management of an upper airway that is shared with the surgeon, (3) need to minimize oral secretions, (4) need for suppression of cough and laryngeal reflexes, (5) need for a relaxed mandible, (6) protection of teeth with a dental guard, and (7) need for rapid awakening with return of protective upper airway reflexes. Cardiac dysrhythmias are frequently associated with the stimulus of endoscopy. In some patients, endoscopy is best performed with the patient awake using local anesthesia. Minimization of oral secretions can usually be effectively accomplished by inclusion of anticholinergics in the preoperative medication. Pulse oximetry is useful in monitoring arterial oxygenation during anesthesia for endoscopy.

Laryngoscopy

General anesthesia for laryngoscopy may be performed with a small (5 mm internal diameter) tracheal tube. This approach permits the use of muscle relaxants to assure optimal surgical working conditions and facilitates ventilation of the lungs. It is usually preferable to tape the tracheal tube to the left side of the mouth as the surgeon will insert the laryngoscope down the right side of the mouth. The disadvantage of using a tracheal tube is interference with the surgeon's view of the larynx, especially the posterior commissure. Intermittent injections or a continuous intravenous infusion of succinylcholine is an effective method to produce skeletal muscle relaxation for these short procedures. General anesthetic techniques in the absence of intubation of the trachea use spontaneous ventilation during the administration of volatile anesthetics in oxygen or intermittent high-pressure insufflation of gases through a ventilating (Sanders) bronchoscope. High-pressure insufflation techniques require profound skeletal muscle relaxation to permit adequate ventilation of the lungs. Small children and patients with bullous lung disease do not tolerate the increased airway pressures associated with this technique. High frequency ventilation is an alternative mode for ventilation of the lungs during laryngoscopy (see Chapter 32).

Laser Surgery

A laser (light amplification by stimulated emission of radiation) is a device capable of producing an intense beam of light that can be focused to produce precisely controlled coagulation, incision, or vaporization of tissues. Edema is minimal and healing is rapid because damage to surrounding tissues is minimal. Laser light is potentially dangerous to personnel present in the vicinity because a misdirected beam of light that strikes unprotected skin or mucous membranes can cause a burn.[16] Corneal burns are a possibility, emphasizing the need for operating room personnel to wear glasses and the need to tape the patient's eyes shut. Patients must remain absolutely immobile as the laser is critically focused on specific target tissues, and any amount of patient movement may divert the beam to adjacent normal tissues.[16] All endotracheal tubes not made from metal may be ignited by the laser beam, particularly in an enriched oxygen atmosphere. For this reason, the inhaled concentrations of oxygen are maintained at the lowest concentrations acceptable (ideally less than 40 percent) and nitrous oxide, which can support combustion, is not administered. Continuous monitoring of arterial oxygenation by pulse oximetry is useful for maintaining the lowest possible inspired concentration of oxygen. Inclusion of helium in the inhaled gases increases the amount of energy required to ignite nonmetal (polyvinylchloride) tracheal tubes.[17] A popular approach is to wrap a red rubber tube with aluminum foil so as to prevent laser-induced ignition of the tracheal tube. Regardless of the tracheal tube selected, the cuff is vulnerable to puncture by the laser beam. When the cuff is inflated with saline instead of air to act as a heat sink for laser energy, it can still be easily perforated by the laser beam but ignition will not occur. The fine spray of saline released by a perforation may serve to quench any possible fire in the airway. Bronchospasm and/or laryngospasm are frequent during and after laser procedures in the larynx and trachea.

Bronchoscopy

Methods of general anesthesia and management of ventilation of the lungs for bronchoscopy do not differ from those for laryngoscopy. Volatile anesthetics are useful to provide adequate suppression of upper airway reflexes and also permit use of high inhaled concentrations of oxygen. Spontaneous ventilation is preferred in cases of foreign body removal because it is theoretically possible that positive airway pressures would push the foreign body deeper into the bronchial tree. Bronchoscopes in current use include the (1) flexible fiberoptic, (2) rigid-ventilating, and (3) rigid-venturi (Sanders injector) type. The flexible fiberoptic bronchoscope offers the advantage of being placed via a large (8.5 mm internal diameter or larger) tracheal tube, permitting reliable ventilation of both lungs during endoscopy. Patient movement or excessive airway pressures during bronchoscopy performed with a rigid bronchoscope may result in a tracheal tear and/or pneumothorax. Trauma associated with bronchoscopy can manifest as airway edema, which may warrant intravenous administration of dexamethasone (0.1 mg·kg^{-1}).

Head and Neck Surgery

Head and neck surgery, such as laryngectomy or radical neck dissection, may last 6 hours to 8 hours and involve substantial blood loss. Patients with carcinoma of the larynx often smoke cigarettes excessively and develop associated chronic obstruc-

tive airways disease. Patency of the upper airway may be compromised by tumor, necessitating placement of a tracheal tube or performance of a tracheostomy before the induction of anesthesia. Surgery near the carotid sinus can elicit vagal responses, manifesting as bradycardia and hypotension. During head and neck surgery, open neck veins create the possibility of venous air embolism. Positive pressure ventilation of the lungs decreases the likelihood of venous air embolism by maintaining an elevated pressure in the veins. Maintenance of blood pressure in a low normal range by varying the inhaled concentrations of volatile anesthetics plus a 10-degree to 15-degree head-up tilt is helpful in minimizing intraoperative blood loss. Blood and intravenous fluids can be warmed to help maintain body temperature during prolonged operations. A catheter placed in the bladder is indicated if large volumes of fluid replacement will be necessary. Cardiac dysrhythmias associated with prolonged Q-T intervals may follow right but not left radical neck dissection, presumably reflecting damage to the cervical autonomic nervous system during surgical dissection (Fig. 25-3).[18]

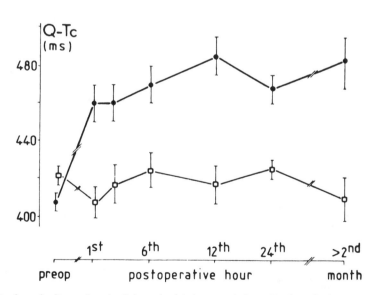

Fig. 25-3. Right radical neck dissection (solid symbols), but not left radical neck dissection (clear symbols), is associated with prolongation of Q-Tc intervals on the electrocardiogram. (From Otteni et al.,[18] with permission.)

Tonsillectomy

Special considerations in the management of anesthesia for tonsillectomy include (1) preoperative evaluation of coagulation, (2) determination of the presence of loose teeth, (3) provision of mandibular and pharyngeal muscle relaxation, (4) suppression of laryngeal reflexes, and (5) rapid awakening and return of protective upper airway reflexes. Blood loss during tonsillectomy averages 4 ml·kg^{-1}, but is usually underestimated due to an undetermined amount of blood draining into the stomach. Maintenance of anesthesia for these short surgical procedures is acceptably achieved with nitrous oxide plus volatile drugs delivered via a tracheal tube. Postoperatively, patients are often placed in the lateral position with the head lower than the hips (tonsil position) so that blood drains out the mouth. As a result, blood loss is less likely to irritate the vocal cords or to be masked by unrecognized accumulation in the stomach.

Reoperation for continued bleeding from the tonsil bed is a major anesthetic challenge. Nearly 90 percent of significant postoperative bleeding, when it does occur, manifests in the first 9 hours postoperatively.[19] These patients are often hypovolemic, as reflected by tachycardia and orthostatic hypotension. Rehydration with lactated Ringer's solution (15 ml·kg^{-1} to 20 ml·kg^{-1}) is mandatory before the induction of anesthesia. Since large volumes of blood may have been swallowed, it is important to treat these patients as if they have a full stomach. A rapid sequence induction of anesthesia using thiopental and succinylcholine plus cricoid pressure is acceptable. Ketamine or etomidate may be selected rather than thiopental, especially if the possibility of hypovolemia exists despite attempts at rehydration. Alternatively, awake intubation of the trachea may be performed. The stomach should be emptied via an orogastric tube after placement of the tracheal tube. After the completion of surgery, protective airway reflexes are allowed to return before the trachea is extubated.

Tracheostomy

Tracheostomy must be regarded as a procedure that is best performed electively in the operating room. Ideally, a translaryngeal tracheal tube should be in place to facilitate ventilation of lungs and permit an unhurried surgical procedure. Cricothyroidotomy can be performed rapidly as a lifesaving procedure when acute upper airway obstruction occurs and translaryngeal intubation of the trachea is not possible. Early complications of tracheostomy include tube displacement, hemorrhage, and pneumothorax.

REFERENCES

1. Myers EF, Krupin T, Johnson M, Zink H. Failure of nondepolarizing neuromuscular blockers to inhibit succinylcholine-induced intraocular pressure—a controlled study. Anesthesiology 1978;48:149–51.
2. Pandey K, Badola RP, Kumar S. Time course of intraocular hypertension produced by suxamethonium. Brit J Anaesth 1972;44:191–5.
3. Miller RD, Way WL, Hickey RF. Inhibition of succinylcholine-induced increased intraocular pressure by nondepolarizing muscle relaxants. Anesthesiology 1968;29:123–6.
4. Kim JW, Smith PH. Timolol-induced bradycardia. Anesth Analg 1980;59:301–3.
5. Bailey PL. Timolol and postoperative apnea in neonates and young infants. Anesthesiology 1984;61:622.
6. Chang J-L, Gonzalez-Abola E, Larson CE. Brain stem anesthesia following retrobulbar block. Anesthesiology 1984;61:789–90.
7. France NK, France TD, Woodburn JD, et al. Succinylcholine alteration of the forced duction test. Ophthalmology 1980;87:1282–5.
8. Abramowitz MD, Oh TH, Epstein BS. Antiemetic effect of droperidol following outpatient strabismus surgery in children. Anesthesiology 1983;59:579–83.
9. Garde JF, Aston R, Endler GC, Sison OS. Racial mydriatic response to belladonna preparations. Anesth Analg 1978;57:572–5.
10. Wolf GL, Capuano C, Hartung J. Nitrous oxide increases intraocular pressure after intravitreal sulfur hexafluoride injection. Anesthesiology 1983;59:547–8.
11. Libonati M, Leahy JJ, Ellison N. The use of succinylcholine in open eye surgery. Anesthesiology 1985;62:637–40.
12. Siffring PA, Poulton TJ. Prevention of ophthalmic complications during general anesthesia. Anesthesiology 1987;66:569–70.
13. Patterson ME, Bartlett PC. Hearing impairment caused by intratympanic pressure changes during general anesthesia. Laryngoscope 1976;86:399–404.
14. Owens WD, Gustave F, Schlaroff A. Tympanic membrane rupture with nitrous oxide anesthesia. Anesth Analg 1978;57:283–6.
15. Man A, Segal S, Ezra S. Ear injury caused by elevated intratympanic pressure during general anesthesia. Acta Anaesth Scand 1980;24:224–6.

16. Sosis M. Anesthesia for laser surgery. In: Stoelting RK, Barash PG, Gallagher TJ, eds. Advances in Anesthesia. Chicago, Year Book Medical Publishers, 1986:175–230.

17. Pashayan AG, Gravenstein JS. Helium retards endotracheal tube fires from carbon dioxide lasers. Anesthesiology 1985;62:272–7.

18. Otteni JC, Pottecher T, Bronner G, Flesch H, Diebolt JR. Prolongation of the Q-T interval and sudden cardiac arrest following right radical neck dissection. Anesthesiology 1983;59:358–61.

19. Crysdale WS. Complications of tonsillectomy and adenoidectomy in 949 children observed overnight. Can Med Assoc J 1986;135:1129–42.

Chapter 26

Obstetrics

Optimal analgesia and/or anesthesia for labor, vaginal delivery, or cesarean section requires an understanding of the physiologic changes in the parturient during pregnancy and labor, the effects of anesthetics on the fetus and neonate, the benefits and risks of various techniques of anesthesia, and the significance of obstetric complications on the management of anesthesia. Unlike the patient scheduled for elective surgery, the parturient is rarely in optimal condition at the time anesthetic care becomes necessary. For example, the parturient must always be considered to represent a full stomach and to be at increased risk for inhalation (pulmonary aspiration) of gastric contents. During labor, emergencies, such as fetal distress, maternal hemorrhage and prolapsed cord, demand immediate anesthesia.

PHYSIOLOGIC CHANGES IN THE PARTURIENT

Pregnancy and subsequent labor and delivery are accompanied by predictable physiologic changes.

Cardiovascular System

Changes in the cardiovascular system during pregnancy provide for the needs of the developing fetus and prepare the mother for events that will occur during labor and delivery. These changes include alterations in (1) the intravascular fluid volume and its constituents, (2) cardiac output, and (3) peripheral circulation (Table 26-1). The supine hypotension syndrome reflects circulatory changes due to the impact of the enlarging gravid uterus.

Intravascular Fluid Volume

The increase in maternal intravascular fluid volume begins in the first trimester and at term results in an average expansion of about 1000 ml. Plasma volume increases 45 percent and the erythrocyte volume increases 20 percent. This disproportionate increase in plasma volume accounts for the relative anemia of pregnancy. The increased intravascular fluid volume offsets the 400 ml to 600 ml blood loss that accompanies vaginal delivery and the average 1000 ml blood loss that accompanies cesarean section. Total plasma protein concentration is reduced, reflecting the dilutional effect of the increased intravascular fluid volume. Nevertheless, protein binding of a drug such as thiopental has not been shown to be altered in the parturient.[1]

Cardiac Output

Cardiac output is increased about 40 percent above nonpregnant levels by the 10th week of gestation and is maintained at this level throughout the second and third trimesters. This augmentation of cardiac output is primarily due to an elevated stroke volume, as heart rate is not greatly in-

369

Table 26-1.   Changes in the Cardiovascular System during Pregnancy

Variable	Compared with Nonpregnant Value
Intravascular fluid volume	Increased 35 percent
Plasma volume	Increased 45 percent
Erythrocyte volume	Increased 20 percent
Cardiac output	Increased 40 percent
Stroke volume	Increased 30 percent
Heart rate	Increased 15 percent
Peripheral circulation	
Systolic blood pressure	No change
Systemic vascular resistance	Decreased 15 percent
Central venous pressure	No change
Femoral venous pressure	Increased 15 percent

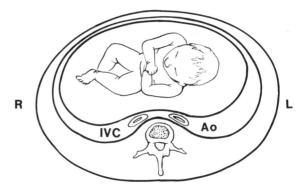

Fig. 26-1. Schematic diagram showing compression of the inferior vena cava (IVC) and abdominal aorta (Ao) by the gravid uterus when the parturient assumes the supine position.

creased. It is likely that placental and ovarian steroids are important in producing and sustaining this increase. Earlier studies suggesting return of cardiac output toward nonpregnant levels during the third trimester were in error. Instead, this decrease reflected reduced venous return due to compression of the inferior vena cava by the gravid uterus when the supine position was assumed.

The onset of labor is associated with further increases in cardiac output, which may reach 45 percent above the prelabor value. The greatest increase in cardiac output occurs immediately after delivery when output is elevated as much as 60 percent above prelabor values. A regional anesthetic is capable of attenuating increases in cardiac output during labor and may therefore be a useful way of protecting a compromised cardiovascular system during the peripartum period. Typically, cardiac output returns to nonpregnant values by 2 weeks postpartum.

Peripheral Circulation

Systolic blood pressure never increases above nonpregnant levels during an uncomplicated pregnancy. Because cardiac output is elevated, the systemic vascular resistance must decrease for the blood pressure to remain normal. There is no change in the central venous pressure during pregnancy, but femoral venous pressure is in-

creased about 15 percent, presumably reflecting compression of the inferior vena cava by the gravid uterus.

Supine Hypotension Syndrome

Reductions in maternal blood pressure associated with the supine position occur in about 10 percent of parturients near term. Diaphoresis, nausea, vomiting, and changes in cerebration may accompany this hypotension. These symptoms are termed the *supine hypotension syndrome.*

The mechanism for the supine hypotension syndrome is decreased venous return due to compression of the inferior vena cava by the gravid uterus when the parturient assumes the supine position (Fig. 26-1). The resulting decrease in venous return leads to a reduction in cardiac output and a decline in blood pressure. Fortunately, the majority (about 90 percent) of parturients are able to initiate compensatory responses on assuming the supine position. These compensatory responses prevent the appearance of the supine hypotension syndrome. For example, increased venous pressure below the level of compression of the inferior vena cava serves to divert venous blood from the lower one-half of the body via the paravertebral venous plexuses to the azygos vein. Flow from the azygos vein enters the superior vena cava and venous return is maintained. This compensatory response means that inadvertent intravascular injection of local anesthetics during an attempted lumbar epidural block can result in bolus delivery of the drug to the heart with resulting profound myocardial depression. An additional compensatory response that offsets inferior vena cava compression by the gravid uterus is an increase in peripheral sympathetic nervous system activity. This increased activity results in elevation of systemic vascular resistance, which permits blood pressure to be maintained despite a diminished cardiac output. It is important to recognize that compensatory increases in systemic vascular resistance are impaired by regional anesthetic techniques. Indeed, arterial hypotension is more common and profound during a regional anesthetic administered to parturients compared with nonpregnant patients.

In addition to compression of the inferior vena cava, the gravid uterus may also compress the lower abdominal aorta (Fig. 26-1). This compression leads to arterial hypotension in the lower extremities, but maternal symptoms or reductions in blood pressure as measured in the arm do not occur.

The significance of aortocaval compression is the associated reduction in uterine and placental blood flow. Even in the presence of a healthy uteroplacental unit, reductions in maternal blood pressure to less than 100 mmHg that persist for longer than 10 minutes to 15 minutes may be associated with progressive fetal acidosis and bradycardia.

The incidence of the supine hypotension syndrome can be minimized by nursing the parturient in the lateral position. Alternatively, left uterine displacement is effective by moving the gravid uterus off the inferior vena cava or aorta. Displacement of the uterus to the left can be accomplished manually or by elevation of the right hip 10 cm to 15 cm with a blanket or foam-rubber wedge (Fig. 26-2).

Respiratory System

Changes in the respiratory system during pregnancy are manifested as alterations in (1) the upper airway, (2) minute ventilation, (3) lung volumes, and (4) arterial oxygenation (Table 26-2).

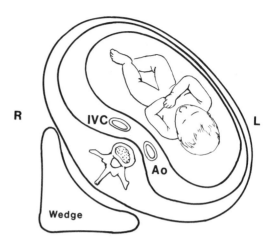

Fig. 26-2. Schematic diagram depicting left uterine displacement by elevation of the parturient's right hip with a foam-rubber wedge. This position moves the gravid uterus off the inferior vena cava (IVC) and aorta (Ao).

Upper Airway

Capillary engorgement of the mucosal lining of the upper respiratory tract accompanies pregnancy and emphasizes the need for gentleness during instrumentation (e.g., suctioning, placement of

Table 26-2. Changes in the Respiratory System

Variable	Compared with Nonpregnant Value
Minute ventilation	Increased 50 percent
Tidal volume	Increased 40 percent
Respiratory rate	Increased 10 percent
Lung volumes	
Expiratory reserve volume	Decreased 20 percent
Residual volume	Decreased 20 percent
Functional residual capacity	Decreased 20 percent
Vital capacity	No change
Total lung capacity	No change
Arterial blood gases and pH	
PaO_2	Increased 10 mmHg
$PaCO_2$	Decreased 10 mmHg
pH	No change
Oxygen consumption	Increased 20 percent

nasal or oral airways, direct laryngoscopy) of the upper airway. It is prudent to select a smaller sized cuffed tracheal tube (6.5 mm to 7.0 mm internal diameter) because the false vocal cords and arytenoids are often edematous.

Minute Ventilation

Minute ventilation is increased about 50 percent above nonpregnant levels during the first trimester and maintained at this elevated level for the remainder of pregnancy. This increased minute ventilation is achieved by an increased tidal volume as breathing rate is not greatly altered (Table 26-2). Increased circulating levels of progesterone are presumed to be the stimulus for increased minute ventilation.

The resting maternal $PaCO_2$ decreases from 40 mmHg to about 30 mmHg during the first trimester as a reflection of increased minute ventilation. Arterial pH, however, remains near normal because of increased renal excretion of bicarbonate ions. Pain associated with labor and delivery results in further hyperventilation, which can be attenuated by lumbar epidural block.

Lung Volumes

Lung volumes, in contrast to the early appearance of increased minute ventilation, do not begin to change until about the fifth month of pregnancy (Table 26-2). With increasing enlargement of the uterus, the diaphragm is forced cephalad. This change is largely responsible for the 20 percent reduction in functional residual capacity present at term. Vital capacity is not significantly changed.

The combintion of increased minute ventilation and decreased functional residual capacity speeds the rate at which changes in alveolar concentrations of inhaled anesthetics can be achieved. Indeed, induction of anesthesia, emergence from anesthesia, and changes in depth of anesthesia are notably faster in parturients.

Arterial Oxygenation

Maternal PaO_2, while breathing room air, normally exceeds 100 mmHg, reflecting the presence of hyperventilation (Table 26-2). Induction of general anesthesia, however, in the parturient may be associated with marked reductions in the PaO_2

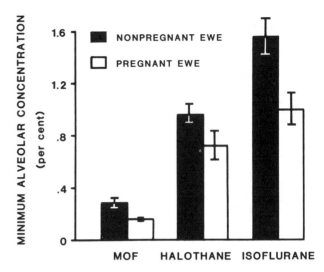

Fig. 26-3. The minimum alveolar concentration (MAC) is reduced in the pregnant ewe as compared with the nonpregnant ewe. (Data from Palahniuk et al.[3])

if apnea, as during intubation of the trachea, is prolonged. This tendency for a rapid decrease in PaO_2 reflects a decreased oxygen reserve secondary to the reduction in functional residual capacity. A reduction in cardiac output due to aortocaval compression and increased oxygen consumption may also contribute to rapid decreases in PaO_2 during apnea. For these reasons, the administration of oxygen (preoxygenation) before any anticipated period of apnea or during a regional anesthetic is important. To maximize fetal benefits of preoxygenation, maternal inhalation of supplemental oxygen may need to be continued for about 6 minutes, as this is the estimated time required for maternal to fetal equilibration.[2] Likewise, it is prudent to routinely monitor arterial oxygen saturations with pulse oximetry and to provide left uterine displacement.

Nervous System Changes

Central nervous system changes during pregnancy are reflected by decreased MAC for volatile anesthetics as demonstrated in animals (Fig. 26-3).[3] It is presumed, but not documented, that similar changes occur in humans. Sedative effects produced by progesterone may be partially responsible for this reduction in anesthesia requirements

(MAC). The important clinical implication of decreased MAC is that alveolar concentrations of inhaled drugs that would not produce unconsciousness in nonpregnant patients may approximate anesthetizing concentrations in parturients. This degree of central nervous system depression may also impair protective upper airway reflexes and subject parturients to the hazards of pulmonary aspiration. Furthermore, the decreased functional residual capacity speeds the rate at which potential excessive alveolar concentrations of anesthetics can be achieved.

Engorgement of epidural veins as intra-abdominal pressure increases with progressive enlargement of the uterus decreases the size of the epidural space and reduces the volume of cerebrospinal fluid in the subarachnoid space. Decreased volume of these spaces facilitates the spread of local anesthetics and is consistent with the 30 percent to 50 percent reduction in dose requirements of local anesthetics necessary for epidural or spinal anesthesia in parturients at term. The observation of exaggerated spread of local anesthetics placed in the epidural space as early as the first trimester suggests a role for biochemical as well as mechanical changes.[4] Indeed, experimental evidence confirms increased sensitivity to local anesthetics in pregnant vs. nonpregnant animals. There are also data that do not demonstrate a difference in the level of sensory anesthesia achieved when equal volumes of local anesthetics are injected into the epidural space of pregnant and nonpregnant patients if care is exercised to prevent aortocaval compression in parturients.[5]

Renal Changes

Renal blood flow and glomerular filtration rate are increased about 50 percent by the fourth month of pregnancy. Therefore, the normal upper limits of the blood urea nitrogen and serum creatinine concentrations are reduced about 50 percent in the parturients.

Hepatic Changes

Serum bilirubin concentrations and hepatic blood flow are unchanged during pregnancy. Nevertheless, most parturients manifest abnormal bromsulfalein excretion tests. Total protein concentrations and plasma cholinesterase (pseudocholinesterase) activity are decreased. Despite the latter, the response of parturients to moderate doses of succinylcholine is not prolonged. For unknown reasons, serum transaminase concentrations and the circulating levels of alkaline phosphatase are often elevated during pregnancy.

Gastrointestinal Changes

Gastrointestinal changes during pregnancy make parturients vulnerable to regurgitation of gastric contents and to the development of acid pneumonitis should pulmonary aspiration occur. For example, the enlarged uterus displaces the pylorus upwards and backwards, which retards gastric emptying. As a result, gastric fluid volume tends to be elevated, even in the fasting state. In addition, gastrin, which is secreted by the placenta, stimulates gastric hydrogen ion secretion such that pH of gastric fluid is predictably low in parturients. Finally, the enlarging uterus changes the angle of the gastroesophageal junction, leading to relative incompetence of the physiologic sphincter mechanism. As a result, gastric fluid reflux into the esophagus and subsequent esophagitis are common in parturients.

Regardless of the time interval since ingestion of food, the parturient in labor must be treated as having a full stomach. Pain, anxiety, and drugs (especially opioids) administered during labor can all significantly retard gastric emptying beyond an already prolonged transit time.

The increased risk for pulmonary aspiration of gastric contents is the reason for recommending the placement of a cuffed tube in the trachea of every parturient who is rendered unconscious by anesthesia. The recognition that the pH of inhaled gastric fluid is important in the production and severity of acid pneumonitis is the basis for the administration of antacids to parturients before the induction of anesthesia. Considering the potential accumulation of antacids in the stomach, particularly if gastric emptying is slowed by opioids, there seems little reason to recommend routine use of antacids at regular intervals during labor.[6] Furthermore, routine use of antacids has not been conclusively proven to reduce morbidity or mortality despite the accepted ability of these drugs to elevate the pH of gastric fluid. It must be appreciated that inhalation of antacids containing particulate matter can produce adverse pulmonary changes. In an attempt to obviate the hazards of inhalation of particulate antacids, the use of the nonparticulate antacid, sodium citrate, has been recommended. Alternatively, histamine H_2-receptor antagonists, such as cimetidine or ranitidine, reliably elevate gastric fluid pH in parturients without producing adverse effects.[7] It must be remembered that H_2-receptor antagonists, unlike antacids, will not alter the pH of gastric fluid already present in the stomach.

Metoclopramide may be useful for reducing gastric fluid volume of parturients in active labor requiring general anesthesia and considered at high risk for elevated gastric fluid volumes (apprehension, opioid analgesia, recent food ingestion, history of heartburn indicative of lower esophageal dysfunction). Gastric hypomotility due to opioids, however, may be resistant to treatment with metoclopramide.

PHYSIOLOGY OF UTEROPLACENTAL CIRCULATION

The placenta provides for the union of maternal and fetal circulations for the purpose of physiologic exchange. Maternal blood is delivered to the placenta by the uterine arteries, and fetal blood arrives via two umbilical arteries. Nutrient-rich and waste-free blood is delivered to the fetus via a single umbilical vein. The most important determinants of placental function are uterine blood flow and the characteristics of substances available for exchange across the placenta.

Uterine Blood Flow

Maintenance of uterine blood flow at term (500 ml·min^{-1} to 700 ml·min^{-1}) is critical as this flow determines the adequacy of placental circulation and fetal well-being. In the presence of a normal placenta, it is estimated that uterine blood flow can decrease about 50 percent before fetal distress, as reflected by acidosis, is detectable.

Uterine blood flow is not autoregulated and is, therefore, directly proportional to mean perfusion pressure across the uterus and inversely proportional to uterine vascular resistance. Therefore, uterine blood flow is reduced by drugs or events that decrease perfusion pressure (decreased systemic blood pressure or increased venous pressure) or increase uterine vascular resistance.

Hypotension

Hypotension due to aortocaval compression or peripheral sympathetic nervous system blockade decreases uterine blood flow by reductions in perfusion pressure. Drugs administered to parturients to produce analgesia and anesthesia during labor and delivery could reduce uterine blood flow via drug-induced changes in blood pressure. For example, when the concentration of volatile anesthetics administered to pregnant ewes exceeds 1 MAC, fetal acidosis develops, suggesting decreased uterine blood flow in association with drug-induced hypotension. Epidural or spinal block do not alter uterine blood flow as long as maternal hypotension is avoided.

Uterine Vascular Resistance

Alpha-adrenergic stimulation produced by methoxamine and metaraminol can increase uterine vascular resistance and decrease uterine blood flow (Fig. 26-4).[8] Conversely, ephedrine is considered a useful sympathomimetic to use to raise blood pressure in parturients because uterine blood flow is maintained in the presence of this vasopressor (Fig. 26-4).[8] Increased uterine vascular resistance with reductions in uterine blood flow can result from maternal stress or pain that stimulates the endogenous release of catecholamines (Fig. 26-5).[9] This response suggests that a regional or general anesthetic may be protective to the fetus. Finally, uterine contractions reduce uterine blood flow secondary to elevated uterine venous pressure.

Placental Exchange

Placental exchange of substances is principally by diffusion from the maternal circulation to the fetus and vice versa. Diffusion of a substance across the placenta to the fetus depends on maternal-to-fetal concentration gradients, maternal protein binding, molecular weight, lipid solubility, and degree of ionization of that substance (Table 26-3). Minimizing the maternal blood concentration of a drug is the most important method for limiting the amount that ultimately reaches the fetus. Further-

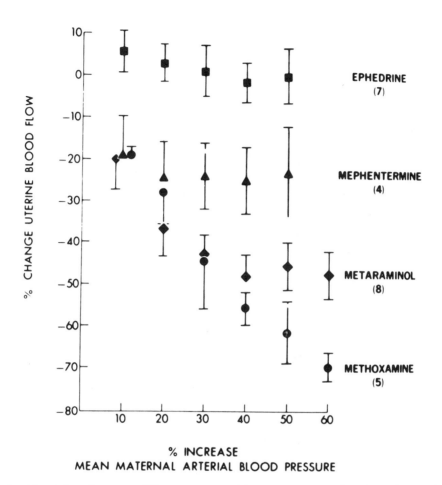

Fig. 26-4. Uterine blood flow (mean ± SE) was measured in pregnant ewes (number of animals studied in parentheses) before and after increases in maternal blood pressure produced by the intravenous administration of sympathomimetics. With the exception of ephedrine, these drugs decreased uterine blood flow despite increasing mean arterial pressure. (From Ralston et al.,[8] with permission.)

more, transfer to the fetus can be decreased by intravenous injection of a drug during a uterine contraction because maternal blood flow to the placenta is markedly reduced at this time.

Maternal Protein Binding

Maternal protein binding of local anesthetics is important because only that portion of the drug not bound to protein is available for diffusion across the placenta. At typical clinical concentrations, 50 percent to 70 percent of lidocaine is bound to protein compared with 95 percent for bupivacaine. The greater degree of protein bind-

ing for bupivacaine could impair placental transfer by reducing the amount of free drug available for diffusion. This is consistent with the observation that the ratio of umbilical vein-to-uterine artery concentration of bupivacaine is lower than the ratio measured for lidocaine. Nevertheless, dissociation of local anesthetics from protein is rapid, and it is questionable whether protein binding of drugs significantly impairs diffusion across the placenta.

Molecular Weight and Lipid Solubility

The large molecular weight and poor lipid solu-

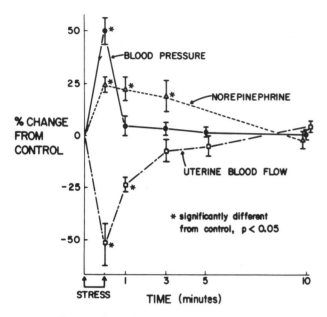

Fig. 26-5. Electrically-induced stress in pregnant ewes lasting 30 seconds to 60 seconds results in increased maternal blood pressure and serum norepinephrine concentrations (mean ± SE). Uterine blood flow is reduced about 50 percent at the time of maximum blood pressure and catecholamine elevation. (From Shnider et al.,[9] with permission.)

bility of nondepolarizing muscle relaxants are consistent with the fact that these drugs cross the placenta only to a limited extent. Succinylcholine has a low molecular weight but is highly ionized and, therefore, does not readily cross the placenta. Conversely, placental transfer of barbiturates, local anesthetics, and opioids is facilitated by the relatively low molecular weight of these substances.

Table 26-3. Determinants of Diffusion across the Placenta

	Rapid Diffusion	Slow Diffusion
Maternal protein binding	Low	High
Molecular weight	<500	>1000
Lipid solubility	High	Low
Ionization	Minimal	Maximum

FETAL UPTAKE AND DISTRIBUTION OF DRUGS

Fetal uptake of a substance that crosses the placenta is facilitated by the lower pH (0.1 unit) of fetal compared with maternal blood. The lower fetal pH means that weakly basic drugs (local anesthetics, opioids) that cross the placenta in the nonionized form will become ionized in the fetal circulation. Since an ionized drug cannot readily cross the placenta back to the maternal circulation, it follows that this drug will accumulate in the fetal blood against a concentration gradient. This phenomenon is known as ion trapping and may explain the higher concentrations of lidocaine found in the fetus when acidosis due to fetal distress is present (Fig. 26-6).[10] Furthermore, conversion of lidocaine to the ionized fraction maintains the concentration gradient from mother to fetus for the continued passage of nonionized lidocaine to the fetus. Despite reduced enzyme activity compared with adults, the neonatal enzyme systems are adequately developed to metabolize most drugs with the possible exception of mepivacaine.

The unique characteristics of the fetal circulation influence the distribution of drugs in the fetus and protect the vital organs of the fetus from exposure to high concentrations of drugs initially present in the umbilical venous blood. For example, about 75 percent of umbilical venous blood passes through the liver such that significant portions of drugs can be metabolized before reaching the fetal arterial circulation for delivery to the heart and brain. Furthermore, drugs in that portion of the umbilical venous blood that enters the inferior vena cava via the ductus venosus will be diluted by drug free blood returning from the lower extremities and pelvic viscera of the fetus.

MATERNAL MEDICATION DURING LABOR

Despite the increasing use of epidural block to provide pain relief during labor and vaginal delivery there is still an occasional role for systemic medications to reduce pain and anxiety. There is no ideal drug as all systemic medications cross the placenta to some extent and produce depressant effects on the fetus. The amount of fetal depres-

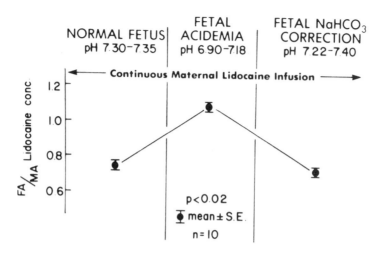

Fig. 26-6. Fetal-to-maternal arterial (FA/MA) lidocaine ratios are higher during fetal acidemia than during control (normal fetus), or during pH correction with sodium bicarbonate. This reflects ion trapping of the ionized fraction of lidocaine in the fetus in the presence of acidosis. (From Biehl et al.,[10] with permission.)

sion depends primarily on the dose of drug and route and time of administration before delivery. Drugs likely to be administered as systemic medications are benzodiazepines, opioids, and ketamine. Barbiturates or scopolamine are no longer popular.

Benzodiazepines

Benzodiazepines readily cross the placenta. When the maternal dose of diazepam exceeds 30 mg, there is associated fetal hypotonia, decreased feeding, and hypothermia. Beat-to-beat variability of the fetal heart rate is decreased with small intravenous doses (5 mg to 10 mg) of diazepam, but there are no detectable adverse effects on the fetus. Therefore, small doses of intravenous diazepam (2.5 mg to 10 mg) or midazolam (1 mg to 3 mg) are acceptable for relieving anxiety as during cesarean section performed with epidural block.

Opioids

Opioids are the most effective systemic medications for the relief of pain during labor and vaginal delivery. All opioids rapidly cross the placenta and

may be responsible for depression of ventilation in the neonate immediately after birth. Meperidine is the most popular opioid used in obstetrics, whereas morphine is rarely administered, primarily because of the apparent greater sensitivity of the medullary ventilatory center of newborns to morphine as compared with meperidine. It should be appreciated that the incidence of neonatal depression associated with maternal administration of intramuscular meperidine (50 mg to 100 mg) is greatest in neonates born 2 hours to 4 hours after injection. Depression of neonates is less when delivery occurs within 1 hour or more than 4 hours after injection. The reason for the apparent safe period with intramuscular meperidine is not known.

Ketamine

Intermittent intravenous doses of ketamine (10 mg to 15 mg) can be titrated to produce the rapid onset of intense analgesia in parturients without resulting in loss of consciousness. This low dose approach is particularly useful for parturients in whom vaginal delivery is imminent or when regional anesthesia is incomplete. Ketamine readily crosses the placenta but in low doses does not cause neonatal depression. Nevertheless, adverse maternal psychological changes may accompany even these low doses of ketamine.

PROGRESS OF LABOR

Progress of labor refers to increasing cervical dilation, effacement, and descent of the fetal presenting part through the vagina with time (Fig. 26-7).[11] The onset of regular contractions signals the beginning of the first stage of labor. This stage is subdivided into the latent and active phases lasting 7 hours to 13 hours in the primigravida and 4 hours to 5 hours in the multigravida. The second stage of labor begins with complete dilation of the cervix. The third stage extends from delivery of the baby until the placenta is expelled.

The progress of labor is unpredictable being influenced by many variables including maternal pain, parity, size and presentation of the fetus, and drugs and techniques used to provide analgesia or anesthesia. Excessive sedation or the pre-

mature initiation of a regional anesthetic is the most common cause for prolongation of the latent phase. Nevertheless, labor can slow during the latent phase in the absence of anesthesia. Furthermore, catecholamine release in response to pain can inhibit uterine contractions such that analgesia provided by appropriate regional anesthetic techniques might even enhance early progress of labor. During the active phase the most likely causes of delayed progress of labor are cephalopelvic disproportion, fetal malposition, and fetal malpresentation.

The impact of anesthesia on the progress of labor is more predictable after labor has become active. For example, during the active phase a T10 sensory level produced by a spinal or epidural block has no significant effect on progress of labor provided fetal malpresentation is absent and hypotension is avoided. However, a regional anesthetic, by removing the reflex urge to bear down, may prolong the second stage of labor. Neverthe-

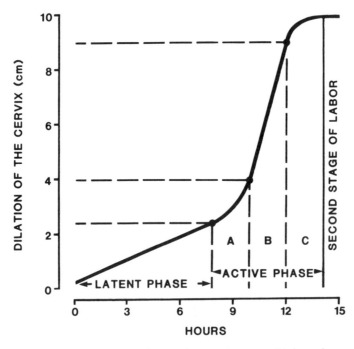

Fig. 26-7. The progress of labor is divided into the first and second stages of labor, depending on the dilation of the cervix. The first stage of labor is further subdivided into a latent and an active phase. The active phase consists of the accelerated phase (A), the phase of maximum slope (B), and the deceleration phase (C). (Adapted from Friedman,[11] with permission.)

less, even if labor is prolonged by a regional anesthetic there is no evidence that this is harmful to the fetus.

Volatile anesthetics produce dose-dependent decreases in uterine activity. Analgesia provided with low inhaled concentrations of halothane (0.5 percent) or enflurane (1 percent) during vaginal delivery does not decrease uterine activity, prolong labor, increase postpartum blood loss, or interfere with the uterine response to oxytocin. Greater inhaled concentrations of volatile anesthetics are the most reliable way of rapidly producing uterine relaxation when necessary.

REGIONAL ANESTHESIA FOR LABOR AND VAGINAL DELIVERY

Compared with analgesia produced by inhaled or parenteral drugs the use of regional anesthetic techniques for labor and vaginal delivery reduces the likelihood of fetal drug depression and maternal pulmonary aspiration. Standards for regional (conduction) anesthesia in obstetrics have been endorsed by the American Society of Anesthesiologists (see Appendix 1).

Regional blocks effective during the first stage of labor include paracervical block, lumbar epidural block and caudal block (Table 26-4). Neuraxial opioids (epidural or subarachnoid injection) have also been evaluated for relief of pain during the first stage of labor. Pain during the second stage of labor is relieved by lumbar epidural block, caudal block, spinal block, and pudendal nerve block (Table 26-4).

Pain During Labor and Delivery

Parturition is associated with two distinct kinds of pain. The first type of pain, visceral in origin, is caused by uterine contractions plus dilation of the cervix. The other type of pain is somatic due to stretching of the vagina and perineum by descent of the fetus. The parturient has an uncontrollable urge to bear down as the presenting fetal part begins its descent through the vagina. It is customary to consider visceral pain as part of the first stage and somatic pain as part of the second stage of labor.

Rational use of regional anesthetic techniques

Table 26-4. Types of Regional Anesthesia for Labor and Vaginal Delivery

Technique	Area of Anesthesia	Type of Pain Blocked
Paracervical block	T10–L1	Visceral
Neuraxial opioids	No distinct sensory loss	Visceral
Lumbar epidural block		
Segmental	T10–L1	Visceral
Standard	T10–S5	Visceral and somatic
Caudal block	T10–S5	Visceral and somatic
Spinal block		
Saddle	S1–5	Somatic
Modified	T10–S5	Visceral and somatic
Pudendal nerve blocks	S2–4	Somatic

requires an understanding of the pathways responsible for the transmission of visceral and somatic pain during labor and vaginal delivery (Fig. 26-8). During the first stage of labor, afferent visceral pain impulses from the uterus and cervix travel in nerves that accompany sympathetic nervous system fibers and enter the spinal cord at T10 to L1. In the late first stage and the second stage of labor, somatic pain impulses originate primarily from receptors in the vagina and perineum and travel via the pudendal nerves to the spinal cord at S2–4.

Paracervical Block

Injection of local anesthetics into the fornix of the vagina lateral to the cervix (3 position and 9 position) eliminates visceral pain by anesthetizing the sensory fibers from the uterus, cervix, and upper vagina. Somatic pain and the urge to bear down are not obtunded. Maternal hypotension does not result because sympathetic nervous system blockade does not occur. Paracervical block is not effective during the second stage of labor because sensory fibers from the perineum are not blocked. The major disadvantage of a paracervical block is the 8 percent to 40 percent incidence of

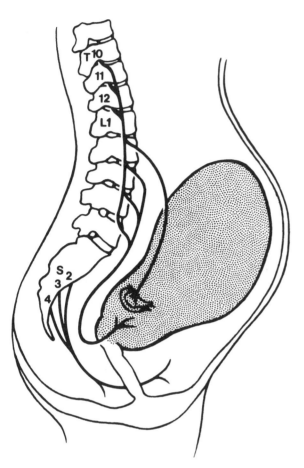

Fig. 26-8. Schematic diagram of pain pathways during parturition. Visceral pain during the first stage of labor is due to uterine contraction and dilation of the cervix. Afferent pain impulses from the uterus and cervix are transmitted by nerves that accompany sympathetic nervous system fibers and enter the spinal cord at T10–L1. Somatic pain during the second stage of labor is vaginal and perineal in origin and impulses travel via the pudendal nerves to S2–4.

fetal bradycardia that develops 2 minutes to 10 minutes after injection of the local anesthetic. The cause of bradycardia is not known but is probably related to decreased uterine blood flow secondary to uterine vasoconstriction from local anesthetics applied in close proximity to the artery plus direct cardiac toxicity due to high fetal blood levels of the local anesthetics. Bradycardia produced by paracervical block is often associated with fetal

acidosis. It would seem prudent to avoid this block in parturients with uteroplacental insufficiency or when there is co-existing fetal distress.

Neuraxial Opioids

The efficacy of epidural or subarachnoid injection of opioids for the relief of pain during the first stage of labor is not well defined. Subarachnoid placement seems to be more effective than epidural injection. Maternal side effects include a high incidence of pruritus, somnolence, and the potential for the delayed onset of depression of ventilation. Neonatal depression does not seem to occur. Opioids administered by epidural or subarachnoid routes are not reliably effective for pain relief during the second stage of labor.

Lumbar Epidural Block

Advantages of a continuous lumbar epidural block via an appropriately placed plastic catheter include the (1) ability to achieve segmental bands of analgesia (T10–L1) during the first stage of labor when total anesthesia is not required, (2) minimal local anesthetic requirements, and (3) maintenance of pelvic muscle tone so that rotation of the fetal head is more easily accomplished. The visceral pain of the first stage of labor can be relieved by injection of 6 ml to 8 ml of 0.25 percent bupivacaine into the lumbar epidural space. Initially, a 2 ml test dose is injected and 3 minutes allowed to elapse before injecting the remaining drug. This small test dose is used to detect an unrecognized subarachnoid injection. Assuming the absence of signs of a spinal block after the test dose, the remaining 4 ml to 6 ml are injected. The low dose of local anesthetic produces a sensory band of analgesia that is unlikely to produce sufficient peripheral sympathetic blockade to result in maternal hypotension. Nevertheless, parturients should be encouraged to remain in the lateral position. Addition of small doses of opioids (50 μg to 150 μg of fentanyl) to low concentrations of bupivacaine (0.125 percent) may accelerate the onset of analgesia. Onset of analgesia, however, does not seem to be enhanced by addition of opioids to higher concentrations of bupivacaine.[12] Blood pressure should be monitored every 1 minute to 2 minutes for the first 10 minutes after injection of local anesthetics, then every 5 minutes to 10 minutes until the block dissipates. During the first 20 minutes after the initial dose of local anesthetics and after any additional doses, the parturient should be under continuous surveillance. If hypotension occurs (systolic blood pressure less than 100 mmHg or greater than a 30 percent decrease in a previously hypertensive parturient), left uterine displacement must be confirmed, intravenous fluids infused rapidly, the parturient placed in a 10 degree to 20 degree head-down position, and oxygen administered via a face mask. If blood pressure is not restored in 1 minute to 2 minutes, ephedrine (5 mg to 10 mg) should be administered intravenously every 1 minute to 2 minutes until an appropriate blood pressure response occurs. Ideally, fetal heart rate is continuously monitored electronically before and after the epidural block is instituted.

Supplemental doses of local anesthetic (about one-half of the initial dose) are administered if the epidural block wanes during the first stage of labor. Additional local anesthetic is injected to provide perineal analgesia as labor progresses. This is accomplished by placing the parturient in the sitting position and injecting slowly 10 ml to 20 ml of local anesthetic solution. Furthermore, an epidural block can be supplemented to provide adequate anesthesia should a cesarean section become necessary.

Institution of a continuous lumbar epidural block is appropriate when the first stage of labor is well established as evidenced by dilation of the cervix (6 cm to 8 cm in a primipara or 4 cm to 6 cm in a multipara) and uterine contractions are strong and regular.

Caudal Block

Caudal block is produced by injection of local anesthetics (10 ml to 12 ml of 0.25 percent bupivacaine) into the sacral epidural space. Compared with a continuous lumbar epidural block, there is a lower incidence of inadvertent dural puncture and perineal analgesia is more profound. Disadvantages of caudal block include difficulty in keeping the sacral area clean, technical difficulties in identifying the sacral hiatus, and accidental injec-

tion of local anesthetics into the fetal head. Finally, it may not be possible to produce a sufficient level of anesthesia with a caudal block should cesarean section become necessary.

Spinal (Saddle) Block

A spinal block is administered immediately before vaginal delivery by injecting small doses of hyperbaric tetracaine (2 mg to 4 mg) or lidocaine (20 mg to 30 mg) into the lumbar subarachnoid space with the parturient in the sitting position. The sitting position is maintained for 2 minutes to 3 minutes to assure that only perineal analgesia (area of the body that would be in contact with a saddle) occurs. A true saddle block does not produce complete pain relief as afferent fibers from the uterus are not blocked.

A modified saddle block is achieved by the subarachnoid injection of 4 mg to 6 mg of tetracaine or 30 mg to 50 mg of lidocaine with the sitting position maintained for 30 seconds. With this approach sensory blockade typically extends to T10, which prevents pain from contractions of the uterus.

The major disadvantage of a spinal block for vaginal delivery is the subsequent appearance of a headache, which is presumably due to loss of fluid through the hole in the dura produced during performance of the block (see Chapter 13).

Pudendal Nerve Block

A pudendal nerve block is typically administered transvaginally by the obstetrician to provide perineal analgesia for delivery. Overlapping innervation of the perineum means the urge to bear down is not completely abolished. Alone, this block provides complete analgesia for episiotomy and repair and is usually sufficient for low forceps delivery. Supplementation with inhalation analgesia is required for mid-forceps delivery. A pudendal nerve block is not associated with peripheral sympathetic nervous system blockade and labor is not prolonged.

INHALATION ANALGESIA FOR VAGINAL DELIVERY

The goal of inhalation analgesia is to maintain the parturient in an awake but comfortable state with intact laryngeal reflexes during the first and second stages of labor. The major risk of inhalation analgesia is loss of protective airway reflexes made more likely by the reduced functional residual capacity and decreased MAC associated with pregnancy. Because all inhaled anesthetics readily cross the placenta, the possibility of neonatal effects must also be considered. However, analgesic concentrations of inhaled anesthetics (about 0.3 MAC to 0.4 MAC) are free from excessive depressant effects on the fetus even if administered for prolonged periods.[13]

An effective form of inhalation analgesia is the continuous administration of 30 percent to 40 percent nitrous oxide. Less satisfactory analgesia results when nitrous oxide is administered only during uterine contractions because about 50 seconds are necessary to achieve an effective analgesic concentration of this drug. Intermittent inhalation of methoxyflurane (0.1 percent to 0.3 percent inhaled) by self-administration or passively from an anesthetic machine is an alternative to the continuous administration of nitrous oxide. It must be appreciated that maternal and neonatal serum fluoride concentrations are increased after the administration of methoxyflurane.[1] Methoxyflurane should not be used in parturients with coexisting renal disease as may accompany toxemia of pregnancy. Enflurane (0.5 percent inspired) provides analgesia during the second stage of labor similar to that achieved with nitrous oxide.[13]

ANESTHESIA FOR CESAREAN SECTION

Cesarean section is one of the most frequent of all surgical procedures. Indications for cesarean section include fetal distress, cephalopelvic disproportion, and failure of labor to progress. The notion that a previous cesarean section mandates the same route of delivery for all subsequent deliveries has been modified and in selected patients (prior low segment transverse uterine incision and cephalic presentation), it is acceptable to allow vaginal delivery.

The decision to select a general or regional anesthetic to provide analgesia for cesarean section depends on the desires of the parturient and the presence or absence of fetal distress. When fetal distress is present, a general anesthetic may be preferable because anesthesia can be established quickly and maternal hypotension is less likely. A regional anesthetic is more often chosen for elective cesarean section, particularly when maternal awareness is desirable. Furthermore, a regional anesthetic minimizes the likelihood of maternal pulmonary aspiration and fetal depression.

General Anesthetic

Preoperative medication often includes pharmacologic attempts to increase gastric fluid pH. It is common practice to administer antacids for this purpose, although H_2-receptor antagonists are also effective for increasing gastric fluid pH (see the section *Gastrointestinal Changes*). Metoclopramide may be useful for decreasing gastric fluid volume before induction of anesthesia, especially if the parturient is in active labor. If anticholinergics are judged to be necessary, glycopyrrolate may be preferred because its quaternary ammonium structure prevents significant transfer across lipid barriers such as the placenta. If the cesarean section is elective, a benzodiazepine may be administered if the parturient is particularly apprehensive.

After preoxygenation, induction of anesthesia is typically accomplished with thiopental (2 $mg \cdot kg^{-1}$ to 4 $mg \cdot kg^{-1}$) plus succinylcholine to facilitate intubation of the trachea with a cuffed tube. Cricoid pressure should be applied until the trachea is protected with the cuffed tube. Administration of small doses of nondepolarizing muscle relaxants (d-tubocurarine 3 mg) before succinylcholine is often used to prevent skeletal muscle fasiculations. Nevertheless, fasiculations are not prominent in parturients, causing some to question the need for prior administration of nondepolarizing muscle relaxants. The fetal brain will not be exposed to high concentrations of thiopental if the maternal dose is limited to about 4 $mg \cdot kg^{-1}$, reflecting clearance of the drug by the fetal liver and dilution by blood from the viscera and lower extremities.

Maintenance of anesthesia until delivery of the fetus is often with nitrous oxide (50 percent to 60 percent inspired) in oxygen plus succinylcholine for skeletal muscle paralysis. The major disadvantage of using only nitrous oxide is parturient awareness during the surgery. Maternal uncon-

Table 26-5. Dose of Local Anesthetic for Spinal Block Before Cesarean Section

Height (cm)	Tetracaine (mg)	Lidocine (mg)
Below 155	7	50
155 to 170	8	60
Above 170	9	70

sciousness can be assured by the administration of about 0.5 MAC of a volatile anesthetic plus nitrous oxide. This low dose of a volatile anesthetic does not increase maternal blood loss, alter the response of the uterus to oxytocin, or produce neonatal depression. Finally, nitrous oxide supplemented with volatile anesthetics is associated with reduced autonomic nervous system responses to surgical stimulation and better maintenance of uterine blood flow. This response is presumed to reflect inhibition of endogenous norepinephrine secretion by the volatile anesthetics. Excessive hyperventilation of the lungs must be avoided as the effects of positive pressure can reduce uterine blood flow.

There is controversy regarding the optimal time for delivery when a general anesthetic is used for cesarean section. More important than duration of anesthesia before delivery is the time to delivery after incision into the uterus. Apgar scores are often decreased when the uterine incision-to-delivery time exceeds 90 seconds, presumably reflecting impaired uteroplacental blood flow.

After delivery, anesthesia can be supplemented with additional volatile drugs or opioids. It would seem reasonable to pass an oral tube into the stomach to evacuate gastric fluid before the conclusion of surgery. The cuffed tube should not be removed from the trachea until it is ensured that maternal laryngeal reflexes have returned.

Spinal Block

Spinal block used for cesarean section must provide a sensory level of T4–6. A convenient guide for judging the appropriate dose of local anesthetic to be injected into the subarachnoid space is based on the height of the parturient (Table 26-5). Addition of morphine (0.2 mg to 0.25 mg) to the local anesthetic solution provides postoperative pain relief for about 24 hours. After injection the parturient is placed supine with leftward displacement of the uterus.

The T4–6 sensory level necessary for cesarean section is associated with significant peripheral sympathetic nervous system blockade and the likelihood of maternal hypotension. Hypotension is hazardous because a decrease in maternal blood pressure is associated with comparable falls in uterine blood flow and placental perfusion leading to fetal hypoxemia and acidosis. The incidence and magnitude of hypotension may be minimized by continuous left uterine displacement, intravenous hydration with 500 ml to 1000 ml of lactated Ringer's solution 15 minutes to 30 minutes before performing the block, and the intramuscular injection of 25 mg to 50 mg of ephedrine approximately 15 minutes before performing the block. If hypotension occurs (systolic blood pressure below 100 mmHg or a 30 percent decrease in a previously hypertensive parturient) despite these measures, an intravenous dose of ephedrine (5 mg to 10 mg) is indicated. Backache is a frequent complaint in parturients and the incidence does not increase after regional anesthesia. Nerve damage is not a risk of spinal block, with the most common neurologic dysfunction in the postpartum period being caused by compression of the lumbosacral trunk between the descending fetal head and the sacrum. Lumbosacral trunk injuries are characterized by foot drop combined with sensory loss.

Lumbar Epidural Block

The sensory level necessary for a cesarean section is more controllable and hypotension less precipitous with a continuous lumbar epidural block. Presumably, the slower onset of peripheral sympathetic nervous system blockade is responsible for the more gradual decrease in blood pressure. Unlike spinal block, anesthesia provided with a lumbar epidural block requires doses of local anesthetics that are associated with significant systemic absorption of the drug. Technically, a lumbar epidural block is more difficult to perform than a spinal block. However, postoperative headache does not occur because the dura is not punctured.

Bupivacaine concentrations must be at least 0.5 percent to assure adequate anesthesia for the surgical stimulus associated with cesarean section. This contrasts with adequate analgesia for vaginal delivery produced by 0.25 percent bupivacaine. Limitation of the concentration of bupivacine to 0.5 percent is recommended to minimize the likelihood of cardiotoxicity should this local anesthetic be accidently injected intravenously (see Chapter 7). An initial 3 ml test dose of local anesthetic containing 1:200,000 epinephrine usually produces maternal tachycardia if administered intravenously and signs of spinal block if it enters the subarachnoid space. Assuming the absence of evidence of a spinal block 3 minutes after the test dose, an additional amount (about 15 ml to 20 ml) of bupivacaine is injected through the lumbar epidural catheter so as to produce a T4–6 sensory level. When a rapid onset of analgesia is necessary, 3 percent 2-chloroprocaine can be used. When chloroprocaine is used, it is imperative that subarachnoid injection be avoided since permanent neurologic damage has been reported after accidental subarachnoid injection of large volumes of this local anesthetic.[14] Lidocaine, 2 percent, is an acceptable alternative to either bupivacaine or chloroprocaine. Analgesia in the postoperative period may be provided by injection of opioids (morphine 3 mg to 5 mg) into the epidural space.[15]

ABNORMAL PRESENTATIONS AND MULTIPLE BIRTHS

Description of fetal position is based on the relationship of the fetal occiput, chin, or sacrum to the left or right side of the parturient. Approximately 90 percent of the deliveries are cephalic presentation in either the occiput transverse or occiput anterior position. All other presentations and positions are considered abnormal.

Persistent Occiput Posterior

During active labor, the occiput undergoes internal rotation to the occiput anterior position. If this rotation does not occur, the persistent occiput posterior position results in prolonged and painful labor. For example, severe back pain reflects pressure on the posterior sacral nerves by the fetal occiput. Regional anesthetic techniques that relax the maternal perineal muscles are often avoided until spontaneous internal rotation of the fetal head occurs.

Breech Presentation

Breech deliveries are associated with increased maternal (cervical lacerations, retained placenta, hemorrhage) and neonatal (intracranial hemorrhage, prolapse of the umbilical cord) morbidity. There is a tendency to deliver breech presentations by elective cesarean section. If cesarean section is planned, either a regional or general anesthetic may be selected. It should be appreciated that during a regional anesthetic, there may be difficulty in extracting the infant through the uterine incision. If uterine hypertonus is the cause, it will be necessary to rapidly induce general anesthesia, intubate the trachea, and administer volatile anesthetics to relax the uterus.

When vaginal delivery is planned for breech presentations, a frequent approach is infiltration of the perineum with local anesthetics plus inhalation analgesia. Rapid induction of general anesthesia and intubation of the trachea may be necessary to permit administration of volatile anesthetics should perineal muscle relaxation be inadequate for delivery of the aftercoming fetal head or if the lower uterine segment contracts and traps the head. An alternative to infiltration and inhalation analgesia is the use of a continuous lumbar epidural block. For example, a lumbar epidural block provides analgesia and maximal perineal relaxation for delivery of the fetal head. The ability of parturients to push during delivery can be preserved by using low concentrations of local anesthetics (0.25 percent bupivacaine) and providing constant maternal encouragement. However, if uterine relaxation is required for facilitation of a breech extraction during vaginal delivery, it will be necessary to induce general anesthesia.

Multiple Gestations

Choice of anesthesia in the presence of multiple gestations must consider the frequent occurrence of prematurity and breech presentation. Inhalation analgesia plus local infiltration or continuous lumbar epidural block are acceptable methods of anesthesia in these patients. Systemic medications, such as opioids, should be minimized, particularly if the fetus is premature.

PREGNANCY AND HEART DISEASE

Detection and evaluation of heart disease in parturients is crucial for planning management of anesthesia during labor and delivery. Increased cardiac output during pregnancy and after delivery may result in congestive heart failure in parturients with co-existing heart disease. For example, each uterine contraction increases cardiac output and central blood volume 10 percent to 25 percent. Subsequent delivery of the fetus and emptying of the uterus relieves compression of the inferior vena cava and aorta, resulting in marked increases in blood volume.

For most types of heart disease, no single technique of anesthesia is specifically indicated or contraindicated. Nevertheless, analgesia produced by a continuous lumbar epidural block can minimize the adverse effects of increased cardiac output, particularly when this increase is exaggerated by pain or anxiety. Inhalation analgesia is usually selected when sudden reductions in systemic vascular resistance and blood pressure would be detrimental.

TOXEMIA OF PREGNANCY

Toxemia of pregnancy refers to either pre-eclampsia or eclampsia. Pre-eclampsia is a syndrome manifesting after the 20th week of gestation characterized by hypertension (above 140/90 mmHg), proteinuria (greater than 2 g·day^{-1}), generalized edema and complaints of headache. Manifestations of pre-eclampsia usually abate within 48 hours after delivery. Eclampsia is present when seizures are superimposed on pre-eclampsia. Eclampsia occurs in about 5 percent of patients with pre-eclampsia and is associated with a maternal mortality of about 10 percent. Cerebral hemorrhage is the most common cause of death.

The etiology of toxemia of pregnancy is un-

known but may involve an antigen-antibody reaction between fetal and maternal tissues in the first trimester that initiates a placental vasculitis. This vasculitis is presumed to decrease placental perfusion, which initiates the release of vasoactive substances (renin, angiotensin, aldosterone) responsible for clinical manifestations of toxemia of pregnancy. An imbalance between the placental production of prostacyclin and thromboxane is consistent with placental ischemia, systemic vasoconstriction, and increased platelet aggregation. Indeed, toxemia of pregnancy involves nearly every system.

Treatment

Definitive treatment of toxemia of pregnancy is delivery of the fetus and placenta. In the interim, magnesium and antihypertensives may be required. A general or regional anesthetic should not be used in attempts to lower blood pressure.

Magnesium

Magnesium is effective in parturients with toxemia of pregnancy by decreasing the irritability of the central nervous system, which reduces the likelihood of seizures. Magnesium also decreases hyperactivity at the neuromuscular junction, presumably by reducing the presynaptic release of acetylcholine as well as by decreasing the sensitivity of postjunctional membranes to acetylcholine. In addition, magnesium relaxes uterine and vascular smooth muscle, which contributes to an increase in uterine blood flow.

Clinically, the therapeutic effects of magnesium therapy are estimated by the responsiveness of deep tendon reflexes. Marked depression of these reflexes is an indication of impending magnesium toxicity. Periodic determination of serum magnesium concentrations is also helpful in adjusting supplemental doses of magnesium so as to keep the level in a therapeutic range of 4 mEq·L^{-1} to 6 mEq·L^{-1}. Serum magnesium levels in excess of this range can lead to severe skeletal muscle weakness, hypoventilation, and cardiac arrest. Intravenous administration of calcium is the antidote for toxic effects of magnesium. Finally, magnesium is

---

Pathophysiology of Toxemia of Pregnancy

Cardiovascular system
    Generalized vasoconstriction
    Increased vascular responsiveness to sympathetic nervous system stimulation
    Decreased colloid oncotic pressure
    Decreased uteroplacental perfusion

Hepatorenal system
    Decreased hepatic blood flow
    Decreased glomerular filtration rate
    Decreased renal blood flow
    Retention of sodium and water

Respiratory system
    Interstitial accumulation of fluid
    Decreased PaO_2
    Exaggerated edema of upper airway and larynx

Central nervous system
    Hyperreflexia
    Cerebral edema
    Seizure activity

Intravascular fluid volume
    Hypovolemia

Coagulation
    Decreased platelet count
    Increased fibrin split products

Uterus
    Hyperactive
    Premature labor

---

excreted by the kidneys and must be used with caution when renal function is impaired.

Potentiation of depolarizing and nondepolarizing muscle relaxants is produced by magnesium. Furthermore, toxemia of pregnancy may be associated with reductions in plasma cholinesterase activity that are greater than those normally associated with pregnancy, resulting in potentiation of the effects of succinylcholine independent of magnesium therapy. This introduces the need for careful titration of the doses of muscle relaxants and monitoring the effects produced by these drugs at the neuromuscular junction. Likewise, doses of sedatives and opioids should be reduced as magnesium can also potentiate their effects. Because magnesium readily crosses the placenta, neonatal muscle tone can be decreased at birth.

Antihypertensives

Antihypertensives are likely to be administered when the diastolic blood pressure exceeds 110 mmHg. Hydralazine is frequently selected because of its rapid onset and ability to maintain or even increase renal blood flow. A continuous intravenous infusion of trimethaphan may be lifesaving in the parturient with a hypertensive crisis. Nitroprusside is not recommended because of the fact that cyanide resulting from the breakdown of this vasodilator can cross the placenta and the theoretical concern that this passage could produce adverse effects on the fetus. The goal is to reduce diastolic blood pressure to about 100 mmHg. Fetal heart rate should be monitored continuously during reduction of maternal blood pressure with drugs to insure an early warning if the uteroplacental circulation is being jeopardized by reduced perfusion pressures.

Management of Anesthesia

Continuous lumbar epidural block is acceptable for vaginal delivery of the pre-eclamptic parturient in good medical control. Epidural block negates the need for maternal opioids and the possible adverse effects of these drugs on a premature fetus. The absence of the maternal urge to bear down reduces the likelihood of associated blood pressure increases. Before the lumbar epidural block is instituted the parturient should be hydrated with intravenous fluids (1 liter to 2 liters of lactated Ringer's solution) as guided by central venous pressure monitoring. Furthermore, coagulation studies should be performed before the placement of the lumbar epidural catheter. Initially, a segmental band of anesthesia (T10–L1) will provide analgesia for uterine contractions. As the second stage of labor is entered, the lumbar epidural block can be extended to provide perineal anesthesia. If hypotension occurs, the hypersensitivity of the maternal vasculature to catecholamines must be considered and reduced intravenous doses of ephedrine (2.5 mg) administered.

Cesarean section is necessary when fetal distress, reflecting deterioration of uteroplacental circulation, accompanies toxemia of pregnancy. A general anesthetic is usually selected because a regional anesthetic would be associated with extensive peripheral sympathetic nervous system blockade. Before induction of anesthesia, an attempt must be made to restore intravascular fluid volume. Continuous monitoring of intra-arterial pressure, cardiac filling pressures, urine output, and fetal heart rate is indicated. Induction of anesthesia is often with thiopental (2 $mg \cdot kg^{-1}$ to 4 $mg \cdot kg^{-1}$) plus succinylcholine to facilitate rapid intubation of the trachea. The use of defasiculating doses of nondepolarizing muscle relaxants before the administration of succinylcholine may not be necessary because magnesium therapy is likely to attenuate skeletal muscle fasiculations produced by the depolarizing drug. Exaggerated edema of the upper airway structures may require the use of smaller tracheal tubes than anticipated. The blood pressure increase elicited by direct laryngoscopy and intubation of the trachea is predictably exaggerated in these parturients. A short duration of direct laryngoscopy is helpful for minimizing the magnitude and duration of the blood pressure increases. Hydralazine (5 mg to 10 mg) administered intravenously 10 minutes to 15 minutes before the induction of anesthesia or intravenous nitroglycerin (1 $\mu g \cdot kg^{-1}$ to 2 $\mu g \cdot kg^{-1}$) just before starting direct laryngoscopy has also been recommended for attenuating these blood pressure responses. Volatile anesthetics can be used to control intraoperative hypertension. The potentiation of all muscle relaxants by magnesium must be remembered and a peripheral nerve stimulator used to monitor the effect of reduced doses of muscle relaxants at the neuromuscular junction.

HEMORRHAGE IN THE PARTURIENT

Hemorrhage in the parturient is the leading cause of maternal mortality. Placenta previa and abruptio placenta are the major causes of bleeding during the third trimester. Uterine rupture can be responsible for uncontrolled hemorrhage that manifests during labor. Postpartum hemorrhage occurs in 3 percent to 5 percent of all vaginal deliveries and is typically due to retained placenta, uterine atony, or cervical or vaginal lacerations.

Placenta Previa

Placenta previa is the abnormally low implantation of the placenta in the uterus. The cardinal symptom of placenta previa is painless vaginal bleeding that typically manifests around the 32nd week of gestation when the lower uterine segment is beginning to form. When this diagnosis is suspected, the position of the placenta should be confirmed by ultrasonography or radioisotope scan. If these tests are not conclusive and vaginal bleeding persists, the diagnosis is made by direct examination of the cervical os. This examination should be done in the delivery room, only after preparations have been taken to replace acute blood loss and to proceed with an emergency cesarean section. Ketamine is a useful drug for induction of anesthesia in the presence of acute hemorrhage due to placenta previa. Maintenance of anesthesia before delivery is typically 50 percent nitrous oxide plus succinylcholine to produce skeletal muscle relaxation. Neonates delivered from parturients in hemorrhagic shock are likely to be acidotic and hypovolemic.

Abruptio Placentae

Abruptio placentae is the separation of a normally implanted placenta after 20 weeks of gestation. When the separation involves only the placental margin, the escaping blood can appear as vaginal bleeding. Alternatively, large volumes of blood loss can remain entirely concealed in the uterus. Severe blood loss from abruptio placentae manifests as maternal hypotension, uterine irritability, and hypertonia plus fetal distress. Clotting abnormalities resembling disseminated intravascular coagulation can occur.

The definitive treatment of abruptio placentae is to empty the uterus. If there are no signs of maternal hypovolemia, clotting abnormalities, or fetal distress, the use of a continuous lumbar epidural block is useful to provide anesthesia for labor and vaginal delivery. However, when the magnitude of hemorrhage is severe, an emergency cesarean section is necessary using a general anesthetic with ketamine for induction of anesthesia and nitrous oxide for maintenance of anesthesia. It is predictable that neonates born under these circumstances will be acidotic and hypovolemic.

Uterine Rupture

Uterine rupture can be associated with separation of a previous uterine scar, rapid spontaneous delivery, or excessive oxytocin stimulation. Overall, however, more than 80 percent of uterine ruptures are spontaneous without an obvious explanation. Manifestations of uterine rupture include complaints of severe abdominal pain, maternal hypotension, and disappearance of fetal heart tones.

Retained Placenta

Retained placenta occurs in about 1 percent of all vaginal deliveries and usually necessitates manual exploration of the uterus. If a lumbar epidural or spinal block was not used for vaginal delivery, manual removal of the placenta may be initially attempted under continuous inhalation analgesia. Induction of general anesthesia with intubation of the trachea and administration of volatile drugs to provide uterine relaxation will be necessary if the uterus remains firmly contracted around the placenta.

Uterine Atony

Uterine atony as a cause of postpartum hemorrhage can occur immediately after delivery or manifest several hours later. Retained placenta is a common accompaniment of uterine atony. Treatment is with synthetic oxytocins (Pitocin, Syntocinon), which do not contain vasopressin. Dilute solutions of synthetic oxytocins exert no cardiovascular effects; but bolus injections may be associated with tachycardia, vasodilation, and hypotension. These cardiovascular effects are avoided by infusion of 10 units to 15 units of synthetic oxytocin in 500 ml of balanced salt solution until uterine contraction is adequate. Finally, synthetic oxytocins, because they lack vasopressin, do not produce exaggerated blood pressure increases in parturients who have been previously treated with sympathomimetics.

AMNIOTIC FLUID EMBOLISM

Amniotic fluid embolism is signalled by the sudden onset of respiratory distress, hypotension, and arterial hypoxemia, reflecting the cardiopulmonary effects of entrance of amniotic fluid into the circulation. Multiparous parturients who experience a tumultuous labor are most likely to experience an amniotic fluid embolism. Definitive diagnosis is made by demonstrating amniotic fluid material in maternal blood that has been aspirated from a central venous catheter. Treatment is directed toward cardiopulmonary resuscitation and correction of arterial hypoxemia. Conditions that can mimic an amniotic fluid embolism include inhalation of gastric contents and pulmonary embolus.

ANESTHESIA FOR NONOBSTETRIC SURGERY DURING PREGNANCY

The objectives for management of anesthesia in parturients undergoing nonobstetric surgery, such as excision of an ovarian cyst or appendectomy, are avoidance of teratogenic drugs, avoidance of intrauterine fetal hypoxia and acidosis, and prevention of premature labor. There is always the possibility that anesthesia may be unknowingly administered in early undiagnosed pregnancy.

Avoidance of Teratogenic Drugs

Most drugs, including anesthetics, have been demonstrated to be teratogenic in at least one animal species. In humans, the critical period of organogenesis is between 15 days and 56 days of gestation. Nevertheless, there is no evidence that anesthetics administered during pregnancy are teratogenic. Sufficient circumstantial evidence exists, however, to warrant caution in the administration of nitrous oxide to women during pregnancy.[16] There is no evidence in humans that drugs administered to produce analgesia during labor and vaginal delivery adversely affect later mental and neurologic development of the offspring.

Avoidance of Intrauterine Fetal Hypoxia and Acidosis

Intrauterine fetal hypoxia and acidosis are prevented by avoiding maternal hypotension, arterial hypoxemia, and excessive changes in the $PaCO_2$.

High inspired concentrations of oxygen do not produce in utero retrolental fibroplasia because high oxygen consumption of the placenta plus uneven distribution of the maternal and fetal blood flow in the placenta prevents fetal PaO_2 from exceeding about 45 mmHg.

Prevention of Premature Labor

The underlying pathology necessitating the surgery and not the anesthetic or technique of anesthesia determines the onset of premature labor. After successful completion of surgery, it is advisable to continue monitoring the fetal heart rate and maternal uterine activity. Premature labor can be treated with beta-2 agonists such as terbutaline or ritodrine. These drugs relax uterine smooth muscle resulting in inhibition of uterine contractions and improved uteroplacental blood flow. Side effects that may accompany beta-2 agonist therapy include maternal hypokalemia and cardiac dysrhythmias and fetal tachycardia and hypoglycemia.

Management of Anesthesia

Elective surgery should always be deferred until after delivery. When surgery is necessary, it is best to delay the operation until the second or third trimester. Emergency surgery in the first trimester is often performed with a lumbar epidural block or spinal block. Spinal block is useful as this technique limits fetal drug exposure to a minimum. Continuous intraoperative monitoring of fetal heart rate, after the 16th week of gestation, is helpful in providing early warning of fetal distress due to impaired uteroplacental perfusion (see the section *Diagnosis and Management of Fetal Distress*). When a general anesthetic is chosen, it should be appreciated that low concentrations of volatile drugs are not associated with significant reductions in uterine blood flow. Regardless of the technique of anesthesia selected, it is recommended that inhaled concentrations of oxygen be at least 50 percent.

DIAGNOSIS AND MANAGEMENT OF FETAL DISTRESS

Fetal well-being is often determined by evaluation of beat-to-beat variability in fetal heart rate as computed from R wave intervals on the fetal electrocardiogram. The fetal electrocardiogram is obtained via an electrode placed on the presenting fetal part or indirectly via ultrasound using a sensor placed on the maternal abdomen. Another useful method for monitoring fetal well-being is evaluation of fetal heart rate decelerations associated with contractions of the uterus. Fetal heart rate decelerations are classified as early, late, and variable. Fetal scalp blood sampling is indicated when abnormal fetal heart rate patterns occur. It has been observed that the fetus is usually depressed when one or more fetal scalp pH values are below 7.2.

Beat-to-Beat Variability

Fetal heart rate varies 5 beats·min^{-1} to 20 beats·min^{-1}, with a normal heart rate ranging between 120 beats·min^{-1} to 160 beats·min^{-1}. This normal variability is thought to reflect the integrity of the neural pathway from the fetal cerebral cortex through the medulla, vagus nerves, and cardiac conduction system. Fetal well-being is assured when beat-to-beat variability is present. Conversely, fetal distress, due to arterial hypoxemia, acidosis, or central nervous system damage is associated with minimal to absent variability of the heart rate. Drugs (local anesthetics used for continuous lumbar epidural block, benzodiazepines, opioids, anticholinergics) administered to parturients may eliminate fetal heart rate variability even in the absence of fetal distress. This drug-induced effect does not appear to be deleterious but may cause difficulty in the interpretation of fetal heart rate monitoring.

Early Decelerations

Early decelerations are characterized by slowing of the fetal heart rate that begins with the onset of the uterine contraction (Fig. 26-9).[17] This deceleration pattern is thought to be caused by vagal stimulation secondary to compression of the fetal head and is not indicative of fetal distress.

Late Decelerations

Late decelerations are characterized by slowing of the fetal heart rate that begins 10 seconds to 30 seconds after the onset of the uterine contraction (Fig. 26-10).[17] This deceleration pattern is associ-

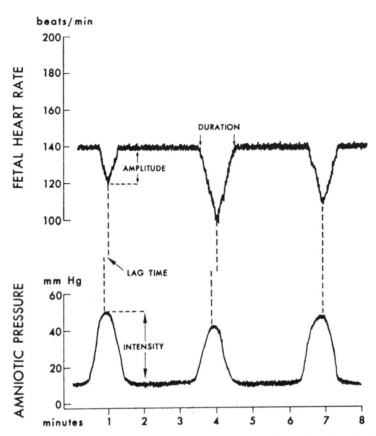

Fig. 26-9. Early decelerations of the fetal heart rate are characterized by a short lag time between the onset of the uterine contraction and the beginning of heart rate slowing. The maximum fetal heart rate slowing occurs at the peak intensity of the contraction. Fetal heart rate is back to normal by the time the contraction has ceased. The most likely explanation for this fetal heart rate slowing is vagal stimulation due to compression of the fetal head. (From Shnider,[17] with permission.)

ated with fetal distress, most likely reflecting myocardial hypoxia secondary to uteroplacental insufficiency as produced by maternal hypotension. Determination of fetal scalp pH is indicated when this pattern persists.

Variable Decelerations

As the designation indicates, these deceleration patterns are variable in magnitude, duration, and time of onset (Fig. 26-11).[17] Variable decelerations are thought to be caused by umbilical cord compression. Unless prolonged beyond 30 seconds or associated with fetal bradycardia less than 70

beats·min^{-1}, they are usually benign. Changing maternal position often lessens or abolishes this pattern.

EVALUATION OF THE NEONATE

The importance of assessment of the neonate immediately after birth is to promptly identify depressed infants who require active resuscitation (see Chapter 27). As a guide to identifying and treating the neonate, the Apgar score has not been surpassed.

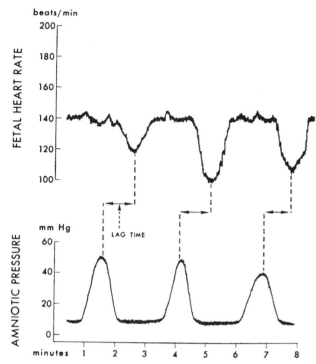

Fig. 26-10. Late decelerations of the fetal heart rate are characterized by a delay between the onset of the uterine contraction and the beginning of fetal heart rate slowing. The fetal heart rate does not return to normal until after the contraction has ceased. Late decelerations indicate uteroplacental insufficiency. (From Shnider,[17] with permission.)

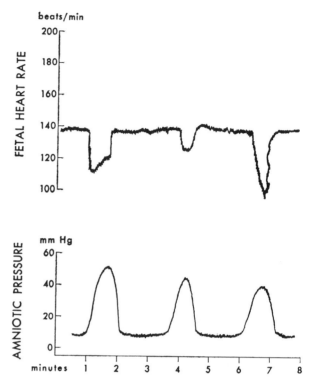

Fig. 26-11. Variable decelerations of fetal heart rate are characterized by varying magnitudes and time of onset of heart rate slowing. This pattern is usually benign but if persistent may reflect compression of the umbilical cord. (From Shnider,[17] with permission.)

Apgar Score

The Apgar score assigns a numerical value to five vital signs measured or observed in neonates 1 minute and 5 minutes after delivery (Table 26-6). Of the five criteria, the heart rate and quality of the respiratory effort are the most important in identifying depressed newborns. A heart rate less than 100 beats·min⁻¹ usually signifies arterial hypoxemia. When Apgar scores are above 7, neonates are either normal or have a mild respiratory acidosis. Mild to moderately depressed infants (scores 3 to 7) frequently improve in response to oxygen administered via a face mask, with or without positive pressure ventilation of the lungs. Intubation of the trachea and perhaps external cardiac massage are indicated when the score is less than 3 (see Chapter 27).

Neurobehavioral Testing

Neurobehavioral testing is able to detect subtle or delayed effects of drugs administered during labor and delivery that are not appreciated by the Apgar score. This testing evaluates the neonate's state of wakefulness, reflex responses, skeletal muscle tone, and responses to sound. Studies of local anesthetics used to provide epidural block have not revealed differences in neurobehavioral scores in neonates exposed to lidocaine or bupivacaine.[18] Compared with spinal blocks, the use of general anesthesia for elective cesarean sections is associated with depression of neurobehavioral testing despite similar Apgar scores in both groups. De-

Table 26-6. Evaluation of the Neonate Using the Apgar Score

Variable	Score		
	Zero	One	Two
Heart rate (beats·min^{-1})	Absent	Below 100	Above 100
Respiratory effort	Absent	Slow	Irregular crying
Reflex irritability	No response	Grimace	Cry
Muscle tone	Limp	Flexion of extremities	Active
Color	Cyanotic	Body pink and extremities cyanotic	Pink

spite this difference, there is no evidence of prolonged adverse effects.[18]

POSTPARTUM TUBAL LIGATION

Postpartum tubal ligation is the most common type of surgery performed in the early postpartum period. Residual epidural anesthesia from the preceding delivery may be used to perform the intraabdominal procedure, which necessitates a T5 level to assure patient comfort. When epidural or spinal blocks have not been used for delivery, it is common to wait 8 hours to 12 hours postpartum before inducing anesthesia for tubal ligation in hopes of improving the likelihood of gastric emptying.

REFERENCES

1. Morgan DJ, Blackman GL, Paull JD, Wolf LJ. Pharmacokinetics and plasma binding of thiopental. II: Studies at cesarean section. Anesthesiology 1981; 54:474–80.
2. Gare DJ, Shime J, Paul WM, Hoskins M. Oxygen administration during labor. Am J Obstet Gynecol 1969;105:954–61.
3. Palahniuk RJ, Shnider SM, Eger EI II. Pregnancy decreases the requirement of inhaled anesthetic agents. Anesthesiology 1974;41:82–3.
4. Fagraeus L, Urban BJ, Bromage PR. Spread of epidural analgesia in early pregnancy. Anesthesiology 1983;58:184–7.
5. Grundy EM, Zamora AM, Winnie AP. Comparison of spread of epidural anesthesia in pregnant and nonpregnant women. Anesth Analg 1979;57:544–6.
6. O'Sullivan GM, Bullingham RE. Noninvasive assignment by radiotelemetry of antacid effect during labor. Anesth Analg 1985;64:95–100.
7. Hodgkinson R, Glassenberg R, Joyce TH, Coombs DW, Ostheimer GW, Gibbs CP. Comparison of cimetidine (Tagamet) with antacid for safety and effectiveness in reducing gastric acidity before elective cesarean section. Anesthesiology 1983;59:86–90.
8. Ralston DH, Shnider SM, deLorimier AA. Effects of equipotent ephedrine, metaraminol, mephentermine, and methoxamine on uterine blood flow on the pregnant ewe. Anesthesiology 1974;40:354–70.
9. Shnider SM, Wright RG, Levinson G, et al. Uterine blood flow and plasma norepinephrine changes during maternal stress in the pregnant ewe. Anesthesiology 1979;50:524–7.
10. Biehl D, Shnider SM, Levinson G, Callender K. Placental transfer of lidocaine. Effects of fetal acidosis. Anesthesiology 1978;48:409–12.
11. Friedman EA. Primigravid labor. A graphicostatistical analysis. Obstet Gynecol 1955;6:567–89.
12. Cohen SE, Tan S, Albright GA, Halpren J. Epidural fentanyl/bupivacaine mixtures for obstetric analgesia. Anesthesiology 1987;67:403–7.
13. Abboud TK, Shnider SM, Wright RG, et al. Enflurane analgesia in obstetrics. Anesth Analg 1981; 60:133–7.
14. Ravindran RS, Bond VK, Tasch MD, Gupta CD, Luerssen TG. Prolonged neural blockade following regional analgesia with 2-chloroprocaine. Anesth Analg 1980;59:447–51.
15. Rosen MA, Hughes SC, Shnider SM, et al. Epidural morphine for the relief of postoperative pain after cesarean delivery. Anesth Analg 1983;62:666–72.
16. Davis AG, Moir DD. Anaesthesia during pregnancy. In: Ostheimer GN, ed. Clinics in Anaesthesiology. London, WB Saunders, 1986;4:233–46.
17. Shnider SM. Diagnosis of fetal distress: Fetal heart rate. In: Shnider SM, ed. Obstetrical anesthesia: Current Concepts and Practice. Baltimore, Williams & Wilkins, 1970; 197–203.
18. Corke BC. Neonatal neurobehavior II: Current clinical status. In: Ostheimer GW, ed. Clinics in Anaesthesiology. London, WB Saunders, 1986;4:219–27.

Chapter 27

Pediatrics

Understanding the physiologic and pharmacologic differences among neonates, infants, children, and adults permits principles used in adult anesthesia to be adapted to pediatric anesthesia. Neonates are defined as being 1 day to 28 days of age, infants are 1 month to 12 months of age, and children are 1 year to puberty.

PHYSIOLOGIC DIFFERENCES

One of the most important differences that physiologically separates neonates and infants from adults is oxygen consumption. Oxygen consumption in neonates may exceed $6 \text{ ml·kg}^{-1} \cdot \text{min}^{-1}$, which is about twice that of adults. To meet this increased demand, there are compensatory changes in the cardiovascular and respiratory systems that distinguish pediatric from adult patients (Tables 27-1 and 27-2).

Cardiovascular

Cardiac output is increased 30 percent to 60 percent in neonates so as to help meet the increased oxygen requirements of this age group. Furthermore, the oxyhemoglobin dissociation curve is shifted to the left, reflecting the presence of fetal hemoglobin. In this regard, both an elevated cardiac output and high hemoglobin concentration (average 17 g·dl^{-1}) are important to offset the decreased release of oxygen from fetal hemoglobin

to tissues. By 4 months to 6 months, oxyhemoglobin dissociation curves approximate those of adults. This change, as reflected by an increase in the P_{50} (arterial partial pressure of oxygen at which 50 percent of hemoglobin is saturated with oxygen) from 19 mmHg to about 26 mmHg, is preceded at 2 months to 3 months of age by a decrease in hemoglobin concentrations to about 11 g·dl^{-1} (physiologic anemia) as fetal hemoglobin is replaced by adult hemoglobin. Anemia sufficient to jeopardize oxygen carrying capacity of the blood is possible when hemoglobin concentrations are less than 13 g·dl^{-1} in the newborn or less than 10 g·dl^{-1} in infants older than 6 months.

Lack of distensibility of the neonate's left ventricle impairs diastolic filling and limits the significance of increasing the stroke volume as a means of increasing cardiac output. As a result, cardiac output in infants is, to a large extent, heart rate dependent.

Arterial blood pressure increases with increasing age. Anatomic closure of the foramen ovale occurs between 3 months and 1 year of age, although 20 percent to 30 percent of adults have probe-patent foramen ovales. Vasoconstrictive responses of neonates to hemorrhage are less than those of adults.

Respiratory

Alveolar ventilation is doubled in neonates compared to adults to help meet increased oxygen requirements of this age group. Carbon dioxide

Table 27-1. Comparison of Cardiovascular Variables

Age	Oxygen Consumption $(ml \cdot kg^{-1} \cdot min^{-1})$	Systolic Arterial Blood Pressure (mmHg)	Heart Rate $(beats \cdot min^{-1})$	Blood Volume $(ml \cdot kg^{-1})$	Hemoglobin $(g \cdot dl^{-1})$
Neonate	6	65	130	85	17
Infant	5	90	120	80	11
1 year	5	95	120	80	12
5 years	6	95	90	75	13
23 years	3	122	77	65	14

production is also increased in neonates, but elevated alveolar ventilation maintains a near normal $PaCO_2$. Because tidal volume on a weight basis is similar for both neonates and adults, increased alveolar ventilation is achieved by increasing the rate of breathing. The PaO_2 increases rapidly after birth, but several days are required to achieve levels comparable to older children. Control of ventilation is immature in neonates, contributing to less predictable responses than adults when hypoxic gas mixtures are inhaled.

Extracellular Fluid Volume

Extracellular fluid volume is equivalent to about 40 percent of the body weight of neonates compared to about 20 percent in adults. By 18 months to 24 months of age, the proportion of extracellular fluid volume relative to body weight is similar to that of adults. Increased metabolic rate characteristic of neonates results in accelerated turnover of extracellular fluid and dictates meticulous attention to intraoperative fluid replacement.

Temperature Regulation

To maintain normal body temperature, infants and children create heat by metabolizing brown fat, crying, and moving more vigorously but, unlike adults, rarely by shivering. Maintaining normal body temperature is more difficult in neonates and infants than in adults because of a larger surface-to-volume ratio, increased metabolic rate, and lack of sufficient body fat for insulation. Therefore, the neonate or infant is more likely than the adult to experience adverse reductions in body temperature when anesthetized in cold operating rooms.

Renal

The kidneys at birth are characterized by decreased glomerular filtration rate, decreased sodium excretion, and decreased concentrating abil-

Table 27-2. Comparison of Respiratory Variables

Age	Weight (kg)	Respiratory Rate $(breaths \cdot min^{-1})$	Tidal Volume $(ml \cdot kg^{-1})$	Vital Capacity $(ml \cdot kg^{-1})$	Alveolar Ventilation $(ml \cdot kg^{-1} \cdot min^{-1})$	Carbon Dioxide Production $(ml \cdot kg^{-1} \cdot min^{-1})$	Functional Residual Capcity $(ml \cdot kg^{-1})$
Neonate	3	35	6	35	130	6	25
Infant	6	30	6				25
1 year	10	24	6				25
5 years	18	20	6				35
23 years	70	15	6	70	60	3	40

ity. Over the first 3 months of life, glomerular filtration rate increases twofold to threefold. Thereafter, the rate of rise is slower until adult values are reached by 12 months to 24 months of age. After fluid restriction, maximum urine osmolarity for term neonates is about 525 mOsm·kg^{-1}. By 15 days to 30 days of age, maximum urine osmolarity may be as high as 950 mOsm·kg^{-1}. Still, it takes 6 months to 12 months before infants are able to concentrate urine as well as adults, emphasizing that this young age group is less able to compensate for extremes of fluid balance.

PHARMACOLOGIC DIFFERENCES

Pharmacologic differences between responses of pediatric and adult patients to drugs is predictable considering differences in extracellular fluid volume, metabolic rate, renal function, and receptor maturity. Specifically, there may be differences in anesthetic requirements and responses to muscle relaxants.

Inhaled Anesthetics

Both the uptake and distribution and potency of inhaled anesthetics differ in neonates and infants as compared to adults.[1-3] In general, the rate at which general anesthesia is induced is shortened in neonates as compared to adults. This is probably because of a smaller functional residual capacity per unit of body weight and a greater tissue blood flow, especially to vessel rich groups (brain, heart, liver, kidneys). For example, the vessel rich group composes approximately 10 percent of total body volume in adults, but 22 percent of total body volume in neonates.[1]

Full-term neonates require lower concentrations of volatile anesthetics than infants. For example, minimum alveolar concentration (MAC) for halothane in neonates is 0.87 percent compared to 1.20 percent in infants (Fig. 27-1).[2] Furthermore, MAC in preterm neonates is less than MAC in full-term neonates (Fig. 27-2).[3] MAC steadily increases until 2 months to 3 months of age. After 3 months of age, MAC progressively declines with aging, although there are slight increases at the time of puberty.

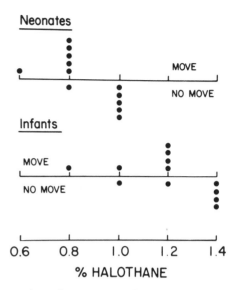

Fig. 27-1. Each circle represents the response (move or no move) of an individual neonate or infant. Halothane anesthetic requirements are reduced in neonates compared to infants. (From Lerman et al.,[2] with permission.)

Injected Anesthetics

An immature blood-brain barrier and decreased ability to metabolize drugs could increase the sensitivity of neonates to effects of barbiturates and opioids. As a result, neonates might require lower doses of these drugs to produce desired pharmacologic effects. Nevertheless, the dose of thiopental required to produce loss of the lid and corneal reflexes is similar in infants, children, and adults (Table 27-3).[4]

Muscle Relaxants and Their Antagonists

Neonates and infants are more sensitive than adults (lower plasma concentrations required to produce pharmacologic effects) to nondepolarizing muscle relaxants. Nevertheless, initial doses of these drugs are similar in both age groups because less drug actually reaches the neuromuscular junction, reflecting the impact of increased extracellular fluid volume and volume of distribution in younger patients (Fig. 27-3).[5] This increased sensitivity combined with reduced glomerular filtration rate (important with d-tubocurarine,

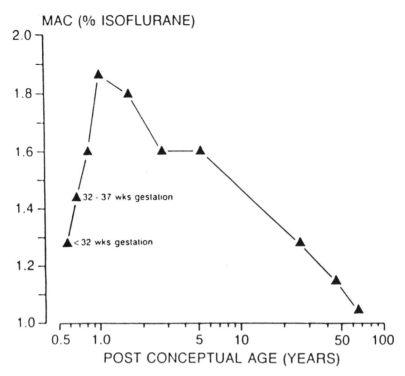

Fig. 27-2. The MAC of isoflurane in preterm neonates (less than 32 weeks gestation) and after 32 weeks to 37 weeks gestation is less (P<0.05) than full-term neonates and infants 1 month to 6 months of age. Values for postconceptual age were obtained by adding 40 weeks to the mean postnatal age for each age group. (From LeDez and Lerman,[3] with permission.)

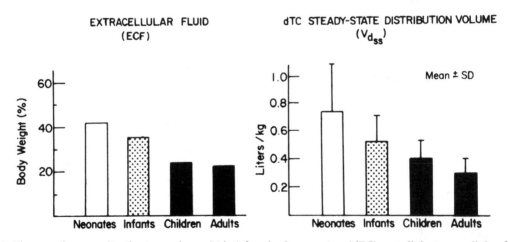

Fig. 27-3. The steady state distribution volume (Vdss) for d-tubocurarine (dTC) parallels extracellular fluid volume in neonates, infants, children, and adults (12 years to 30 years). The increased dilutional volume in neonates and infants masks an increased sensitivity of these age groups to nondepolarizing muscle relaxants. (From Fisher et al.,[5] with permission.)

Table 27-3. Thiopental Dose Response

	Dose that Produces Loss of Reflex ($mg \cdot kg^{-1}$) in 90% of Patients
Lid reflex	
Infants[a]	6.4
Young children	5.3
Adults	6.0
Corneal reflex	
Infants	7.0
Young children	6.9
Adults	6.1

[a] Infants 1 month to 11 months; young children 1 year to 4 years; adults 18 years to 42 years.
(Data from Brett and Fisher[4].)

metocurine, and pancuronium) may result in unexpected intense pharmacologic effects after administration of these drugs (Fig. 27-4).[5] In addition, decreased hepatic clearance can result in prolongation of the duration of action of vecuronium in neonates.[6] The dose of neostigmine required to antagonize nondepolarizing muscle relaxants is actually lower in pediatric patients (Fig. 27-5).[7] In clinical practice, however, it is not necessary to alter the doses of neostigmine administered to infants and children compared to adults.

Neonates and infants require more succinylcho-line on a body weight basis than older children to produce comparable degrees of skeletal muscle paralysis. For example, pediatric patients require $2 \ mg \cdot kg^{-1}$ succinylcholine administered intravenously to provide conditions for intubation of the trachea similar to those produced by $1 \ mg \cdot kg^{-1}$ administered to adults. Presumably, this increased dose requirement reflects dilutional effects of the increased extracellular fluid volume and volume of distribution characteristic of younger patients.

THE IMMEDIATE PREOPERATIVE PERIOD

Preoperative Evaluation

The purpose of the preoperative evaluation is to obtain the history, perform a physical examination, evaluate laboratory data, and to establish rapport with the child and parents. Pediatric anesthesia differs from adult anesthesia in that the history frequently must be obtained from the parent rather than the patient. This requires coordination between the anesthesia team and the hospital ward to ensure that the parents are available during the preanesthetic evaluation. The history should elicit congenital anomalies, allergies, bleeding tendencies, or a recent exposure to a communicable disease. Also, the medications the child is taking

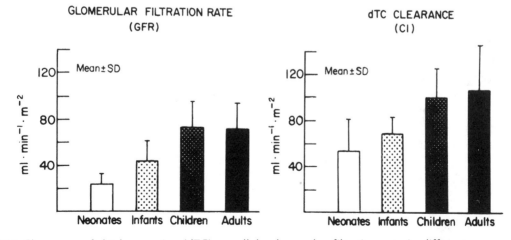

Fig. 27-4. Clearance of d-tubocurarine (dTC) parallels glomerular filtration rate in different age groups. (From Fisher et al.,[5] with permission.)

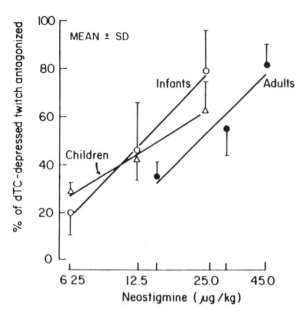

Fig. 27-5. Dose response curves demonstrate that infants and children require less neostigmine than adults to antagonize nondepolarizing neuromuscular blockade produced by d-tubocurarine (dTC). (From Fisher et al.,[7] with permission.)

should be determined. Finally, experiences with previous anesthetics should be sought.

Physical examination includes evaluation of the heart, lungs, and evidence of upper respiratory infections (fever, coryza). Recent upper respiratory infections can be reasons for delaying elective surgery because of secretions and increased airway reactivity. Also, the presence of loose teeth should be determined and dangerously loose teeth removed if necessary. The skin should be examined for evidence of dehydration or cyanosis (Table 27-4).

Laboratory data should seek evidence of hypoglycemia, hypocalcemia, or clotting disorders, which frequently occur in preterm infants or infants who have undergone asphyxia during birth. Also, if a history of vomiting or excessive fluid losses from diarrhea is evident, serum electrolytes, pH, and an assessment of extracellular fluid volume should be sought. If the hemoglobin is less than 10 g·dl^{-1}, the reason should be determined. Although hemoglobin concentrations below 10

Table 27-4. Changes Associated with Dehydration

Variable	Degree of Hydration (% decrease in body weight)		
	5	10	15
Skin turgor	↓	↓ ↓	↓ ↓ ↓
Sunken fontanelle	↓	↓ ↓	↓ ↓ ↓
Skin color	Pale	Gray	Mottled
Mucous membranes	Dry	Very dry	Parched
Urine	↓	↓ ↓	Anuria
Heart rate	No change	↑	↑ ↑

Symbols: ↓, slight decrease; ↓ ↓, moderate decrease; ↓ ↓ ↓, severe decrease; ↑, slight increase; ↑ ↑, moderate increase.

gl·dl^{-1} per se are not reasons for delaying elective operations, often previously unknown abnormalities will be detected.

Preoperative Medication

Obviously, the best preoperative medication scheme is a friendly, reassuring visit from the anesthesiologist. By answering questions and describing the operative procedure (sometimes with animated illustrations), the need for preoperative medication may be decreased. Still, barbiturates, opioids, and sedative-hypnotics are frequently administered for preoperative medication. Intramuscular injections can be avoided by administering drugs orally with water, or rectally 1 hour to 2 hours before surgery. Oral administration of 0.25 ml·kg^{-1} of a solution containing diazepam, meperidine, and atropine decreases the incidence of children crying on arriving in the operating room and does not delay recovery from anesthesia.[8] Rectally administered methohexital 10 mg·kg^{-1} to 25 mg·kg^{-1} can be given in a 10 percent solution. An 8 French 15-cm long catheter can be inserted approximately 3 cm into the rectum. The parents can hold the child while the drug is being administered and until the child falls asleep, which is usually in 5 minutes to 7 minutes. Once asleep, the patient can be transferred to the operating room. In many instances, pharmacologic preoperative medication is not necessary (see Chapter 10).

Pediatric Anesthetic Breathing Systems

The three most commonly used anesthetic breathing systems for pediatric anesthesia are the circle breathing system, the Ayre's T piece, and the Bain system (see Chapter 11). Heated and humidified anesthetic gases can reduce operative heat loss and possibly postoperative complications in neonates undergoing major abdominal or thoracic surgery. Therefore, whatever anesthetic breathing system is chosen, heated, humidified gases probably should also be used.

INDUCTION AND MAINTENANCE OF ANESTHESIA

An inhalation induction of anesthesia is very common for elective procedures in children and is especially easy to perform with halothane as compared to enflurane or isoflurane because the former has a less pungent smell. Sometimes, the induction of anesthesia can be facilitated by initially breathing 70 percent nitrous oxide with the gradual introduction of volatile anesthetics. Rapid increases in anesthetic concentrations should be avoided because it can be irritating to the respiratory tract, resulting in coughing and even laryngospasm. A constant monotone conversation by the anesthesiologist is conducive to a rapid induction of anesthesia. If an intravenous catheter is in place, anesthesia can be induced by conventional induction drugs including thiopental, methohexital, or ketamine. If an intravenous catheter is not in place, ketamine can be given intramuscularly with or without succinylcholine.

Intubation of the trachea is commonly facilitated by the intravenous administration of succinylcholine. Pretreatment with atropine administered intravenously protects against succinylcholine-induced heart rate slowing that may be particularly prominent in pediatric patients. Appreciation of anatomic differences between pediatric and adult patients is essential in performance of direct laryngoscopy for intubation of the trachea and selection of appropriately sized tracheal tubes (see Chapter 12). Indeed, postintubation laryngeal edema is unlikely if the size of the tube in the trachea is such that an audible air leak occurs around it during positive airway pressures equivalent to 15 cm H_2O to 25 cm H_2O. Treatment of postintubation laryngeal edema is with humidification of inspired gases and aerosolized racemic epinephrine.

Anesthesia should be maintained with concentrations of volatile anesthetics, which cause the fewest physiologic changes and still offer adequate surgical conditions (usually in the range of 1.1 MAC to 1.4 MAC). The signs of anesthesia required for adequate surgical conditions for neonates, infants, and children are similar to those for adults, such as movement and increases in heart rate and arterial pressure. A guide to depth of anesthesia in neonates and infants is loss of the sucking reflex. This can be tested by placing a finger in the patient's mouth, which would normally elicit sucking. In the absence of a sucking reflex, anesthetic concentrations are probably sufficient for surgery. Hypotension that accompanies administration of volatile anesthetics to neonates and infants most likely reflects unrecognized hypovolemia.[2,3]

When and How Should an Intravenous Infusion be Started?

Other than for very short surgical procedures, an intravenous infusion should be initiated in all children who are to be anesthetized. In many instances, an intravenous infusion is difficult to start preoperatively. After induction of anesthesia, however, especially with inhaled anesthetics, such as halothane, the peripheral veins dilate and movement of the child ceases, making placement of intravenous catheters much easier. Fluids are ideally delivered from a calculated drip chamber to assure that an excessive amount of fluid is not accidentally given intravenously.

Monitoring

Monitoring of pediatric patients should be the same as for adult patients undergoing comparable types of surgery (see Chapter 16). Arterial blood pressure, electrocardiogram, heart and breath sounds with an esophageal or precordial stethoscope, body temperature, and systemic oxygenation (transcutaneous oxygen electrode or pulse oximeter) should be monitored routinely in all infants and children undergoing surgery. Monitoring end-tidal carbon dioxide concentrations is useful but false low readings may occur because of small tidal volumes and relatively high inspired gas flows. Selection of the proper width blood pressure cuff (greater than one-third of the circumference of the limb) is important. For example, a cuff that is too small will produce an artificially elevated blood pressure, whereas one that is too large will produce a falsely low reading.

In seriously ill children who may be undergoing more extensive surgery, especially when hemorrhage or large shifts in extracellular fluid are expected, blood pressure probably should be monitored continuously via a catheter inserted into a peripheral artery. Monitoring of central venous pressure may aid in determining the adequacy of intravascular fluid volume. Central venous pressure can be measured via an umbilical vein catheter in neonates and either the internal jugular, external jugular, or subclavian vein in infants or children. Catheterization of the bladder and monitoring of urinary output also are helpful when blood loss or shifts in extracellular fluid volume are expected. Urinary output should probably exceed $0.5 \ ml \cdot kg^{-1} \cdot hr^{-1}$ and should have a specific gravity below 1.010. Analysis of arterial blood gases and pH is often helpful during extensive surgery. Acidosis is not uncommon during pediatric anesthesia. Also, the PaO_2 should be determined in premature infants in view of the risk of developing retinopathy of prematurity (see the section *Retinopathy of Prematurity*).

Hypoglycemia and hypocalcemia frequently occur in seriously ill infants. In these infants, blood glucose concentrations should be determined during surgery. If hypoglycemia occurs, $1 \ ml \cdot kg^{-1}$ to $3 \ ml \cdot kg^{-1}$ of a 20 percent glucose solution should be infused intravenously over a 5-minute period. Blood glucose concentrations should again be determined 15 minutes later to ensure that adequate glucose has been given. Conversely, excessive glucose levels should be avoided because osmotic diuresis and dehydration may result. Hypocalcemia can result in hypotension, poor peripheral perfusion, and cardiac failure, especially if the serum calcium levels are below $4.5 \ mEq \cdot L^{-1}$. If so, calcium gluconate, $100 \ mg \cdot kg^{-1}$, should be infused into a central vein while the electrocardiogram is being continuously monitored.

Fluid Maintenance and Replacement

Intraoperative fluid replacement may be considered as maintenance and replacement fluids (Table 27-5). Recommended fluids often contain glucose, although the notion that pediatric patients are more prone than adults to hypoglycemia is not a consistent observation. Maintenance fluids are best correlated with metabolic rate; replacement fluid requirements should be based on the underlying disease process, extent of surgery, and anticipated fluid translocation. Maintenance fluid requirements for the first 24 hours of life are about 80 $ml \cdot kg^{-1}$. In general, blood replacement is considered when the hematocrit decreases below 30 percent or when estimated blood loss exceeds 10 percent of the calculated blood volume of 80 $ml \cdot kg^{-1}$. The following formula can be used to estimate the acceptable blood loss before hematocrit reaches 30 percent and replacement is necessary.[9]

Acceptable blood loss = (estimated erythrocyte mass* − estimated erythrocyte mass when hematocrit is 30 percent)

For example, if a 4 kg infant has a preoperative hematocrit of 35 percent, approximately 50 ml of blood could be lost before the hematocrit would decrease to 30 percent. This formula, however, does not consider the dilutional aspect of crystalloid solution administration. Therefore, blood probably should be replaced when 30 ml to 35 ml of blood has been lost. If blood loss is to be replaced by crystalloid solution, then a volume of three times the estimated blood loss needs to be given, usually in the form of 0.9 percent saline or lactated Ringer's solution.

REGIONAL ANESTHESIA

Traditionally, regional anesthesia has not commonly been performed in pediatric patients.

---

* erythrocyte mass = blood volume ($80 \ ml \cdot kg^{-1}$) × hematocrit.

Table 27-5. Guidelines for Intraoperative Fluid Infusion Rates

	Lactated Ringer's Solution Plus Glucose $(ml \cdot kg^{-1} \cdot hr^{-1})$		
	Maintenance	Replacement	Total
Minor surgery (herniorrhaphy)	4	2	6
Moderate surgery (pyloromyotomy)	4	4	8
Extensive surgery (bowel resection)	4	6	10

Nevertheless, caudal anesthesia has been used to provide anesthesia and postoperative analgesia for lower abdominal, genitourinary, and rectal procedures. It is important to remember that the dural sac extends more caudad in children than in adults. Intravenous and axillary blocks have been used for repair of tendon laceration or fractures of one of the extremities. The administration of ketamine intramuscularly or intravenously may be used to facilitate the child's cooperation during regional anesthesia. Penile nerve block is easily performed and provides analgesia to the newborn undergoing circumcision.

NEWBORN RESUSCITATION

In a severely depressed newborn, immediate resuscitative efforts should take place. Although they are similar to adult resuscitative efforts, differences do exist, which need to be emphasized (see Chapter 34). In the immediate period of initial evaluation, the mouth and nose should be suctioned. Once breathing is established and the umbilical cord has stopped pulsating, the cord can be cut and the newborn taken to the resuscitative area. Stripping blood from the umbilical cord to the newborn increases blood volume, breathing rate, and pulmonary artery pressure. Indeed, early clamping of the cord may deprive the newborn of up to 30 $ml \cdot kg^{-1}$ of blood. The newborn should be placed in a radiantly heated resuscitation bed.

Apgar Scores

The Apgar source (0 to 10) determined 1 minute after birth can be used to guide the extent to which resuscitation is necessary (see Chapter 26).

8 to 10

Most newborns fall into this category, which requires little treatment other than suctioning of the pharynx and wrapping in a warm blanket.

5 to 7

Usually, these newborns have suffered mild asphyxia before birth. They usually respond to vigorous stimulation and blowing of oxygen over the face. If they do not respond in 1 minute to 2 minutes, ventilation of the lungs should be instituted via a bag and mask.

3 to 6

These newborns are moderately depressed, cyanotic, and have poor breathing efforts. It may be necessary to control ventilation of the lungs via a bag and mask. Ventilation of the lungs may be difficult because airway resistance is increased, which may cause gas to enter the esophagus, stomach, and gastrointestinal tract, leading to gastric distension and vomiting. If breathing has not started spontaneously, the trachea should be intubated and blood obtained from a doubly clamped segment of the umbilical cord for analysis of arterial blood gases and pH.

0 to 2

These newborns are severely asphyxiated and require prompt resuscitative efforts. The trachea should be immediately intubated and ventilation of the lungs controlled at a rate of 30 breaths to 60 breaths·min^{-1}. An occasional breath should be held for 2 seconds to 3 seconds to expand atelectatic areas. Also, positive end-expiratory pressure to 1 mmHg to 3 mmHg is often useful. The adequacy of ventilation of the lungs is best determined by physical examination and analysis of arterial blood gases. Both sides of the chest should rise equally and simultaneously. If one side rises before the other, the tip of the tracheal tube may have entered the bronchus or pneumothorax or (rarely) a diaphragmatic hernia may be present. An airway pressure greater than 25 cm H_2O should not be used. If the heart rate is less than 60 beats·min^{-1} external cardiac compressions are instituted.

The trachea should be suctioned before ventilation of the lungs, especially in infants born with meconium staining of the amniotic fluid. If meconium is distributed into the periphery of the lungs, a substantial number of these infants will develop pulmonary dysfunction in the first few days of life.

Vascular Resuscitation

If the response to ventilation of the lungs and stimulation is not immediate, an umbilical artery catheter should be inserted to permit analysis of arterial blood gases, pH, and blood pressure; to expand blood volume; and to administer drugs. The umbilical cord stump should be held straight up with a clamp and the abdomen and cord sterilized with an iodine-containing solution. The stump can then be tied near the base and the cord cleanly cut with a scalpel, leaving 1 cm to 2 cm of stump. The umbilical artery can then be dilated with a curved forcep. A 3.5-gauge to 5.0-gauge French umbilical artery catheter is advanced into the dilated vessel and connected to a three-way stopcock. Before injecting anything from the catheter, blood must be withdrawn to clear air from the catheter. Hypovolemic newborns are usually hypotensive (mean arterial pressure below 50 mmHg), pale, and have poor capillary filling and perfusion. Their extremities are cold and their pulses weak or absent. Hypovolemia is treated with blood, plasma, or crystalloid solutions. At times, the volume of fluid required may exceed 50 percent of the blood volume. On the other hand, care must be taken not to overexpand the intravascular fluid volume and cause hypertension.

UNUSUAL DISEASES THAT AFFECT PEDIATRIC PATIENTS

Diaphragmatic Hernia

Diaphragmatic hernia results from incomplete embryologic closure of the diaphragm such that intestinal contents occupy the chest (most often the left thorax) with associated hypoplasia of the lung on that side. The incidence of this defect is about 1 in every 5000 live births. Approximately 30 percent of cases of diaphragmatic hernia are associated with polyhydramnios. Manifestations at birth include a scaphoid abdomen and profound arterial hypoxemia. Radiographs of the chest demonstrate loops of intestine in the thorax and a shift of the mediastinum to the opposite side. Pulmonary hypertension and congenital heart disease are common.

Immediate treatment of the neonate is decompression of the stomach via a gastric tube and administration of oxygen, most often via a tracheal tube. Positive pressure ventilation of the lungs via a mask could further compromise pulmonary function if any gas passes via the esophagus to further increase gastric volume. Pneumothorax on the side opposite the hernia is a hazard if airway pressures exceed 25 cm H_2O during controlled ventilation of the lungs. Nitrous oxide should be avoided during anesthesia for surgical correction, as this gas could diffuse into the loops of intestine in the chest (see Chapter 2). Arterial oxygenation should be monitored, as these neonates may be at risk for developing retinopathy of prematurity. After reduction of the hernia, attempts to expand the hypoplastic lung are not recommended, as damage to the normal lung can occur from excessive positive airway pressure. The hypoplastic lung will gradually expand over several days with inspiratory pressures that do not exceed 25 cm H_2O.

Tracheoesophageal Fistula

Tracheoesophageal fistula is often first suspected soon after birth when an oral catheter cannot be passed into the stomach or when infants develop cyanosis and coughing during oral feedings. Pulmonary aspiration is likely to occur. Initial treatment is a gastrostomy using local anesthesia. This provides a vent for excess gas that may enter the stomach through the fistula as during mechanical ventilation of the lungs. During corrective surgery, it is important to place the tracheal tube below the level of the fistula while at the same time guarding against endobronchial intubation. There is an increased incidence of congenital heart disease in these neonates, and the incidence of prematurity approaches 40 percent.

Pyloric Stenosis

Pyloric stenosis occurs in about 1 of every 500 live births and usually manifests at 2 weeks to 5 weeks of age. Persistent vomiting results in loss of hydrogen ions, with compensatory attempts by the kidney to maintain a normal pH by exchanging potassium for hydrogen. The result is a dehydrated infant with hypokalemic, hypochloremic metabolic alkalosis. Surgery is performed electively (not as an emergency) after 24 hours to 48 hours of intravenous fluid therapy including sodium and potassium chloride.

The likelihood of aspiration of gastric fluid is increased in these patients during induction of anesthesia. Therefore, the stomach should be emptied as completely as possible with a large-bore catheter before induction of anesthesia. Postoperative depression of ventilation (possibly due to cerebrospinal fluid alkalosis) is often seen in these patients, emphasizing the need for close monitoring in the early hours after surgery.

Trisomy 21 (Down's Syndrome)

Trisomy 21 occurs in about 0.15 percent of all live births. Correction of associated congenital anomalies (atrial or ventricular septal defects, duodenal atresia) or the need to provide dental care may be the reasons these patients undergo surgery. In this regard, the need to reduce excessive upper airway secretions with anticholinergics and provide se-

Table 27-6. Comparison of Epiglottitis and Laryngotracheobronchitis

	Epiglottitis	Laryngotracheobronchitis
Age	2–6 yr	2 yr or less
Cause	Bacterial	Viral
Onset	Rapid over 24 hr	Gradual over 24 hours to 72 hours
Signs and symptoms	Inspiratory stridor	Inspiratory stridor
	Fever often greater than 39°C	Fever rarely above 39°C
	Drooling	Croupy cough
	Lethargic to restless	Rhinorrhea
	Tachypnea	
	Insist on sitting	
	Cyanosis	
Treatment	Oxygen	Oxygen
	Urgent intubation of the trachea	Aerosolized racemic epinephrine
	Antibiotics	Humidity

dation for an often uncooperative patient must be considered in the preoperative medication. Patency of the upper airway may be difficult to maintain after the onset of unconsciousness, reflecting the short neck, small mouth, and large tongue characteristic of these patients. Intubation of the trachea, however, is usually not difficult. Manipulation of the head and neck during intubation of the trachea must be performed cautiously, as many of these patients have asymptomatic atlantoaxial instability.

Epiglottitis

Epiglottitis typically manifests as an acute onset of difficulty in swallowing, high fever, and inspiratory stridor in children 2 years to 6 years old. Differentiation of epiglottitis from laryngotracheobronchitis (croup) may be difficult; but characteristically the latter occurs in younger patients, the onset is slower, the fever is lower, and airway obstruction less severe (Table 27-6). It is mandatory that children with suspected epiglottitis be admitted to the hospital, as sudden total upper airway obstruction can occur at any time. Treatment of epiglottitis is with antibiotics, such as ampicillin (causative bacteria is *Haemophilus influenzae*), and intubation of the trachea. An attempt to visualize the epiglottis should not be undertaken until the child is in the operating room and preparations are completed for intubation of the trachea and possible emergency tracheostomy. Induction and maintenance of anesthesia for intubation of the trachea is with a volatile anesthetic, most often halothane, in oxygen. Muscle relaxants are not administered as onset of skeletal muscle paralysis in the presence of upper airway obstruction may result in total airway obstruction. Resolution of epiglottitis usually requires 48 hours to 96 hours. Extubation of the trachea is performed in the operating room only after direct laryngoscopy has confirmed the resolution of the swelling of the epiglottis.

Bronchopulmonary Dysplasia

Bronchopulmonary dysplasia is a chronic pulmonary disorder that typically afflicts infants and children who required increased concentrations of oxygen and mechanical ventilation of the lungs at birth to treat respiratory distress syndrome. Speculated causes of bronchopulmonary dysplasia include pulmonary oxygen toxicity and damage due to high airway pressures (greater than 35 cm H_2O) during mechanical ventilation of the lungs (see Chapter 31). Characteristic findings include increased airway resistance, decreased arterial oxygenation due to mismatch of ventilation to perfusion, and recurrent pulmonary infections. Pulmonary dysfunction in these patients will be most marked in the first year of life.

Retinopathy of Prematurity (Retrolental Fibroplasia)

Retinopathy of prematurity reflects neovascularization and scarring of retinal vasculature that may result in visual impairment. Arterial hyperoxia is an important risk factor in development of neovascularization but prematurity (especially birth weights less than 1500 grams) must also be present. The risk of developing retinopathy is negligible after 44 weeks postconception (i.e., preterm neonates born at 36 weeks of gestation remain at risk until 8 weeks of age). During anesthesia, it is important to adjust inhaled concentrations of oxygen so as to maintain PaO_2 between 60 mmHg and 80 mmHg.

Apnea Spells

Apnea spells (cessation of breathing lasting at least 20 seconds and resulting in cyanosis and bradycardia) occur in 20 percent to 30 percent of premature neonates in the first month of life.[10] Since inhaled and injected anesthetics affect control of breathing, it is likely that the risk of apnea spells will be increased during the postoperative period, especially in preterm infants less than 60 weeks postconceptual age.[11] For this reason, it has been recommended that apnea monitoring be used for 12 hours to 24 hours after surgery in infants less than 60 weeks postconceptual age. The risk of apnea spells precludes outpatient surgery in susceptible patients (see Chapter 29).

Sepsis

Sepsis in neonates is associated with a high mortality rate, presumably reflecting the presence of an immature immune system. Signs of sepsis are nonspecific but often include lethargy and tachypnea. Fever and leukocytosis, in contrast to adults, may not be present in septic neonates.

Thermal (Burn) Injuries

About one-half of all thermal injuries occur in children and one-third of related deaths occur in children less than 15 years of age. Associated pathophysiologic responses include catecholamine release, acute hypovolemia, ileus, and myocardial depression. After the initial 24 hours of fluid resuscitation, the circulatory system enters a hyperdynamic state often accompanied by hypertension. Urine output is a useful guide to the adequacy of fluid replacement. Thermal injuries of the upper airway manifesting as hoarseness and tachypnea may require emergency intubation of the trachea. An increase in serum potassium concentrations due to tissue necrosis and hemolysis is common during the early postburn period. Carbon monoxide poisoning often complicates burns that occur in closed spaces and is the most common immediate cause of death from fire. Management of anesthesia in these patients may be complicated by absence of access sites for placement of intravascular catheters or monitors due to thermal injury, perioral scarring and contractures, potassium release after administration of succinylcholine, and resistance to the effects of nondepolarizing muscle relaxants.[12]

Malignant Hyperthermia

Malignant hyperthermia is an inherited disease that manifests most often, but not exclusively, in children. The incidence of this syndrome is approximately 1 in 12,000 pediatric anesthetics and 1 in 40,000 adult anesthetics. The pathophysiologic defect appears to be in the excitation-contraction coupling of skeletal muscles, and the concentration of calcium in the myoplasm. Exposure to triggering drugs, such as the volatile anesthetics, and/or succinylcholine, results in sustained high levels of calcium in the myoplasm and persistent skeletal muscle contraction. Susceptible patients may develop spasm of the masseter muscles after administration of succinylcholine, making it impossible to open the mouth to perform direct laryngoscopy for intubation of the trachea.[13] Sustained skeletal muscle contraction results in signs of hypermetabolism including tachycardia, arterial hypoxemia, metabolic and respiratory acidosis, and profound elevations in body temperature. Unexplained tachycardia or elevations in the exhaled concentrations of carbon dioxide are early manifestations of malignant hyperthermia, whereas elevations in body temperature may be a late sign. Intravenous administration of dantrolene (up to 10 mg·kg^{-1}) is the drug of choice for the treatment of malignant hyperthermia. In addition, aggressive attempts to lower body temperature, including gastric lavage with iced saline and immersion of the patient in ice water, should be considered.

Patients known to be susceptible to malignant hyperthermia should receive intravenous dantrolene, 2.5 mg·kg^{-1}, 15 minutes to 30 minutes before induction of anesthesia. Drugs known to trigger the syndrome are avoided in the management of anesthesia. Although no anesthetic regimen is completely safe, drugs considered to be acceptable for use during anesthesia in these patients include opioids, benzodiazepines, barbiturates, ketamine, ester and amide local anesthetics, pancuronium, vecuronium, and atracurium. Nitrous oxide is also probably safe. Regional anesthesia is an attractive selection in susceptible patients.

Identification of malignant hyperthermia-susceptible patients before anesthesia has obvious advantages. In this regard, a detailed medical and family history with particular reference to previous anesthetic experiences, should be obtained. Prior uneventful anesthetics, however, do not necessarily indicate that individuals are not susceptible. Only about 70 percent of malignant hyperthermia-susceptible patients have elevations of resting concentrations of creatine kinase. The absence of such an elevation, therefore, does not rule out malignant hyperthermia susceptibility. The definitive diagnosis of malignant hyperthermia susceptibility requires skeletal muscle biopsy and in vitro isometric contracture testing in the presence of caffeine, halothane, or both.

REFERENCES

1. Eger EI II, Bahlman SH, Munson ES. The effect of age on the rate of increase of alveolar anesthesia concentration. Anesthesiology 1971;35:365–72.
2. Lerman J, Robinson S, Willis MM, Gregory GA. Anesthetic requirements for halothane in young children 0–1 month and 1–6 months of age. Anesthesiology 1983;59:421–4.
3. LeDez KM, Lerman J. The minimum alveolar concentration (MAC) of isoflurane in preterm neonates. Anesthesiology 1987;67:301–7.
4. Brett CM, Fisher DM. Thiopental dose-response relations in unpremedicated infants, children and adults. Anesth Analg 1987;66:1024–7.
5. Fisher DM, O'Keefe C, Stanski DR, Cronnelly R, Miller RD, Gregory GA. Pharmacokinetics and pharmacodynamics of d-tubocurarine in infants, children and adults. Anesthesiology 1982;57:203–8.
6. Fisher DM, Miller RD. Neuromuscular effects of vecuronium (ORG NC45) in infants and children during N_2O, halothane anesthesia. Anesthesiology 1983;58:519–23.
7. Fisher DM, Cronnelly R, Miller RD, Sharma M. The neuromuscular pharmacology of neostigmine in infants and children. Anesthesiology 1983;59:220–5.
8. Brzustowicz RM, Nelson DA, Betts EK, Rosenberry KR, Swedlow DB. Efficacy of oral premedication for pediatric outpatient surgery. Anesthesiology 1984;60:475–7.
9. Furman EB, Roman DG, Lemmer LAS, Hairabet J, Jasinski M, Laver MB. Specific therapy in water,

electrolyte and blood-volume replacement during pediatric surgery. Anesthesiology 1975;42:187–93.

10. Gregory GA, Steward DJ. Life-threatening perioperative apnea in the ex-"premie." Anesthesiology 1983;59:495–98.

11. Kurth CD, Spitzer AR, Broennle AM, Downes JJ. Postoperative apnea in preterm infants. Anesthesiology 1987;66:483–8.

12. Martyn J. Clinical pharmacology and drug therapy in the burned patient. Anesthesiology 1986;65:67–75.

13. Rosenberg H, Fletcher JE. Masseter muscle rigidity and malignant hyperthermia susceptibility. Anesth Analg 1986;65:161–4.

Chapter 28

Elderly Patients

Elderly patients, who are arbitrarily defined as over 65 years of age (i.e., a chronologic rather than biologic distinction) are becoming an increasingly important segment of society, accounting for more than 10 percent of the population in the United States. Approximately one-half of patients who reach 65 years of age will require surgery before they die. Elderly patients are more vulnerable to adverse effects of anesthesia because of their generalized decline in organ function, which may manifest only with the added stress of the perioperative period (Fig. 28-1).[1] For example, cardiac function sufficient for a sedentary life style may become inadequate with the stress of intraoperative blood loss or postoperative infection.

An important concept, which is often unappreciated, is to distinguish between the normal attrition of organ function that occurs in all patients with increasing age and loss of function that marks the onset of pathologic changes from one or more of the diseases frequently encountered in elderly patients. The cells of the body normally replicate about 45 times to 50 times before they cease to function. The average natural life span is 85 years, with a standard deviation of 4 years. The actual life expectancy is less than 85 years because of superimposed diseases (e.g., hypertension, diabetes mellitus) or other factors (e.g., drugs, trauma).

Psychological, physiologic, and pharmacologic changes that must be taken into account when anesthetizing elderly patients must be added to the concomitant disease processes that may also exist. Although morbidity and mortality of surgery in elderly patients is higher than that for their younger counterparts, these problems are usually due to concomitant disease processes, such as heart disease, diabetes mellitus, or renal failure, rather than aging per se.[2] Emergency surgery, which allows little time for control of co-existing diseases, may be particularly harzardous in elderly patients. It is likely that age-related diseases play a more important role than age itself in increasing the risk of anesthesia and surgery in elderly patients.

PSYCHOLOGICAL FACTORS

All patients, independent of age, evidence psychological concerns about upcoming surgery. In this respect, the elderly do not differ from other surgical patients who have a variety of concerns about a proposed surgical experience. However, certain stresses, including the fear of the loss of function and independence, concerns about the possibility of impending death, and the fear that their current illness may result in long-term institutionalization and dependency, impinge on the elderly to a greater extent. In addition, especially with respect to the elderly, there is the impact of social and sensory isolation.

Before surgery, one may see an increasing preoc-

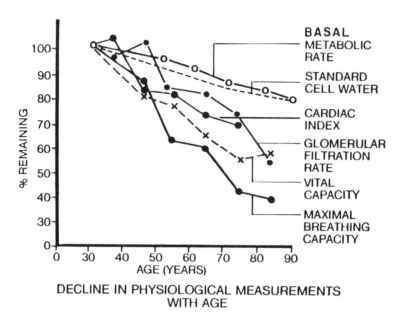

DECLINE IN PHYSIOLOGICAL MEASUREMENTS WITH AGE

Fig. 28-1. Aging is associated with progressive reductions in function (1 percent to 1.5 percent annually) of major organ systems. (From Evans, [1] with permission.)

cupation with events of the past. This may reflect a life review, a summing up. Listening to the process of a life review by the patient before surgery may be helpful in preparation for surgery. If, however, the elderly patient becomes preoccupied with an event or experience in the past that may seem trivial to the examiner, it may represent a symptom of significant depression. The elderly do have a higher incidence of psychiatric disturbances.

Before surgery, it is important to identify the existence of depression and to distinguish between long-term, endogenous versus short-term, reactive depression. Patients with endogenous depression are associated with a higher preoperative and postoperative risk. Depression in the elderly may not present itself with profound melancholy, but rather with persistent somatic complaints that do not have any basis, as well as weakness, lethargy, and problems in concentration. The patient with endogenous depression is more likely to have poor appetite, weight loss, agitation, lack of energy, and recurrent thoughts of suicide.

Recognition of the intellectually impaired older adult is especially important. These patients also present a significant risk for postoperative mor-

bidity and are at a greater risk of developing postoperative delirium that tends to be reversible, although some do not return to their prior level of functioning. It is important to carry out a intellectual assessment in the intellectually impaired elderly patient to differentiate those with a pre-existing, chronic, organic deficit from those with a reaction to the surgery and anesthesia.

Elderly patients with personality disorders may present significant problems preoperatively. They may be manipulative, histrionic, hypochondriacal, attention demanding, or theatrical. It is important that they be recognized early in order to set firm limits, which for most is very therapeutic.

If endogenous depression, cognitive impairment, or personality disorder is strongly suspected, psychiatric help should be sought. Because postoperative complications and overall outcome are related to preoperative psychiatric status, such help may be beneficial both mentally and physically.

PHYSIOLOGY

The generalized decline in organ function that accompanies aging may be characterized as a decreased margin of reserve for adaptation, especially with the introduction of acute stresses such as accompany the perioperative period (Fig. 28-1).[1]

Central Nervous System

Progressive declines in central nervous system activity and loss of neurons, especially in the cerebral cortex, accompany aging. Conduction velocity in peripheral nerves slows, and there may be reduced numbers of fibers in spinal cord tracts. These changes may manifest as decreased dose requirements for drugs that act on the central nervous system (MAC) or peripheral nervous system (see the section Pharmacology).

Cardiovascular System

Systolic blood pressure increases with aging, reflecting development of poorly compliant arterial walls. Heart rate decreases with advancing age, suggesting an increase in activity of the parasympathetic nervous system. Furthermore, degenerative changes that accompany aging can involve the sinus node and/or cardiac conduction systems, resulting in atrioventricular heart block. Drug-induced heart rate changes (atropine isoproterenol, propranolol) are less and reflex-induced increases via the carotid sinus in response to hypotension (hypovolemia, anesthetic drug overdose) are attenuated in elderly patients.

Cardiac output decreases about 1 percent·yr^{-1} after 30 years of age, reflecting reductions in oxygen requirements for aging tissues. Cerebral, coronary, and skeletal muscle blood flow are relatively maintained, however, emphasizing that these organs may receive a greater percentage of blood flow in elderly patients. Furthermore, cardiac output does not decrease in all elderly patients, especially those who maintain physical fitness.[3]

Stroke volume is relatively unaffected by aging, although the ability to increase myocardial contractility in response to stress is impaired. Conceivably, drug-induced myocardial depression may be exaggerated in elderly patients.

Pulmonary system changes that accompany aging are characterized by deterioration of gas exchange and changes in the mechanics of breathing. For example, PaO_2 decreases about 0.5 mmHg·yr^{-1} after 20 years of age and the $AaDO_2$ increases (Fig. 28-2).[4] These changes reflect mis-

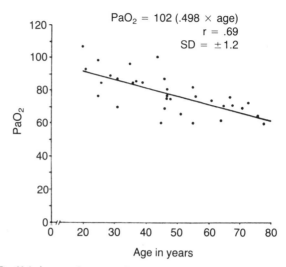

Fig. 28-2. Increasing age is associated with progressive declines in the resting awake PaO_2. Note the formula should indicate that (.498 × age) is subtracted from 102. (From Wahba,[4] with permission.)

matching of ventilation to perfusion due principally to reductions in cardiac output and degenerative changes (loss of alveolar septae) in the lungs. Aging alone does not alter the $PaCO_2$, although the $AaDCO_2$ may increase due to ventilation of unperfused alveoli (i.e., increased physiologic dead space).

Mechanical ventilatory function is impaired because of decreased elasticity of the lungs and increased stiffness of the thorax. Vital capacity and forced exhaled volume in 1 second decrease with aging whereas residual volume and functional residual capacity increase. Maximum breathing capacity is substantially reduced (up to 50 percent) in elderly patients.

Although asymptomatic at rest, elderly patients may become symptomatic with the stress of surgery as pulmonary changes interfere with optimum ability to oxygenate blood and clear airway secretions. Pneumonia occurs with increased frequency in elderly patients reflecting decreased pulmonary reserve and an increased incidence of aspiration of pharyngeal sections often compounded by colonization in the pharynx because of poor oral hygiene and general depression of the immune system.

Renal System

Aging is associated with progressive declines in renal blood flow (parallels reductions in cardiac output), glomerular filtration rate, and urine concentrating ability. These changes combined with reduced cardiac function make elderly patients more vulnerable to fluid overload. In addition, prolonged and exaggerated responses to certain drugs (digoxin, antibiotics) are predictable in the presence of reduced renal clearance characteristic of aging (see the section *Pharmacology*). Ability to conserve sodium is reduced, making elderly patients vulnerable to hyponatremia, whereas decreased renin activity with associated reductions in plasma concentrations of aldosterone may contribute to development of hyperkalemia. Despite reduced renal function, plasma concentrations of creatinine do not increase, reflecting decreased skeletal muscle mass and accompanying declines in production of creatinine.

Hepatic System

Hepatic blood flow decreases with aging in proportion to reductions in cardiac output. Decreased activity of hepatic microsomal enzymes is predictable, but it is likely that reduced hepatic blood flow is more important in delayed drug clearance observed in elderly patients. Production of albumin is also reduced, resulting in decreased plasma protein binding of some drugs.

Gastrointestinal System

There is a general decrease in esophageal and intestinal motility, which results in delayed gastric emptying. Also, gastroesophageal sphincter tone is frequently decreased. As a result of these changes, elderly patients probably represent an increased risk for pulmonary aspiration when rendered unconscious by general anesthesia.

Endocrine System

Diabetes mellitus and hypothyroidism are potential accompaniments of increased aging (see Chapter 23).

Skin and Musculoskeletal Systems

Atrophy of the epidermis with loss of collagen and decreases in elasticity makes elderly patients more vulnerable to decubitus ulcers or damage due to

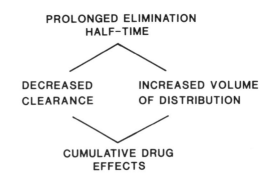

Fig. 28-3. Age-related changes in pharmacokinetics most often manifest as a prolonged elimination half-time due to decreased clearance or increased volume of distribution of drugs. Cumulative drug effects are likely to occur with repeated doses.

incorrect positioning during surgery (see Chapter 15). Damage from removal of tape or monitoring electrodes may result in unexpected injury to the underlying skin. Osteoarthritis, rheumatoid arthritis, and osteoporosis have obvious implications for upper airway management and for positioning of elderly patients during surgery. Skeletal muscle atrophy predictably accompanies aging.

PHARMACOLOGY

Pharmacokinetics (distribution and elimination of drugs) and pharmacodynamics (responsiveness of receptors to drugs) change with increasing age.

Pharmacokinetics

Age-related changes in pharmacokinetics most often manifest as prolongation of elimination half-times of drugs, making elderly patients particularly vulnerable to cumulative drug effects and adverse drug interactions (Fig. 28-3). Increased elimination half-times of drugs can reflect decreased clearance and/or increases in the volume of distribution. Age-induced decreases in renal and hepatic clearance have modest effects on clearance of nondepolarizing muscle relaxants from the plasma.[5] However, when associated diseases are superimposed on age-related changes, clearance of muscle relaxants, and other drugs can be quite pro-

---

Causes of Increased Elimination Half-Times of Drugs

Decreased Clearance
    Renal blood flow
    Glomerular filtration rate
    Hepatic blood flow
    Hepatic microsomal enzyme activity

Increased volume of distribution
    Body fat content
    Protein binding

---

longed.[6] Reduced hepatic clearance mechanisms are most likely responsible for prolonged elimination half-times of opioids in elderly patients.[7] Prolonged elimination half-times of diazepam in elderly patients are consistent with increased tissue storage of this lipid-soluble drug in the greater fraction of adipose tissue relative to body weight that accompanies aging. Decreases in total body water content are predictable considering the anhydrous characteristics of adipose tissue.

Pharmacodynamics

Confirmation of pharmacodynamic changes is demonstration of increases or decreases in plasma concentrations of drugs required to produce specific pharmacologic effects. For example, age-related decreases in anesthetic requirements (MAC) for inhaled drugs most likely reflects pharmacodynamic changes (Fig. 28-4).[8] Conversely, plasma concentrations of nondepolarizing muscle relaxants necessary to produce comparable degrees of twitch response suppression are similar in young and elderly adults, suggesting that changes in the neuromuscular junction do not accompany aging.[5,6] Likewise, doses of thiopental or etomidate necessary to produce equivalent pharmacologic effects are not changed with aging (Fig. 28-5).[9,10] A speculated decrease in numbers of receptors with aging is not supported by demonstrations that density of beta adrenergic receptors does not change in elderly patients.[11] Instead, the affinity of these receptors for adrenergic agonists declines with aging, explaining the reduced responsiveness

of the cardiovascular system to drugs acting on the autonomic nervous system.

MANAGEMENT OF ANESTHESIA

Preoperative Evaluation and Preparation

Preoperative evaluation of elderly patients must consider the likely presence of co-existing diseases (hypertension, coronary artery disease, peripheral vascular disease, chronic obstructive airways disease, diabetes mellitus, arthritis, anemia) and decreases in major organ function that accompany aging independent of the reason for surgery (Fig. 28-1).[1] Even in the absence of symptoms, it is likely that many elderly patients have significant coronary artery disease. The likelihood of adverse drug interactions is increased by known alterations in pharmacokinetics and pharmacodynamics characteristic of aging. Furthermore, elderly patients are likely to be taking several different drugs (Table 28-1) that may contribute to adverse drug interactions. A drug history is particularly important because of the numerous abnormalities and drug interactions that may occur in elderly patients. Unfortunately, elderly patients can become confused and forget not only what drugs they are taking, but how much and when the last dose was taken. Close consultation with the family and physician is essential in these cases. Often, merely asking the patient to show you what drugs they are taking and how frequently they take them can alleviate some of the problems in taking an accurate history.

In awake patients, orthostatic hypotension associated with increases in heart rate suggests decreased intravascular fluid volume. Conversely, orthostatic hypotension not accompanied by increases in heart rate is suggestive of a sympathetic nervous system that is not functioning properly due to aging or drugs (antihypertensives). Changes in mental status that occur with extension and rotation of the head may reflect vertebrobasilar arterial insufficiency or cervical osteoarthritis. If maintenance of anesthesia with a face mask is anticipated, edentulous patients can keep their dentures in place. Careful preoperative evaluation and correction of electrolyte derangements (e.g.,

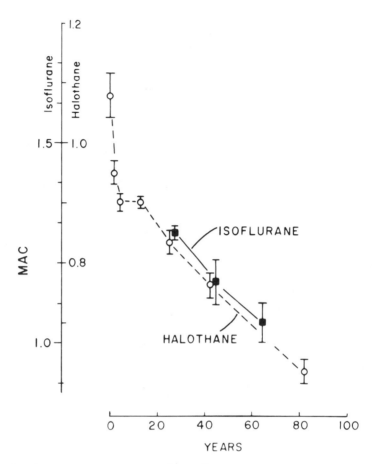

Fig. 28-4. Minimum alveolar concentration (MAC) for isoflurane and halothane decreases with increasing age. (From Quasha et al.,[8] with permission.)

diuretics and hypokalemia) and pulmonary dysfunction may reduce the likelihood of perioperative complications.

Simplified bedside pulmonary function testing is often helpful in the preoperative evaluation of elderly patients. These values can determine whether chest physiotherapy might be beneficial preoperatively or can be used for comparison when assessing pulmonary function postoperatively. Because of the high incidence of pulmonary complications postoperatively, preoperative teaching of incentive spirometry and chest physiotherapy, along with the use of bronchodilators, may reduce the incidence of postoperative respiratory complications. Preoperative medication with drugs is used sparingly in elderly patients with a detailed expla-

nation of events to anticipate in the perioperative period serving as a useful substitute for drug-induced anxiety relief and sedation. Attempts to increase gastric fluid pH and reduce gastric fluid volume in selected patients may be useful, considering the potential vulnerability to aspiration produced by changes (i.e., prolonged gastric emptying, decreased glottic reactivity) associated with aging.

Regional Anesthesia

Regional anesthesia is appropriate for selected operations (e.g., lower abdominal, orthopaedic procedures) in alert and cooperative elderly pa-

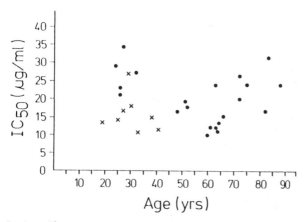

Fig. 28-5. Plasma concentrations of thiopental necessary to produce early burst suppression on the electroencephalogram do not change with age. Solid circles represent surgical patients who underwent arterial sampling, and x symbols represent volunteer subjects who underwent venous blood sampling. (From Homer and Stanski,[9] with permission.)

Mechanical Changes Associated with Aging
Edentulous or poor dental hygiene
Arthritis
Weak posterior membranous portion of trachea
Senile atrophy of skin
Decreased airway reactivity
Decreased gastroesophageal sphincter tone

---

tients. Elderly patients may be more sensitive to spinal anesthesia than younger adults, manifesting as prolonged duration of action (perhaps reflecting decreased vascular absorption) and exaggerated

Table 28-1. Drugs Often Taken by Elderly Patients that May Contribute to Adverse Effects or Drug Interactions

Drug	Response
Diuretics	Hypokalemia Hypovolemia
Centrally-acting antihypertensive drugs	Decreased autonomic nervous system activity Decreased anesthetic requirements
Beta-adrenergic antagonists	Decreased autonomic nervous system activity Bronchospasm Bradycardia
Cardiac antidysrhythmias	Prolonged effects of muscle relaxants
Lithium	Cardiac dysrhythmias Prolonged effects of muscle relaxants
Antibiotics	Prolonged effects of muscle relaxants

reductions in blood pressure (perhaps reflecting reduced reflex compensatory responses mediated via the sympathetic nervous system). Although a debatable practice, some anesthesiologists administer a prophylactic intramuscular dose of ephedrine before institution of a spinal anesthetic in attempts to attenuate its hypotensive effects. Epidural anesthesia is an acceptable alternative to spinal anesthesia, with the possible advantage of a more gradual reduction in blood pressure than that which accompanies spinal anesthesia. Doses of local anesthetics required to achieve epidural anesthesia decrease with aging, perhaps reflecting progressive occlusion of intervertebral foramina, with connective tissue resulting in greater epidural spread of the local anesthetics.[12] In adults less than 60 years old, about 1 ml to 1.6 ml of local anesthetic per segment is required for epidural anesthesia assuming 1.5 percent to 2 percent lidocaine or its equivalent is used. This dose should be reduced by 25 percent to 50 percent in the elderly.

General Anesthesia

Changes associated with aging can cause mechanical problems during general anesthesia. In the edentulous patient or the patient with poor dental hygiene, it is difficult to obtain a proper mask fit, and the chance of dislodging a loose tooth is enhanced. The presence of arthritis, especially in the cervical areas, may make intubation of the trachea difficult. Furthermore, the weak posterior membranous portion of the trachea increases the possibility of tracheal trauma. The anesthesiologist should be especially careful when using a stylet to perform an endotracheal intubation when the trachea is not easily visualized. Probing with the stylet in place can cause trauma and, in rare cases, create a false passage that will result in inadequate ventilation of the lungs and production of mediastinal emphysema. Senile atrophy makes the skin more sensitive to injury from adhesive tape and monitoring pads as used for the electrocardiogram. The combination of arthritis and sensitive skin makes the problems associated with poor positioning of the elderly patient particularly important so as to avoid pressure necrosis and neuropathies (see Chapter 15). There is no evidence that specific inhaled or injected anesthetics are preferable for induction of anesthesia or maintenance of anesthesia in elderly patients, remembering that these patients may require lower doses and be more susceptible to depressant and or prolonged effects than their younger counterparts (see the section *Pharmacology*). Reduced reactivity of the glottic opening plus decreased tone of the gastroesophageal sphincter probably place the elderly patient at increased risk for regurgitation or aspiration during induction of anesthesia. This possibility, however, does not routinely justify the rapid intravenous induction of anesthesia with drugs such as thiopental and succinylcholine. On occasion, an awake intubation of the trachea preceded by topical anesthesia and light sedation may be indicated (see Chapter 12).

Mechanical ventilation of the lungs with supplemental oxygen is useful, considering predictable changes in the pulmonary system that accompany aging. As with anesthetic drugs, the initial doses of muscle relaxants probably should be decreased because of the reduced skeletal muscle mass and altered renal clearance mechanisms that are likely to accompany aging. Nevertheless, clearance of atracurium is largely independent of hepatic and renal mechanisms, and its duration of action is not significantly influenced by aging.[13] Vecuronium shows detectable but modest prolongation of duration of action in elderly compared with younger patients.[6,13] Reversal of nondepolarizing muscle

relaxants with anticholinesterases does not seem to introduce any unique risks in elderly patients, except that the incidence of cardiac dysrhythmias may be greater in the elderly, probably reflecting a different pharmacologic relationship between neostigmine and atropine (or glycopyrrolate) in the elderly as compared with younger adults.[14] Likewise, monitoring of elderly patients does not introduce unique risks, although complications from insertion of catheters into peripheral arteries could be greater in elderly patients with associated arteriosclerosis. Considering predictable reductions in organ function, monitoring cardiac filling pressures, the electrocardiogram, urine output, and body temperature may assume increased importance in elderly patients. Postoperatively, early ambulation is desirable to decrease the likelihood of pulmonary infection or development of venous thrombi.

REFERENCES

1. Evans TI. The physiological basis of geriatric anaesthesia. Anaesth Intensive Care 1973;1:319–28.
2. Halbrecht TJ, Garrison RN, Fry DE. Role of infection in increased mortality associated with age in laparotomy. Am Surg 1983;49:173–8.
3. Craig DB, McLeskey CH, Mitenko PA, Thomson IR, Janis KM. Geriatric anaesthesia. Can J Anaesth 1987;34:156–67.
4. Wahba W. Body build (age) and preoperative arterial oxygen tension. Can Anaesth Soc J 1975;22:653–8.
5. Matteo RS, Backus WW, McDaniel DD, Brotherton WP, Abraham R, Diaz J. Pharmacokinetics and pharmacodynamics of d-tubocurarine and metocurine in the elderly. Anesth Analg 1985;64:23–9.
6. Rupp SM, Castagnoli KP, Fisher DM, Miller RD. Pancuronium and vecuronium pharmacokinetics and pharmacodynamics in young and elderly adults. Anesthesiology 1987;67:45–9.
7. Bentley JB, Borel JD, Nenad RE, Gillespie TJ. Age and fentanyl pharmacokinetics. Anesth Analg 1982;61:968–71.
8. Quasha AL, Eger EI II, Tinker JH. Determination and applications of MAC. Anesthesiology 1980;53:315–34.
9. Homer TD, Stanski DR. The effect of increasing age on thiopental disposition and anesthetic requirement. Anesthesiology 1985;62:714–24.
10. Arden JR, Holley FO, Stanski DR. Increased sensitivity to etomidate in the elderly: Initial distribution versus altered brain response. Anesthesiology 1986;65:19–27.
11. Feldman RD, Limbird LE, Nadeau J, Robertson D,

Wood AJJ. Alterations in leukocyte beta-receptor affinity with aging. A potential explanation for altered beta-adrenergic sensitivity in the elderly. N Engl J Med 1984;310:815–9.

12. Finucane BT, Hammonds WD, Welch MB. Influence of age on vascular absorption of lidocaine from the epidural space. Anesth Analg 1987;66:843–6.

13. D'Hollander AA, Luyckx C, Barivais L, DeVille A. Clinical evaluation of atracurium besylate requirement for a stable muscle relaxation during surgery: Lack of age-related effects. Anesthesiology 1983; 59:237–40.

14. Owens WD, Waldbaum LS, Stephen CR. Cardiac dysrhythmias following reversal of neuromuscular blocking agents in geriatric patients. Anesth Analg 1978;57:186–90.

Chapter 29

Outpatient Surgery

Outpatient (ambulatory) surgery offers an alternative to the traditional sequence of hospitalization before elective operations requiring anesthesia. It is likely that nearly 50 percent of all operations will someday be performed as outpatient surgery. Compared with inpatient surgery, advantages of performing the same operation as an outpatient procedure include a decrease in medical costs, increased availability of beds for patients who require hospitalization, protection from hospital-acquired infections, and avoidance of disruption of the family unit attendant upon hospitalization. Cost savings extend beyond the actual medical expenses as patients can return to daily activity sooner, reducing financial loss due to absence from work or need to provide for outside child care. Another cost saving results from the decreased need to build expensive hospital facilities, as existing beds become available for inpatients. The short separation time from family provided by outpatient surgery is especially important for children, as this reduces the number of postoperative psychological problems caused by separation-induced anxiety, which may persist long after completion of surgery.

An alternative to the same-day admission and discharge outpatient surgery concept is a prospectively planned overnight admission to the hospital following surgery. This approach, which has been designated "*AM admit*" preserves the advantages of the same-day admission but eliminates any physician concerns regarding the ability to optimally manage potential anesthetic or operative complications in the early postoperative period.

FACILITIES

Outpatient surgical facilities are either in a hospital or a free-standing clinic (Surgicenter). The free-standing clinic must have a transfer and admission agreement with a nearby hospital should unexpected hospitalization be required after surgery. Less than 3 percent of patients, however, will require hospitalization after outpatient surgery. Protracted nausea and vomiting are the most frequent reasons for admission to the hospital. The incidence of hospitalization because of life-threatening complications after outpatient surgery is very low, being estimated as 0.007 percent.[1]

The operating rooms, monitors, anesthetic equipment, and postoperative recovery room facilities used for outpatient surgery should not differ from those used for inpatients. The recovery room must be large enough to permit patients to remain for several hours after surgery without overtaxing the facilities. Outpatient surgical facilities should have a physician director, usually an anesthesiologist, who is responsible for the daily administrative decisions, including the final judgments regarding whether a given procedure should be performed on an outpatient basis.

SELECTION

Selection of individuals for outpatient surgery is determined by the characteristics of the patient and the type of operation.

Characteristics of the Patient

The patient must desire to have surgery performed as an outpatient and be in otherwise good general health or have a systemic disease (diabetes mellitus, essential hypertension, congenital heart disease) that is medically controlled. The patient or a responsible adult must be reasonably intelligent and reliable to assure compliance with preoperative and postoperative instructions. Patients with a previous history of prolonged postoperative nausea and vomiting or in whom it is unlikely that pain will be relieved by oral analgesics are not likely candidates for outpatient surgery. Ideally, the driving distance to the outpatient facility should not exceed 1 hour in order to ensure rapid return to the hospital should serious postoperative complications develop.

Patients prone to hospital-acquired infections (infants, immunosuppressed patients) may benefit from having their surgery performed as outpatients. For example, about one in five infants admitted as inpatients for elective inguinal hernia repair develop an upper respiratory tract or enteric infection.[1] The incidence of these types of infections is 50 percent to 70 percent less when the surgery is performed on an outpatient basis.

Age is usually not a factor in the selection of patients for outpatient surgery. Nevertheless, pediatric patients probably benefit most from outpatient surgery. Premature neonates less than 44 weeks postconceptual age, however, are at increased risk for outpatient surgery because of the frequent presence of anemia in these patients plus the potential for immaturity of the respiratory center. Indeed, these neonates are prone to become apneic in the perioperative period.[2,3] For these reasons, it is probably reasonable to delay nonessential surgery for premature neonates until they are beyond 44 weeks postconceptual age (see Chapter 27). Other infants who may be at increased risk for outpatient surgery are those who required treatment of respiratory distress syn-

---

Examples of Operations that Can Be Performed as Outpatient Procedures

Extraocular muscle resection
Dental and oral surgical procedures
Bronchoscopy and esophagoscopy
Tonsillectomy and adenoidectomy
Nasal polypectomy
Rhinoplasty
Myringotomy
Breast biopsy
Augmentation mammoplasty
Laparoscopy with or without tubal ligation
Inguinal hernia repair
Dilation and curettage
Circumcision
Cystoscopy
Vasectomy
Superficial procedures on extremities

---

drome after birth. These infants may develop bronchopulmonary dysplasia associated with abnormal blood gases and an increased incidence of pulmonary infections in the first 6 months to 12 months after termination of ventilator therapy (see Chapter 27). Despite these qualifications, performance of infant inguinal hernia repair is a well-accepted outpatient surgical procedure. In elderly patients, acceptability for outpatient surgery is influenced by physical status and the ability to be cared for by a competent adult at home.

Type of Operation

Types of operations acceptable as outpatient procedures are often established on an evolutionary basis. Traditionally, those operations of short duration (less than 2 hours) that are associated with minimal bleeding, postoperative pain, or physiologic derangement are considered suitable for outpatient surgery. Nevertheless, there is no evidence that recovery time parallels anesthesia time. This suggests that arbitrary limits placed on the type of outpatient surgery permitted based on the anticipated duration of the procedure are unwarranted.[4] Finally, the surgery should not be associated with the risk of airway obstruction or interfere with early postoperative ambulation. These recommendations, however, are only guidelines as emphasized by the frequent performance as outpatient procedures of (1) tonsillectomy and adenoidectomy, which may be accompanied by postoperative hemorrhage; and (2) laparoscopy, which invades the peritoneal cavity. Indeed, the incidence of bleeding after tonsillectomy and adenoidectomy performed as an outpatient procedure may be lower (1.73 percent) than the incidence of this complication when surgery was performed on inpatients (4.35 percent).[1]

Infected cases are rarely considered for outpatient surgery because of the need for separate operative and recovery facilities. Likewise, emergency surgery is not likely to be an outpatient procedure, as this would disrupt the elective schedule. Furthermore, it is difficult to adequately evaluate patients requiring emergency surgery as outpatients.

PREOPERATIVE PREPARATION AND INSTRUCTIONS TO THE PATIENT

The surgeon is responsible for scheduling outpatient surgery, obtaining a medical history, performing a physical examination, initiating the necessary preoperative laboratory studies, and providing instructions to the patient or responsible parent. It is not possible or convenient for the anesthesiologist to see every patient at the time of scheduling surgery. Therefore, it may be necessary for the surgeon to describe and explain the preoperative anesthetic requirement to the patient. If questions related to anesthesia arise that cannot be adequately answered by the surgeon, it is reasonable to ask the anesthesiologist for a consultation at this time. Otherwise, it is satisfactory for the patient to be seen by the anesthesiologist on the day of surgery.

Laboratory Data Required Preoperatively

The laboratory data required preoperatively will depend on the patient's age, history, physical examination, and current drug therapy (see Chapter 9). Most guidelines for outpatient surgery require a recent (within 30 days of surgery) hemoglobin determination. The hemoglobin concentration should exceed 10 g·dl.$^{-1}$ This minimum hemoglobin requirement is based on the concept that anemia is associated with medical diseases that could influence postoperative outcome. For patients over 40 years of age, it may be appropriate to determine blood glucose concentrations and blood urea nitrogen concentrations preoperatively. Determination of serum glutamic oxalacetic transaminase concentrations, as routine screening tests for the detection of unsuspected hepatocellular disease may be considered for adult patients. Serum potassium concentrations should be measured routinely if patients are being treated with potassium-losing diuretics. A pregnancy test may be indicated in certain patients. Routine urinalysis offers little or no new information and in many respects only duplicates the blood chemistry measurements. In the absence of positive findings on the history or physical examination, it is not necessary to obtain routine preoperative electrocardiograms or radiographs of the chest in patients less than 40 years of age.

Written Instructions

Written instructions describing outpatient surgery requirements should be given to the patient or parents by the surgeon at the time of scheduling of the surgical procedure. The surgeon should verbally explain to the patient the reasons for these requirements and the patient or parents should then sign the written instructions. Explaining the reasons for not eating or drinking before surgery is particularly important.

ARRIVAL ON THE DAY OF SURGERY

After the patient arrives for outpatient surgery, compliance with the written instructions is verified, particularly as they relate to fasting. It is especially important that clandestine liquid or food intake by pediatric patients be considered and confirmed not to have occurred. The anesthesiologist should review the patient's medical record and laboratory data at this time. In addition, the pertinent areas to be pursued by the anesthesiologist include questions regarding previous anesthetics, current drug therapy, allergies, and previous adverse responses

---

Information Provided on Written Instruction Sheet Given to Patient when Outpatient Surgery Is Scheduled

1. Make sure requested laboratory tests are completed
2. Nothing to eat or drink up to 8 hours before surgery (traditionally nothing by mouth after midnight)
3. A child less than 1 year of age may receive clear liquids up to 4 hours before surgery
4. Wear minimal to no cosmetics or jewelry
5. Where and when to report for surgery and estimate of discharge time
6. Must be accompanied by an adult to provide transportation home
7. Notify surgeon if there is a change in the patient's medical condition before surgery
8. After surgery resume eating when hungry, starting with clear liquids and progressing to soups and then regular diet
9. Do not drive an automobile or make important decisions for at least 24 hours to 48 hours after anesthesia
10. Telephone number to contact physician regarding significant postoperative complications

---

such as postoperative vomiting. An examination of the upper airway, including dentition and evaluation of the peripheral nervous system if regional anesthesia is anticipated, is performed. Finally, the anesthesiologist should elicit any change in the medical condition (fever, cough, sputum production, diarrhea) that may have developed since the outpatient surgery was scheduled. Pediatric patients must be thoroughly evaluated for any evidence of an upper respiratory tract infection that has manifested since scheduling. Indeed, rhinorrhea poses an enigma in pediatric patients scheduled for outpatient surgery. Benign rhinorrhea is usually an allergic rhinitis that does not contraindicate elective surgery, assuming there is no associated history of asthma. If there is any doubt, rhinorrhea

should be assumed to be an upper respiratory tract infection and elective surgery should be delayed. In this regard, the temperature pattern can be useful in differentiating between an infectious and noninfectious process. For example, a temperature above 38° Celsius in children is highly suggestive of an upper respiratory tract infection.

PREOPERATIVE MEDICATION

Preoperative medication with drugs to reduce anxiety or produce sedation before outpatient surgery is often avoided for fear of delaying the return to wakefulness after anesthesia and surgery.[4] Opioids may be avoided in attempts to minimize drug-induced vomiting. Droperidol may be useful for outpatients undergoing operations associated with a high incidence of postoperative nausea and vomiting. Reassurance by the anesthesiologist and surgeon is a potent antidote to preoperative anxiety in most patients (see Chapter 10). Nevertheless, pharmacologic premedication may be desirable in mentally retarded or hyperactive patients. Barbiturates or benzodiazepines can be administered orally to these patients before they leave home. If this is not possible, the patient should arrive at the outpatient facility at least 2 hours before scheduled surgery to allow administration (ideally orally) of the preoperative medication and production of desirable effects before induction of anesthesia. Alternatively, intravenous administration of short-acting opioids (alfentanil, fentanyl) before induction of anesthesia may be useful as preoperative medication. For pediatric patients, oral administration of diazepam or a combination of diazepam, meperidine, and atropine does not delay recovery.[5]

Compared with adult inpatients, those scheduled for outpatient surgery have been shown to have increased volumes of acidic gastric fluid (Fig. 29-1).[6] Because inhalation of acidic gastric fluid is a major hazard associated with drug-induced depression or unconsciousness, it may be reasonable to administer drugs orally in the preoperative period to reduce gastric fluid volume (metoclopramide) and increase gastric fluid pH (antacids, H_2 antagonists). Nevertheless, the value or need for these drugs as a routine in the management

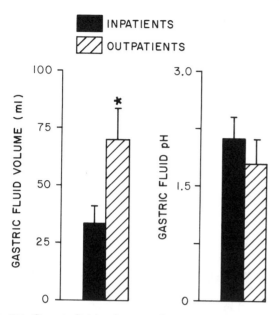

Fig. 29-1. Gastric fluid volume and pH (mean ± SD) were determined for inpatients (n-21) and outpatients (n-21) undergoing minor surgery. Gastric fluid volume was significantly greater for outpatients (P<0.05) than inpatients despite similar periods (12 hours and 15 hours, respectively) of fasting. Gastric fluid pH did not differ significantly between groups. (Based on data in Ong et al.,[6].)

of patients scheduled for inpatient or outpatient surgery has not been documented. More important than pharmacologic attempts to alter gastric fluid volume and pH is rapid and skillful protection of the airway by placement of a cuffed tube in the trachea of appropriate patients.

Routine intramuscular administration of anticholinergics as preoperative medication is not necessary, with the possible exception of patients in whom administration of ketamine is planned (anticipated excessive salivation) or those scheduled for oral endoscopies. In these latter patients, excessive oral secretions may interfere with the production of topical anesthesia. Otherwise, the discomfort of a dry mouth and throat and the possibility of residual mydriasis and difficulty focusing are undesirable in adult outpatients. Furthermore, pediatric patients may be susceptible to increases in body temperature secondary to anti-

cholinergic effects on sweating. If bradycardia develops intraoperatively, atropine can be administered intravenously.

TECHNIQUE OF ANESTHESIA

All techniques of anesthesia and drugs used to produce anesthesia for inpatients can be considered for use in outpatients. However, use of techniques and/or drugs that permit a prompt and nearly complete recovery with minimal side effects (absence of sedation, nausea, vomiting, orthostatic hypotension) is mandatory for optimal safety of patients who will be discharged from the hospital within a few hours after surgery. Local infiltration anesthesia is preferable when the planned operative procedure permits. Alternatives to local anesthesia are general anesthesia, regional anesthesia, or peripheral nerve block (see Chapter 9). Regardless of the technique of anesthesia selected, a catheter should probably be inserted into a peripheral vein before the institution of anesthesia. This catheter is necessary to allow administration of fluids (5 ml·kg^{-1} to 7 ml·kg^{-1} of lactated Ringer's solution with 5 percent glucose) to offset dehydration associated with preoperative fasting. The other important reason for placing an intravenous catheter is administration of drugs to produce anesthesia or to treat adverse intraoperative events, such as bradycardia, cardiac dysrhythmias, or hypotension. Nevertheless, placement of an intravenous catheter in every patient may be unnecessary when technical difficulties outweigh the advantages of having an intravenous infusion site and/or the surgery will be very short (less than 15 minutes) and only superficial tissues are involved.

General Anesthesia

General anesthesia is most frequently selected for outpatient surgery. Induction of anesthesia is pleasantly achieved with the intravenous administration of conventional induction drugs. Methohexital is alleged to have a shorter duration of action than thiopental or thiamylal and, for this reason, is a popular drug for induction of anesthesia for outpatients. Nevertheless, it must be appreciated that repeated rejections of any barbiturate can lead to cumulative effects and delayed postoperative awakening. Etomidate, like methohexital, is associated with rapid awakening but the increased incidence of myoclonic movements, nausea, and vomiting detracts from its use. Propofol produces rapid induction of anesthesia and recovery is prompt, with minimal residual psychomotor effects. Benzodiazepines are not popular for induction of anesthesia in outpatients because of their prolonged duration of action. Furthermore, intense amnesia, particularly after administration of midazolam, could interfere with patients remembering postoperative instructions after they return home. Availability of a specific benzodiazepine antagonist may negate these undesirable effects.

Pediatric patients may prefer an inhalation induction to the needle stick required for an intravenous induction of anesthesia, but even this alternative should be discouraged; as a small-gauge catheter can be placed with minimal discomfort. Furthermore, the discomfort associated with local infiltration can be obviated by using a 30-gauge needle and wiping the alcohol prep solution from the site with a dry gauze before puncturing the skin. When an inhalation induction of anesthesia is planned, however, the most frequently selected drug is halothane. Compared with halothane, induction of anesthesia with enflurane or isoflurane is associated with more patient excitement, breath-holding, coughing, and laryngospasm. In uncontrollable patients, induction of anesthesia can be achieved with administration of rectal methohexital (10 mg·kg^{-1} to 25 mg·kg^{-1}), which produces unconsciousness in 7 minutes to 10 minutes. The disadvantage of rectal methohexital is delayed awakening after surgery.

Placement of a tube in the trachea is often facilitated by skeletal muscle relaxation produced by intravenous administration of succinylcholine or short-acting nondepolarizing muscle relaxants. A significant disadvantage of succinylcholine for use in outpatients is the occurrence of postoperative myalgia. The incidence of myalgia may be reduced by prior administration of subparalyzing doses of nondepolarizing muscle relaxants (Table 29-1).[7] Short-acting nondepolarizing muscle relaxants are alternatives, but their onset of action will likely be slower than succinylcholine and residual neuromuscular blockade at the conclusion of surgery may require pharmacologic antagonism.

Table 29-1. Myalgia 24 Hours After Elective Dilation and Curettage

	Incidence (%)
No succinylcholine (n − 20)	0
Succinylcholine 1 mg·kg^{-1} (n − 20)	40
d-Tubocurarine 0.04 mg·kg^{-1} Succinylcholine 1 mg·kg^{-1} (n − 20)	0

(Data from Stoelting and Peterson[7].)

Intubation of the trachea should not be avoided because the surgery is being performed as an outpatient procedure. Use of a small diameter tube and care to avoid trauma, however, during direct laryngoscopy are particularly important for outpatients. Pediatric patients are probably the most vulnerable to airway edema after intubation of the trachea because of the small diameter of their glottic opening. Nevertheless, the incidence of laryngotracheal edema (croup) after 1 hour to 4 hours of tracheal intubation was only 5 percent in children 1 year to 7 years of age.[8] Furthermore, symptoms of laryngotracheal edema are most likely to occur in the first hour after extubation of the trachea when the patient is still in the recovery room.

Maintenance of anesthesia is often with nitrous oxide and volatile anesthetics or short-acting opioids. Intravenous administration of short-acting opioids (alfentanil 1 μg·kg^{-1} to 3μg·kg^{-1}) reduces anesthetic requirements for volatile drugs and may reduce the need for postoperative analgesics. The incidence of postoperative nausea and vomiting, however, may be greater after administration of opiods. There is no important difference among halothane, enflurane, and isoflurane with respect to awakening times, which are rapid after discontinuance of all three drugs. Halothane is the most commonly used drug for pediatric outpatient anesthesia. Unlike halothane, enflurane and isoflurane significantly enhance the effects of nondepolarizing muscle relaxants or alone may provide sufficient skeletal muscle relaxation to negate the need for muscle relaxants. Continuous intravenous infusions of propofol or alfentanil may be associated with more rapid awakening after short surgical procedures than that which occurs after administration of volatile anesthetics.[9] Nitrous oxide is a principal component of all general anesthetic techniques used for outpatient surgery. In this regard, the role of nitrous oxide as a causative factor for postoperative nausea and vomiting is unresolved, with studies showing an association offset by others that fail to document this effect.[10] Ketamine is seldom used to anesthetize adults for outpatient surgery because of prolonged recovery and the occasional occurrence of unpleasant postoperative dreams. In contrast, ketamine has been extensively used for outpatient pediatric procedures without overt behavioral problems or hallucinations.

At the conclusion of surgery, infiltration of the incision with long-acting local anesthetics, such as bupivacaine, may decrease the need for postoperative analgesics. Severe postoperative pain may be treated by intravenous administration of short-acting opioids such as alfentanil or fentanyl. Nausea, vomiting, and sedation may accompany administration of opioids for this purpose. Conversely, nausea and vomiting often accompany pain and can be relieved when analgesia is provided by intravenous administration of opioids. Droperidol administered intravenously in doses of $10~\mu \cdot kg^{-1}$ to $30~\mu g \cdot kg^{-1}$ is useful in the treatment of patients with persistent postoperative nausea and vomiting, remembering that higher doses of droperidol may cause sedation and delay discharge from the recovery room.

Regional Anesthesia

A disadvantage of regional anesthesia (lumbar epidural or spinal block) for outpatient surgery is residual sympathetic nervous system blockade that produces orthostatic hypotension and prevents early postoperative ambulation. The possibility of headache after a spinal block further detracts from the use of this technique of anesthesia for outpatient surgery. Despite these disadvantages, regional anesthesia can be successfully used for outpatient surgery in selected patients. Furthermore, there is no evidence that early ambulation increases the incidence of postspinal headache. In younger patients or those in whom the potential

for headache may be unacceptably high, epidural block is a suitable alternative to spinal block.

Peripheral Nerve Block

Peripheral nerve blocks are useful for operations on the extremities. An intravenous block is appropriate for superficial surgery on the extremities. Brachial plexus block is necessary when other than superficial surgery is performed on the arm.

DISCHARGE FROM RECOVERY ROOM

Discharge from the recovery room is based on documentation that residual effects of anesthesia are dissipated. Recovery from anesthesia is evidenced by the presence of stable and normal vital signs, a level of consciousness similar to preoperative status, and the ability to ambulate without assistance. If regional anesthesia was employed, it is important to document complete return of both sensory and motor function. Nausea, vomiting, and vertigo should be absent and the patient should not be in excessive pain. The ability to tolerate fluids (water, carbonated drinks, popsicles) should be determined. Hoarseness or stridor in a patient in whom a tracheal tube was inserted must be watched carefully. Significant laryngeal edema typically manifests within the first hour after tracheal intubation. Most of these patients respond to conservative measures and can be discharged without overnight hospitalization. As a precaution, however, these patients should be observed for 3 hours to 4 hours after extubation of the trachea to assure that symptoms are not progressing. Otherwise, most patients are ready for discharge from the recovery room to an adult escort within 1.5 hours after surgery. The decision to discharge patients is most often the responsibility of the anesthesiologist in consultation, when appropriate, with the surgeon.

Patients should be reminded that mental clarity and dexterity may remain impaired for as long as 24 hours to 48 hours despite an overall feeling of well-being. Therefore, important decisions, driving an automobile, or operation of complex equipment should not be attempted during this period. Ingestion of alcohol or depressant drugs should be cautioned against, as additive responses with residual anesthetic effects are possible. Diet should initially consist of clear liquids progressing to soup, cereal, crackers, and ice cream as tolerated. Oral analgesics, such as acetaminophen, should be provided for those likely to require such medication. Finally, patients should be provided with a telephone number of a physician familiar with their case, as well as instructions for symptoms (bleeding, difficulty breathing, fever) that should be reported to the doctor and a list of possible complications (sore throat, myalgia, incisional pain, headache) that do not require physician consultation. A nurse or physician at the outpatient facility should call the patient the next day to assure that recovery is proceeding without complications.

REFERENCES

1. Natof HE. Complications associated with ambulatory surgery. JAMA 1980;244:1116–8.
2. Welborn LG, Ramirez N, Oh TH, et al. Postanesthetic apnea and periodic breathing in infants. Anesthesiology 1986;65:658–61.
3. Kurth CD, Spitzer AR, Broennle MD, et al. Postoperative apnea in former premature infants. Anesthesiology 1985;63:A475.
4. Meridy HW. Criteria for selection of ambulatory surgical patients and guidelines for anesthetic management: A retrospective study of 1553 cases. Anesth Analg 1982;61:921–6.
5. Brzustowicz RM, Nelson DA, Betts EK, Rosenberry KR, Swedlow DB. Efficacy of oral premedication for pediatric outpatient surgery. Anesthesiology 1984;60:475–7.
6. Ong BY, Palahniuk RJ, Cumming M. Gastric volume and pH in outpatients. Can Anaesth Soc J 1978;25:36–9.
7. Stoelting RK, Peterson C. Adverse effects of increased succinylcholine dose following d-tubocurarine pretreatment. Anesth Analg 1975;54:282–8.
8. Smith FK, Deputy BS, Berry FA. Outpatient anesthesia for children undergoing extensive dental treatment. J Dis Child 1978;45:142–5.
9. Zuurmond WWA, vanLeeuwen L. Alfentanil v. isoflurane for outpatient arthroscopy. Acta Anaesthesiol Scand 1986;30:329–32.
10. Korttila K, Hovorka J, Erkola O. Nitrous oxide does not increase the incidence of nausea and vomiting after isoflurane anesthesia. Anesth Analg 1987;66:761–5.

Recovery Period

Chapter 30

Recovery Room

The recovery room (postanesthesia care unit, PACU) is that area designated for the monitoring and care of patients who are recovering from the immediate physiologic derangements produced by anesthesia and surgery. Standards for postanesthesia care have been endorsed by the American Society of Anesthesiologists (see Appendix 2). This room should be staffed with specially trained nurses skilled in the prompt recognition of postoperative complications. Location of the recovery room in close proximity to the operating rooms assures rapid access to physician consultation and assistance. Specifically, an anesthesiologist should be readily available and responsible for ensuring safe recovery from anesthesia. Equipment and drugs must be available to provide routine care (supplemental oxygen, suction, monitoring of vital signs, pulse oximeter, electrocardiogram) and advanced organ support (ventilators, transducers to monitor intravascular pressures, devices for continuous infusion of drugs). An electrical defibrillator and appropriate drugs to assist in the optimal provision of cardiopulmonary resuscitation must be available. The recovery room should have good access to radiographic and arterial blood gas services. The size of the recovery room is determined by the number and type of operative procedures, with approximately 1.5 recovery room beds being necessary for every operating room. Discharge of patients from the recovery room is the responsibility of a physician, most often an anesthesiologist. Administratively, an anesthesiologist usually serves as the medical director of the recovery room.

RECOVERY FROM ANESTHESIA

Recovery from anesthesia is usually uneventful and routine, beginning with discontinuation of the administration of anesthetic drugs and extubation of the trachea while the patient is still in the operating room. The rate of reduction in the alveolar concentration (partial pressure) of an inhaled anesthetic as a reflection of recovery is dependent on the patient's alveolar ventilation, the lipid solubility of the anesthetic drug, the magnitude of metabolism of the anesthetic drug, and the duration of anesthesia (see Chapter 2).[1] Patients are likely to begin responding to verbal stimuli when alveolar anesthetic concentrations are reduced to about one-half the minimum alveolar concentration (MAC) value for the volatile drug.[2] This value is designated MAC awake. Recovery from the anesthetic effects of injected drugs depends on the dose administered; the time since the last injection; and the drug's lipid solubility, hepatic inactivation, and/or renal excretion. If muscle relaxants have been administered, it is important to assess the residual activity of these drugs using a peripheral nerve stimulator. This assessment should be made in the operating room

425

Information Given to Nurse at the Time of Admission to the Recovery Room

Patient's name and age

Surgical procedure

Preoperative medication and anesthetic drugs used

Other intraoperative drugs—anticholinesterases, opioid antagonists, benzodiazepine antagonists, diuretics, cardiac dysrhythmics

Preoperative vital signs

Co-existing medical diseases and associated defects

Preoperative drug therapy

Allergies

Intraoperative estimated blood loss and measured urine output

Intraoperative fluid and blood replacement

Anesthetic and surgical complications

Special medications or procedures that will be necessary in the recovery room

---

before allowing the return of spontaneous ventilation or considering extubation of the trachea.

ADMISSION TO THE RECOVERY ROOM

Upon arrival in the recovery room, the anesthesiologist provides the nurse with pertinent details of the patient's history, medical condition, anesthetic, and surgery. Supplemental inspired oxygen is routinely provided in many instances, regardless of the duration or type of surgery. Ideally, a nurse is responsible for the care of only one patient in the recovery room. Vital signs should be recorded at least every 15 minutes while the patient is in the recovery room. The vital signs and other pertinent information are recorded on a separate

sheet that becomes part of the patient's medical record (Fig. 30-1). While in the recovery room, the patient is encouraged by the nurse to cough, deep breathe, and change position. Before discharge from the recovery room, the patient is evaluated by a physician (usually an anesthesiologist), who writes a note in the patient's medical record describing pertinent aspects of the anesthetic and recovery room period. This note serves as a source of information to the anesthesiologist who may be responsible for administration of anesthesia to this patient in the future. Although criteria for discharge from the recovery room are not standardized, they typically include (1) absence of adverse events associated with surgery, such as continued bleeding; (2) a level of consciousness consistent with the return of protective upper airway reflexes; (3) the ability to maintain a patent upper airway; (4) the presence of stable vital signs; and (5) acceptable cardiac, pulmonary, and renal function. The recovery room nurse should give a full description of the patient's intraoperative and immediate postopertaive course to the ward nurse at the time the patient is returned to the ward.

PHYSIOLOGIC DISORDERS IN THE RECOVERY ROOM

Physiologic disorders that must be diagnosed and treated in the recovery room during emergence from the immediate effects of anesthesia and surgery include pulmonary complications, circulatory complications, agitation, pain, renal dysfunction, bleeding abnormalities, and decreased body temperature.

Pulmonary Complications

Pulmonary complications associated with the early postoperative period include upper airway obstruction, arterial hypoxemia, alveolar hypoventilation, and inhalation (aspiration) of gastric contents.

Upper Airway Obstruction

Upper airway obstruction in the recovery room is most often due to occlusion of the pharynx by the tongue. Laryngeal obstruction is less common but can occur secondary to laryngospasm or can be caused by direct airway injury. Obstruction of the pharynx or larynx can occur after head and neck

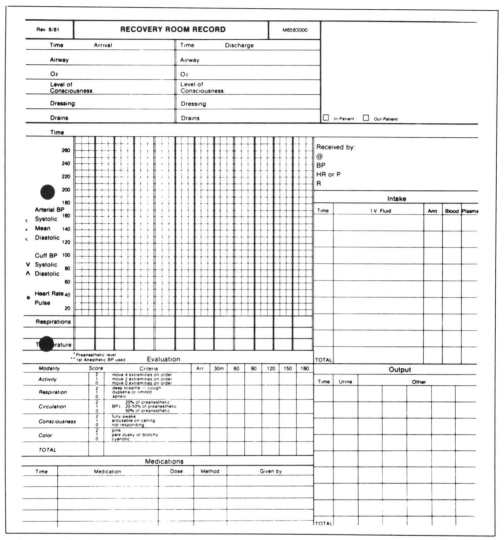

Fig. 30-1. An example of a postanesthesia recovery room record.

surgery when the head cannot be positioned optimally to maintain a patent upper airway.

Physical examination of patients with upper airway obstruction reveals flaring of the nares, retraction at the suprasternal notch (tracheal tug) and intercostal spaces, and vigorous diaphragmatic and abdominal contractions. The most effective method of eliminating airway obstruction due to occlusion of the pharynx by the tongue is extension of the head with or without anterior displacement of the mandible (head tilt-jaw thrust method) (see Chapter 34). This maneuver stretches muscles attached to the tongue, serving to pull the tongue away from the posterior pharyngeal wall. If upper airway obstruction is not immediately reversible by this maneuver, a nasopharyngeal or oropharyngeal airway can be inserted. A nasopharyngeal airway is better tolerated by patients awakening from general anesthesia and thus is the preferred initial selection. An oropharyngeal airway placed in the semiconscious patient may stimulate gagging and vomiting, as well as laryngospasm. Treatment of laryngospasm is initially extension of the head and anterior displacement of the mandible plus application of positive airway pressure with a bag and mask delivering pure oxygen. If laryngospasm is incomplete, this treatment is satisfactory until the spasm spontaneously dissipates. Complete laryngospasm that persists despite these maneuvers should be rapidly treated with intravenous administration of succinylcholine (0.15 mg·kg^{-1} to 0.3 mg·kg^{-1}). Direct laryngoscopy and intubation of the trachea with a cuffed tube is indicated when upper airway obstruction persists despite proper head positioning and use of an artificial airway. Should intubation of the trachea be technically impossible, the placement of a 12-gauge to 14-gauge extracath needle (catheter over-needle) through the cricothyroid membrane (cricothyroidotomy) will provide temporary oxygenation until a more definitive procedure, such as tracheostomy, can be performed.

Upper airway obstruction due to laryngeal edema may be treated by humidifying the inhaled gases and administering nebulized racemic epinephrine. Intravenous administration of dexamethasone (0.15 mg·kg^{-1}) has been used for treatment of laryngeal edema, but the efficacy of this therapy has not been confirmed. In children, laryngeal edema can rapidly progress to complete upper airway obstruction, emphasizing the importance of close surveillance in the recovery room.

Arterial Hypoxemia

Arterial hypoxemia in the immediate postoperative period most likely reflects the impact of anesthetic drugs and/or events occurring intraoperatively. Decreases in the PaO$_2$ are common, particularly after upper abdominal or thoracic surgery.[3] For example, the PaO$_2$ decreases about 20 mmHg after upper abdominal or thoracic surgery. The decrease in PaO$_2$ is much less after lower abdominal (10 mmHg) or peripheral surgery (6 mmHg).

Etiology. Factors leading to postoperative arterial hypoxemia are multiple. Probably the most common cause of postoperative arterial hypoxemia is an increase in right-to-left intrapulmonary shunting due to atelectasis. Atelectasis may be segmental due to bronchial obstruction with secretions or diffuse, reflecting decreased lung volumes. Mismatching of ventilation to perfusion is accentuated by mechanical abnormalities of the lungs such as decreases in the functional residual capacity (FRC). Reductions in cardiac output can contribute to

---

Factors Leading to Postoperative Arterial Hypoxemia

Right-to-left intrapulmonary shunt (atelectasis)

Mismatching of ventilation to perfusion (decreased functional residual capacity)

Decreased cardiac output

Alveolar hypoventilation (residual effects of anesthetics and/or muscle relaxants)

Inhalation of gastric contents (aspiration)

Pulmonary embolus

Pulmonary edema

Pneumothorax

Posthyperventilation hypoxia

Increased oxygen consumption (shivering)

Elderly

Obese

---

decreases in the PaO$_2$ in patients with mismatching of ventilation to perfusion or intrapulmonary shunts. In the absence of supplemental inspired oxygen, the accumulation of carbon dioxide in the alveoli due to drug-induced hypoventilation may lead to arterial hypoxemia. Inhalation of acidic gastric fluid results in rapid onset of profound arterial hypoxemia due to (1) reflex airway closure, (2) loss of surfactant activity leading to atelectasis, and (3) loss of capillary integrity manifesting as noncardiogenic pulmonary edema. A pulmonary embolus, occurring in the immediate postoperative period, can cause profound arterial hypoxemia, although the exact physiologic explanation for the hypoxemia is unclear. This diagnosis should be suspected in any patient who develops acute dyspnea and tachypnea in the recovery room. Pulmonary edema due to left ventricular failure is usually preceded by systemic hypertension and typically occurs in the first hour after surgery (Fig. 30-2).[4] Arterial hypoxemia due to a pneumothorax

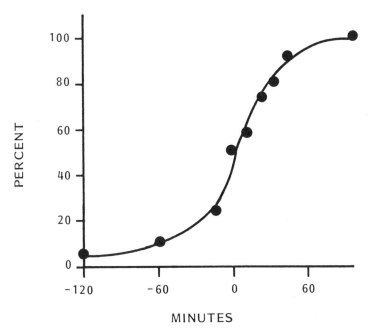

Fig. 30-2. Perioperative pulmonary edema is most likely to occur (percent) within 60 minutes after surgery (O). (From Cooperman and Price,[4] with permission.)

reflects compression of alveoli producing a right-to-left intrapulmonary shunt. Patients undergoing radical neck dissection, mastectomy, or nephrectomy are particularly vulnerable to the development of a pneumothorax. A pneumothorax of over 20 percent in spontaneously breathing patients or any pneumothorax in the presence of mechanical ventilation of the lungs should be treated by insertion of a chest tube. If circulatory depression accompanies a tension pneumothorax, emergency treatment is placement of a 12-gauge to 14-gauge extracath needle (catheter overneedle) into the second anterior intercostal space. Posthyperventilation hypoxia reflects compensatory hypoventilation in attempts to replenish body stores of carbon dioxide that have been depleted by intraoperative hyperventilation.[3] Arterial hypoxemia due to this compensatory hypoventilation is prevented by increasing the inhaled concentrations of oxygen. Diffusion hypoxia as a cause of arterial hypoxemia in the recovery room is unlikely because the early dilutional effect of nitrous oxide on the alveolar partial pressures of oxygen is

prevented by only a few breaths of oxygen at the conclusion of the anesthetic (see Chapter 2). Postoperative shivering can result in substantial increases in oxygen consumption but only rarely contributes to arterial hypoxemia.[5] Finally, advanced age and obesity are likely to be associated with exaggerated reductions in arterial oxygenation in the postoperative period.

Diagnosis. Diagnosis of arterial hypoxemia in the recovery room requires measurement of the PaO_2. Monitoring arterial oxygen saturation with a pulse oximeter is useful for facilitating early recognition of excessive declines in PaO_2. Arterial hypoxemia is considered to be present when the PaO_2 is less than 60 mmHg. Clinical signs of arterial hypoxemia (hypertension, hypotension, tachycardia, bradycardia, cardiac dysrhythmias, agitation) are nonspecific. A lowered hemoglobin concentration may impair detection of cyanosis. Furthermore, circulatory and ventilatory responses to arterial hypoxemia are attenuated by the effects of residual anesthetics. For example, sedative concentrations

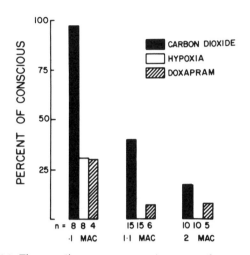

Fig. 30-3. The ventilatory response (percent of consciousness) to carbon dioxide, hypoxia, and doxapram was depressed in a dose-related manner by halothane administered to volunteers without pulmonary disease. For example, 0.1 MAC halothane reduced the ventilatory response to hypoxia by about 75 percent as compared with the conscious response. The ventilatory response to hypoxia was absent at 1.1 MAC halothane. (From Knill and Gelb,[6] with permission.)

Factors Leading to Postoperative Alveolar Hypoventilation

Drug-induced central nervous system depression (volatile anesthetics, opioids)

Residual effects of muscle relaxants

Suboptimal ventilatory muscle mechanics

Increased production of carbon dioxide

Co-existing chronic obstructive airways disease

---

of volatile anesthetics (0.1 MAC) nearly abolish the usual increase in ventilation produced by arterial hypoxemia (Fig. 30-3).[6] Thus, arterial hypoxemia is unlikely to stimulate ventilation in postoperative patients who have received a volatile anesthetic.

Treatment. Treatment of arterial hypoxemia in the recovery room is with supplemental oxygen. Supplemental oxygen does not eliminate the cause of arterial hypoxemia but may symptomatically alleviate it while concomitant corrective measures are employed. For example, if arterial hypoxemia is due to hypoventilation from excessive residual effects of opioids, specific pharmacologic antagonism with naloxone is indicated. Mismatching of ventilation to perfusion decreases with coughing, deep breathing, and eventually ambulation.

Indications for supplemental oxygen in the recovery room are not specific. Indeed, almost every patient demonstrates a reduction in PaO_2 after anesthesia and surgery and will therefore benefit from supplemental oxygen. Supplemental oxygen should never be withheld in the postoperative period for fear of abolishing the hypoxic drive to ventilation that may be present in patients with chronic obstructive airways disease. In the presence of chronic obstructive airways disease associated with carbon dioxide retention, graded doses of supplemental oxygen can be administered via an air-entrainment (Venturi) mask while following the patient's oxygenation with measurement of the PaO_2. Indeed, inhaled concentrations of oxygen of 24 percent to 28 percent are often sufficient to raise the patient's PaO_2 to acceptable levels. If arterial hypoxemia persists despite administration of pure oxygen or if hypercapnia accompanies supplemental oxygen therapy, the trachea should be intubated and the patient's lungs mechanically ventilated. In such patients, ventilation of the lungs using positive end-expiratory pressure (PEEP) will increase the FRC and result in an increased PaO_2. Furthermore, ventilation of the lungs using PEEP often allows a reduction in the inspired concentrations of oxygen without decreases in the PaO_2.

Alveolar Hypoventilation

Alveolar hypoventilation leading to hypercarbia is a frequent occurrence in the early postoperative period.

Etiology. Factors leading to postoperative alveolar hypoventilation are multiple. A frequent cause, however, is inadequate central stimulation to ven-

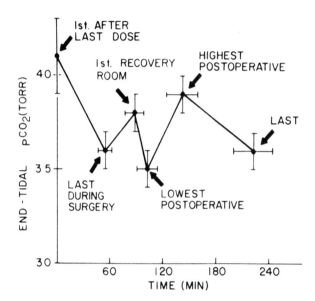

Fig. 30-4. Recurrent fentanyl-induced depression of ventilation is evidenced by elevations of the end-tidal PCO_2 after arrival in the recovery room. (From Becker et al.,[7] with permission.)

tilation due to residual effects of inhaled and/or injected anesthetic drugs. Anesthetic-induced depression of ventilation is evidenced by a shift of the carbon dioxide response curve to the right with or without a concomitant increase in the $PaCO_2$. Ventilatory depression produced by inhaled anesthetics decreases with time. In contrast, opioids, such as fentanyl, can produce biphasic ventilatory depression. For example, drug-induced depression may dissipate with the increased external stimulation provided by the transport and admission to the recovery room only to be followed by a second period of respiratory depression as external stimulation wanes (Fig. 30-4).[7] Residual effects of muscle relaxants may interfere with optimal activity of respiratory muscles leading to accumulation of carbon dioxide. Persistent neuromuscular blockade may reflect (1) prior inadequate pharmacologic antagonism, (2) delayed excretion of the muscle relaxant due to renal disease, or the (3) potentiation of these drugs by other mechanisms (aminoglycoside antibiotics, hypermagnesemia, hypothermia). It should be appreciated that both respiratory acidosis and hypokale-

mia inhibit reversal of neuromuscular blockade with anticholinesterases. Conceivably, alveolar hypoventilation in the recovery room could lead to respiratory acidosis and an unmasking of residual neuromuscular blockade, leading to further carbon dioxide retention. Evidence of residual neuromuscular blockade is best detected with a peripheral nerve stimulator. In addition, the ability to sustain head lift for at least 5 seconds, vigorous hand grasp, tongue protrusion for several seconds, vital capacity above 10 ml·kg^{-1}, and maximal inspiratory force of at least -20 cm H_2O can be used as evidence of adequate recovery from the effects of the muscle relaxant. Suboptimal ventilatory mechanics may be related to the patient's position, obesity, gastric dilation, and the site of the surgical incision. For example, the site of surgical incision affects the ability to take a deep breath as measured by vital capacity. Patients undergoing thoracic or upper abdominal surgery have the greatest reduction in vital capacity, showing as much as a 60 percent reduction on the day of surgery. Postoperative pain can limit tidal volume. Increased production of carbon dioxide is rare but may be a consideration when hyperalimentation solutions are being administered or body temperature is elevated. Finally, chronic obstructive airways disease associated with preoperative hypercarbia is predictably accompanied by a similar finding postoperatively.

Diagnosis. Diagnosis of alveolar hypoventilation in the recovery room requires measurement of the $PaCO_2$. Alveolar hypoventilation is considered to be present when the $PaCO_2$ exceeds 44 mmHg. Signs of carbon dioxide retention, such as tachycardia and hypertension, are not reliably present in postoperative patients.

Measurement of the vital capacity and maximal inspiratory force are good guides to the ability of postoperative patients to breathe spontaneously and maintain adequate alveolar ventilation. The vital capacity should be at least 15 ml·kg^{-1} (about double the predicted tidal volume) and the inspiratory force greater than -20 cm H_2O. Inspiratory force can be tested in the absence of consciousness, whereas measurement of vital capacity requires patient cooperation. If these minimum values cannot be generated, ventilation of the lungs should be mechanically provided.

Treatment. If alveolar hypoventilation is due to residual effects of inhaled anesthetics but the patient remains capable of generating an inspiratory force greater than -20 cm H_2O, it is permissible to allow spontaneous emergence from anesthesia combined with a regimen to keep the patient alert. If not, controlled ventilation of the lungs via a cuffed tube in the trachea will be necessary to maintain normocarbia and accelerate elimination of the inhaled drugs. If alveolar hypoventilation is due to residual effects of opioids, the intravenous administration of incremental doses of naloxone (0.1 $\mu g \cdot kg^{-1}$) is an appropriate consideration. It must be appreciated, however, that the duration of naloxone is brief such that alveolar hypoventilation may recur. Disadvantages of naloxone include sudden reversal of analgesia and associated activation of the sympathetic nervous system, which has been associated with hypertension and cardiac dysrhythmias, particularly when a tracheal tube is in place. Irreversible ventricular fibrillation has also been reported after the administration of naloxone in the early postoperative period.[8] When residual neuromuscular blockade is responsible for alveolar hypoventilation, treatment is either administration of additional anticholinesterase drugs or mechanical ventilation of the lungs until the effects of the muscle relaxants dissipate spontaneously.

Circulatory Complications

Circulatory complications associated with the early postoperative period include hypotension, hypertension, and cardiac dysrhythmias.

Hypotension

Etiology. Multiple causes must be considered in the differential diagnosis of hypotension in the recovery room. The most likely cause of hypotension, however, is decreased venous return and reduced cardiac output due to hypovolemia. Indeed, residual effects of anesthetic drugs are likely to attenuate peripheral vasoconstrictor responses leading to hypotension as an early manifestation of hypovolemia. Hypovolemia is usually a reflec-

---

Factors Leading to Postoperative Hypotension
Hypovolemia
Decreased myocardial contractility
Sepsis
Pulmonary embolus
Pneumothorax
Cardiac tamponade

---

tion of inadequately replaced blood loss or third space loss during surgery. Unrecognized continuing hemorrhage as a cause of hypovolemia and hypotension must also be considered. Reductions in myocardial contractility as a cause of hypotension in the recovery room may be due to residual effects of anesthetics, co-existing ventricular dysfunction, or an acute myocardial infarction. Indeed, most patients with confirmed postoperative myocardial infarction are found to have experienced a period of unexplained hypotension with or without premature ventricular contractions in the recovery room. Angina pectoris occurs in only about one-fourth of these patients, possibly reflecting masking of pain by residual analgesic effects of anesthetics. Sepsis leading to vasodilation and capillary fluid leakage may be responsible for hypotension, particularly after surgery on the genitourinary tract. Other causes of hypotension in the recovery room include pulmonary embolus, pneumothorax, and cardiac tamponade.

Diagnosis and Treatment. Before any therapy of hypotension is instituted, it is important to confirm the accuracy of the blood pressure measurement. Artifactual blood pressure readings can be due to an improperly placed or sized blood pressure cuff, an inaccurately calibrated transducer, or positioning of the transducer above the level of the right atrium (midaxillary line). For example, the measured pressure is falsely reduced about 0.7 mmHg for every centimeter the transducer is elevated above heart level in supine patients.

Oliguria (less than 0.5 $ml \cdot kg^{-1} \cdot hr^{-1}$) is a useful guide to the presence of hypovolemia or decreased myocardial contractility. Inncreased urine output after a fluid challenge with 3 ml·kg^{-1} to 6 ml·kg^{-1} of lactated Ringer's solution suggests the presence of hypovolemia rather than decreased myocardial contractility. A low hematocrit plus evidence of bleeding at the operative site should suggest inadequate surgical hemostasis. Elevation of the legs and administration of a sympathomimetic to maintain perfusion pressure until hypovolemia can be corrected is prudent treatment.

If hypotension persists despite fluid replacement, an estimate of right atrial pressure is indicated. In the presence of normal left ventricular function, central venous pressure will be a reasonable reflection of intravascular fluid volume. In the presence of selective left ventricular dysfunction or co-existing chronic obstructive airways disease, the central venous pressure may not be an accurate guide and pressures measured via a pulmonary artery catheter are necessary for an accurate diagnosis. Hypovolemia as a cause of hypotension is suggested by a low pulmonary artery occlusion pressure (less than 10 mmHg), a normal to low cardiac index (normal above 2.5 L·min^{-1}·m^{-2}) and a normal to elevated calculated systemic vascular resistance (normal 900 dynes–sec·cm^5 to 1400 dynes–sec·cm^5). Decreased myocardial contractility as the etiology of hypotenssion is characterized by high pulmonary artery occlusion pressures (above 15 mmHg) and a low cardiac output. After optimizing intravascular fluid volume, the treatment of hypotension due to decreased myocardial contractility is with inotropes (see Chapter 3). Sepsis as a cause of hypotension is characterized by low pulmonary artery occlusion pressures, elevated cardiac output, and decreased systemic vascular resistance. Replacement of fluid loss with crystalloid solutions (colloid can leak into tissues drawing fluid with it) and maintenance of coronary perfusion pressures with alpha agonists, such as phenylephrine, are indicated in the immediate treatment of hypotension due to sepsis.

Hypertension

Etiology. Hypertension that develops in the immediate postoperative period is most often due to the stimulation provided by sensation of pain as emergence from anesthesia occurs. When hypertension does develop during recovery from anesthesia, it usually manifests in the first 30 minutes after surgery (Fig. 30-5).[9] Preoperative hypertension is present in over one-half of patients who develop hypertension in the recovery room. Postoperative hypertension can be exaggerated if antihypertensives were withdrawn preoperatively. Other causes to consider when hypertension occurs in the recovery room include fluid overload, arterial hypoxemia, and hypercarbia. Excessive and sustained elevations in blood pressure can lead to left ventricular failure with pulmonary edema, myocardial ischemia due to increased myocardial oxygen requirements, cardiac dysrhythmias, and cerebral hemorrhage.

Diagnosis and Treatment. Management of acute hypertension begins with identification and correction of the initiating cause. When pain is the etiology of acute hypertension, the immediate treatment is the intravenous administration of opioids until adequate pain relief is achieved (see the section *Pain*). Hypertension that persists in the absence of a known etiology is best managed by the continuous intravenous infusion of vasodilators such as nitroprusside. The arterial blood pressure is titrated to a desired level by adjusting the infusion rate of nitroprusside. The infusion rate should not exceed 10 μg·kg^{-1}·min^{-1} or a total dose of 1.5 mg·kg^{-1} for a 1-hour to 3-hour administration. Even when these dose recommendations are followed, it is important to measure the arterial pH hourly to detect the appearance of acidosis due to the metabolism of nitroprusside to cyanide. Should metabolic acidosis appear, nitroprusside must be discontinued immediately and an alternative vasodilator, such as trimethaphan, administered. Hydralazine in 2.5 mg to 5 mg increments administered intravenously is also an effective treatment for postoperative hypertension. Disadvantages of hydralazine include a delayed onset (5 minutes to 15 minutes) and baroreceptor-mediated tachycardia when the blood pressure decreases. Regardless of the drug selected to produce normotension, it is important to reliably monitor blood pressure often via a catheter in a peripheral artery.

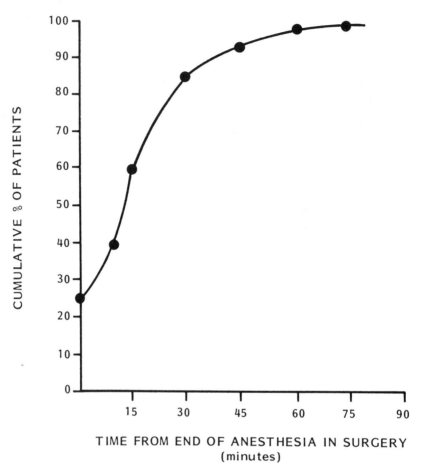

Fig. 30-5. Hypertension that develops postoperatively typically manifests in the first 30 minutes after the end of surgery. (From Gal and Cooperman,[9] with permission.)

Cardiac Dysrhythmias

Etiology. Cardiac dysrhythmias in the immediate postoperative period have multiple causes. Arterial hypoxemia should be the first cause considered when cardiac dysrhythmias manifest initially in the recovery room. Sinus tachycardia is a common occurrence in the early postoperative period. This rhythm should suggest the possible presence of arterial hypoxemia, hypovolemia, or pain. Sinus bradycardia accompanies arterial hypoxemia and decreases in body temperature and may reflect effects of anticholinesterases administered earlier to reverse nondepolarizing muscle relaxants. The appearance of premature ventricular contractions should suggest the presence of arterial hypoxemia, myocardial ischemia, electrolyte abnormalities, or respiratory acidosis. Hypertension may increase myocardial irritability, leading to premature ventricular contractions. The appearance of cardiac dysrhythmias in patients receiving digitalis preparations should arouse suspicion of digitalis toxicity.

Treatment. Most cardiac dysrhythmias occurring in the recovery room do not require treatment other than correcting the underlying cause. Regardless of the type of cardiac dysrhythmia, the first priority is to assure the patency of the upper airway and the adequacy of arterial oxygenation.

Factors Leading to Postoperative Cardiac Dysrhythmias

Arterial hypoxemia

Hypovolemia

Pain

Hypothermia

Anticholinesterases

Myocardial ischemia

Electrolyte abnormalities
  Hypokalemia
  Hypocalcemia

Respiratory acidosis

Hypertension

Digitalis intoxication

Preoperative cardiac dysrhythmias

Specific drug therapies to treat hemodynamically significant cardiac dysrhythmias include intravenous administration of atropine (3 $\mu g \cdot kg^{-1}$ to 6 $\mu g \cdot kg^{-1}$) to increase heart rate, verapamil (75 $\mu g \cdot kg^{-1}$ to 150 $\mu g \cdot kg^{-1}$ infused over 1 minute to 3 minutes) to slow heart rate, and lidocaine (1 $mg \cdot kg^{-1}$ to 1.5 $mg \cdot kg^{-1}$) to suppress premature ventricular contractions. Electrical cardioversion is necessary to treat hemodynamically significant atrial or ventricular tachydysrhythmias that are unresponsive to drug therapy.

Agitation (Emergence Delirium)

A small number of patients awaken from anesthesia in an agitated state, which may require physical restraint. The incidence of this behavior seems to be increased in young patients who are apprehensive about the findings at operation as well as in individuals who fear pain. Arterial hypoxemia and/or hypercapnia as a cause of agitation must be initially considered. The perception of pain in patients who have not regained full consciousness and self-control may manifest as agitation. Other causes of agitation include unrecognized gastric dilation, urinary retention, and pneumothorax. The incidence of postoperative agitation is increased in patients who have received scopolamine as preoperative medication, particularly when this drug is administered in the absence of opioids (see Chapter 10). Agitation can also follow the administration of atropine, but the incidence is less than that associated with scopolamine. Intravenous administration of physostigmine 15 $\mu g \cdot kg^{-1}$ to 45 $\mu g \cdot kg^{-1}$ (often combined with glycopyrrolate to prevent peripheral cholinergic effects) will reverse agitation associated with anticholinergics. Presumably, physostigmine (a tertiary amine anticholinesterase) crosses the blood-brain barrier and acts to increase levels of acetylcholine, which then displaces anticholinergics from central receptor sites. Physostigmine may also reverse prolonged somnolence due to central nervous system effects of anticholinergics. Benzodiazepine-induced prolonged somnolence is reversible with intravenous administration of a specific antagonist, flumazenil.

Pain

Pain is a predictable response as the effects of anesthetic drugs wane in the early postoperative period.

Etiology

Many factors influence the incidence and severity of postoperative pain. Infants and elderly patients seem to experience less pain than middle-aged patients. The need for postoperative pain medication is reduced when the anesthesiologist visits patients preoperatively and provides detailed explanations of postoperative events, including the occurrence of pain (Fig. 30-6).[10] Inclusion of opioids in the preoperative medication or use of opioids during maintenance of anesthesia usually delays the first postoperative request for pain medication. Preoperative traits, such as a neurotic personality or fear of pain, tend to increase postoperative pain. The site of operation influences the severity of postoperative pain, with thoracotomy and upper abdominal and orthopaedic surgery being the most painful.

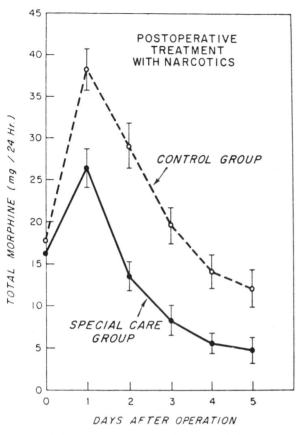

Fig. 30-6. Adult patients (n-97) undergoing abdominal surgery were divided into two groups. Both groups were visited preoperatively by the anesthesiologist, but only the special care group received a detailed explanation regarding the character, intensity, and management of pain in the postoperative period. The normal occurrence of postoperative pain was stressed to these patients. The value of this explanation was evidenced by the decreased total dose of morphine administered to the special care patients compared with the control group. (From Egbert et al.,[10] with permission.)

Treatment

Treatment of postoperative pain is usually with incremental doses of morphine (15 $\mu g \cdot kg^{-1}$ to 40 $\mu g \cdot kg^{-1}$) administered intravenously every 15 minutes to 30 minutes until adequate pain relief is achieved. Indeed, intravenous titration of opioids often results in analgesia sooner than do

larger doses administered intramuscularly. Continuous or intermittent (patient-controlled analgesia [PCA]) intravenous infusions of low doses of opioids may provide more consistent and optimal analgesia with minimal cardiorespiratory depression. In the future, transdermal administration of opioids may provide a route of administration that allows sustained maintenance of therapeutic plasma concentrations of drugs. Continuous thoracic or lumbar block with long-acting local anesthetics, such as bupivacaine, is an effective method for providing postoperative analgesia, especially in patients with chronic pulmonary disease who may be vulnerable to opioid-induced ventilatory depression. Disadvantages of epidural block include skeletal muscle weakness and orthostatic hypotension due to peripheral sympathetic nervous system blockade. Both of these adverse effects interfere with early postoperative ambulation. Intercostal nerve blocks are particularly useful for management of postcholecystectomy pain. Pneumothorax is a rare but possible side effect of these blocks. Placement of opioids into the epidural space or subarachnoid space (i.e., neuraxial opioids) is useful in providing prolonged postoperative analgesia. Significant depression of ventilation, either immediate or delayed for up to 6 hours to 12 hours and requiring treatment with naloxone, occurs in less than 1 percent of patients. Most important, adequate analgesia, regardless of how it is provided, allows the patient to take deep breaths and cough, thus reducing the likelihood of postoperative atelectasis and pneumonia.

Evolution of effective pain management techniques, especially PCA and neuraxial administration of opioids, has led to the development of anesthesiology-based Acute Pain Management Services (Fig. 30-7).[11] The Acute Pain Management Service may assume complete responsibility for postoperative pain relief.

Renal Dysfunction

Oliguria (less than 0.5 $ml \cdot kg^{-1} \cdot hr^{-1}$) that manifests in the recovery room most likely reflects reduced renal blood flow due to hypovolemia or decreased cardiac output (see the section *Hypotension*). An indwelling urinary catheter is important

PCA STANDARD ORDERS

1. Drug
   _____ MORPHINE (1 mg/ml)
   _____ MEPERIDINE (10 mg/ml)
   _____ OTHER _____ Concentration _____
2. Loading dose (optional) _____ mg   Time_____
3. Incremental dose _____mg, *i.e.,* _____ml
4. Lockout interval—8 minutes
5. Four-hour limit (ml) _____ (max = 30 ml/4 hours)
6. If pain not controlled after one hour, increase
   incremental dose by _____ mg, *i.e.,* _____ ml,
   one time only.
7. If pain still not controlled after one additional hour,
   reduce lockout interval by _____ minutes, one time only.
8. *No systemic narcotics* to be given except by order of
   Acute Pain Management Service.
9. Monitoring:
   Respiratory rate, analgesic level, sedation level—
   q2h for 8 hours, then q4h.
10. Documentation:
    Record drug use on vital signs sheet at each
    monitoring interval and 8 hour totals on medication
    sheet.
11. Treatment of side effects:
    A. DROPERIDOL 0.25 mg for nausea/vomiting.
       MR × 1.
    B. "In and out" bladder catheter prn for urinary
       retention.
    C. NALOXONE 0.1 mg IV stat for respiratory rate
       < 8. MR × 3. Call Acute Pain Management
       Service.
12. For inadequate analgesia or other problems related to
    PCA, call the Acute Pain Management Service.

Dr. _____ of the Acute Pain Management
Service was notified about this patient at _____ (hours).
Date _____ _____, M.D.

EPIDURAL NARCOTIC STANDARD ORDERS

1. Initial dose: Drug _____ mg _____ Time _____
2. Drug for continuing analgesia:
   A. PF MORPHINE (1 mg/ml) _____ mg q 6–12 hours.
   B. FENTANYL (5 µg/ml) Infuse _____ µg
      (_____ ml)/hour with infusion controller.
   C. OTHER: Drug/Conc _____ Dose _____
      Interval _____
3. Maintain IV access (drip, heparin lock) for 24 hours after
   last dose of epidural narcotic.
4. NALOXONE 0.4 mg at bedside.
5. *No systemic narcotics* to be given except as ordered by
   Acute Pain Management Service.
6. Monitoring:
   A. Respiratory rate and sedation scale q1h for first 24
      hours. Sedation scale q1h for second 24 hours.
      After 48 hours, sedation scale q4h.
   B. Respiratory monitor for first 24 hours. Yes _____
      No _____
7. Nausea/vomiting prophylaxis:
   METOCLOPRAMIDE 10 mg IV slowly q8h × 3; then
   q8h prn for nausea/vomiting.
8. Treatment of side effects:
   A. RR < 10/min, —call Acute Pain Management Service.
      RR < 8/min, —NALOXONE 0.4 mg IV stat. MR prn.
      Call Acute Pain Management Service.
   B. NALOXONE 0.1 mg IV for severe itching. MR q
      10 min. × 5
   C. DROPERIDOL 0.25 mg IV if metoclopramide
      ineffective for nausea/vomiting. MR × 1.
   D. NALOXONE 0.1 mg IV for urinary retention. MR q
      10 min. × 5. If ineffective, "in and out" bladder
      catheter.
9. For inadequate analgesia or other problems related to
   epidural, call Acute Pain Management Service.

Dr. _____ of the Acute Pain Management
Service was notified about this patient at _____ (hours).
Date _____ _____, M.D.

Fig. 30-7. Acute Pain Management Service: Typical postoperative orders. (From Ready et al.,[11] with permission.)

<table>
<tr><td colspan="2" align="center">Patients at High Risk for Postoperative
Renal Dysfunction</td></tr>
<tr><td colspan="2">Co-existing renal disease</td></tr>
<tr><td colspan="2">Major trauma</td></tr>
<tr><td colspan="2">Sepsis</td></tr>
<tr><td colspan="2">Advanced age</td></tr>
<tr><td colspan="2">Multiple intraoperative blood transfusions</td></tr>
<tr><td colspan="2">Prolonged intraoperative hypotension</td></tr>
<tr><td colspan="2">Cardiac or vascular operations</td></tr>
<tr><td colspan="2">Biliary tract surgery in presence of obstructive jaundice</td></tr>
</table>

Table 30-1. Laboratory Tests for Evaluation of Postoperative Bleeding Abnormalities

Test	Abnormal in Presence of
Platelet count	Dilutional thrombocytopenia Disseminated intravascular coagulation
Bleeding time	Platelet-inhibiting drugs (acetylsalicyclic acid-containing drugs)
Prothrombin time	Disseminated intravascular coagulation Vitamin K deficiency Hepatic disease Warfarin
Partial thromboplastin time	Deficiencies of factor V and/or factor VIII Heparin Hemophilia
Fibrinogen	Disseminated intravascular coagulation
Fibrin split products	Disseminated intravascular coagulation

for the early recognition of oliguria in postoperative patients at high risk for renal failure.

Bleeding Abnormalities

Bleeding abnormalities in the postoperative period most often reflect hemorrhage secondary to inadequate surgical hemostasis. Alternatively, postoperative bleeding may be due to coagulopathies, which can be diagnosed using specific laboratory tests (Table 30-1) (see Chapter 18). While awaiting the results of laboratory tests, the whole blood clotting test can be performed at the bed side to evaluate both clot formation (forms in less than 12 minutes), retraction (platelet function), and lysis.

A platelet count is useful in evaluation of bleeding after massive transfusions of blood (see Chapter 18). A qualitative platelet defect may be due to drugs ingested preoperatively, such as aspirin. This problem is recognized by demonstration of prolonged bleeding times despite normal platelet counts. In these situations, the administration of platelets will reverse thrombocytopenia and also return bleeding times to normal. Disseminated intravascular coagulation is suggested by thrombocytopenia, prolonged prothrombin time, reduced serum concentrations of fibrinogen, and increased circulating levels of fibrin split products.

Dilution of factors V and VIII by massive transfusions of whole blood or inadequate reversal of heparin will manifest as a prolonged partial thromboplastin time. Fresh frozen plasma will reverse prolongation in the prothrombin time and partial thromboplastin time when due to liver disease or factor V or VIII deficiency. Protamine reverses heparin-induced prolongation of the partial thromboplastin time.

Decreased Body Temperature

Decreased body temperature is a complication of operations performed in cold operating rooms. Compensatory mechanisms to offset heat loss (peripheral vasoconstriction, shivering) are prevented by anesthetics and muscle relaxants. Loss of body heat intraoperatively is minimized by maintaining the operating room temperature near 21° Celsius and warming of the inhaled gases. The reduced basal metabolic rate associated with decreased body temperature can manifest in the recovery room as slow awakening from anesthesia. When shivering develops in postoperative patients, it is important to provide supplemental inspired oxygen to offset the marked increases (300 percent to 400 percent) in oxygen consumption that accompany increased skeletal muscle activity.

PROPHYLACTIC VENTILATION

Spontaneous ventilation is often rapid and shallow after surgery. Lung volumes are likely to be decreased, resulting in reduced pulmonary compliance, increased airway resistance, and an increased work of breathing. This restrictive pattern of breathing is accentuated by pain and the surgical incision, which may interfere with normal chest and abdominal wall function. All these changes lead to the accumulation of secretions in alveoli and often the development of atelectasis and pneumonia. For these reasons, postoperative mechanical ventilation of the lungs via a tracheal tube in selected at risk patients (especially those with coexisting chronic obstructive airways disease undergoing upper abdominal or thoracic operations) will serve to reduce the likelihood of significant pulmonary complications. Equally important is provision of adequate postoperative analgesia (see the section *Pain*).

Criteria for extubation of the trachea after surgery must be individualized. Useful criteria include (1) state of consciousness, (2) vital capacity greater than 15 ml·kg^{-1}, (3) inspiratory force greater than -20 cm H_2O, and (4) acceptable arterial blood gases and pH (see Chapter 32). The directional change of these measurements is more important than a single value. Extubation of the trachea is performed after suctioning the patient's pharynx and trachea. The patient then inhales deeply or the lungs are passively expanded with oxygen, the cuff on the tracheal tube is deflated, and the tube is removed from the trachea at maximum lung inflation. This sequence assures that the initial gas flow is outward and permits secretions to be forcefully exhaled rather than inhaled as the tracheal tube is removed.

REFERENCES

1. Carpenter RL, Eger EI II, Johnson BH, Unadkat JD, Sheiner LB. Pharmacokinetics of inhaled anesthetics in humans: Measurements during and after the simultaneous administration of enflurane, halothane, isoflurane, methoxyflurane, and nitrous oxide. Anesth Analg 1986;65:575–82.
2. Stoelting RK, Longnecker DE, Eger EI II. Minimum alveolar concentrations in man on awakening from methoxyflurane, halothane, ether and fluroxene anesthesia: MAC awake. Anesthesiology 1970;33:5–9.
3. Marshall BE, Wyche MQ. Hypoxemia during and after anesthesia. Anesthesiology 1972;37:178–209.
4. Cooperman LH, Price HR. Pulmonary edema in the operative and postoperative period: Review of 40 cases. Ann Surg 1970;172:883–91.
5. Bay J, Nunn JF, Prys-Roberts C. Factors influencing arterial PO_2 during recovery from anesthesia. Br J Anaesth 1968;40:398–407.
6. Knill RL, Gelb AW. Ventilatory responses to hypoxia and hypercapnia during halothane sedation and anesthesia in man. Anesthesiology 1978;49:244–51.
7. Becker LD, Paulson BA, Miller RD, Severinghaus JW, Eger EI II. Biphasic respiratory depression after fentanyl-droperidol or fentanyl alone used to supplement nitrous oxide anesthesia. Anesthesiology 1976;44:291–6.
8. Andree RA. Sudden death following naloxone administration. Anesth Analg 1980;59:782–4.
9. Gal TJ, Cooperman LH. Hypertension in the immediate postoperative period. Br J Anaesth 1975;47:70–4.
10. Ebgert LD, Battit GE, Welch CE, Bartlett MK. Reduction of postoperative pain by encouragement and instruction of patients. N Engl J Med 1964;270:825–7.
11. Ready LB, Oden R, Chadwick HS, et al. Development of an anesthesiology-based postoperative pain management service. Anesthesiology 1988;68:100–6.

Section VI

Consultant Anesthetic Practice

Chapter 31

Respiratory Therapy

Respiratory therapy includes oxygen therapy, humidification and aerosol therapy, bronchial hygiene, and prophylaxis against the development of postoperative pulmonary complications. The anesthesiologist must possess a thorough knowledge of these various modalities of respiratory therapy, their efficacy, limitations, and potential complications. The value of respiratory therapy has been increased by an improved understanding of the pathophysiology of pulmonary disease and the predictable impact of anesthesia and operation on pulmonary function. In addition, the measurement of arterial blood gases and pH has provided a reliable means both to determine the need and to assess the value of respiratory therapy.

OXYGEN THERAPY

Oxygen therapy administered as increased inhaled concentrations of oxygen (supplemental oxygen) is indicated when the PaO_2 decreases below 60 mmHg. The shape of the oxyhemoglobin dissociation curve is such that marked reductions in saturation of hemoglobin with oxygen occur with even small decreases in the PaO_2 below 60 mmHg (90 percent saturation). This marked reduction in saturation of hemoglobin with oxygen decreases the arterial content of oxygen and jeopardizes tissue oxygen availability.

The routine administration of supplemental oxygen to postoperative patients is often beneficial and seldom hazardous. Oxygen therapy is usually delivered by nasal cannula or face mask.

Nasal Cannula

Supplemental oxygen can be administered via a nasal cannula with minimal patient discomfort. A nasal cannula incorporates two prongs that extend about 1 cm into the patient's nares and is held in place by an adjustable elastic head strap. Inspired oxygen concentrations achieved with a nasal cannula depend on the flow rate of oxygen ($L \cdot min^{-1}$) as well as the patient's tidal volume, breathing rate, inspiratory flow rate, and volume of the nasopharynx. As a guideline, the inhaled oxygen concentration is increased about 4 percent for each $L \cdot min^{-1}$ of oxygen delivered. Oxygen flow rates above 6 $L \cdot min^{-1}$ (inhaled oxygen concentrations about 44 percent) do not predictably further increase the inhaled concentrations of oxygen because the volume of the nasopharynx is already filled. Excessive flow rates of oxygen may result in air swallowing and gastric distention. Mouth breathing does not ablate the effectiveness of oxygen therapy delivered by nasal cannula because inspiratory airflow through the posterior pharynx entrains (Bernoulli effect) oxygen from the nose.

Face Mask

Face masks used for oyxgen therapy are categorized as simple, partial rebreathing, nonrebreathing and air-entrainment (Fig. 31-1A–D).[1]

Simple

A simple face mask does not include a valve or oxygen reservoir bag. This mask can provide an inhaled concentration of oxygen between 35 percent and 60 percent with oxygen flow rates of 5 $L \cdot min^{-1}$ to 8 $L \cdot min^{-1}$ (Fig. 31-1A).[1] Variations in the patient's ventilatory parameters alter the inhaled concentrations of oxygen. In adults, the oxygen flow rate should always be at least 5 $L \cdot min^{-1}$ to assure the absence of rebreathing of carbon dioxide. A simple face mask affords little, if any, advantage over a nasal cannula in terms of delivering constant inhaled concentrations of oxygen.

Partial Rebreathing

A partial rebreathing face mask is a valveless system that includes an oxygen reservoir bag (Fig. 31-1B).[1] With oxygen flows greater than 10 $L \cdot min^{-1}$, the inhaled concentrations of oxygen are between 50 percent and 65 percent.

Nonrebreathing

A nonrebreathing face mask includes a unidirectional valve plus an oxygen reservoir bag (Fig 31-1C).[1] Inhaled concentrations of oxygen can be increased to near 100 percent using this face mask. It is difficult, however, to provide a sufficiently tight mask fit to completely eliminate entrainment of room air. The flow rate of oxygen into this system should be sufficient to maintain an inflated reservoir bag.

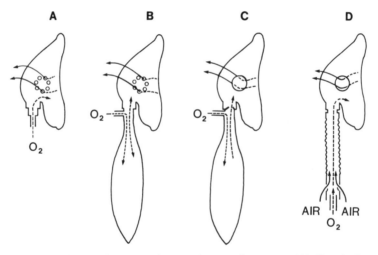

Fig. 31-1. Examples of face masks used to provide supplemental oxygen. (A) Simple face mask. Oxygen flows directly into the mask and exhaled gases leave through holes at the side of the mask. (B) Partial rebreathing face mask. Because there are no valves, the initial portion of the exhaled gases, which contains little or no carbon dioxide (dead space gas), is free to mix with the oxygen in the reservoir bag. As the reservoir bag fills and the pressure in the bag increases, the gases exhaled during the last part of exhalation, which contain carbon dioxide (alveolar gas), are forced out through the holes at the side of the mask. This preferential loss of alveolar gas means that carbon dioxide rebreathing is unlikely. (C) Nonrebreathing face mask. A unidirectional valve prevents dilution of inhaled gases containing oxygen with room air or rebreathing of exhaled gases containing carbon dioxide. (D) Air-entrainment face mask. Oxygen flow through an air injector entrains varying volumes of room air, producing predictable (24 percent to 40 percent) and unchanging inhaled concentrations of oxygen. (From Dripps et al.,[1] with permission.)

Table 31-1. Air-Entrainment (Venturi) Face Masks

Inhaled Concentration of Oxygen (%)	Oxygen Flows (L·min^{-1})	Air Entrainment (L·min^{-1})
24	2–4	50–100
28	4–6	40–60
31	5–8	56
35	8	40
40	8–12	24–36

Air-Entrainment

An air-entrainment (Venturi) face mask employs the Bernoulli principle to entrain large volumes of room air (up to 100 L·min^{-1}) to mix with oxygen flowing through an injector (2 L·min^{-1} to 12 L·min^{-1}) (Fig. 31-1D).[1] The resultant mixture of gases produces stable inhaled concentrations of oxygen between 24 percent and 40 percent, depending on the bore of the oxygen injector (Table 31-1).[2] Furthermore, the high flow of gas into the face mask results in constant inhaled concentrations of oxygen despite changes in the characteristics of the patient's ventilation.

Hazards of Oxygen Therapy

Hazards of oxygen therapy include retrolental fibroplasia, carbon dioxide retention, adsorption atelectasis, and pulmonary oxygen toxicity.

Retrolental Fibroplasia

Retrolental fibroplasia is a hazard of oxygen therapy administered to neonates, especially those of low birth weight (below 1500 g) and gestational age less than 44 weeks (see Chapter 27).

Carbon Dioxide Retention

Carbon dioxide retention may be exacerbated when patients with chronic obstructive airways disease dependent on hypoxic stimulation to maintain ventilation receive supplemental oxygen. In these patients, chronic elevation of the $PaCO_2$ has resulted in normalization of arterial and cerebrospinal fluid pH. Such individuals may thus be insensitive to carbon dioxide as a respiratory stimulant. As a result, removal of the hypoxic stimulus to maintain ventilation by increasing the PaO_2 above 60 mmHg with supplemental inhaled oxygen can result in profound alveolar hypoventilation and hypercarbia. Nevertheless, supplemental oxygen should never be withheld when the PaO_2 is less than 50 mmHg, remembering, however, that there may be little to gain by increasing the PaO_2 above 60 mmHg.

Adsorption Atelectasis

Adsorption atelectasis reflects oxygen uptake from alveoli that exceeds delivery of oxygen by ventilation. Normally, nitrogen in alveoli is in equilibrium with that in the pulmonary capillary blood such that loss of nitrogen from alveoli is unlikely. As a result, nitrogen maintains alveolar volume acting as an internal splint. When high concentrations of oxygen (greater than 60 percent) are substituted for room air, the nitrogen is diluted or washed out of the alveoli, and absorption atelectasis occurs if oxygen uptake exceeds delivery. Oxygen uptake in excess of delivery is likely to occur in selected alveoli that are poorly ventilated due to the presence of peribronchiolar edema and/or secretions in the bronchioles supplying these alveoli.

Adsorption atelectasis is most common in the dependent regions of the lungs because edema fluid and secretions tend to accumulate in these areas and the alveoli are relatively small. The impact on arterial oxygenation of low ventilation to these alveoli is exaggerated because gravity favors the distribution of pulmonary blood flow to dependent regions.

Pulmonary Oxygen Toxicity

It is well established that prolonged exposure of alveoli to high inspired partial pressures of oxygen results in pulmonary damage. This damage is characterized by the formation of fibrin (hyaline) membranes, alveolar and septal thickening, endothelial destruction, and necrosis of membranous pneumocytes. Other pulmonary effects of pure oxygen include depression of the ability of alveolar macrophages to kill phagocytosed bacteria, depression of mucociliary clearance, tracheitis after only 6 hours of exposure, decreased pulmonary compliance, increased airway resistance, and decreased diffusing capacity.

It is unlikely that pulmonary oxygen toxicity develops in humans breathing less than 50 percent oxygen at 1 atmosphere even for prolonged periods.[3] Certainly, sufficient inspired oxygen should always be delivered to prevent the persistence of arterial hypoxemia. When greater than 50 percent inspired oxygen is needed to maintain a satisfactory PaO_2, however, it is important to consider the use of positive end-expiratory pressure (PEEP) in attempts to reduce inspired concentrations of oxygen below 50 percent without adversely affecting the PaO_2.

HUMIDIFICATION AND AEROSOL THERAPY

Humidity describes the water content of inhaled gases. Absolute humidity is the mass of water vapor contained in a volume of gas at a given temperature. Relative humidity is the ratio of absolute humidity to the maximum mass of water vapor that a gas could contain at a given temperature expressed as a percent. At 37° Celsius and 100 percent relative humidity, a liter of gas contains 43.8 mg of water, which exerts a vapor pressure of 47 mmHg. Alveolar gases have a relative humidity of 100 percent at 37° Celsius. When the inhaled gases contain less than 43.8 mg $H_2O \cdot L^{-1}$, the vapor pressure exerted by water is less than 47 mmHg and there is a vapor pressure gradient between the inhaled gases and respiratory mucosa. The amount of moisture given up by the respiratory mucosa is directly proportional to this gradient. For example, at 20° Celsius and 50 percent relative humidity, inhaled gases contain 9.3 mg $H_2O \cdot L^{-1}$. For each liter of these gases inhaled, 34.5 mg of water (43.8 mg minus 9.3 mg) must be vaporized from the respiratory mucosa to achieve 100 percent relative humidity in the alveoli at a body temperature of 37° Celsius. Resulting dehydration of respiratory mucosa increases the viscosity of the mucous secretions and reduces the effectiveness of the mucociliary system in removing these secretions. Retained secretions produce an inflammatory response of respiratory mucosa, whereas narrowing of small airways by partial obstruction with mucus results in increased airway

resistance and maldistribution of ventilation to perfusion. Arterial hypoxemia may reflect maldistribution of ventilation to perfusion, whereas atelectasis is predictable with total occlusion of the bronchioles by mucus.

Warming, filtration, and humidification of inhaled gases normally occurs in the upper respiratory tract. When dry gases are inhaled or the natural conditioning system (nose) is bypassed by a tracheal tube or a tracheostomy tube, the lower airways must provide the additional moisture. In these situations, artificial humidifying devices, such as humidifiers or nebulizers, should be considered. Humidifiers are often used when dry gases are inhaled via a natural airway in an attempt to provide a water content similar to that normally present in room air. When the upper airway is bypassed, a humidifier is often inadequate, and the water deficit must be made up by use of a more efficient device, the nebulizer.

Humidifiers

Humidifiers are categorzied as pass-over and bubble-through (cascade).

Pass-Over Humidifiers

Pass-over humidifiers depend on evaporation to add water vapor to gases that pass over the water surface. Relative humidity of the effluent gases is dependent on gas flow and the temperature of both the water and gases. Inability to predictably deliver 90 percent to 100 percent relative humidity at 37° Celsius limits the usefulness of these types of humidifiers.

Bubble-Through Humidifiers

Bubble-through humidifiers that break up the delivered gases into small bubbles as they pass through a heated water reservoir are frequently used to humidify inhaled gases delivered by mechanical ventilators. Heating the water is important as the capacity of gases to hold moisture is greatly increased when temperatures are increased. The water in the humidifier can be heated to body temperature, but as gases travel through the delivery tubing, they cool and water collects ("rains out") in the tubing. Elevation of the water temperature above body temperature to assure delivery of gases at body temperature is acceptable. Temperature of the inhaled gases, however, should be monitored at the proximal airway to provide an early warning should these gases reach a temperature capable of producing respiratory mucosa burn. Ideally, inhaled gases should be 36° Celsius to 37° Celsius so as to ensure a relative humidity near 100 percent.

Nebulizers

An aerosol is a suspension of particles in a carrier gas. Devices used to generate aerosols are nebulizers. Nebulizers are categorized as jet (pneumatic) and ultrasonic.

Jet Nebulizers

Jet nebulizers are the most frequently used type of aerosol generators. High pressure gas enters the nebulizer chamber through a restricted orifice that produces a jet stream of high velocity. This jet stream is directed across one end of a small diameter tube that is immersed in the liquid to be nebulized and subambient pressure (Bernoulli effect) immediately adjacent to the tube is produced, resulting in pulling of surface liquid into the tube. When the liquid reaches the top of the tube, it is aerosolized by the jet stream to particles usually less than 30 μm in diameter.

Jet nebulizers are used in respiratory therapy to humidify inspired gases, decrease the viscosity of airway secretions, and deliver bronchodilator drugs directly to the airways.

Humidify Inspired Gases. The particulate water produced by jet nebulizers evaporates as the inhaled gases are warmed in the respiratory tract. This evaporation reduces or eliminates the vapor pressure gradient for water between the inhaled gases and respiratory mucosa. In contrast to humidifiers, jet nebulizers are more likely to provide sufficient relative humidity at 37° Celsius.

Decrease Viscosity of Airway Secretions. Aerosol administration of water is an efficient method to decrease the viscosity of airway secretions and thus facilitate mucus clearance by normal mucociliary activity. In addition to aerosolized water, acetylcysteine and hypertonic saline have been used to enhance mucus clearance. Acetylcysteine is a mu-

colytic agent that disrupts the disulfide bonds in mucoproteins and reduces mucus viscosity. This drug is extremely irritating to airways and should be administered with a bronchodilator to prevent or minimize bronchospasm. Hypertonic saline results in an osmotic flux that dilutes and increases the mucus volume and promotes expectoration. Like acetylcysteine, saline aerosols increase airway resistance and are thus undesirable in patients with chronic obstructive airways disease.

Deliver Bronchodilator Drugs. Bronchodilator drugs (racemic epinephrine, isoproterenol, selective beta-2 agonists) are most often administered as aerosols to reduce airway resistance due to bronchoconstriction (see Chapter 30). Bronchodilation reflects beta-2 agonist effects of these drugs. Systemic absorption of racemic epinephrine and isoproterenol can produce adverse beta-1 agonist effects (tachycardia, hypertension, cardiac dysrhythmias). Selective beta-2 agonists with minimal to absent beta-1 agonist effects are useful drug selections for patients with bronchoconstriction and underlying heart disease. Likewise, these drugs are useful for administration to patients anesthetized with halothane, which can sensitize the heart to the dysrhythmogenic effects of beta-1 stimulation.

Racemic epinephrine is a mixture of the d-isomers and l-isomers of epinephrine. In theory, inhalation of the racemic mixture compared to the l-isomer (50 times more active than the d-isomer) is less likely to produce systemic effects. Therapeutic aerosols are most efficacious when particles of 0.5 μm to 3 μm in diameter are administered. Particles with a diameter less than 0.5 μm are so stable that they are exhaled while those greater than 3 μm in diameter are likely to be deposited ("rain out") in the upper airways.

Aerosolized racemic epinephrine is used more for its alpha agonist (vasoconstrictive) than its beta agonist (bronchodilator) effects. For example, racemic epinephrine is effective in reducing laryngeal edema as follows intubation of the trachea particularly in pediatric patients. The recommended dose is 0.25 ml to 0.5 ml of 2.25 percent racemic epinephrine in 5 ml of water or normal saline administered as an aerosol every 1 hour to 4 hours until stridor wanes.

Albuterol is administered via a device placed in the inspiratory limb of the anesthesia delivery circuit. Each puff of albuterol delivered into the breathing circuit provides about 100 μg of the drug with 400 μg being the maximum dose usually necessary to produce desirable effects on the airways.

Ultrasonic Nebulizers

Ultrasonic nebulizers convert alternating current into ultrahigh frequency oscillations that are transmitted to the fluid container of the nebulizer producing fragmentation of the liquid into small particles. The mean particle diameter produced by an ultrasonic nebulizer is 2.8 μm (1 μm to 10 μm). Fluid overload is a potential problem as ultrasonic nebulizers can nebulize up to 6 ml $H_2O \cdot min^{-1}$. Inhaled ultrasonic aerosols are also irritating to the airways, causing bronchoconstriction and increased airway resistance.

Nosocomial Pulmonary Infections

Sterile, pyrogen-free water should be used for all humidifiers and nebulizers so as to avoid the possibility of the water reservoir becoming a source of hospital acquired (nosocomial) infections. All aerosol and mechanical ventilator circuits should be changed every 24 hours. Most oxygen therapy humidifiers are now provided as sterile and disposable single patient units.

BRONCHIAL HYGIENE

Bronchial hygiene depends on optimal removal of secretions from the lungs by mucociliary clearance, coughing, tracheal suctioning, and chest physiotherapy.

Mucociliary Clearance

Cilia located on epithelial cells lining the respiratory mucosa are responsible for moving respiratory tract secretions (10 $ml \cdot day^{-1}$ to 100 $ml \cdot day^{-1}$) towards the glottic opening. Cilia beat in a whiplike manner at rates up to 20 $times \cdot sec^{-1}$ and are able to move mucus cephalad at a rate of 2 $cm \cdot min^{-1}$. Depression of ciliary activity and an associated retention of secretions is produced by inhaled anesthetics, tracheal tubes, inhalation of cold and dry gases, high inhaled concentrations of oxygen, and pulmonary infections. Ciliary activity may be depressed up to 6 days postoperatively, depending on the duration of the anesthetic.[4]

Coughing

Coughing is a major mechanism for removal of secretions from large airways. An effective cough requires a maximal inhalation followed by closure of the glottis and contraction of the muscles of the chest and abdomen to create subglottic pressures of up to 200 cm H_2O. As the glottis opens, the flow of exhaled air may exceed 600 $L \cdot min^{-1}$. High air-flow velocities necessary to propel secretions from the upper airways are generated most effectively at large lung volumes. Rapid shallow breathing patterns and decreased lung volumes characteristic of postoperative patients with pain limit the effectiveness of coughing.

Tracheal Suctioning

Orotracheal or nasotracheal suctioning should be performed only when there is evidence during auscultation of the chest of retained secretions that do not clear with coughing. Tracheal suctioning should not be prophylactic or routine. For example, mechanical irritation by the catheter during tracheal suctioning may cause trauma to the respiratory mucosa and predispose to bacterial colonization. Mechanical stimulation of the trachea or carina by the catheter may evoke a vasovagal response with resultant bradycardia and hypotension.[5] Tracheal suctioning also predisposes to significant arterial hypoxemia because of aspiration of pulmonary gases with associated small airway closure and alveolar collapse. Arterial hypoxemia during tracheal suctioning is minimized by (1) administration of pure oxygen before suctioning, (2) selection of a suction catheter that is no greater than one-half the internal diameter of the trachea, (3) limitation of the duration of suctioning to less than 15 seconds, and (4) manual inflation of the lungs with oxygen after suctioning.

Chest Physiotherapy

Chest physiotherapy consists of postural drainage, percussion, vibration, deep breathing, and assisted coughing. These maneuvers aid in the removal of airway secretions and improve inflation of poorly ventilated alveoli. Indeed, improved ciliary clearance of airway secretions and a decreased incidence of postoperative atelectasis have been attributed to properly performed chest physiotherapy.

POSTOPERATIVE RESPIRATORY THERAPY

Postoperative respiratory therapy is designed to prevent events that lead to pneumonia and arterial hypoxemia that characterize postoperative pulmonary complications (Fig. 31-2). The severity of postoperative pulmonary complications parallels the magnitude of reduction in lung volumes. Presumably, decreases in vital capacity (VC) and functional residual capacity (FRC) interfere with the generation of an effective cough and contribute to the collapse of alveoli. The net effect of these changes is a decreased clearance of secretions from the airways and atelectasis, leading to pneumonia and arterial hypoxemia. Atelectasis is likely to accompany shallow breathing ("splinting") that is a result of postoperative incisional pain. Likewise, a cough may be excruciatingly painful. Failure to prevent the postoperative reduction in FRC by totally relieving incisional pain suggests that trauma from the surgical procedure also interferes with the optimal function of the chest wall by changing the normal relation of the diaphragm, intercostal muscles, and abdominal muscles.[6] Nevertheless, relief of pain as provided by nerve blocks (intercostal blocks, epidural block) or administration of opioids (neuraxial opioids, patient controlled analgesia) contributes to optimal performance of therapies designed to restore FRC (see Chapter 20).

The frequency of postoperative pulmonary complications is greatest after thoracic and upper abdominal surgery.[6] For example, significant postoperative atelectasis occurs in 20 percent to 40 percent of patients undergoing these types of surgery. This incidence parallels the 60 percent reduction of VC on the day after upper abdominal surgery. Lower abdominal surgery is associated with a lesser incidence of postoperative pulmonary complications and a smaller reduction in VC as compared with the observed decrease after upper abdominal surgery. In addition to the site of surgery, other factors that influence the incidence of postoperative pulmonary complications include co-existing pulmonary disease, a history of cigarette smoking, obesity, and increasing age. The choice of drugs or techniques used to produce anesthesia does not seem to alter predictably the incidence of postoperative pulmonary infections. A subcostal versus transverse upper abdominal incision, as for a cholecystectomy, probably does not alter the incidence of postoperative pulmonary complications.[7]

The identification of FRC as the most important lung volume in the postoperative period provides a specific goal for respiratory therapy after surgery. Specific therapies designed to increase FRC include voluntary deep breathing and ambulation, intermittent positive pressure breathing, incentive spirometry, and exhalation maneuvers.

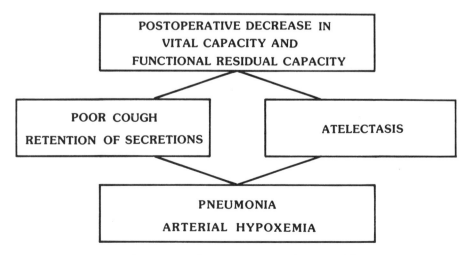

Fig. 31-2. Pathogenesis of postoperative pulmonary infections.

Voluntary Deep Breathing and Ambulation

Voluntary deep breathing with maintenance of inspiration at peak inflation for 3 seconds to 5 seconds creates a large transpulmonary pressure gradient and facilitates re-expansion of collapsed alveoli and restoration of lung volumes. A motivated patient and adequate postoperative analgesia are necessary to assure optimal deep breathing.

Ambulation and the associated changes in position have great therapeutic benefit in the prevention of postoperative pulmonary complications. Presumably, this therapeutic benefit reflects increased lung volumes, particularly FRC.

Intermittent Positive Pressure Breathing

Intermittent positive pressure breathing (IPPB) as a method to reduce the incidence of postoperative pulmonary complications is controversial.[8] Certainly, postoperative IPPB therapy does not need to be routine. When IPPB is prescribed, the emphasis should be an achievement of an optimal tidal volume rather than creation of a peak airway pressure.

Patients scheduled for surgical procedures associated with a high incidence of postoperative pulmonary complications, such as upper abdominal or thoracic surgery, should have a preoperative measurement of inspiratory capacity (IC). Postoperatively, the IC should again be measured and, if less than 80 percent of the preoperative value, IPPB therapy instituted. Ideally, patients should inhale three times to six times the predicted tidal volume for IPPB treatment to be effective. This inhaled tidal volume should be monitored with a spirometer placed at the exhalation valve of the IPPB delivery circuit. Nevertheless, there is no evidence that IPPB treatment is better than voluntary deep breathing and ambulation in altering the incidence or severity of postoperative pulmonary complications.

Incentive Spirometry

Incentive spirometry is a form of voluntary deep breathing in which patients are given an inhaled volume as a goal to achieve. When the use of incentive spirometry is anticipated, a preoperative baseline IC should be obtained and the patient instructed in the use of the device. The preoperative IC should be the postoperative goal. Incentive spirometry therapy also emphasizes holding the inhaled volume to provide a sustained inflation important for expanding collapsed alveoli. The major disadvantage of this therapy is the need for patient cooperation, which may be limited in the presence of postoperative pain.

Exhalation Maneuvers

Exhalation maneuvers, such as inflating balloons, using blow-bottles or performing a forced VC are not recommended because their performance causes the patient to exhale below the FRC, leading to atelectasis and increased airway resistance. Indeed, the only therapeutic benefit elicited by exhalation maneuvers is the deep breath that must be taken initially.

REFERENCES

1. Dripps RD, Eckenhoff JE, Vandam LD, eds. Inhalation therapy and pulmonary physiotherapy. In: Introduction to Anesthesia. The Principles of Safe Practice. Philadelphia, WB Saunders, 1988:469–76.
2. Cohen JL, Demers RR, Saklad M. Air-entrainment masks: A performance evaluation. Resp Care 1977; 22:277–82.
3. Cheney FW Jr, Huang TW, Gronka R. The effects of 50% oxygen on resolution of experimental lung injury. Am Rev Resp Dis 1980;122:373–9.
4. Gamsu G, Singer MM, Vincent HH. Postoperative impairment of mucus transport in the lung. Am Rev Resp Dis 1976;114:673–9.
5. Harken AH. A routine for safe, effective endotracheal suctioning. Am Surg 1975;41:398–404.
6. Craig DB. Postoperative recovery of pulmonary function. Anesth Analg 1981;60:46–52.
7. Williams CD, Brenowitz JB. Ventilatory patterns after vertical and transverse upper abdominal incisions. Am J Surg 1975;130:725–8.
8. Inverson LIG, Ecker RR, Fox HE, May IA. A comparative study of IPPB, the incentive spirometer, and blow bottles: The prevention of atelectasis following cardiac surgery. Ann Thoracic Surg 1978;25:197–200.

Chapter

32

Critical Care Medicine

Evolution of critical care medicine as a legitimate and important area of specialization reflects the contributions of many clinicians, particularly anesthesiologists. Indeed, 10 of the 28 founding members of the Society of Critical Care Medicine were anesthesiologists. A certificate of Special Qualifications in Anesthesiology Critical Care Medicine is available to Diplomates of the American Board of Anesthesiology who spend 1 year of additional postgraduate training in critical care medicine beyond primary training requirements and subsequently achieve a passing score on a written examination administered by the American Board of Anesthesiology.

The training of anesthesiologists in the management of anesthesia is a useful beginning for subsequent development of additional skills required for the care of critically ill patients with multiple organ system dysfunction. For example, no other specialty provides day-to-day experience in airway management, ventilation of the lungs, intravenous administration of potent and rapidly acting drugs, blood and fluid administration, and both noninvasive and invasive monitoring of vital organ function.

Examples of organ system failure occurring alone or in combination in an intensive care unit and requiring treatment by specialists in critical care medicine include acute respiratory failure, congestive heart failure, septic shock, brain injury, acute renal failure, and acute liver failure. Nutrition is likely to require medical intervention in critically ill patients. Ethical and legal considerations, as well as cost effectiveness, are important issues in management of patients in intensive care units. Hospital ethics committees are useful to evaluate individual cases and make nonbinding recommendations to primary physicians regarding treatment.

ACUTE RESPIRATORY FAILURE

Acute respiratory failure is not a single disease entity but instead is a combination of pathophysiologic derangements that can arise from a variety of etiologic insults. Nevertheless, manifestations of acute respiratory failure are sufficiently similar to be considered as a single entity designated the adult respiratory distress syndrome (ARDS).

Diagnosis

Arterial hypoxemia (PaO_2 below 60 mmHg) despite supplemental inhaled oxygen is an invariable accompaniment of ARDS. Mismatching of ventilation to perfusion is the most likely cause for arterial hypoxemia. In its most extreme form, this mismatching may be right-to-left intrapulmonary shunting in which unventilated alveoli continue to be perfused. Also contributing to this mismatching is a reduction in functional residual capacity (FRC)

Etiology of Acute Respiratory Failure

Primary pulmonary dysfunction
  Obstructive airways disease
  Restrictive pulmonary disease
  Pneumonia
  Inhaled toxins—gastric fluid, meconium,
    smoke
  Oxygen toxicity
  Embolization-blood, fat, amniotic fluid
  Pulmonary contusion
  Near-drowning
  Hyaline membrane disease

Cardiovascular dysfunction
  Hemorrhagic shock
  Sepsis
  Congestive heart failure
  Massive blood transfusion
  Disseminated intravascular coagulation
  Postcardiopulmonary bypass

Central nervous system dysfunction
  Hypothalamic injury
  Depressant drug overdose

Neuromuscular dysfunction
  Myasthenia gravis
  Spinal cord transection
  Guillain-Barré
  Tetanus
  Drug-induced-muscle relaxants,
    antibiotics

Miscellaneous
  Acute pancreatitis
  Uremia
  Morbid obesity

and decreased pulmonary compliance. Loss of pulmonary capillary integrity is reflected by pulmonary edema despite pulmonary artery occlusion pressures less than 15 mmHg. Increased pulmonary vascular resistance and pulmonary hypertension are likely to develop when ARDS persists. Patients in whom ARDS develops may develop elevated complement proteins (C5a) before appearance of overt clinical manifestations.[1]

Acute respiratory failure is often distinguished from chronic respiratory failure on the basis of the relationship of the $PaCO_2$ to the pH. For example, acute respiratory failure is associated with an abrupt increase in the $PaCO_2$ and a corresponding decrease in pH. Conversely, in the presence of chronic respiratory failure, the pH is near normal, reflecting compensation by virtue of renal tubular reabsorption of bicarbonate ions.

Serial measurement of arterial blood gases and pH is necessary to establish the diagnosis of ARDS, determine the need for mechanical support of ventilation, assess the effects of therapy, and confirm when the patient no longer needs mechanical support of ventilation.

Treatment

Treatment of ARDS is directed at supporting pulmonary function until the lungs can recover from the insult that initiated pulmonary dysfunction. In addition to administration of supplemental oxygen and maintenance of intravascular fluid volume, it is usually necessary to intubate the trachea and provide mechanical ventilation of the lungs, including the use of positive end-expiratory pressure (PEEP) or an end-inspiratory plateau.

Mechanical Ventilation of the Lungs

Mechanical ventilation of the lungs is provided by machines known as ventilators. Ventilators may be classified as pressure-cycled, volume-cycled, or time-cycled, depending on the mechanism responsible for terminating the inspiratory phase of the mechanical breath. Mechanical ventilators may change from the expiratory to inspiratory phase by being set to deliver assisted ventilation, controlled ventilation, high frequency positive pressure ventilation (HFPPV), assisted-controlled ventilation, or intermittent mandatory ventilation (IMV).

Pressure-cycled ventilators terminate the inspiratory phase of the mechanical breath when a preselected pressure is achieved in the ventilator circuit. Therefore, tidal volume and inspiratory time are directly related to pulmonary compliance and inversely related to airway resistance. Significant leaks in the delivery circuit may prevent development of sufficient airway pressure to cycle the ventilator to exhalation. Conversely, decreased pulmonary compliance or increased airway resistance may result in attainment of the predetermined airway pressure before a sufficient tidal volume has been delivered to the patient. Most pressure-cycled ventilators are incapable of providing the constant tidal volume and unchanging inhaled concentration of oxygen necessary for the management of critically ill patients. Therefore, these types of ventilators are most often used for intermittent positive pressure breathing (IPPB) therapy and short-term ventilatory support in the recovery room.

Volume-cycled ventilators terminate the inspiratory phase of the mechanical breath after delivery of a preselected volume of gas to the delivery circuit. Flow generators maintain a uniform gas flow rate throughout the inspiratory phase that is independent of the airway pressure. Changes in pulmonary compliance or airway resistance are unlikely to alter the flow characteristics of the ventilator, insuring a more constant tidal volume with changing clinical conditions. For this reason, most ventilators used for critical care are volume-cycled.

It is a common misconception that the tidal volume delivered by volume-cycled ventilators is constant regardless of changes in the patient's pulmonary compliance and airway resistance. In fact, a portion of the tidal volume generated by the ventilator is compressed within the ventilator breathing circuit and does not reach the patient. This lost compression volume is dependent on the compliance of the entire ventilator-patient circuit and the peak inspiratory pressure. For most ventilators, the compression volume of the delivery circuit is 3 ml·cm H_2O^{-1} to 5 ml·cm H_2O^{-1}. For example, a volume-cycled ventilator (equally true for all other types of ventilators) with a preset tidal volume of 700 ml, a peak inspiratory pressure of 20 cm H_2O, and a compression factor of 4 ml·cm H_2O^{-1} will deliver 620 ml (700 ml minus compression volume) to the patient. If the patient's pulmonary compliance further decreases, the peak

inflation pressure will increase and the delivered tidal volume will be further reduced. Compression volume is particularly important to consider in setting the tidal volume delivered to children. For example, a ventilator set to deliver a tidal volume of 10 ml·kg^{-1} to a 10 kg child would deliver only 20 ml, assuming a peak inspiratory pressure of 20 cm H_2O and a compression factor of 4 ml·cm H_2O^{-1}. Consideration of compression volume loss may indicate the need to measure exhaled tidal volume with a spirometer in selected patients.

Time-cycled ventilators terminate the inspiratory phase of the mechanical breath after a preselected time interval has elapsed. The tidal volume delivered by time-cycled ventilators is determined by the inspiratory time and inspiratory flow rate.

Assisted Ventilation. Ventilators capable of assisted (patient-triggered) mechanical ventilation of the lungs respond to a decrease in airway pressure caused by the patient's spontaneous breathing effort, which causes the ventilator to switch to the inspiratory mode. The magnitude of the decreased airway pressure necessary to trigger mechanical augmentation of a spontaneously initiated tidal volume is adjustable by means of a sensitivity control on the ventilator.

Controlled Ventilation. Controlled mechanical ventilation of the lungs provides automatic cycling of the ventilator at a preselected rate independent of the patient's effort to breathe. This mode of ventilation is used primarily to assure delivery of a predictable minute ventilation to patients being treated for ARDS. Initiation and/or maintenance of controlled ventilation of the lungs may require depression of the patient's own spontaneous ventilatory effort by the administration of sedatives or opioids, muscle relaxants, or deliberate hyperventilation to lower the $PaCO_2$ below the apneic threshold. Deliberate hyperventilation produces respiratory alkalosis that may be physiologically deleterious (see Chapter 17).

The initial ventilator settings typically include a respiratory rate of 6 breaths·min^{-1} to 10 breaths·min^{-1}, tidal volume 10 ml·kg^{-1} to 15 ml·kg^{-1}, and an inhaled concentration of oxygen near 50 percent. A slow ventilator rate combined with a large tidal volume optimizes the distribution of ventilation relative to perfusion, particularly in the presence of regional differences in airway resistance. Subsequent adjustments of the ventilator settings and the inhaled concentration of oxygen are based on the measurement of arterial blood gases and pH. The goal is to achieve a PaO_2 between 60 mmHg and 100 mmHg, $PaCO_2$ between 36 mmHg and 44 mmHg, and pH between 7.36 and 7.44.

High frequency positive pressure ventilation (HFPPV) is an alternative mode of controlled ventilation that has been used to treat ARDS and to manage patients with a bronchopleural fistula.[2] Not all reports, however, demonstrate advantages of HFPPV over more traditional approaches in the management of patients with these conditions.[3] Characteristics of HFPPV include (1) ventilatory frequency 60 breaths·min^{-1} to 100 breaths·min^{-1}, (2) small tidal volumes that result in a low mean positive airway pressure during inspiration, and (3) provision of continuous positive intratracheal pressure throughout the ventilator cycle. An important advantage ascribed to this form of ventilation is the failure of airway resistance and pulmonary compliance to influence the efficacy of ventilation. In addition, maintenance of a low mean airway pressure results in minimal effects on cardiac output or intracranial pressure, and the likelihood of pulmonary barotrauma is reduced. Furthermore, HFPPV produces reflex suppression of spontaneous ventilation, allowing mechanical support without the use of drugs or deliberate hyperventilation. The mechanism by which HFPPV produces acceptable alveolar ventilation and arterial oxygenation delivering tidal volumes less than the patient's calculated anatomic dead space is unknown.

High frequency jet ventilation is similar to HFPPV, using ventilatory frequencies of 60 breaths·min^{-1} to 600 breaths·min^{-1}. The distinguishing feature of this form of ventilation is gas entrainment such that the tidal volume and inhaled concentration of oxygen are difficult to quantitate. Also closely related to HFPPV is high frequency oscillation, which uses ventilatory frequencies as high as 15 Hz or 900 cycles·min^{-1}.

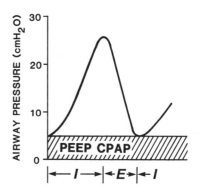

Fig. 32-1. Schematic diagram of airway pressures during the inspiratory phase (I) and expiratory phase (E) of a mechanical breath. Airway pressure does not decrease below 5 cm H_2O during I and E, reflecting positive end-expiratory pressure (PEEP). Spontaneous breathing in which airway pressure does not decrease to zero during I and E is commonly referred to as continuous positive airway pressure (CPAP).

Assisted-Controlled Ventilation. A ventilator used to provide assisted-controlled ventilation is set such that the cycling rate is slightly less than the patient's breathing rate. If the patient stops breathing, the ventilator will convert to the controlled ventilation mode at the present respiratory frequency.

Intermittent mandatory ventilation (IMV) is a ventilation mode that may be incorporated into ventilators. This mode of ventilation finds its greatest use during weaning (see the section *Cessation of Mechanical Inflation of the Lungs*).

Positive End-Expiratory Pressure

Positive end-expiratory pressure (PEEP) is produced by applying positive pressure to the exhalation valve at the conclusion of the mechanical exhalation phase (Fig. 32-1). Alternatively, the exhalation valve can be depressurized gradually to provide resistance (retard) to exhalation (Fig. 32-2). Retardation of expiratory gas flow rate serves to maintain patency of peripheral airways.

Mechanism of Beneficial Effect. It is presumed that PEEP increases arterial oxygenation, pulmonary compliance, and the FRC by expanding previously collapsed but perfused alveoli. As a result, the matching of ventilation to perfusion is improved

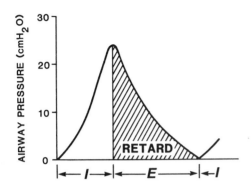

Fig. 32-2. Schematic diagram of airway pressure during the inspiratory phase (I) and expiratory phase (E) of a mechanical breath. The exhalation valve is depressurized slowly so as to "retard" or slow the rate at which airway pressure decreases towards zero during E.

and the magnitude of right-to-left intrapulmonary shunting of blood is reduced. It should be recognized that PEEP is unlikely to improve the PaO_2 when arterial hypoxemia is due to hypoventilation or is associated with a normal or even increased FRC.

Institution of Positive End-Expiratory Pressure. Institution of PEEP is often recommended when the PaO_2 cannot be maintained above 60 mmHg despite inhaled concentrations of oxygen that exceed 50 percent. Short-term administration of greater than 50 percent oxygen to maintain adequate arterial oxygenation is acceptable, but it must be recognized that pulmonary oxygen toxicity is a hazard when inhaled concentrations of oxygen exceed 50 percent for more than 24 hours.

Initially, PEEP is added in 2.5 cm H_2O to 5 cm H_2O increments until the PaO_2 is greater than 60 mmHg while the patient is breathing less than 50 percent oxygen. The goal is to deliver the amount of PEEP that maximally improves the PaO_2 without substantially reducing cardiac output or increasing the risk of pulmonary barotrauma. Typically, maximum improvement of PaO_2 is achieved with less than 15 cm H_2O of PEEP. Refractory arterial hypoxemia, however, may require PEEP up to 30 cm H_2O before improvement in arterial oxygenation is produced.

Hazards of Positive End-Expiratory Pressure. Hazards of PEEP include (1) decreased cardiac output, (2) pulmonary barotrauma, (3) increased extravascular lung water, and (4) redistribution of pulmonary blood flow.

The reduction in cardiac output produced by PEEP is due to interference with venous return and a leftward displacement of the ventricular septum that restricts filling of the left ventricle. It is conceivable that improvements in PaO_2 produced by PEEP could be offset by reductions in cardiac output. The potential for PEEP to reduce cardiac output is exaggerated in the presence of decreased intravascular fluid volume and/or normal lungs, which permit maximal transmission of increased airway pressures.[4] A pulmonary artery catheter is helpful in guiding fluid replacement and for monitoring the impact of PEEP on cardiac output. Levels of PEEP that exceed about 10 cm H_2O can interfere with the interpretation of the pulmonary artery occlusion pressure as a monitor of left atrial pressure. This reflects transmission of intra-alveolar pressure to the pulmonary capillaries, which is then measured as the pulmonary artery occlusion pressure.

Pneumothorax, pneumomediastinum, and subcutaneous emphysema are examples of barotrauma due to overdistension of alveoli by PEEP. An abrupt deterioration of PaO_2 and cardiovascular function during PEEP should arouse suspicion of pulmonary barotrauma, especially pneumothorax.

Increased intravascular lung water associated with PEEP may reflect obstruction to pulmonary lymph flow as well as alterations in permeability characteristics of the pulmonary capillaries.

The adverse effects of PEEP on distribution of pulmonary blood flow are complex but presumably reflect, in part, overdistension of alveoli. When overdistension of alveoli occurs, pulmonary blood flow is likely to be shunted to areas with less resistance to flow, such as less distended or even collapsed alveoli. The net effect of this alveolar overdistension is increased mismatching of ventilation to perfusion, manifesting as a reduction of PaO_2.

End-inspiratory plateau (EIP) is characterized by sustained positive pressure for about 1.5 seconds at no flow. The rationale for EIP is to offset the impact of variations in pulmonary time constants (airway resistance times pulmonary compliance) between lung compartments that prevent homogeneity of gas distribution. Presumably, EIP promotes distribution of gas to lung units with high resistance to flow. The net effect is an improved matching of ventilation to perfusion and inflation of collapsed alveoli in patients with ARDS. This inspiratory pattern may also be of benefit in the ventilator management of neonatal respiratory distress syndrome.

Monitoring of Treatment

Monitoring of treatment of ARDS depends on evaluation of pulmonary gas exchange and cardiac function. Measurements of arterial and venous blood gases, pH, cardiac output, cardiac filling pressure and intrapulmonary shunt, and calculation of systemic and pulmonary vascular resistance are used to monitor the adequacy of treatment of ARDS. A pulmonary artery catheter is useful for making many of the measurements and calculations.

Arterial Oxygenation

The adequacy of treatment of ARDS that is directed toward relieving arterial hypoxemia is reflected by the PaO_2 (normal 60 mmHg to 100 mmHg). The efficiency of the exchange of oxygen across the capillary membrane is reflected by the difference between the calculated alveolar partial pressure of oxygen (PAO_2) and the measured PaO_2. Calculation of the alveolar-to-arterial difference for oxygen ($AaDO_2$) when patients are breathing pure oxygen provides an estimate of the magnitude of right-to-left intrapulmonary shunting of blood (see Chapter 17). One of the difficulties with the use of the $AaDO_2$ is that the normal range changes with variations in the inhaled concentration of oxygen. With this in mind, a more useful calculation may be the ratio of the PaO_2 to PAO_2, which is less influenced by the inhaled concentrations of oxygen (see Chapter 17).

Ventilation

The adequacy of alveolar ventilation during treatment of ARDS is monitored by measurement of the $PaCO_2$ (normal 36 mmHg to 44 mmHg). The efficiency of the transfer of carbon dioxide across the alveolar capillary membrane is reflected by the ratio of dead space ventilation to tidal volume (VD/VT) (see Chapter 17). Normally, the VD/VT is less than 0.3 but may increase to greater than 0.6 in patients with ARDS.

Tissue Oxygenation

The mixed venous partial pressure of oxygen (PvO_2), as measured in blood obtained from the pulmonary artery, reflects tissue extraction of oxygen (see Chapter 17). A PvO_2 below 30 mmHg indicates the need to increase cardiac output so as to assure adequate tissue oxygenation.

Acidemia

Measurement of pH is necessary to detect metabolic and/or respiratory acidosis that commonly accompanies ARDS. For example, metabolic acidosis predictably accompanies arterial hypoxemia and inadequate delivery of oxygen to the tissues. Respiratory acidosis reflects alveolar hypoventilation and the resulting acute increase of the $PaCO_2$. Cardiac dysrhythmias, increased pulmonary vascular resistance, and decreased responsiveness to catecholamines are adverse effects of acidosis.

Cardiac Output and Filling Pressures

Measurement and maintenance of a normal cardiac output (above $2.5 \ L \cdot min^{-1} \cdot m^{-2}$) is essential for assuring adequate delivery of oxygen to tissues during treatment of ARDS. Cardiac output is most frequently measured by the thermodilution technique using a pulmonary artery catheter. Measurement of left and right atrial filling pressures combined with the value for cardiac output permits construction of ventricular function curves for use in guiding fluid administration and drug therapy. Likewise, systemic and pulmonary vascular resistance can be calculated using appropriate pressure measurements and the cardiac output.

Cessation of Mechanical Support of Ventilation

Cessation of mechanical support of ventilation of the lungs in patients being treated for ARDS can be considered in the presence of (1) measurements that are compatible with spontaneous ventilation, (2) cardiovascular stability, and (3) a favorable

---

Guidelines that Suggest the Likelihood of Successful Cessation of Mechanical Inflation of the Lungs

Vital capacity above 15 ml·kg^{-1}

Alveolar-to-arterial difference for oxygen less than 350 mmHg (FIO$_2$ = 1.0)

Arterial/alveolar partial pressure of oxygen above 0.75

Arterial partial pressure of oxygen above 60 mmHg (FIO$_2$ below 0.5)

Arterial pH above 7.3

Arterial partial pressure of carbon dioxide below 50 mmHg

Maximal inspiratory pressure greater than minus 20 cm H$_2$O

Dead space/tidal volume less than 0.6

Conscious and oriented

Stable cardiac function

Optimal intravascular fluid volume and electrolyte status

Absence of infection

Good nutritional status

---

clinical impression of the patient's condition. Weaning can be considered to occur in three stages: cessation of mechanical inflation of the lungs (weaning), followed by removal of the tracheal tube (extubation), and finally elimination of the need for supplemental oxygen.

Cessation of Mechanical Inflation of the Lungs

Guidelines that suggest the likely success of weaning include serial measurements and calculations of several parameters. Ultimately, the decision to attempt weaning must be individualized considering not only the status of pulmonary function but also the co-existence of other organ system abnormalities.

T-tube and IMV are the two methods employed in weaning patients from mechanical support of ventilation of the lungs.

T-Tube

T-tube weaning is initiated by connecting the tube in the trachea of the patient to a device (T-tube) through which humidified and oxygen-enriched gases are delivered. In addition, 2.5 cm H$_2$O to 5 cm H$_2$O of continuous positive airway pressure (CPAP) is often delivered via the T-tube to the airway. The use of CPAP prevents the decrease in FRC associated with cessation of positive pressure ventilation of the lungs.[5] Indeed, incompetence of the glottic opening produced by the presence of a tracheal tube seems to interfere with the maintenance of a normal FRC. Initially, the patient is allowed to breathe spontaneously for 5 minutes to 10 minutes each hour. Tachycardia, tachypnea (greater than 35 breaths·min^{-1}), or alterations in the level of consciousness during the brief period of spontaneous ventilation confirm that weaning has been premature and mechanical support of ventilation is immediately reinstituted. When pulmonary function has recovered to the extent that weaning is appropriate, it will be possible to lengthen gradually the periods of spontaneous ventilation to 2 hours or longer.

Intermittent Mandatory Ventilation. Periodic mechanical inflation of the lungs during periods of spontaneous ventilation is described as IMV. The intermittent mechanical breath can be provided as a mandatory breath at a preset interval (nonsynchronous) or as a synchronized breath (SIMV) initiated by the spontaneous ventilatory effort of the patient. There is no evidence to substantiate an advantage of SIMV over IMV.

Weaning using IMV is initiated by gradually decreasing the number of mechanical breaths delivered each minute. Ideally, the IMV rate is sequentially decreased as long as the PaCO$_2$ remains near the patient's normal level, the pH is 7.36 to 7.44, and tachypnea is absent.

Removal of the Tracheal Tube

Extubation of the trachea should be considered when the patient tolerates 2 hours of spontaneous ventilation during T-tube weaning or an IMV rate of 1 breath·min^{-1} to 2 breaths·min^{-1} without deterioration of (1) arterial blood bases, (2) pH, (3) consciousness, or (4) cardiac status. In addition, the patient should have active laryngeal reflexes and the ability to generate an effective cough so as to clear secretions from the airway.

Elimination of the Need for Supplemental Oxygen

Supplemental inhaled oxygen is often needed for a period of time despite recovery from ARDS sufficient to permit spontaneous ventilation. This need for supplemental oxygen most likely reflects persistence of mismatching of ventilation to perfusion. Weaning from supplemental oxygen is accomplished by the gradual reduction in the inhaled concentration of oxygen, as guided by monitoring the PaO_2. It is probably not necessary to increase the PaO_2 above 60 mmHg using supplemental inhaled oxygen. Furthermore, a PaO_2 above 60 mmHg can eliminate the hypoxic stimulus to ventilation in patients with chronic obstructive airways disease associated with chronic carbon dioxide retention. This loss of hypoxic stimulation of ventilation in these patients could result in unacceptable hypercarbia despite an acceptable level of oxygenation.

CONGESTIVE HEART FAILURE

Congestive heart failure characterized by decreased cardiac output requires pharmacologic treatment with inotropes and/or vasodilators guided by information obtained from a pulmonary artery catheter. Drug-induced increases in cardiac output are reflected as reductions in atrial filling pressures, improved arterial oxygenation, and increased PvO_2. Dopamine, dobutamine, and epinephrine are examples of inotropes that are used to increase myocardial contractility and cardiac output (see Chapter 3).

In certain patients, reductions in systemic vascular resistance produced by vasodilator drugs, such as nitroprusside, are used to improve forward left ventricular stroke volume. Reductions in systemic blood pressure with associated decreases in coronary perfusion pressure, however, limit the usefulness of vasodilator therapy of congestive heart failure. Maintenance of an optimal intravascular fluid volume as guided by cardiac filling pressures will minimize reductions in blood pressure produced by nitroprusside. Nitrolgycerin is an alternative to nitroprusside and is particularly useful in patients with coronary artery disease, as it selectively redistributes coronary blood flow to subendocardial areas. Reductions in systemic vascular resistance are less predictable with nitroglycerin because this drug, in contrast to nitroprusside, acts predominantly on venules.

Intra-aortic balloon counterpulsation may be helpful in some patients who develop cardiogenic shock after a myocardial infarction. The intra-aortic balloon is programmed to the electrocardiogram so as to deflate just before systole and to inflate during diastole. The presystolic deflation of the balloon diminishes systemic blood pressure and afterload, which reduces cardiac work and myocardial oxygen requirements. Inflation of the balloon during diastole increases diastolic blood pressure and thus improves coronary blood flow and myocardial oxygen delivery.

SEPTIC SHOCK

Septic shock occurs most frequently after trauma or operative procedures on the genitourinary tract. About 70 percent of cases are due to gram-negative bacteremia. Septic shock can be divided into an early (hyperdynamic) and late phase.

Early Phase

The early phase (first 24 hours) of septic shock is characterized by vasodilation and hypotension associated with reductions in systemic vascular resistance and increased cardiac output. Vasodilation is presumed to be due to an endotoxin derived from cell walls of bacteria. Fever and hyperventilation are frequently present.

Late Phase

After about 24 hours, vasoconstriction replaces vasodilation and lactic acidosis now accompanies a decreased cardiac output. Oliguria is characteristically present. Hematologic abnormalities suggestive of disseminated intravascular coagulation (decreased platelets, prolonged prothrombin and partial thromboplastin time, increased concentrations of fibrin split products) typically accompany the late phase of septic shock.

Treatment

Treatment of septic shock is with intravenous antibiotics and repletion of intravascular fluid volume. Antibiotics should be started immediately after the drawing of blood for culture and sensitivity. Most often two antibiotics are selected, with one (clindamycin) effective against gram-positive and another (aminoglycoside derivative) against gram-negative bacteria. Antibiotics can be changed if necessary following the results of the blood culture. Fluid replacement must be aggressive and guided by measurement of right and/or left atrial filling pressures and urine output. Dopamine is an effective inotrope when pharmacologic support of both cardiac output and renal function is necessary. Administration of large doses of corticosteroids have not been shown to be beneficial in the treatment of septic shock.[6]

Surgical intervention may be necessary to treat the source of bacteremia. No anesthetic drug has been shown to be ideal in the presence of septic shock. Nevertheless, ketamine would seem an acceptable drug for induction of anesthesia in patients requiring emergency surgery in the presence of hypotension due to bacteremia.

BRAIN INJURY

Critical care of the brain-injured patient is based on the recognition and treatment of hazardous elevations of the intracranial pressure (ICP). Cerebral protection and resuscitation have been most successful in patients who experience head injury. Institution of deliberate hyperventilation of the lungs plus administration of diuretics and corticosteroids are the recommended initial interventions to reduce ICP. Administration of barbiturates is recommended when the ICP remains elevated despite traditional therapy.

Intracranial Pressure

A catheter placed through a burr hole into a cerebral ventricle or a transducer placed on the surface of the brain is used to monitor ICP. High risk patients including those with head injury, large

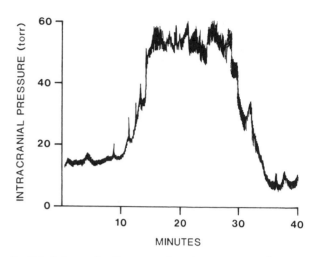

Fig. 32-3. Schematic diagram of a plateau wave characterized by an abrupt and sustained (10 minutes to 20 minutes) increase in intracranial pressure followed by a rapid reduction in pressure, often to levels below those present before the onset of the wave.

brain tumors, cerebral aneurysms, and hydrocephalus should probably have their ICP monitored. A normal ICP pressure wave is pulsatile and varies with the cardiac impulse and respiration. The mean ICP should remain below 15 mmHg. An abrupt increase in the ICP observed during continuous monitoring is known as a plateau wave (Fig. 32-3). Painful stimulation in an otherwise unresponsive patient can initiate a plateau wave. Hence, the liberal use of analgesics to avoid pain is indicated even in unresponsive patients.

Treatment

Methods to decrease ICP include posture; deliberate hyperventilation; and administration of osmotic and/or renal tubular diuretics, corticosteroids, barbiturates, and institution of cerebrospinal fluid drainage. A frequent recommendation is to treat sustained increases of ICP above 20 mmHg. Treatment may be indicated when ICP is less than 20 mmHg if the appearance of an occasional plateau wave suggests a low intracranial compliance.

Posture. Elevation of the head to about 30 degrees is essential in the care of brain-injured patients so as to encourage venous outflow from the brain and thus lower ICP. It should also be appreciated that extreme flexion or rotation of the head can obstruct the jugular veins and restrict venous outflow from the brain. The head-down position as used to place central catheters via the external or internal jugular vein must be avoided, as this position can markedly increase ICP.

Hyperventilation. Deliberate hyperventilation of the lungs of adults to a $PaCO_2$ between 25 mmHg to 30 mmHg is an effective and rapid method to lower ICP. Further reductions in the $PaCO_2$ in previously normocapnic patients do not provide additional benefits, and excessive alkalosis might result in cerebral ischemia. Presumably, beneficial effects of hyperventilation of the lungs on ICP reflect decreased cerebral blood flow and resulting reductions in intracranial blood volume. Children with higher cerebral blood flows than adults are treated with more aggressive hyperventilation of the lungs to lower the $PaCO_2$ to between 20 mmHg to 25 mmHg. The duration of the efficacy of hyperventilation for reducing ICP is unknown. In volunteers, however, the effect of hyperventilation wanes with time, as evidenced by a return of cerebral blood flow to normal after about 6 hours.[7] Furthermore, if the cerebral vessels are damaged (e.g., trauma) or diseased (e.g., tumor), their reactivity may be diminished.

Osmotic Diuretics. Intravenous administration of hyperosmotic drugs, such as mannitol (0.25 g·kg^{-1} to 1 g·kg^{-1} over 15 minutes to 30 minutes), reduces ICP by producing a transient increase in the osmolarity of plasma, which acts to draw water from tissues, including the brain. However, if the blood-brain barrier is disrupted, mannitol may pass into the brain and cause cerebral edema by drawing water into the brain. The duration of the hyperosmotic effect of mannitol is about 6 hours. It is important to note that mannitol is not associated with a high incidence of rebound increase in ICP after this time. The brain eventually adapts to sustained elevations in plasma osmolarity such that chronic use of hyperosmotic drugs is likely to become less effective.

Diuresis induced by mannitol may result in acute hypovolemia and adverse electrolyte changes (hy-

pokalemia, hyponatremia), emphasizing the need to replace intravascular fluid volume with infusions of crystalloid and colloid solutions. A rule of thumb is to replace urine output with an equivalent volume of crystalloids, most often lactated Ringer's solution. Glucose and water solutions are not recommended because they are rapidly distributed in total body water including the brain. If the blood glucose concentrations decrease more rapidly than brain glucose, the brain water becomes relatively hyperosmolar, and water enters the central nervous system and exaggerates existing cerebral edema.

Tubular Diuretics. Rapid intravenous administraljtion of furosemide (0.5 mg·kg^{-1} to 1 mg·kg^{-1}) is particularly useful in lowering an excessively elevated ICP that is associated with increased intravascular fluid volume. Advantages of furosemide compared with mannitol include the failure of furosemide to significantly increase serum osmolarity or decrease the plasma concentrations of potassium and sodium.

Corticosteroids. Corticosteroids such as dexamethasone or methylprednisolone are effective in lowering ICP and reducing mortality associated with acute head injury and intracranial tumors. The mechanism for the beneficial effect of corticosteroids is not known but may involve stabilization of capillary membranes and/or reductions in the production of cerebrospinal fluid.

Barbiturates. Administration of barbiturates may be recommended when the ICP remains elevated despite deliberate hyperventilation of the lungs, drug-induced diuresis, and administration of corticosteroids. This recommendation is based on the predictable ability of these drugs to reduce ICP, presumably by decreasing cerebral blood volume secondary to cerebral vascular vasoconstriction and decreased cerebral blood flow. The goal of barbiturate therapy is to maintain the ICP below 20 mmHg without the occurrence of plateau waves. An effective regimen is the intravenous administration of an initial dose of pentobarbital (3 mg·kg^{-1} to 5 mg·kg^{-1}) followed by a continuous rate of infusion to maintain the blood concentration of barbiturate between 3 mg·dl^{-1} to 6 mg·dl^{-1}.[8] An alternative to measuring the blood concentration of pentobarbital every 12 hours to 24 hours is to adjust the infusion rate to maintain an isoelectric electroencephalogram, which confirms the presence of maximum drug-induced depression of cerebral metabolic requirements for oxygen. Discontinuation of barbiturate infusion can be considered when the ICP has remained in a normal range for 48 hours. Failure of barbiturates to lower the ICP is a grave prognostic sign. Even when barbiturates are effective, the overall morbidity and mortality in head trauma patients has not been shown to be improved by the use of these drugs as compared with patients treated aggressively with deliberate hyperventilation of the lungs, drug-induced diuresis, and administration of corticosteroids.[9]

A hazard of barbiturate therapy as used to lower the ICP is hypotension, which can jeopardize the maintenance of an adequate cerebral perfusion pressure. Such hypotension is particularly likely in the presence of decreased intravascular fluid volume. Dopamine or dobutamine may be necessary if barbiturate-induced hypotension due to myocardial depression occurs.

Cerebrospinal Fluid Drainage. Cerebrospinal fluid drainage, either from the lateral cerebral ventricles or lumbar subarachnoic space, effectively reduces ICP and intracranial volume. Lumbar cerebrospinal fluid drainage, however, is not often recommended because herniation of the cerebellum through the foramen magnum might occur.

ACUTE RENAL FAILURE

The best treatment of acute renal failure is prevention by maintenance of an optimal intravascular fluid volume and cardiac output (see Chapter 22). A pulmonary artery catheter is helpful in achieving these goals. A relative fluid overload, resulting in pulmonary edema, may be necessary to prevent oliguria and the risks of acute renal failure. Treatable iatrogenic pulmonary edema is an acceptable complication if the fluids responsible for this adverse response help prevent oliguric renal failure. When acute renal tubular necrosis develops, however, the only treatment is hemodialysis.

ACUTE HEPATIC FAILURE

Regardless of the etiology, acute hepatic failure is associated with a poor prognosis. Hyperventilation is a constant feature of early hepatic failure and most likely reflects stimulation of ventilation by ammonia. Hypoglycemia is frequent. Cardiac output tends to be elevated, reflecting decreased systemic vascular resistance and increased arteriovenous shunting. Most patients with acute hepatic failure develop a bleeding diathesis resembling disseminated intravascular coagulation. Renal failure, arterial hypoxemia, hypotension, and hepatic encephalopathy accompanied by increased ICP are frequent terminal events. Treatment of acute hepatic failure is symptomatic and supportive, including the use of neomycin and/or lactulose to decrease the production of ammonia.

REFERENCES

1. Yeston N. Complement-induced respiratory dysfunction. A story. Curr Rev Respir Ther 1984;6:83–9.
2. O'Rourke PP, Crone RK. High frequency ventilation. JAMA 1982;250:2845–7.
3. Brichant JF, Rouby JJ, Viars P. Intermittent positive pressure ventilation with either positive end-expiratory pressure or high frequency jet ventilation (HFJV), or HFJV alone in human acute respiratory failure. Anesth Analg 1980;65:1135–42.
4. Trichet B, Falke K, Togut A, Laver MB. The effect of preexisting pulmonary vascular disease on the response to mechanical ventilation with PEEP following open-heart surgery. Anesthesiology 1975;42:56–67.
5. Annest SJ, Gottlieb M, Paloski WH, et al. Detrimental effects of removing end-expiratory pressure prior to endotracheal extubation. Ann Surg 1980;191:539–45.
6. Bone RC, Fisher CJ, Clemmer TP, et al. A controlled clinical trial of high-dose methylprednisolone in the treatment of severe sepsis and septic shock. N Engl J Med 1987;317:653–8.
7. Raichle ME, Posner JB, Plum F. Cerebral blood flow during and after hyperventilation. Arch Neurol 1970;23:394–403.
8. Rockoff MA, Marshall LF, Shapiro HM. High dose barbiturate therapy in humans: A clinical review of 60 patients. Ann Neurol 1979;6:194–9.
9. Miller JD. Barbiturates and raised intracranial pressure. Ann Neurol 1979;6:189–93.

Chapter 33

Management of Chronic Pain

Ironically, pain, which is probably the most common symptom in medicine, remains difficult to treat and poorly understood. Although cardiovascular disease and cancer are dramatic and life-threatening diseases, chronic pain can be the cause of months or years of discomfort with a resultant poor quality of life. Furthermore, chronic pain has the potential of interfering with an individual's livelihood and interaction with key people in his or her life, such as family members. Although accurate statistics have not been accumulated, chronic pain probably costs society millions of dollars in medical services and loss of work productivity. Often patients are exposed to a high risk of iatrogenic complications from improper therapy, including opioid addiction or multiple and often unsuccessful surgical procedures.

Unlike acute pain, chronic pain is frequently unrelated to activation of nociceptors. Chronic pain may occur in the absence of noxious stimulation. Autonomic nervous system dysfunction may be present. Psychological factors can alter sensitivity to somatic stimuli and can lead to intense pain despite a mild sensory stimulus.

ROLE OF THE ANESTHESIOLOGIST IN THE DIAGNOSIS AND TREATMENT OF CHRONIC PAIN

Depending on the level of commitment, at one extreme an anesthesiologist may be a full-time member of a pain clinic or, at the other extreme,

may provide occasional diagnostic and therapeutic nerve blocks in the role of a consultant.

Pain Clinic

A pain clinic consists of a group of a physicians from different specialties, including anesthesiology, who interact to solve the problem of chronic pain by evaluating the nociceptive and psychological aspects of the problem.[1] Anesthesiologists are frequently directors of pain clinics. Patients are usually referred to the clinic by their primary physician. Comprehensive records should be collected that document the activities and pain levels of the patient. After arriving at the pain clinic, patients undergo medical and psychological examinations and evaluation by a social worker who documents significant social problems. After this information has been collected, the multidisciplinary pain clinic physicians discuss the case and arrive at an appropriate diagnosis as to the most likely origin of the pain. A decision is then reached as to what further evaluation or treatment is necessary, such as drug detoxification if drug dependency exists, referral to an orthopaedic or neurosurgical physician if neural deficits are present, or performance of a nerve block by an anesthesiologist.[2]

Consultant

The anesthesiologist whose primary commitment is in areas other than the diagnosis and treatment of chronic pain may be asked to perform diagnostic

Diagnostic and Therapeutic Nerve Blocks Used in Management of Chronic Pain
Subarachnoid (spinal) block
Epidural block
Stellate ganglion block
Brachial plexus block
Intercostal nerve block
Intravenous regional block
Lumbar sympathetic block
Celiac plexus block

Chronic Pain Interview
1. What has been the duration, intensity, and location of the pain?
2. What precipitates or exacerbates the pain?
3. What other symptoms, if any, accompany the pain?
4. What have been the effects of the pain on sleep, employment, and social and interpersonal relationships?
5. What medications is the patient currently taking?
6. What treatment or medications have been previously tried without success?
7. Is there litigation or some form of financial compensation that would be jeopardized if the pain was successfully treated?

or therapeutic nerve blocks. Of prime importance is that the anesthesiologist recognize personal limitations. Expertise in performing a diagnostic or therapeutic nerve block does not imply an equivalent amount of expertise in the overall evaluation of chronic pain. For example, has a patient who has chronic back pain undergone complete evaluation before the epidural injection of corticosteroids? Has a spinal cord tumor been ruled out? Diagnostic and therapeutic nerve blocks should only be performed after a thorough medical evaluation has been performed to ensure that an important disease process is not being overlooked.

APPROACH TO THE PATIENT WITH CHRONIC PAIN

The anesthesiologist's initial patient contact is an interview to determine whether a nerve block or other pain-removing procedure will be helpful in the diagnosis or treatment of chronic pain. The interview should be constructed to answer several types of questions.[2]

Certain guidelines indicate how satisfied a patient may be if the pain were removed. Patients who are socially happy with adequate family support may continue their occupation despite the pain. These same patients who are unhappy taking analgesics and who have had pain for several months, rather than years, are more likely to be motivated to want to remove their pain.

Psychological Tests

Psychological testing is helpful for detecting psychopathology that may initiate or aggravate pain complaints and for determining the psychological impact of chronic pain. The State-Trait Anxiety Inventory evaluates the patient's level of anxiety, with high scores suggesting suicidal intent. The McGill Pain Questionnaire is a list of words describing pain syndromes that the patient selects to best fit the symptoms. Selection of words not typical of the presumed diagnosis may suggest a strong psychological component to the patient's pain. The Minnesota Multiphasic Personality Inventory (MMPI) is commonly used but takes over an hour to complete and contains questions that some patients find objectionable.

Regardless of sophisticated psychological testing, the clinician must resist the temptation to label patients with chronic pain as malingerers. Patients with chronic pain often are despairing, demoralized, worried, and sometimes hostile. Neurotic behavior is a natural and normal response to chronic pain. In fact, one may become suspicious of a patient who has chronic debilitating pain and yet appears to be a happy, well-adjusted individual. Patients should not be excluded from treatment because of their personality profiles. Neurotic patients are entitled to the same pain relief as "normal" patients.

Measurement of Pain

Although several methods of measuring pain exist, the "pain estimate" is probably the most useful method for the clinician who occassionally performs diagnostic or therapeutic nerve blocks. With the pain estimate, the patient assigns a number to the intensity of the pain. The patient is asked to rank the pain on a visual analog scale of zero to 10 where "zero" refers to no pain and "10" refers to pain so severe that suicide may be considered. Several numbers may be assigned each day; for example, one number might be the average pain per day, and another number might be the worse pain. Patients can record these numbers before and after a nerve block to assess the magnitude and duration of pain relief.

Physical Examination

A routine physical examination should be performed, with special emphasis on a thorough neurologic examination. In addition, the following areas require special attention during the physical examination.

Map Out the Painful Area

If the area is not too tender, the painful area can be outlined with a felt-tipped pen. If possible, the painful area should be identified according to the peripheral nerve or dermatome areas.

Skin

The characteristics of the skin often provide a clue as to sympathetic nervous system function. Warm, dry, smooth skin with coarse hair is evidence of vasodilation. Vasoconstricted skin is blanched, clammy, cool, thin, and glistening, with thin or sparse hair.

Muscle and Joint

Evidence of guarding, wasting, deformity, swelling, and temperature changes should be noted and will give a clue as to how active a painful area

has been. For example, a muscular hand and arm with a preliminary diagnosis of causalgia should be highly suspect because the evidence is that the patient has been using that arm extensively.

Maneuvers That Alter Pain

An assessment of maneuvers that relieve and cause the pain may include locally applied pressure (especially on a trigger point), leg raising to elicit lumbar root irritation, and changes in temperature.

DIAGNOSTIC NERVE BLOCKS

Diagnostic nerve blocks can be used to (1) anatomically define the pain pathway, (2) differentiate pharmacologically the size of the fibers that mediate the pain, (3) differentiate central pain from peripheral pain, and (4) determine whether a neurolytic block or surgical resection of a nerve should be performed.

If a specific pathway of pain can be localized, a neurolytic nerve block might be considered. Furthermore, the diagnostic block allows the patient to undergo a "trial run" without permanent change. Sometime, the numbness or lack of sensation is more unpleasant for the patient than is the pain itself. Also, by using different concentrations of local anesthetics, the size of the nerve fiber mediating the pain can be better defined (e.g., small diameter sympathetic nerve fibers versus larger somatic nerve fibers).

Nerve blocks can sometimes be used to detect drug addiction. If a patient with chronic pain still requires a normal dose of opioid during the effective period of a successful nerve block, then addiction should be suspected.

Placebo

Placebo injection is the administration of a solution without known analgesic action. For example, a small amount of saline may be injected rather than a local anesthetic for a diagnostic nerve block. An inexperienced clinician might assume that a patient does not have an organic basis for pain if a placebo relieves the discomfort. A placebo, however, may relieve pain (often very transient) 30 percent to 40 percent of the time in any one patient.[3] Therefore, a patient may have an organic basis for pain but still achieve partial relief from a placebo injection. Accordingly, interpretation of a placebo response may be difficult, which limits its value to the clinician who occasionally attempts to evaluate the results of a diagnostic nerve block when a placebo has been injected.

Differential Nerve Block

Because fiber size is an important factor that governs susceptibility of a nerve to be blocked by local anesthetics, differential nerve blocks can be used to distinguish placebo, sympathetic, and somatic sensory sources of pain. The most commonly used differential nerve block is a graduated spinal block technique.[4] After a lumbar subarachnoid puncture is performed, the following solutions are injected in a four-step procedure:

1. Seven milliliters of "artificial cerebrospinal fluid" with no preservatives (placebo).
2. Seven milliliters of 0.2 percent procaine (sympathetic nerve blockade).
3. Seven milliliters of 0.5 percent procaine (sensory blockade).
4. Seven milliliters of 1.0 percent procaine (motor blockade).

Pain is judged to be psychogenic if relief occurs with the placebo injection. If relief occurs with a 0.2 percent procaine injection, a sympathetic nervous system pathway of transmission is usually assigned as the cause. If pain persists after 1.0 percent procaine has been administered, a more central origin, or psychogenic pain, should be considered.

Unfortunately, the differential spinal approach has many drawbacks. A patient cannot move during a differential spinal anesthetic to perform the maneuvers that elicit the pain. Insertion of an epidural catheter may provide more flexibility in this regard. Also, the placebo may itself cause relief of pain of organic basis. Hypotonic solutions injected into the cerebrospinal fluid have been known to result in blockade of pain conduction. Thus, a slow withdrawal of cerebrospinal fluid and then reinjection 5 minutes later is a preferable technique. Also, it is assumed that 0.2 percent

procaine only blocks sympathetic nerves without sensory involvement. Although the dominant block probably is sympathetic, sensory fibers are undoubtedly blocked to a limited extent. Thus, if a sympathetic nervous system origin for the pain is suspected, a more specific stellate ganglion or lumbar sympathetic block can be performed (see Chapter 14).

THERAPEUTIC NERVE BLOCKS

Therapeutic nerve blocks may be performed with local anesthetics, neurolytics, or neuraxial placement of opioids.

Local Anesthetics

Although nerve blocks with local anesthetics can be very valuable in a diagnostic manner, they also can be used in a therapeutic manner in patients with chronic pain. For example, reflex sympathetic dystrophy can be interrupted with local anesthetics. Second, a temporary local anesthetic-induced nerve block may allow physical therapy to be performed in areas that are normally painful. Third, the inflammatory response can be reduced by a local anesthetic nerve block, usually in combination with a corticosteroid injection. Fourth, occasionally chronic pain can be relieved with one or more local anesthetic nerve blocks on a prolonged, or even a permanent basis; however, these situations are very rare. Finally, by performing a sympathetic nerve block with a local anesthetic, vascular supply in an ischemic area in patients with vascular disease can be improved.

Neurolytic Block

In those patients with persistent chronic pain, nerve destruction with neurolytics, such as alcohol, phenol, or ammonium sulfate, may be useful. The use of alcohol or phenol probably should be restricted to clinicians with special expertise and experience in the injection of these drugs. Furthermore, the use of neurolytics probably is only indicated in those patients with short life expectancy, such as those individuals with pain from terminal cancer. The use of alcohol or phenol on peripheral nerves is frequently followed by the appearance of a denervation hypersensitivity type of pain, which may be worse than the original pain. For this reason, injection of alcohol and phenol probably should be restricted to the epidural or subarachnoid spaces. There is little difference in the efficacy between alcohol and phenol, although initial responses are very different. For example, alcohol causes intense pain on injection and produces neurolysis promptly. In contrast, phenol in glycerine produces no pain on injection but requires several minutes to produce its neurolytic effects. When used for intrathecal neurolysis, it must be recognized that alcohol is hypobaric (inject with patient positioned so the affected sensory roots are uppermost) and phenol is hyperbaric. Patient movement during or shortly after the injection can result in unwanted spread of the neurolytic solutions. Indeed, the principal disadvantage of neurolytic nerve blocks is the difficulty in preventing the spread of destructive effects to surrounding normal tissues or impairment of bowel and bladder activity. For somatic nerve blocks, 100 percent alcohol is used. Blockade of smaller diameter sympathetic nerve fibers is with 50 percent alcohol. Phenol is used in concentrations ranging from 5 percent to 20 percent for peripheral nerves.

One problem with neurolytics is that alcohol or phenol rarely produces an analgesic state as intense as did the diagnostic local anesthetic block. Therefore, patients are frequently disappointed that the neurolytic block has not produced as much pain relief as did the diagnostic local anesthetic block. The patient should, therefore, be cautioned about the effectiveness of a neurolytic block. Furthermore, "permanent" neurolytic blocks are really not permanent, and recovery of sensation of pain occurs in a matter of weeks or months, emphasizing their usefulness in patients with a short life expectancy.

Ammonium sulfate, usually a 10 percent solution, is a neurolytic drug, which is less effective than alcohol or phenol, but is associated with few, if any, complications. It dehydrates the nerve and is effective in relieving pain from unmyelinated (i.e., C fibers) nerves. Intercostal neuralgia is probably the most common pain syndrome treated with ammonium sulfate.

Neuraxial Opioids

Chronic pain, especially pain due to cancer, is effectively relieved by neuraxial (subarachnoid or epidural) administration of opioids, most often morphine[5]. Effectiveness of neuraxial opioids reflects the presence of opioid receptors in the substantia gelatinosa of the spinal cord. Advantages of neuraxial opioids for relief of pain include prolonged duration of action and absence of sympathetic nervous system blockade or skeletal muscle paralysis. Delayed depression of ventilation (up to 12 hours after drug injection) and other side effects of neuraxial opioids (pruritus, sedation, urinary retention, nausea, and vomiting) are less likely to occur after administration of neuraxial opioids for the treatment of cancer pain than when this approach is used to treat acute postoperative pain in patients who are not tolerant to opioids. Because pain relief is usually less than 36 hours, it is unrealistic to expect to repeat subarachnoid or epidural injections for prolonged periods. In this regard, the use of implanted infusion devices, which consists of a percutaneously refillable reservoir for the opioid and a mechanism for pumping the drug from the reservoir through the catheter in the subarachnoid or epidural space, may be useful.[6] Unfortunately, progressive tolerance to morphine develops when subarachnoid infusion of morphine is prolonged beyond about 7 days. When tolerance to opioids develops, responsiveness of opioid receptors may be restored by replacing neuraxial opioids with local anesthetics for several days. Neuraxial injections of clonidine may also be useful when opioid tolerance develops.[7] Conversely, abrupt discontinuation of chronic neuraxial opioid infusions may be followed by an opioid withdrawal syndrome.

EVALUATION OF A NERVE BLOCK

Especially to the clinician who only infrequently interacts with a patient with chronic pain, caution should be applied to the evaluation of a diagnostic and/or therapeutic nerve block. In fact, evaluation of a patient's physiologic and psychological responses to a nerve block is often more difficult than the technical procedure required to produce

Table 33-1. Clinical Results with Intrathecally Applied Morphine

	Age (years), Sex	Number of Injections	Agent and Dose (mg)	Pain	
				Mean Change in Intensity (Scale of 0 to 10)	Mean Duration of Relief (Hours)
Patient 1	56, M	3	Morphine (0.5)	7, 1	18
		2	Saline Solution	6, 1	6
Patient 2	60, M	2	Morphine (0.5)	7, 1	12
		2	Saline Solution	8, 8	No relief
Patient 3	57, F	2	Morphine (0.5)	5, 0	22
		1	Saline Solution	6, 5	No relief
Patient 4	68, M	2	Morphine (1.0)	5, 0	20
		2	Saline Solution	5, 4	No relief
Patient 5	66, M	2	Morphine (0.5)	5, 1	14
		1	Saline Solution	6, 7	No relief
Patient 6	71, M	2	Morphine (0.5)	3, 1	10
		1	Saline Solution	3, 1	8
Patient 7	51, M	3	Morphine (1.0)	4, 0	24
		2	Saline Solution	5, 4	No relief
Patient 8	62, M	1	Morphine (0.5)	4, 0	21
		1	Saline Solution	5, 5	No relief

(From Wang et al.,[5] with permission.)

the block. For example, the use of a local anesthetic block to predict the success of a neurolytic block or surgical resection of a nerve is difficult. It is incorrect to assume that if the diagnostic block relieves the pain, then a neurolytic block or a surgical resection certainly will be successful. As indicated previously, local anesthetic blocks frequently produce a more intense relief of pain than neurolytics. Furthermore, if a surgical procedure is performed, the pain may return, either due to regeneration of the nerve or a denervation hypersensitivity type of reaction. Also, even though diagnostic nerve blocks allow the patient to experience the numbness and side effects that could be permanent from nerve ablation techniques, they are not always accurate predictors of long-term pain relief. For example, diagnostic nerve blocks provide little help in evaluating the influence of pain relief on psychological factors, such as family interactions and financial gain (e.g., litigation).

Evaluation of results from therapeutic nerve blocks requires more thorough questioning than

"Is your pain gone?" First, the frequency and intensity of the pain should be recorded, including the number of hours in bed and the number of hours spent standing and reclining daily. The patient should record his or her estimate as to the abililty to walk, bend, and work. Perhaps the number of activities (e.g., making the bed, washing the car) that can be performed before versus after a nerve block should be recorded. Furthermore, the influence on recreational and social activities should be documented. Last, and perhaps most important, an accurate list of medications taken daily should be made. Only after this type of evaluation can the true effectiveness of a therapeutic nerve block be evaluated.

TRANSCUTANEOUS ELECTRICAL NERVE STIMULATION

Transcutaneous electrical nerve stimulation (TENS) is the patient activated delivery of pulsed electrical current to skin overlying the painful area. Presumably, this electrical current activates large afferent fibers, resulting in stimulation of inhibitory dorsal horn neurons and/or release of endorphins. Reliable effectiveness of TENS in chronic pain management has not been substantiated.

PATIENT-CONTROLLED ANALGESIA

Patient-controlled analgesia (PCA) is the use of a special programmable pump that allows the patient to self-administer small intravenous doses of opioids. This approach permits maintenance of sustained therapeutic plasma concentrations of opioids that are not possible with intramuscular injections separated by 4 hours to 6 hours. PCA has limited application in treatment of chronic pain, finding its greatest usefulness in the management of acute postoperative pain[8] (see Chapter 30).

COMMON PAIN PROBLEMS ALL ANESTHESIOLOGISTS SHOULD BE ABLE TO MANAGE

Although the clinician should refer most chronic pain problems to physicians who are involved with pain clinics, there are a few pain problems with which all anesthesiologists should be capable of managing, at least in the initial stages of diagnosis and/or treatment.

Causalgia and Reflex Sympathetic Dystrophy

Causalgia occurs after nerve injury, whereas reflex sympathetic dystrophy typically follows a trivial injury without apparent neurologic damage. Often, however, these terms are used interchangeably. Both are accompanied by similar manifestations, which include chronic, severe burning pain; localized autonomic nervous system dysfunction; and atrophic changes. In addition, the pain is characterized as aching, intense, and/or agonizing and is usually enhanced by mechanical stimulation, movement, and application of heat or cold. Initially, vascular changes, probably resulting from altered sympathetic nervous system activity, lead to a warm, erythematous, dry, swollen extremity. Later, the extremity will be cool, pale, and/or cyanotic; and there will be atrophy of skin and skeletal muscles and decreased density of bones.

The diagnosis can be established and treatment initiated by performing a stellate ganglion block for causalgia of the upper extremity or a lumbar sympathetic block for causalgia of the lower extremity (see Chapter 14). If sympathetic nerve blockade clearly produces relief of pain, then the diagnosis of causalgia is established Brachial plexus block will relieve pain due to sympathetic nervous origin, but it is likely that unnecessary blockade of sensory and even motor fibers may also occur.

It is hoped that the duration of pain relief will exceed the expected duration of local anesthetic action when performing a sympathetic block. Furthermore, subsequent blocks may provide progressively longer pain-free intervals. Up to five to seven stellate ganglion or lumbar sympathetic nerve blocks can be performed on alternate days, with the goal that ultimately a prolonged period of pain relief will result, lasting several weeks or months.

Dramatic relief of pain and increase in skin temperature has been reported in several patients in whom sympathetic nerve blockade was performed by infusing a sympatholytic drug intravenously into an extremity isolated from the general circulation by a tourniquet.[9] Specifically, guanethidine, 10 mg to 20 mg, or reserpine, 1 mg to 2 mg in 20 ml to 25 ml of normal saline, is injected intravenously through an indwelling needle into the extremity. The extremity is isolated from the circulation for 10 minutes to allow the binding of guanethidine or reserpine to the tissues. Then the tourniquet is slowly released. This intravenous regional sympathetic nerve block technique is used most often when stellate ganglion or lumbar sympathetic blocks have been ineffective. Furthermore, this approach appears to be useful in patients who show signs of returning sympathetic nervous system function despite apparently adequate surgical excision of the sympathetic ganglia.

Chronic Back Pain

Chronic back pain represents a significant health problem, with various conservative and surgical treatments frequently being ineffective. The result is chronic pain, loss of productivity, and occasionally disability. Patients who have a lumbar radiculopathy usually have pain as a result of inflammation of the nerve root or through compression of the dorsal root ganglion. Pain arising from inflammation surrounding the nerve root is frequently responsive to the epidural administration of corticosteroids such as triamcinolone or methylprednisolone. Before proceeding with this treatment, it is mandatory to rule out the presence of infection or a space-occupying lesion. Finally, an epidural injection of corticosteroids should not be performed until a careful diagnostic evaluation (including consultation with a neurosurgeon or an orthopaedic surgeon) has been performed and the patient is advised of the possible benefits and complications of corticosteroid injections, including the distinct possibility that no relief from the injections may occur. All information given and received should be recorded in the patient's chart.

The patient is placed in the lateral position and 3 ml to 4 ml of 1 percent lidocaine (other local anesthetics could be used) is injected. The local anesthetic provides temporary relief of pain, confirming that the tip of the needle is in the epidural space. Then, methylprednisolone, 80 mg to 100 mg, is injected. The patient is asked to remain in the lateral position for 15 minutes. If the radicular pain has been present for more than 6 months, the success of epidural corticosteroids is markedly decreased. This is probably due to proliferation of scar and fibrous tissue around the damaged tissue surrounding the nerve root.

Intercostal Neuralgia

Intercostal neuralgia, following thoracotomy or rib fracture, is characterized by paresthesias and pain in response to touch or movement of the thorax. Although the pain usually subsides within 2 weeks, it can persist for several months or years, requiring active treatment. In most cases, destructive nerve blocks with alcohol, phenol, ammonium sulfate, or surgical removal of a neuroma or rhizotomy offer little help. Alcohol or phenol injections are usually followed by a 10 percent to 50 percent incidence of postblock neuritis, in which the pain is worse than before the block was performed. One approach is to perform local anesthetic intercostal or paravertebral nerve blocks. During the pain-free time, physical therapy can be performed. Repeated efforts of this kind occasionally will result in prolonged relief of pain. In severe cases, 10 percent

ammonium sulfate has been used. Although this is not effective in all cases, ammonium sulfate is not associated with complications such as postblock neuritis.[10]

Postherpetic Neuralgia

After an acute infection of herpes zoster, a syndrome called "postherpetic neuralgia" can exist for an extended period of time, especially in elderly or immunosuppressed patients. After the acute infective period in which the cutaneous lesions (most often T1–8 dermatomes) gradually disappear in 2 weeks to 4 weeks, the pain usually subsides. Pain and scarring, however, may persist. Local anesthetic, alcohol, and phenol intercostal nerve blocks are not predictably effective in relieving the pain. Early cases (less than 3 months) sometimes can be effectively treated with sympathetic nerve blocks with local anesthetic. Oral administration of a phenothiazine (fluphenazine) and a tricyclic antidepressant (amitriptyline) can occasionally relieve the pain. In elderly patients, however, complications, such as orthostatic hypotension, can occur after the use of these drugs. Also, patients may become sleepy and lose their appetite, leading to increasing debilitation. Another approach has been the subcutaneous intralesional injection of local anesthetics and corticosteroids. Specifically, 20 ml to 30 ml of a solution of triamcinolone (2 mg·ml^{-1}) and bupivacaine (0.25 percent) is injected under the painful skin area. Although several clinicians are enthusiastic about this approach, others find that this treatment has produced only limited success.

Myofascial Pain Syndrome

Many chronic pain states of obscure origin depend on feedback cycles from myofascial trigger points. The trigger point concept has been difficult for many physicians to accept because precise neuroanatomic connections between the trigger point and the pain are not present. The clinician should always examine a patient with chronic pain for the possibility of a trigger point. There often are multiple painful areas with multiple trigger points in the same patient. On examination of such patients, the painful muscular areas have been described as feeling like a rope. A positive "jump sign" has been described, whereby the trigger area is palpated, and the patient "jumps away" from the pain. Detection of a trigger point to palpation makes it relatively easy for a successful treatment regimen to be instituted. For example, topical application of a vapor coolant spray and a follow-up of the localized analgesic effect with active and passive physiotherapy can be useful. Also, weak local anesthetic concentrations, such as 0.5 percent lidocaine or 0.25 percent bupivacaine, can be injected into the trigger point. By including a small dose of corticosteroids (cortisol 25 mg) with the local anesthetic solution, more extended relief of pain can sometimes result. Trigger point injections can be repeated as necessary every 3 days to 7 days.

Pancreatic Cancer

Neurolytic celiac plexus block is useful for relief of pain associated with pancreatic cancer and other upper abdominal malignancies. This reflects the fact that the celiac plexus carries sensory and autonomic nervous system fibers from all the abdominal viscera except the left colon and the pelvic organs. Typically, neurolytic block is with 30 ml to 50 ml of 50 percent alcohol or 6 percent phenol injected through needles whose proper position has been verified (radiography, computed tomography) to minimize the risk of accidental subarachnoid injection.[11] Analgesics are necessary to offset the pain produced by injection of alcohol and intravenous administration of fluids (10 ml·kg^{-1} to 15 ml·kg^{-1}) reduces the likelihood of symptomatic postblock orthostatic hypotension owing to splanchnic vasodilation. Although this type of pain has been classified as an example of a problem that all anesthesiologists should be able to manage, neurolytic celiac plexus block should be performed only by those with experience in this technique.

REFERENCES

1. Kroening RJ. Pain clinics structure and function. Semin Anesth 1985;4:231–7.
2. Carron H. Management of the patient with chronic pain. Resident and Staff Physician 1981;6:46–54.
3. Taub A. Factors in the diagnosis and treatment of chronic pain. J Autism Child Schizophr 1975;5:1–12.
4. Miller RD, Munger WL, Power PE. Chronic pain and local anesthetic neural blockade. In: Cousins MJ, Bridenbaugh PO, eds. Neural blockade. Philadelphia, JB Lippincott, 1988;616–37.
5. Wang JK, Naus LA, Thomas JE. Pain relief by intrathecally applied morphine in man. Anesthesiology 1979;50:149–51.
6. Coombs DW, Saunders RL, Gaylor MS, Pageau MG. Epidural narcotic infusion reservoir: Implantation techniques and efficacy. Anesthesiology 1982;56:469–73.
7. Coombs DW, Saunders RL, Lachance D, et al. Intrathecal morphine tolerance. Use of intrathecal clonidine, DADLE, and intraventricular morphine. Anesthesiology 1985;62:358–63.
8. White PF. Patient-controlled analgesia: A new approach to the management of postoperative pain. Semin Anesth 1985;4:255–62.
9. Hannington-Kiff G. Intravenous regional sympathetic block with guanethidine. Lancet 1974;1:1019–20.
10. Miller RD, Johnston RR, Hosobuchi Y. Treatment of intercostal neuralgia with 10 percent ammonium sulfate. J Thorac Cardiovasc Surg 1975;69:476–8.
11. Brown DL, Bulley CK, Quiel EL. Neurolytic celiac plexus block for pancreatic cancer pain. Anesth Analg 1987;66:869–73.

Chapter 34

Cardiopulmonary Resuscitation

Cardiopulmonary resuscitation (CPR) applies many of the skills unique to the practice of anesthesiology. As a result, anesthesiologists are involved in the provision and teaching of all aspects of CPR (Table 34-1). Furthermore, new advances and concepts in CPR often reflect basic research by anesthesiologists.

CPR is categorized as Basic Life Support (BLS) and Advanced Cardiac Life Support (ACLS). BLS consists of provision of a patent upper airway (A-airway), exhaled air ventilation (B-breathing), and circulation of blood by closed chest cardiac compression (C-circulation). The A,B,C's of BLS may be instituted by trained lay persons, as well as by physicians, without the need for specialized equipment. ACLS includes use of specialized equipment to maintain the airway, external defibrillation, drug therapy, and postresuscitation management. The highest survival rates and quality of survival are attained when BLS is initiated within 4 minutes from the time of cardiac arrest and when ACLS is initiated within 8 minutes.[1]

Management of CPR is a team effort and coordination of the team is the responsibility of the team leader, ideally a physician skilled in airway management. It is the responsibility of the team leader to (1) ensure the quality of BLS, (2) facilitate early use of electrical defibrillation, and (3) direct and monitor adequacy of drug therapy.[2] Ulti-mately, the team leader may also decide when resuscitation efforts should cease.

PROVISION OF A PATENT UPPER AIRWAY

Methods to provide a patient upper airway after a cardiac arrest are designed to relieve obstruction due to the tongue falling against the posterior pharynx. Extension of the head and displacement of the mandible anteriorly serves to stretch the muscles attached to the tongue and thus pull the tongue off the posterior pharynx. This maneuver is known as the head tilt-jaw thrust method and is identical to the recommended procedure for securing a patent airway in the patient rendered unconscious by anesthetic drugs (Fig. 34-1). The jaw thrust maneuver without head tilt is the recommended method for opening the airway in a victim with a suspected neck injury.

EXHALED AIR VENTILATION

Exhaled air ventilation (mouth-to-mouth) when performed properly provides adequate alveolar ventilation. However, delivered oxygen concentrations using this technique are only 16 percent to 17 percent such that the maximum alveolar PO_2 obtainable is about 80 mmHg. The PaO_2 will be even lower (i.e., arterial hypoxemia is predictable), reflecting increased venous admixture and low

Table 34-1. Comparative Resuscitation Techniques

	Infant	Child (1 year to 8 years old)	Adult
Ventilation method	Mouth-to-mouth and nose	Mouth-to-mouth and nose	Mouth-to-mouth
Check for pulse	Bracheal artery at midforearm	Carotid artery	Carotid artery
Sternal depression method	Encircle chest with both hands and depress midsternum with thumbs	Depress sternum with three fingers	Depress sternum with heel of hand on lower third of sternum
Sternal depression depth	1.3 cm to 2.5 cm	2.5 cm to 3.8 cm	3.8 cm to 5 cm
Sternal depression rate	At least $100 \cdot min^{-1}$	$80 \cdot min^{-1}$ to $100 \cdot min^{-1}$	$80 \cdot min^{-1}$ to $100 \cdot min^{-1}$
Sternal depression to ventilation ratio	5:1	5:1	15:2 if one rescuer, 5:1 if two rescuers
Management of an obstructed upper airway due to a foreign body	Back blows followed by chest (not abdominal) thrusts Finger probe under vision if unconscious	Abdominal thrusts	Abdominal thrusts Chest thrusts in selected patients Blind finger probes if unconscious

cardiac output present during CPR. Gastric distension often accompanies exhaled air ventilation, particularly if high airway pressures due to an incompletely patent upper airway are required. Even with a patent upper airway, some gas is likely to enter the stomach when inflation pressures exceed 15 cm H_2O. Manual pressure applied over the victim's epigastrium to relieve gastric distension is not recommended as this maneuver may produce regurgitation of gastric contents.[2] Nevertheless, gastric distension that impairs ventilation of the lungs must be relieved by any method available, including manual pressure over the epigastrium.

CLOSED CHEST (EXTERNAL) CARDIAC COMPRESSION

Optimal blood flow produced by closed chest cardiac compression depends on the proper placement of the rescuer's hands on the victim's sternum, the position of the rescuer's body in relation to the victim, and the depth and the rate of depression of the sternum.

The heel of the rescuer's hand is placed over and parallel to the lower third of the adult victim's sternum so as to provide maximum compression of the underlying cardiac ventricles (Fig. 34-2).[2]

Pressure over the xyphoid process or rib cage must be avoided so as to minimize the likelihood of damage to abdominal organs, particularly the liver or the production of rib fractures with damage to the heart and lungs. The rescuer should kneel next to the victim so that the upper body is over the victim's chest. The rescuer's elbows are kept straight and the shoulders positioned directly over the hands. This position enables the rescuer to use the weight of the upper body for compression, which must depress the sternum of an adult victim 3.8 cm to 5 cm.[2] Relaxation on the sternum must be complete at the end of each compression to permit the heart to fill. The rescuer's hands, however, must maintain contact with the victim's sternum or correct hand position may be lost. Properly performed closed chest cardiac compression can produce systolic blood pressure peaks of more than 100 mmHg, but diastolic blood pressure is low and mean arterial pressure in the carotid arteries seldom exceeds 40 mmHg. Carotid artery blood flow resulting from closed chest compressions is usually less than one-third of normal. The recommended minimum compression rate is $80 \cdot min^{-1}$, whereas the duration of each compression is ideally 50 percent of the cycle time. Achieve-

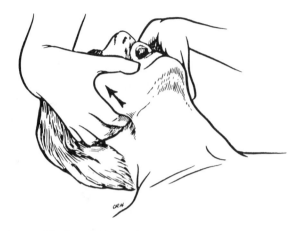

Fig. 34-1. The head tilt-jaw thrust maneuver provides a patent upper airway by stretching muscles attached to the tongue, thus pulling the tongue away from the posterior pharynx. Forward displacement of the mandible is accomplished by grasping the angles of the mandible and lifting with both hands, serving to displace the mandible forward while tilting the head backward.

ment of the proper ratio of compression time to relaxation time requires a pause at the point of maximal sternal depression. This is the reason for avoidance of quick, bouncing compressions. When a single rescuer is present, external cardiac compression and exhaled air ventilation are provided at a compression-to-breath ratio of 15:2 each minute. When two rescuers are available, the compression rate is $80 \cdot min^{-1}$ to $100 \cdot min^{-1}$, and a breath is delivered during the upstroke of every fifth compression (a ratio of 5:1). The effectiveness of closed chest cardiac compressions should be verified by palpation of peripheral pulses.

The mechanism responsible for blood flow during closed chest cardiac compression is traditionally attributed to compression of the cardiac ventricles between the sternum and the spine, resulting in an increase in pressure within the ventricles and closure of the mitral and tricuspid valves (cardiac pump mechanism). This pressure was thought to cause antegrade flow into the pulmonary artery and aorta. In addition, increases in intrathoracic pressure that accompany closed chest cardiac compressions are important for producing antegrade flow (thoracic pump mechanism). Conceptually, the heart is like a balloon in a closed box such that increases in intrathoracic pressure squeeze blood from the heart. Indirect evidence for the thoracic pump mechanism is the observation that patients who develop acute ventricular fibrillation remain conscious for several seconds if they cough vigorously.[3] Presumably, cough-in-

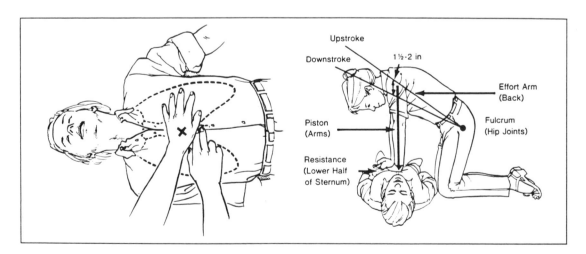

Fig. 34-2. Proper hand and body position for performance of closed chest cardiac compression in an adult. (From Standards and guidelines for cardiopulmonary resuscitation and emergency cardiac care,[2] with permission.)

duced increases in intrathoracic pressure provide antegrade blood flow.

The potential exists for increases in intrathoracic pressure produced by CPR to elicit elevations in intracranial pressure (ICP), particularly in patients with co-existing decreases in intracranial compliance. If this is true, cerebral perfusion pressure (blood pressure minus ICP) may remain low despite apparently adequate CPR as suggested by systolic blood pressure. Indeed, data suggest that CPR is of limited effectiveness in providing adequate cerebral blood flow.[4] Consistent with this observation is the extremely poor neurologic prognosis if adequate spontaneous cardiovascular function is not achieved within 15 minutes despite apparently adequate CPR.

Variations in conventional techniques of CPR are being studied in attempts to improve blood pressure and blood flow during the resuscitation sequence. These variations include (1) simultaneous chest compression and ventilation of the lungs using high airway pressures, (2) abdominal compressions interposed between sternal depressions, (3) continuous abdominal binding, and (4) use of antishock trousers.[2]

SPECIALIZED EQUIPMENT TO MAINTAIN THE AIRWAY

Supplemental oxygen and adjuncts for airway management must be instituted as promptly as possible during CPR. Adjuncts for use in airway management are designed to assure control of the airway, improve ventilation and oxygenation, and isolate the trachea from the gastrointestinal tract. A pocket face mask is the simplest advancement beyond mouth-to-mouth ventilation. Exhaled air ventilation may be provided via this mask. Alternatively, a reservoir bag with a one-way valve may be attached to this mask to permit manual ventilation of the lungs. Another advantage of a reservoir bag is the ability to deliver oxygen for ventilation of the lungs. For example, a 10 $L \cdot min^{-1}$ flow of oxygen will provide inhaled oxygen concentrations of about 50 percent. This mask should be transparent so that regurgitated gastric contents may be recognized promptly. Oropharyngeal or nasopharyngeal airways may be useful, remembering that oral airways may evoke vomiting

or laryngospasm if introduced into conscious or semiconscious victims. Incorrect placement of an oral airway can displace the tongue back into the pharynx and result in airway obstruction.

The best method for maintenance of a patent upper airway is placement of a cuffed tube in the trachea using direct laryngoscopy in the presence of cricoid pressure. This tracheal tube permits (1) optimal adjustment of tidal volume and breathing rate, (2) reliable addition of supplemental oxygen to the inhaled gases, and (3) protection of the lungs from inhalation of gastric contents when the cuff is inflated with air to provide a seal against the tracheal mucosa. An alternative to placement of a cuffed tube in the trachea is blind insertion of a solid cuffed tube known as an esophageal obturator airway (EOA) into the esophagus. Inflation of the cuff on the EOA with 30 ml of air occludes the esophagus to reduce the likelihood of gastric regurgitation into the pharynx, whereas openings in the proximal end of the tube, which remains in the pharynx, are a route for administration of oxygen and ventilation of the lungs. The length of the EOA has been standardized so that insertion into the esophagus of an adult until the mask rests properly on the victim's face will result in positioning of the esophageal cuff below the carina. Thus, when the cuff is inflated with the proper amount of air, it will not compress the posterior membranous wall of the trachea. The major hazards of the EOA are esophageal perforation and unrecognized placement in the trachea. In addition, regurgitation invariably follows removal of the EOA, emphasizing the need to have a cuffed tube in the trachea before extubation of the esophagus. A modification of the EOA incorporates a lumen (esophageal gastric tube airway [EGTA]) through which a gastric tube can be passed and the stomach suctioned without interfering with ventilation of the lungs.

Mechanical ventilators are not reliably effective during CPR. For example, pressure-cycled ventilators will prematurely cease to deliver gas flow when the sternum is depressed, whereas volume-cycled ventilators will not be able to deliver a reliable tidal volume during this time. Alternatively, manually triggered oxygen-powered breathing devices are available for ventilation of the lungs via a face mask, tracheal tube, or esophageal airways. Using these devices, the instantaneous development of a high flow rate of oxygen (100 L·min^{-1}) and maximum pressures of 50 cm H_2O by manual depression of the control button allows the rescuer to interpose breaths at the desired time during external cardiac compressions.

EXTERNAL DEFIBRILLATION

External defibrillation is the definitive treatment of ventricular fibrillation. The most important determinant of the success of external defibrillation and the survival of the victim is the length of

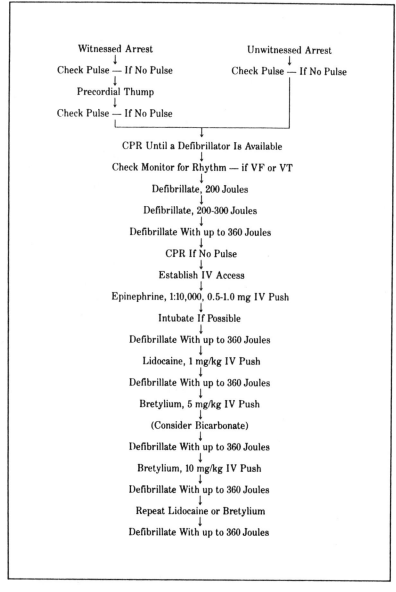

Fig. 34-3. Treatment of ventricular fibrillation (VF) or pulseless ventricular tachycardia (VT) in an adult. The pulse and cardiac rhythm should be checked after each defibrillation attempt. Epinephrine is repeated every 5 minutes during the resuscitation. (From Standards and guidelines for cardiopulmonary resuscitation and emergency cardiac care,[2] with permission.)

the interval from cardiac arrest to application of countershock.[1] Current recommendations are to apply external defibrillation as soon as ventricular fibrillation is identified and a defibrillation is available (Fig. 34-3).[2] An initial defibrillation setting of approximately 200 joules (watt-sec) is recommended for adult victims regardless of body weight. If this initial attempt is unsuccessful, a second attempt should be made using an energy setting of 200 joules to 300 joules, remembering that thoracic impedance decreases modestly after the first shock. As a result, a second attempt at the same energy level may deliver more current to the heart than with the first attempt. Should the first two shocks fail to defibrillate, a third shock not to exceed 360 joules should be delivered immediately. If ventricular fibrillation recurs, defibrillation should be reinitiated at the energy level that had previously resulted in successful defibrillation. It is important to minimize the current delivered to the heart to reduce the likelihood of damage to the myocardium.

Paddle electrodes used to deliver current from the defibrillator must be placed in positions that will maximize current flow through the myocardium. Standard placement is with one electrode to the right of the upper sternum and below the

clavicle and with the other electrode at the level of the apex of the heart in the midaxillary line (Fig. 34-4). The paddles for the electrodes should be applied to the chest with firm pressure equivalent to about 10 kg. In the presence of a permanent pacemaker, care should be taken to avoid placing the electrodes too near (not closer than 10 cm to 12 cm) to the pacemaker generator because defibrillation can cause artificial cardiac pacemaker malfunction. Electrodes 8 cm to 10 cm in diameter are appropriate for adults, and electrodes 4.5 cm in diameter are adequate for infants and children.

DRUG THERAPY

An essential part of ACLS is prompt establishment of an intravenous infusion site for reliable delivery of drugs and fluids into the circulation (Table 34-2). Peripheral venous injection sites are associated with delayed delivery of drugs to the heart during CPR, emphasizing the importance of administration of drugs via a centrally placed catheter (subclavian vein, internal jugular vein) when possible. A period of 1 minute to 2 minutes should be allowed for drugs to reach the central circulation when they are injected via a peripheral vein. Despite advantages of central venous placement, it is mandatory not to delay or interrupt early resuscitation efforts to place a central catheter in preference to peripheral venous placement (antecubital vein), which can be accomplished without interruption of CPR. If a tracheal tube is in place and there is a delay in achieving venous access, it is important to remember that epinephrine, lidocaine, and atropine are absorbed across tracheal and bronchial mucosa when injected into the tracheal tube.

Epinephrine

Epinephrine is effective in the treatment of cardiac arrest because this drug produces alpha-adrenergic effects, manifesting as peripheral vasoconstriction. As a result, external cardiac compressions produce increased blood pressure. The increased perfusion pressure leads to improved myocardial blood flow. Evidence of improved myocardial blood flow and myocardial oxygenation is conver-

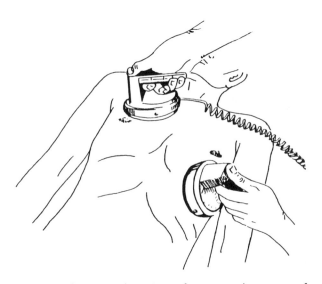

Fig. 34-4. Schematic depiction of proper placement of paddle electrodes in an adult.

Table 34-2. Drug Therapy During CPR

	Indications	Dose
Oxygen	Arterial hypoxemia	100 percent
Epinephrine	Ventricular fibrillation Cardiac asystole Electromechanical dissociation	5 μg·kg^{-1} to 10 μg·kg^{-1} IV 1 mg in 10 ml into tracheal tube (TT)
Sodium bicarbonate	Not recommended except in selected patients for treatment of metabolic acidosis with or without hyperkalemia	1 mEq·kg^{-1} IV initially 0.5 mEq·kg^{-1} IV every 10 minutes of continued CPR or as dictated by pH
Lidocaine	Recurrent or refractory ventricular fibrillation Ventricular tachycardia	1 mg·kg^{-1} IV or TT, then continuous IV infusion of 15 μg·kg^{-1}·min^{-1} to 60 μg·kg^{-1}·min^{-1} (1 mg·min^{-1} to 4 mg·min^{-1} to 70 kg adult)
Procainamide	When lidocaine not effective	0.75 mg·kg^{-1} over 5 minutes not to exceed 1 g in an adult
Bretylium	When lidocaine and procainamide not effective	5 mg·kg^{-1} IV every 5 minutes not to exceed 30 mg·kg^{-1} in an adult
Atropine	Bradycardia Third-degree atrioventricular heart block Cardiac asystole	70 μg·kg^{-1} IV or TT not to exceed 3 mg in an adult
Isoproterenol	When atropine not effective	0.03 μg·kg^{-1}·min^{-1} to 0.3 μg·kg^{-1}·min^{-1} (2 μg·min^{-1} to 20 μg·min^{-1} to a 70 kg adult)
Verapamil	Paroxysmal supraventricular tachycardia	70 μg·kg^{-1} IV initially followed in 15 minutes to 30 minutes by 140 μg·kg^{-1} if cardiac dysrhythmias persist
Calcium chloride	Not recommended except in selected patients for treatment of hypocalcemia or hyperkalemia	

sion of fine ventricular fibrillation to coarse ventricular fibrillation as manifested on the electrocardiogram (ECG). Coarse ventricular fibrillation reflects a well-oxygenated myocardium that is more susceptible than fine ventricular fibrillation to termination with external defibrillation.

The recommended dose of epinephrine is 5 μg·kg^{-1} to 10 μg·kg^{-1} (0.5 mg to 1 mg or 5 ml to 10 ml of a 1:10,000 solution to an adult) administered intravenously every 5 minutes during the resuscitation sequence. Epinephrine should not be administered in the same intravenous line as alkaline solutions. Delivery of epinephrine to the tracheobronchial mucosa via an endotracheal tube (1 mg or 10 ml of a 1:10,000 solution) is followed by prompt systemic absorption (Fig. 34-5).[5] This route of administration should be used if a tracheal tube is in place before establishing intravenous access. Intracardiac injection of epinephrine is recommended only when the intravenous or tracheal route is not available. Hazards of intracardiac injection of epinephrine include pneumothorax, coronary artery laceration, cardiac tamponade, and interruption of external cardiac compressions. Furthermore, inadvertent injection of the epinephrine into the cardiac muscle can produce intractable ventricular fibrillation.

Sodium Bicarbonate

Accumulation of lactic acid and the development of metabolic acidosis during cardiac arrest reflect anaerobic metabolism due to arterial hypoxemia. Ensuring adequate alveolar ventilation is the most important factor in control of acid base balance during CPR. Hyperventilation corrects respiratory acidosis by removing carbon dioxide, which is

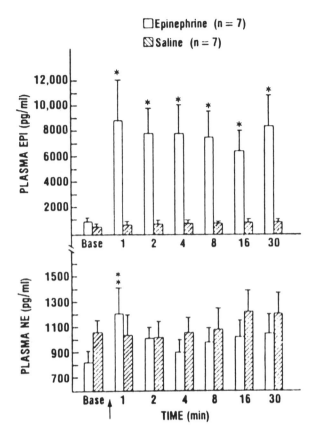

Fig. 34-5. Plasma epinephrine (EPI) and norepinephrine (NE) concentrations before (base) and after endotracheal administration (arrow) of epinephrine (5 ml of 1:10,000) or saline (5 ml) to baboons. (From Chernow et al.,[5] with permission.)

freely diffusable across cell membranes. Administration of sodium bicarbonate in the absence of pH measurements is not recommended during cardiac arrest considering the effectiveness of alveolar ventilation in maintaining an acceptable pH and the potential adverse effects associated with administration of sodium bicarbonate.[2] Indeed, data indicate that treatment with sodium bicarbonate does not improve ability to defibrillate or improve survival rates in experimental animals. Furthermore, mixed venous blood may be a more reliable indicator than arterial blood of acid-base

---

Adverse Effect Associated with Administration of Sodium Bicarbonate

Shift of the oxyhemoglobin dissociation curve to the left

Hypernatremia

Hyperosmolarity

Paradoxical intracellular acidosis due to production of carbon dioxide

Extracellular alkalosis

May inactivate simultaneously administered catecholamines

---

balance during CPR (Fig. 34-6).[6] In certain circumstances, such as patients with co-existing acidosis with or without hyperkalemia, intravenous administration of sodium bicarbonate may be of benefit. When sodium bicarbonate is used, the initial dose is 1 mEq·kg^{-1} and no more than half this dose should be repeated every 10 minutes during the resuscitation sequence.

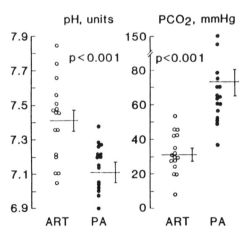

Fig. 34-6. Arterial (ART) and mixed venous (PA) pH and PCO_2 were measured during cardiopulmonary resuscitation in patients. Mixed venous blood most accurately reflects acid-base status during resuscitation. (From Weil et al.,[6] with permission.)

Lidocaine

The rapid onset and absence of adverse effects on myocardial contractility or conduction of cardiac impulses make lidocaine the drug of choice for suppression of ventricular dysrhythmias in patients with refractory or recurrent ventricular tachycardia or fibrillation. Lidocaine may suppress ventricular dysrhythmias by (1) slowing the rate of spontaneous depolarization so as to decrease automaticity, (2) elevating the fibrillation threshold, and (3) inhibiting re-entry pathways. Prevention of re-entry is probably the most important mechanism by which lidocaine prevents ventricular dysrhythmias. It should be appreciated that administration of lidocaine to patients with third-degree atrioventricular heart block is hazardous, as drug-induced suppression of the ectopic ventricular pacemaker could cause ventricular arrest.

Therapeutic blood levels of lidocaine (1.5 $\mu g \cdot ml^{-1}$ to 6 $\mu g \cdot ml^{-1}$) are most predictably obtained with an initial rapid intravenous injection of 1 mg $\cdot kg^{-1}$ followed by a continuous infusion of 15 $\mu g \cdot kg^{-1} \cdot min^{-1}$ to 60 $\mu g \cdot kg^{-1} \cdot min^{-1}$. Lidocaine is metabolized by the liver and its rate of metabolism is dependent on hepatic blood flow. When an intravenous route of administration is not immediately available, it should be remembered that lidocaine injected via a tracheal tube will undergo significant systemic absorption across the tracheobronchial mucosa.

Procainamide

Procainamide may be useful in suppressing ventricular ectopy when lidocaine is not effective. Phases 4 depolarization is slowed and re-entry pathways are blocked, but unlike lidocaine this drug depresses interventricular conduction of cardiac impulses. The dose of procainamide is 0.75 mg $\cdot kg^{-1}$ administered intravenously over 5 minutes until the ventricular dysrhythmia is suppressed or signs of toxicity (hypotension, widening of the QRS) appear on the ECG. The maximum recommended dose of procainamide is 1 gram.

Bretylium

Bretylium is indicated for treatment of (1) refractory ventricular dysrhythmias, including ventricular tachycardia, that are unresponsive to lidocaine or procainamide; and (2) persistent ventricular fibrillation despite multiple attempts at external defibrillation. This drug has effects on the autonomic nervous system (stimulation of norepinephrine release) and cell membranes (elevation of the ventricular fibrillation threshold, increased duration of the cardiac action potential, and prolonged effective refractory period). Prolongation of the cardiac action potential and effective refractory period of normal cardiac muscle make it less likely that irritable foci in ischemic myocardium will initiate re-entry circuits. Bretylium, in contrast to lidocaine or procainamide, does not slow phase 4 depolarization.

The initial intravenous dose of bretylium is 5 mg $\cdot kg^{-1}$ infused over 5 minutes followed by attempted external defibrillation. If ventricular fibrillation persists, additional doses can be administered every 15 minutes to 30 minutes to a total dose not to exceed 30 mg $\cdot kg^{-1}$ to an adult. Bretylium can also be administered as a continuous intravenous infusion at a rate of 1 mg $\cdot min^{-1}$ to 2 mg $\cdot min^{-1}$. An adverse effect of bretylium is hypotension, presumably due to block of the sympathetic nervous system. The dose of bretylium should be reduced in patients with severe renal disease because most of this drug is excreted unchanged by the kidneys.

Atropine

Atropine is the initial drug for treatment of hemodynamically significant bradycardia or atrioventricular heart block. The parasympatholytic action of atropine is responsible for acceleration of conduction of cardiac impulses through the atrioventricular node. Atropine 70 $\mu g \cdot kg^{-1}$ should be given intravenously every 5 minutes until the desired heart rate is achieved or until a total dose of 3.0 mg has been administered. Atropine is also absorbed into the systemic circulation when administered via the tracheal tube into the trachea.

Isoproterenol

Isoproterenol administered as a continuous intravenous infusion of 0.03 $\mu g \cdot kg^{-1} \cdot min^{-1}$ to 0.3 $\mu g \cdot kg^{-1} \cdot min^{-1}$ is indicated for the treatment of atropine-refractory bradycardia or third-degree atrioventricular heart block associated with hemodynamic depression. Beta agonist effects of isoproterenol are responsible for the desirable increases in systolic blood pressure, heart rate, and myocardial contractility produced by this drug. These advantages, however, may be offset by associated increases in myocardial oxygen requirements. Furthermore, vasodilation due to beta stimulation of vascular receptors leads to decreased diastolic blood pressure, which decreases coronary blood flow and myocardial oxygen delivery. For these reasons, isoproterenol should be administered only until a transvenous artificial cardiac pacemaker can be inserted.

Verapamil

Verapamil is a calcium entry blocking drug that is particularly useful in the treatment of paroxysmal supraventricular tachycardia. The initial intravenous dose is 70 $\mu g \cdot kg^{-1}$ followed in 15 minutes to 30 minutes by 140 $\mu g \cdot kg^{-1}$ if tachycardia persists and an adverse response to the initial dose did not occur. Bradycardia, hypotension, facilitated accessory pathway conduction of cardiac impulses, and myocardial depression may follow its administration.

Calcium

Studies in the cardiac arrest setting have not demonstrated benefit from the administration of calcium despite the important role this ion plays in myocardial contractility and cardiac impulse formation.[2] Considering the possible detrimental role that may accompany high plasma concentrations of calcium in the postresuscitation period, it seems logical to avoid administration of calcium except for specific indications (hyperkalemia, hypocalcemia, excessive myocardial depression due to calcium entry blocker therapy) (see the section *Postresuscitation Management*). When indicated, calcium chloride is administered intravenously in doses of 2 $mg \cdot kg^{-1}$ to 4 $mg \cdot kg^{-1}$ and repeated as necessary.

CARDIAC ASYSTOLE

Cardiac asystole is a less frequent cause of cardiac arrest than ventricular fibrillation, and the prognosis for resuscitation is poor, often reflecting extensive myocardial ischemia from prolonged periods of inadequate coronary perfusion. It may be difficult to differentiate cardiac asystole from ventricular fibrillation, emphasizing the need to review two different lead configurations to confirm the ECG diagnosis. If the cardiac rhythm is unclear, the recommendation is to apply electrical defibrillation (Fig. 34-7).[2] If cardiac asystole is present, the treatment is continued CPR, drug therapy, and consideration of transvenous artificial cardiac pacemaker insertion (Fig. 34-7).[2]

ELECTROMECHANICAL DISSOCIATION

Electromechanical dissociation is present when a normal ECG persists in the absence of an effective stroke volume as evidenced by the disappearance of peripheral pulses and blood pressure. The prognosis is grave and mandates aggressive therapy and an intense search for correctable causes (Fig. 34-8).[2]

VENTRICULAR TACHYCARDIA

Treatment of ventricular tachycardia depends on the hemodynamic significance of the cardiac dysrhythmia (Fig. 34-9).[2] Cardioversion requires less energy than defibrillation but must be synchronized to avoid delivering the shock during the relative refractory portion of the cardiac cycle, which could result in ventricular fibrillation.

PAROXYSMAL SUPRAVENTRICULAR TACHYCARDIA

Emergency treatment of paroxysmal supraventricular tachycardia (PSVT) depends on the hemodynamic stability of the patient and the presence of underlying disease (Fig. 34-10).[2] Distinction between sinus tachycardia, ventricular tachycardia, and PSVT may be difficult to distinguish on the ECG.

MANAGEMENT OF THE OBSTRUCTED AIRWAY

An airway that is obstructed due to the lodgement of a foreign body in the glottic opening will not be effectively managed by maneuvers, such as the head tilt-jaw thrust method, designed to pull the

If Rhythm Is Unclear and Possibly Ventricular
Fibrillation, Defibrillate as for VF. If Asystole is Present
↓
Continue CPR
↓
Establish IV Access
↓
Epinephrine, 1:10,000, 0.5 - 1.0 mg IV Push
↓
Intubate When Possible
↓
Atropine, 1.0 mg IV Push (Repeated in 5 min)
↓
(Consider Bicarbonate)
↓
Consider Pacing

Fig. 34-7. Treatment of cardiac asystole in adults. Epinephrine is repeated every 5 minutes during the resuscitation. (From Standards and guidelines for cardiopulmonary resuscitation and emergency cardiac care,[2] with permission.)

Continue CPR
↓
Establish IV Access
↓
Epinephrine, 1:10,000, 0.5 - 1.0 mg IV Push
↓
Intubate When Possible
↓
(Consider Bicarbonate)
↓
Consider Hypovolemia,
Cardiac Tamponade,
Tension Pneumothorax,
Hypoxemia,
Acidosis,
Pulmonary Embolism

Fig. 34-8. Treatment of electromechanical dissociation in adults. Epinephrine is repeated every 5 minutes during the resuscitation. (From Standards and guidelines for cardiopulmonary resuscitation and emergency cardiac care,[2] with permission.)

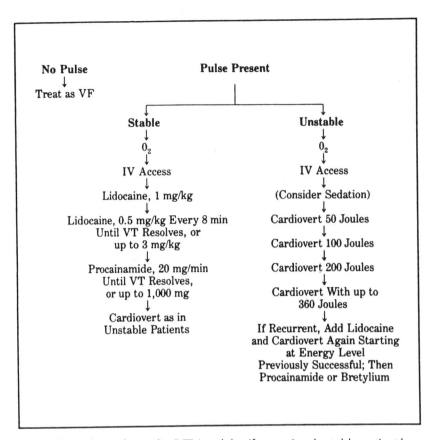

Fig. 34-9. Treatment of ventricular tachycardia (VT) in adults. If a previously stable patient becomes unstable (systolic blood pressure less than 90 mmHg, angina pectoris, dyspnea, unconsciousness), treatment shifts to the unstable column. Once VT has resolved, it is common to begin a continuous intravenous infusion of the cardiac antidysrhythmic that aided in resolution of the VT. (From Standards and guidelines for cardiopulmonary resuscitation and emergency cardiac care,[2] with permission.)

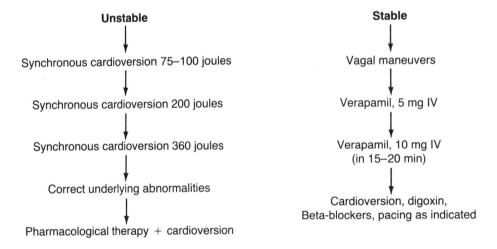

If conversion occurs but PSVT recurs, repeated electrical cardioversion is *not* indicated. Sedation should be used as time permits.

Fig. 34-10. Treatment of paroxysmal supraventricular tachycardia in adults. (From Standards and guidelines for cardiopulmonary resuscitation and emergency cardiac care,[2] with permission.)

tongue away from the posterior pharynx (Fig. 34-1). In this situation, the recommended treatment in both conscious and unconscious victims is delivery of manual pressure to the abdomen or chest to increase airway pressure. For example, manual inward and upward depression over the victim's epigastrium (abdominal thrust, external subdiaphragmatic compression or Heimlich maneuver) forces the diaphragm cephalad, compressing the lungs and raising airway pressures.[7] Increased airway pressures produced by the abdominal thrust forces ("pops") the obstructing particle out of the glottic opening into the pharynx. The abdominal thrust maneuver can be used in awake and unconscious victims and is equally effective in the supine or standing position (Fig. 34-11).[2] Complications of this maneuver include rib fractures and rupture or laceration of thoracic or abdominal viscera. The chest thrust (i.e., manual compression over the mid or lower sternum) is an alternative to abdominal compression in morbidly obese or near term parturients experiencing foreign body airway obstruction. In the unconscious victim, delivery of a precordial thump (see the section *Precordial Thump*) or external cardiac compression creates airway pressures similar to those produced by a chest thrust. Finally, in the unconscious victim, a blind finger examination of the pharynx is indicated if these previous maneuvers have not been successful.

Cricothyroidotomy

Cricothyroidotomy is a method to provide emergency oxygenation and ventilation of the lungs when upper airway obstruction cannot be relieved by supraglottic intubation of the trachea. A 12-gauge to 14-gauge catheter mounted over a needle (extracath) is inserted through the relatively avascular cricothyroid membrane (palpable transverse indentation between the thyroid and cricoid cartilages into the lumen of the trachea (Fig. 34-12).[8] Entrance into the tracheal lumen is recognized by aspiration of air into an attached syringe (Fig. 34-

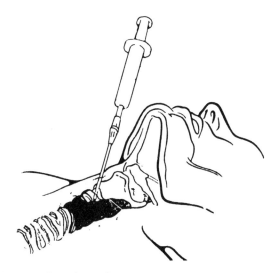

Fig. 34-12. Cricothyroidotomy is accomplished by passing a 12-gauge to 14-gauge catheter mounted over a needle (extracath) through the cricothyroid membrane into the trachea. Entrance into the tracheal lumen is recognized by aspiration of air into an attached syringe. Subsequent advancement of the catheter into the trachea and attachment to an oxygen delivery system permits oxygenation and ventilation of the lungs. (From Textbook of Advanced Cardiac Life Support,[8] with permission.)

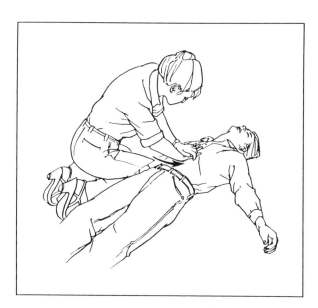

Fig. 34-11. Management of an obstructed airway by delivery of subdiaphragmatic abdominal thrusts. (Heimlich maneuver) delivered to an unconscious adult. (From Standards and guidelines for cardiopulmonary resuscitation and emergency cardiac care,[2] with permission.)

12).[8] The catheter is threaded over the needle into the trachea and attached to an oxygen delivery system using appropriate connectors (15 mm endotracheal tube connector or tubing for intravenous fluid delivery systems). If the upper airway is obstructed, exhalation must occur through the ventilatory catheter that is intermittently disconnected from the oxygen source and opened to the atmosphere. In fact, elevated airway pressures may cause a partially obstructing foreign body to be expelled from the glottic opening into the pharynx.

PRECORDIAL THUMP

Precordial thump is a forceful blow delivered with the fleshy part of the rescuer's fist to the midportion of the victim's sternum. A single precordial thump is recommended only for initial treatment of (1) monitored ventricular fibrillation or tachycardia, and (2) cardiac asystolle due to third-degree atrioventricular heart block. The precordial thump may serve as mechanical defibrillation or cardioversion or as a mechanism to produce cardiac contraction until a transvenous artificial cardiac pacemaker can be inserted. Precordial thump is not recommended for pediatric patients.

RESUSCITATION OF INFANTS AND CHILDREN

Techniques of CPR as applied to infants (less than 1 year old) differ in some instances from those of children (1 year to puberty) or adults (Table 34-1). These differences relate to airway management, ventilation of the lungs, closed chest cardiac compression, external defibrillation, and drug therapy. Furthermore, the most readily palpable pulse in infants up to 1 year of age is the brachial artery at the mid-upper arm in contrast to the carotid artery in children and adults.

Airway Management and Ventilation of the Lungs

Excessive extension of the infant's head may obstruct the upper airway. The infant's tongue is large, however, in relation to the mouth such that moderate extension of the head is useful for opening the upper airway. The rescuer seals his or her mouth over the infant's mouth and nose to provide exhaled air ventilation. This approach is easier than mouth-to-mouth ventilation because of the disparate sizes of the structures involved. In addition, the lungs of the infant under 9 months of age are more easily ventilated through the nose than through the mouth due to the cephalad position of the infant's larynx (C1 to C3) and the proximity of the epiglottis to the palate. After 1 year of age, mouth-to-mouth ventilation is acceptable.

The optimal method for management of airway obstruction in children is controversial. In children, the recommendation is to use subdiaphragmatic abdominal compressions.[2] In children less than 1 year of age, the risk of intra-abdominal injury from this maneuver is the reason for recommending the combination of back blows and chest thrusts. Blind finger probes are avoided in infants and children because the foreign body may be pushed further into the airway, causing greater airway obstruction.

Airway adjuncts for adults are available in smaller sizes for infants and children with the exception of the EOA and EGTA, which are not recommended for victims less than 16 years old. Tracheal tubes without cuffs are often used in children less than 5 years of age.

Closed Chest Cardiac Compression

Differences in size and anatomy of infants, children, and adults dictate differences in the technique of external cardiac compression for these various age groups. In infants, the cardiac ventricles are positioned more cephalad in the chest such that external compression is performed on the midsternum rather than the lower sternum. The recommended rate of sternal compression is a rate of at least 100 min^{-1} and the depth of sternal depression is 1.3 cm to 2.5 cm.[2] The rescuer's hands should encircle the infant's chest, and the thumbs are used to depress the sternum against the heart. Depression of the sternum may be achieved with three fingers in young children and the heel of one hand in older children.

External Defibrillation and Drug Therapy

The energy setting for successful external defibrillation in children is directly related to body weight.[2] An initial energy setting of 2 joules·kg^{-1}

should be selected and if this is unsuccessful a second attempt may be made using 4 joules·kg^{-1}. If a second attempt is unsuccessful, the recommendation is to re-evaluate the adequacy of BLS and the possible need for drug therapy rather than increasing the energy setting above 4 joules·kg^{-1}. Paddles 4.5 cm in diameter are suitable for infants and those 8 cm in diameter are used for children.

POSTRESUSCITATION MANAGEMENT

Postresuscitation management begins after establishment of a spontaneous cardiac output in the victim of a cardiac arrest. The patient who is awake and breathing spontaneously needs only to be monitored closely in an intensive care unit. Supplemental oxygen and a radiograph of the chest should be routine after CPR. Drug therapy may be necessary to optimize vital organ function and survival (Table 34-3). For example, a continuous intravenous infusion of lidocaine is often maintained for the first 24 hours. Optimal adjustment of the intravascular fluid volume and support of the circulation as facilitated by monitoring with a pulmonary artery catheter may be necessary. Renal failure may necessitate hemodialysis.

Restoration of a spontaneous cardiac output after 12 or more minutes of cerebral ischemia is accompanied by an initial hyperperfusion of the brain followed within 15 minutes to 90 minutes by

Table 34-3. Postresuscitation Drug Therapy

Drug	Indications
Lidocaine	Cardiac ventricular irritability
Dopamine	Decreased myocardial contractility associated with oliguria
Dobutamine	Same as dopamine but not specific for increasing renal blood flow
Furosemide	Increased intracranial pressure
Barbiturates Diazepam Phenytoin	Central nervous system seizure activity
Nitroprusside	Systemic hypertension

profound reductions of cerebral blood flow to levels (5 percent to 40 percent of normal) often incompatible with neuronal viability.[9] This "no reflow phenomenon" is not accompanied by intravascular clotting or changes in ICP. Presumably, massive increases in cerebral small vessel resistance, possibly due to the accumulation of vasoconstrictor prostaglandins, are responsible for decreased cerebral blood flow. Furthermore, ischemia is accompanied by decay of the normal calcium gradients across cell membranes. Rapid shifts of calcium into arterial walls can also result in vascular spasm and possible neuronal damage. For this reason, there is interest in exploring the use of calcium entry blockers, such as nimodipine, to ameliorate postischemic brain injury.[10] Moreover, the routine administration of calcium during management of cardiac arrest may not be beneficial if neuronal calcium overloading is a result of cellular ischemia.

The ability of barbiturate therapy to reduce ICP is accepted (see Chapter 32). The efficacy of barbiturate therapy, however, for improving brain survival after global cerebral ischemia due to cardiac arrest is both unlikely and unproven. Certainly, barbiturate protection will occur only when the ischemic insult did not interfere with basal cellular metabolism as evidenced by continued presence of electrical activity on the electroencephalogram. During cardiac arrest (i.e., global ischemia) the electroencephalogram becomes flat in 20 seconds to 30 seconds, and subsequent administration of barbiturates would not be expected to improve neurologic outcome. Possibly, the most beneficial effect of barbiturates or other drugs, such as diazepam or phenytoin, is to suppress seizure activity and associated increases in cerebral oxygen requirements in the postresuscitation period. Advantages of nonbarbiturate therapy (diazepam, phenytoin) would be less cardiovascular depression, which often limits the total dose of barbiturates that can be administered, particularly if hypovolemia is present. Certainly, there is no evidence to support the routine administration of barbiturates to patients who have been resuscitated from a cardiac arrest.[2] Furthermore, there is no evidence that hypothermia or corticosteroids instituted after cardiac arrest improve survival or neurologic outcome. Mild hypothermia present at the time of cardiac arrest, however, may offer some degree of cerebral protection.

Hyperglycemia at the time of cardiac arrest is related to a less favorable neurologic outcome when compared with patients who are normoglycemic. Presumably, this reflects lactate production and intracellular acidosis due to anaerobic glycolysis of glucose. It remains uncertain if infusion of glucose containing solutions should be avoided in the postresuscitation period.

Monitors specific for the central nervous system in the cardiac arrest victim with residual neurologic dysfunction include (1) ICP monitoring devices, (2) the electroencephalogram, (3) computed tomography of the cerebral ventricles, (4) cortical evoked potentials, (5) measurement of total and/or regional cerebral blood flow, and (6) frequent neurologic examination. Resuscitation and protection of the brain that has experienced potential ischemic damage includes (1) maintenance of systemic blood pressure at normal levels, (2) prevention of increased ICP by mild hyperventilation of the lungs ($PaCO_2$ 25 mmHg to 30 mmHg), (3) drug-induced diuresis, (4) avoidance of hyperthermia, and (5) elevation of the head 30 degrees to increase cerebral venous drainage (see Chapter 32).

REFERENCES

1. Cobb LA, Hallstrom AP. Community based cardiopulmonary resuscitation: What have we learned? Ann NY Acad Sci 1982;382:330–42.
2. Standards and guidelines for cardiopulmonary resuscitation and emergency medical care. JAMA 1986;255:2841–3044.
3. Neimann JT, Rosborough J, Hausknecht M, Brown D, Criley JM. Crough-CPR. Documentation of systemic perfusion in man and in an experimental model: A "window" to the mechanism of blood flow in external CPR. Crit Care Med 1980;8:141–6.
4. Roberts MC, Weisfeldt ML, Traystan RJ. Cerebral blood flow during cardiopulmonary resuscitation (Editorial). Anesth Analg 1981;60:73–5.
5. Chernow B, Holbrook P, D'Angona DS, et al. Epinephrine absorption after intratracheal administration. Anesth Analg 1984;63:829–32.
6. Weil MH, Rackow EC, Trevino R, Grundler W, Falk JL, Griffel MI. Difference in acid-base state between venous and arterial blood during cardiopulmonary resuscitation. N Engl J Med 1986;315:153–6.
7. Heimlich HJ. A life-saving maneuver to prevent food-choking. JAMA 1975;234:398–401.
8. Textbook of Advanced Cardiac Life Support. American Heart Association, Dallas, 1987:34.
9. White BC, Wiegenstein JG, Winegar CD. Brain ischemic anoxia. Mechanisms of injury. JAMA 1984;251:1586–90.
10. Steen PA, Gisvold SE, Milde JH, et al. Nimodipine improves outcome when given after complete cerebral ischemia in primates. Anesthesiology 1985;62:406–14.

Appendix 1
Standards For Conduction Anesthesia in Obstetrics*

(Approved by House of Delegates on October 12, 1988)

These standards apply to the use of major conduction anesthesia administered to the parturient during labor and delivery. These standards may be exceeded based on the judgment of the responsible anesthesiologist. They are intended to encourage high quality patient care, but cannot guarantee any specific patient outcome. They are subject to revision from time to time as warranted by the evolution of technology and practice.

STANDARD I

Major conduction anesthesia, (lumbar or caudal epidural, subarachnoid or bilateral lumbar sympathetic block) shall be initiated and maintained only in locations in which appropriate resuscitation equipment and drugs are immediately available to manage procedurally related problems (e.g., hypotension, respiratory depression, convulsions and myocardial depression).

Resuscitation equipment shall include: sources of oxygen and suction, equipment to maintain an airway and perform endotracheal intubation, and a means to provide positive pressure ventilation. Drugs and equipment for cardiopulmonary resuscitation shall be immediately available.

STANDARD II

Major conduction blocks in obstetrics shall be initiated and maintained by or under the direction of a physician with appropriate privileges.

Physicians must be approved, through the institutional credentialing process, to administer or supervise the administration of obstetric anesthesia and must be qualified to manage procedurally related complications.

STANDARD III

Major conduction anesthesia should not be administered until the patient has been examined, and the fetal status and progress of labor evaluated by a qualified physician who is readily available to supervise the labor and to deal with any obstetric complications that may arise.

* Also see Chapter 26.

STANDARD IV

An intravenous infusion shall be established before initiation and maintained throughout the duration of major conduction block.

STANDARD V

A qualified individual shall monitor continually† the parturient's oxygenation, ventilation and circulation.

Anesthetic techniques, drugs, and maternal vital signs shall be documented in the medical record.

STANDARD VI

Qualified personnel, other than the anesthesiologist attending the mother, should be immediately available to assume responsibility for resuscitation of the depressed newborn.

The primary responsibility of the anesthesiologist is to provide care to the mother. If the anesthesiologist is also requested to provide brief assistance in the care of the newborn, the benefit to the child must be compared to the risk of temporarily leaving the mother.

STANDARD VII

All patients recovering from major conduction anesthesia shall receive appropriate postanesthesia care.

1. A postanesthesia care unit (PACU) shall be available to receive patients. The design, equipment and staffing shall meet requirements of the facility's accrediting and licensing bodies.
2. When the PACU is not available, equivalent postanesthesia care shall be provided in a suitable location.

STANDARD VIII

A physician with appropriate privileges shall remain in the facility to manage anesthetic complications until the patient is accepted by the PACU or equivalent area.

STANDARD IX

There shall be a policy to ensure the availability in the facility of a physician capable of managing anesthetic complications and providing cardiopulmonary resuscitation for patients in the PACU.

---

† Note that "continual" is defined as "repeated regularly and frequently in steady rapid succession" whereas "continuous" means "prolonged without any interruption at any time".

Appendix 2
Standards for Postanesthesia Care

(Approved by House of Delegates on October 12, 1988)

These standards apply to postanesthesia care in all locations. These standards may be exceeded based on the judgment of the responsible anesthesiologist. They are intended to encourage high quality patient care, but cannot guarantee any specific patient outcome. They are subject to revision from time to time as warranted by the evolution of technology and practice.

STANDARD I

All patients who have received general anesthesia, regional anesthesia, or monitored anesthesia care shall receive appropriate postanesthesia management.

1. A postanesthesia care unit (PACU) or an area which provides equivalent postanesthesia care shall be available to receive patients after surgery and anesthesia. All patients who receive anesthesia shall be admitted to the PACU except by specific order of the anesthesiologist responsible for the patient's care.
2. The medical aspects of care in the PACU shall be governed by policies and procedures that have been reviewed and approved by the Department of Anesthesiology.
3. The design, equipment, and staffing of the PACU shall meet requirements of the facility's accrediting and licensing bodies.
4. The nursing standards of practice shall be consistent with those approved in 1986 by the American Society of Post Anesthesia Nurses (ASPAN).

STANDARD II

A patient transported to the PACU shall be accompanied by a member of the anesthesia care team who is knowledgeable about the patient's condition. The patient shall be continually evaluated and treated during transport with monitoring and support appropriate to the patient's condition.

STANDARD III

Upon arrival in the PACU, the patient shall be re-evaluated and a verbal report provided to the responsible PACU nurse by the member of the anesthesia care team who accompanies the patient.

1. The patient's status on arrival in the PACU shall be documented.
2. Information concerning the preoperative condition and the surgical/anesthetic course shall be transmitted to the PACU nurse.
3. The member of the Anesthesia Care Team shall remain in the PACU until the PACU nurse accepts responsibility for the nursing care of the patient.

STANDARD IV

The patient's condition shall be evaluated continually in the PACU.

1. The patient shall be observed and monitored by methods appropriate to the patient's medical condition. Particular attention should be given to monitoring oxygenation, ventilation and circulation. While qualitative clinical signs may be adequate, quantitative methods are encouraged.
2. An accurate written report of the PACU period shall be maintained. Use of an appropriate PACU scoring system is encouraged for each patient on admission, at appropriate intervals prior to discharge, and at the time of discharge.
3. General medical supervision and coordination of patient care in the PACU should be the responsibility of the anesthesiologist.
4. There shall be a policy to assure the availability in the facility of a physician capable of managing complications and providing cardiopulmonary resuscitation for patients in the PACU.

STANDARD V

A physician is responsible for the discharge of the patient from the PACU.

1. When discharge criteria are used, they must be approved by the Department of Anesthesiology and the medical staff. They may vary depending upon whether the patient is discharged to a hospital room, to the ICU, to a short stay unit, or home.
2. In the absence of the physician responsible for the discharge, the PACU nurse shall determine if the patient meets the discharge criteria. The name of the physician accepting responsibility for discharge shall be noted on the record.

Index

Page numbers followed by f represent figures; those followed by t represent tables.